# CRITICAL CARE NEUROLOGY
## PART I

# HANDBOOK OF CLINICAL NEUROLOGY

*Series Editors*

MICHAEL J. AMINOFF, FRANÇOIS BOLLER, AND DICK F. SWAAB

VOLUME 140

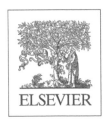

ELSEVIER

# CRITICAL CARE NEUROLOGY
## PART I

*Series Editors*

MICHAEL J. AMINOFF, FRANÇOIS BOLLER, AND DICK F. SWAAB

*Volume Editors*

EELCO F.M. WIJDICKS AND ANDREAS H. KRAMER

VOLUME 140

3rd Series

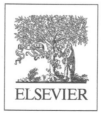

ELSEVIER

ELSEVIER

Radarweg 29, PO Box 211, 1000 AE Amsterdam, Netherlands
The Boulevard, Langford Lane, Kidlington, Oxford OX5 1GB, United Kingdom
50 Hampshire Street, 5th Floor, Cambridge, MA 02139, United States

**Notices**

Knowledge and best practice in this field are constantly changing. As new research and experience broaden our understanding, changes in research methods, professional practices, or medical treatment may become necessary.

Practitioners and researchers must always rely on their own experience and knowledge in evaluating and using any information, methods, compounds, or experiments described herein. In using such information or methods they should be mindful of their own safety and the safety of others, including parties for whom they have a professional responsibility.

With respect to any drug or pharmaceutical products identified, readers are advised to check the most current information provided (i) on procedures featured or (ii) by the manufacturer of each product to be administered, to verify the recommended dose or formula, the method and duration of administration, and contraindications. It is the responsibility of practitioners, relying on their own experience and knowledge of their patients, to make diagnoses, to determine dosages and the best treatment for each individual patient, and to take all appropriate safety precautions.

To the fullest extent of the law, neither the Publisher nor the authors, contributors, or editors, assume any liability for any injury and/or damage to persons or property as a matter of products liability, negligence or otherwise, or from any use or operation of any methods, products, instructions, or ideas contained in the material herein.

**British Library Cataloguing-in-Publication Data**
A catalogue record for this book is available from the British Library

**Library of Congress Cataloging-in-Publication Data**
A catalog record for this book is available from the Library of Congress

ISBN: 978-0-44-463600-3

For information on all Elsevier publications
visit our website at https://www.elsevier.com/

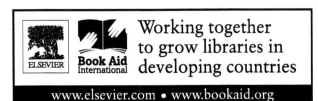

Working together
to grow libraries in
developing countries

www.elsevier.com • www.bookaid.org

*Publisher:* Mara Conner
*Editorial Project Manager:* Kristi Anderson
*Production Project Manager:* Sujatha Thirugnana Sambandam
*Cover Designer:* Alan Studholme

Typeset by SPi Global, India

**Handbook of Clinical Neurology 3rd Series**

*Available titles*

Vol. 79, The human hypothalamus: basic and clinical aspects, Part I, D.F. Swaab, ed. ISBN 9780444513571
Vol. 80, The human hypothalamus: basic and clinical aspects, Part II, D.F. Swaab, ed. ISBN 9780444514905
Vol. 81, Pain, F. Cervero and T.S. Jensen, eds. ISBN 9780444519016
Vol. 82, Motor neurone disorders and related diseases, A.A. Eisen and P.J. Shaw, eds. ISBN 9780444518941
Vol. 83, Parkinson's disease and related disorders, Part I, W.C. Koller and E. Melamed, eds. ISBN 9780444519009
Vol. 84, Parkinson's disease and related disorders, Part II, W.C. Koller and E. Melamed, eds. ISBN 9780444528933
Vol. 85, HIV/AIDS and the nervous system, P. Portegies and J. Berger, eds. ISBN 9780444520104
Vol. 86, Myopathies, F.L. Mastaglia and D. Hilton Jones, eds. ISBN 9780444518996
Vol. 87, Malformations of the nervous system, H.B. Sarnat and P. Curatolo, eds. ISBN 9780444518965
Vol. 88, Neuropsychology and behavioural neurology, G. Goldenberg and B.C. Miller, eds. ISBN 9780444518972
Vol. 89, Dementias, C. Duyckaerts and I. Litvan, eds. ISBN 9780444518989
Vol. 90, Disorders of consciousness, G.B. Young and E.F.M. Wijdicks, eds. ISBN 9780444518958
Vol. 91, Neuromuscular junction disorders, A.G. Engel, ed. ISBN 9780444520081
Vol. 92, Stroke – Part I: Basic and epidemiological aspects, M. Fisher, ed. ISBN 9780444520036
Vol. 93, Stroke – Part II: Clinical manifestations and pathogenesis, M. Fisher, ed. ISBN 9780444520043
Vol. 94, Stroke – Part III: Investigations and management, M. Fisher, ed. ISBN 9780444520050
Vol. 95, History of neurology, S. Finger, F. Boller and K.L. Tyler, eds. ISBN 9780444520081
Vol. 96, Bacterial infections of the central nervous system, K.L. Roos and A.R. Tunkel, eds. ISBN 9780444520159
Vol. 97, Headache, G. Nappi and M.A. Moskowitz, eds. ISBN 9780444521392
Vol. 98, Sleep disorders Part I, P. Montagna and S. Chokroverty, eds. ISBN 9780444520067
Vol. 99, Sleep disorders Part II, P. Montagna and S. Chokroverty, eds. ISBN 9780444520074
Vol. 100, Hyperkinetic movement disorders, W.J. Weiner and E. Tolosa, eds. ISBN 9780444520142
Vol. 101, Muscular dystrophies, A. Amato and R.C. Griggs, eds. ISBN 9780080450315
Vol. 102, Neuro-ophthalmology, C. Kennard and R.J. Leigh, eds. ISBN 9780444529039
Vol. 103, Ataxic disorders, S.H. Subramony and A. Durr, eds. ISBN 9780444518927
Vol. 104, Neuro-oncology Part I, W. Grisold and R. Sofietti, eds. ISBN 9780444521385
Vol. 105, Neuro-oncology Part II, W. Grisold and R. Sofietti, eds. ISBN 9780444535023
Vol. 106, Neurobiology of psychiatric disorders, T. Schlaepfer and C.B. Nemeroff, eds. ISBN 9780444520029
Vol. 107, Epilepsy Part I, H. Stefan and W.H. Theodore, eds. ISBN 9780444528988
Vol. 108, Epilepsy Part II, H. Stefan and W.H. Theodore, eds. ISBN 9780444528995
Vol. 109, Spinal cord injury, J. Verhaagen and J.W. McDonald III, eds. ISBN 9780444521378
Vol. 110, Neurological rehabilitation, M. Barnes and D.C. Good, eds. ISBN 9780444529015
Vol. 111, Pediatric neurology Part I, O. Dulac, M. Lassonde and H.B. Sarnat, eds. ISBN 9780444528919
Vol. 112, Pediatric neurology Part II, O. Dulac, M. Lassonde and H.B. Sarnat, eds. ISBN 9780444529107
Vol. 113, Pediatric neurology Part III, O. Dulac, M. Lassonde and H.B. Sarnat, eds. ISBN 9780444595652
Vol. 114, Neuroparasitology and tropical neurology, H.H. Garcia, H.B. Tanowitz and O.H. Del Brutto, eds. ISBN 9780444534903
Vol. 115, Peripheral nerve disorders, G. Said and C. Krarup, eds. ISBN 9780444529022
Vol. 116, Brain stimulation, A.M. Lozano and M. Hallett, eds. ISBN 9780444534972
Vol. 117, Autonomic nervous system, R.M. Buijs and D.F. Swaab, eds. ISBN 9780444534910
Vol. 118, Ethical and legal issues in neurology, J.L. Bernat and H.R. Beresford, eds. ISBN 9780444535016
Vol. 119, Neurologic aspects of systemic disease Part I, J. Biller and J.M. Ferro, eds. ISBN 9780702040863
Vol. 120, Neurologic aspects of systemic disease Part II, J. Biller and J.M. Ferro, eds. ISBN 9780702040870
Vol. 121, Neurologic aspects of systemic disease Part III, J. Biller and J.M. Ferro, eds. ISBN 9780702040887
Vol. 122, Multiple sclerosis and related disorders, D.S. Goodin, ed. ISBN 9780444520012
Vol. 123, Neurovirology, A.C. Tselis and J. Booss, eds. ISBN 9780444534880

# Foreword

Modern hospitals in the developed countries have changed remarkably in character over the last quarter-century, no longer serving as a hospice for the chronically sick. Instead, their focus is now primarily on surgical patients requiring perioperative care, patients requiring a procedural intervention, and patients with critical illnesses requiring care in the intensive care unit because of the complexity of their disorders. In the same manner as many other medical disciplines, neurology has become for the most part an outpatient specialty. Patients requiring surgery or with complex neurologic disorders necessitating a multidisciplinary approach and constant monitoring now make up a large component of the patients admitted to hospital and seen by neurologists. It was with this in mind that we felt the need to include critical care neurology within the embrace of the *Handbook of Clinical Neurology* series. To this end, we approached two leaders in the field to develop the subject, and are delighted that they agreed to do so and with what they have achieved.

Eelco Wijdicks is professor of neurology and chair of the division of critical care neurology at the Mayo Clinic College of Medicine, Rochester, Minnesota, and is a well-known author and the founding editor of the journal *Neurocritical Care*. Andreas H. Kramer is a clinical associate professor in the departments of critical care medicine and clinical neurosciences at the Hotchkiss Brain Institute of the University of Calgary, in Alberta, Canada. Both are leaders in the field of neurointensive care, with wide experience in patient management and an international record in developing evidence-based guidelines for optimizing patient care. Together they have developed two volumes of the *Handbook* to cover the pathophysiology and treatment of patients with acute neurologic or neurosurgical disorders requiring care in the intensive care unit (Volume 140), or with neurologic complications that have arisen in the setting of a medical or surgical critical illness (Volume 141).

Forty-one chapters deal with all aspects of these disorders, including ethical and prognostic considerations. Many of the management issues that are discussed in these pages are among the most difficult ones faced by contemporary clinicians, and the availability of these authoritative reviews – buttressed by the latest advances in medical science – will increase physician confidence by providing the most up-to-date guidelines for improving patient care. We are grateful to Professors Wijdicks and Kramer, and to the various contributors whom they enlisted as coauthors, for crafting two such comprehensive volumes that will be of major utility both as reference works for all practitioners and as practical guides for those in the front line.

As series editors, we reviewed all of the chapters in these volumes, making suggestions for improvement as needed. We believe that all who are involved in the care of critically ill patients in the hospital setting will find them a valuable resource. The availability of the volume electronically on Elsevier's Science Direct site should increase their accessibility and facilitate searches for specific information.

As always, we extend our appreciation to Elsevier, our publishers, for their continued support of the *Handbook* series, and warmly acknowledge our personal indebtedness to Michael Parkinson in Scotland and to Mara Conner and Kristi Anderson in California for their assistance in seeing these volumes to fruition.

Michael J. Aminoff
François Boller
Dick F. Swaab

# Preface

New subspecialties in neurology continue to germinate, and critical care neurology (also known as neurocritical care) is one of the more recent ones. The field has matured significantly over the last two decades, and a neurointensivist is a recognizable and legitimate specialist. The field involves primarily the care of patients with an acute neurologic or neurosurgical disorder. These disorders are life-threatening because the main injury may damage critical structures and often affects respiration and even the circulation. A neurologic complication may also appear *de novo* in the setting of a medical or surgical critical illness. These two clinical situations form the pillars of this field and therefore justify two separate volumes. In these two books we include traditional sections focused on epidemiology and pathophysiology, but others are more tailored towards management of the patient, sections we think are informative to the general neurologist. Therapeutic interventions and acute decisions are part of a daily commitment of a neurointensivist. We assumed that a focus on management (and less on diagnostics) will be most useful for the reader of this handbook series. The immediacy of management focuses on prevention of further intracranial complications (brain edema and brain tissue shift, increased intracranial pressure, and seizures) and systemic (cardiopulmonary) insults.

We have written extensively on many of these topics but in these two volumes we let other practitioners write about their practice, experiences, and research. They have all made a name for themselves and we are pleased they were able to contribute to this work. Although the major topics are reviewed, we realize some may have been truncated or not covered because we tried to avoid a substantial overlap with other volumes in the series.

This is a contributed book with all its inherent quirks, stylistic mismatches, and inconsistencies, but we hope we have edited a text that is more than the sum of its parts. We appreciate the fact that the series editors of the *Handbook of Clinical Neurology* recognized this field of neurology. Herein, we are making the argument that delivery of care by a neurointensivist is an absolute requirement and its value for the patient is undisputed. Still, the best way to achieve this is through integrated care, and neurointensivists can only function in a multidisciplinary cooperative practice. The new slate of neurointensivists in the USA can be certified in neurology, neurosurgery, internal medicine, anesthesiology, or other critical care specialties and time will tell if this all-inclusiveness will dilute or strengthen the specialty. One fact is clear: our backgrounds are different and this significantly helped in shaping this volume.

We thank the editors of the series – Michael Aminoff, Francois Boller, and Dick Swaab – for inviting us three years ago to prepare these volumes. We must particularly thank Michael Parkinson and Sujatha Thirugnana Sambandam, who steered the books to fruition.

I—Eelco Wijdicks—know the series very well and when I did my neurology residency in Holland in the early 1980s it was known as "Vinken and Bruyn," and residents and staff would always look there first to find a solution for a difficult patient, to read up on an usual disorder or to understand a mechanism. I admired the beautiful covers and authoritative reviews and I remember it had a special place in our library. I was thrilled to see the complete series in the Mayo Neurology library when I arrived in the USA.

We are both honored to have contributed to this renowned series of clinical neurology books.

Eelco F.M. Wijdicks
Andreas H. Kramer

# Contributors

**M.M. Adil**
Ochsner Neuroscience Center, New Orleans, LA, USA

**A. Balofsky**
Department of Anesthesiology, University of Rochester Medical Center, Rochester, NY, USA

**J. Bösel**
Department of Neurology, University of Heidelberg, Heidelberg, Germany

**M.C. Brouwer**
Department of Neurology, Center for Infection and Immunity, Academic Medical Center, University of Amsterdam, Amsterdam, The Netherlands

**D.A. Brown**
Department of Neurological Surgery, Mayo Clinic, Rochester, MN, USA

**M. Czosnyka**
Department of Clinical Neurosciences, University of Cambridge, Cambridge, UK

**A. Ercole**
Division of Anaesthesia, University of Cambridge and Neurosciences/Trauma Critical Care Unit, Addenbrooke's Hospital, Cambridge, UK

**N. Etminan**
Department of Neurosurgery, University Hospital Mannheim, University of Heidelberg, Mannheim, Germany

**E.P. Flanagan**
Department of Neurology, Mayo Clinic, Rochester, MN, USA

**J. George**
Department of Neurology, University of Rochester Medical Center, Rochester, NY, USA

**D.M. Greer**
Department of Neurology, Yale School of Medicine, New Haven, CT, USA

**M.N. Hadley**
Department of Neurosurgery, University of Alabama, Birmingham, AL, USA

**J.J. Halperin**
Overlook Medical Center, Summit, NJ, and Sidney Kimmel Medical College of Thomas Jefferson University, Philadelphia, PA, USA

**J.C. Hemphill III**
Department of Neurology, University of California, San Francisco, CA, USA

**S. Hocker**
Division of Critical Care Neurology, Mayo Clinic, Rochester, MN, USA

**D.Y. Hwang**
Division of Neurocritical Care and Emergency Neurology, Department of Neurology, Yale School of Medicine, New Haven, CT, USA

**T. Jacobs**
Department of Neurosurgery, University of Michigan, Ann Arbor, MI, USA

**G. Korbakis**
Department of Neurosurgery, UCLA David Geffen School of Medicine, Los Angeles, CA, USA

**M. Kottapally**
Department of Neurology, University of Miami, Miami, FL, USA

**A.H. Kramer**
Departments of Critical Care Medicine and Clinical Neurosciences, Hotchkiss Brain Institute, University of Calgary and Southern Alberta Organ and Tissue Donation Program, Calgary, AB, Canada

**D. Larriviere**
Division of Neuromuscular Medicine, Ochsner
Neuroscience Center, New Orleans, LA, USA

**V.H. Lee**
Section of Cerebrovascular Diseases, Department of
Neurological Sciences, Rush University Medical Center,
Chicago, IL, USA

**R.L. Macdonald**
Division of Neurosurgery, St. Michael's Hospital,
Toronto, Ontario, Canada

**C.B. Maciel**
Division of Neurocritical Care and Emergency
Neurology, Department of Neurology, Yale School of
Medicine, New Haven, CT, USA

**J. Mantia**
Clinical Neurophysiology Unit, Sunnybrook Health
Sciences Centre, Toronto, Ontario, Canada

**M. McDermott**
Stroke Program, University of Michigan, Ann Arbor,
MI, USA

**D.K. Menon**
Division of Anaesthesia, University of Cambridge and
Neurosciences/Trauma Critical Care Unit,
Addenbrooke's Hospital, Cambridge, UK

**L. Morgenstern**
Stroke Program, University of Michigan, Ann Arbor,
MI, USA

**P. Nyquist**
Departments of Anesthesiology and Critical Care
Medicine, Neurology and Neurosurgery, and General
Internal Medicine, Johns Hopkins University School of
Medicine, Baltimore, MD, USA

**N.D. Osteraas**
Section of Cerebrovascular Diseases, Department of
Neurological Sciences, Rush University Medical Center,
Chicago, IL, USA

**P. Papadakos**
Departments of Anesthesiology, Neurology, Surgery and
Neurosurgery, University of Rochester Medical Center,
Rochester, NY, USA

**M. Pichler**
Department of Neurology, Mayo Clinic, Rochester,
MN, USA

**J.D. Pickard**
Department of Clinical Neurosciences, University of
Cambridge, Cambridge, UK

**S.J. Pittock**
Department of Neurology and Department of
Laboratory Medicine and Pathology, Mayo Clinic,
Rochester, MN, USA

**L. Rivera-Lara**
Department of Anesthesiology and Critical Care
Medicine and Neurology, Johns Hopkins University
School of Medicine, Baltimore, MD, USA

**D.B. Seder**
Department of Critical Care Services, Maine Medical
Center, Portland, ME and Tufts University School of
Medicine, Boston, MA, USA

**C.D. Shank**
Department of Neurosurgery, University of Alabama,
Birmingham, AL, USA

**K. Sharma**
Division of Neurosciences Critical Care, Johns
Hopkins University School of Medicine, Baltimore,
MD, USA

**L.A. Steiner**
Department for Anesthesia, Surgical Intensive Care,
Prehospital Emergency Medicine and Pain Therapy,
University Hospital of Basel, Basel, Switzerland

**R.D. Stevens**
Division of Neurosciences Critical Care, Johns
Hopkins University School of Medicine, Baltimore,
MD, USA

**A.M. Thabet**
Department of Neurology, University of California,
San Francisco, CA, USA

**D. van de Beek**
Department of Neurology, Center for Infection and
Immunity, Academic Medical Center, University of
Amsterdam, Amsterdam, The Netherlands

**P.M. Vespa**
Departments of Neurosurgery and Neurology, UCLA
David Geffen School of Medicine, Los Angeles,
CA, USA

**B.C. Walters**
Department of Neurosurgery, University of Alabama,
Birmingham, AL, USA

**E.F.M. Wijdicks**
Division of Critical Care Neurology, Mayo Clinic and
Neurosciences Intensive Care Unit, Mayo Clinic
Campus, Saint Marys Hospital, Rochester, MN, USA

**G.B. Young**
Departments of Clinical Neurological Sciences and
Medicine (Critical Care), Western University, London,
Ontario, Canada

**W. Ziai**
Departments of Anesthesiology and Critical Care
Medicine, and Neurology and Neurosurgery, Johns
Hopkins University School of Medicine, Baltimore, MD,
USA

# Contents of Part I

# Contents of Part II

# Section 1

# Care in the neurosciences intensive care unit

*Handbook of Clinical Neurology*, Vol. 140 (3rd series)
*Critical Care Neurology, Part I*
E.F.M. Wijdicks and A.H. Kramer, Editors
http://dx.doi.org/10.1016/B978-0-444-63600-3.00001-5

Chapter 1

# The history of neurocritical care

E.F.M. WIJDICKS*

*Division of Critical Care Neurology, Mayo Clinic and Neurosciences Intensive Care Unit, Mayo Clinic Campus, Saint Marys Hospital, Rochester, MN, USA*

## Abstract

Critical care medicine came into sharp focus in the second part of the 20th century. The care of acutely ill neurologic patients in the USA may have originated in postoperative neurosurgical units, but for many years patients with neurocritical illness were admitted to intensive care units next to patients with general medical or surgical conditions. Neurologists may have had their first exposure to the complexity of neurocritical care during the poliomyelitis epidemics, but few were interested. Much later, the development of neurocritical care as a legitimate subspecialty was possible as a result of a new cadre of neurologists, with support by departments of neurosurgery and anesthesia, who appreciated their added knowledge and expertise in care of acute neurologic illness. Fellowship programs have matured in the US and training programs in certain European countries. Certification in the USA is possible through the American Academy of Neurology United Council of Neurologic Specialties. Most neurointensivists had a formal neurology training. This chapter is a brief analysis of the development of the specialty critical care neurology and how it gained strength, what it is to be a neurointensivist, what the future of care of these patients may hold, and what it takes for neurointensivists to stay exemplary. This chapter revisits some of the earlier known and previously unknown landmarks in the history of neurocritical care.

Modern medicine provides intensive care when necessary, but a need to manage acute serious illness in a satisfactory fashion through close attention to detail has always been an important goal. The care of highly complex deteriorating patients intensified in the second part of the 20th century (Relman, 1980; Reynolds and Tansey, 2011b), and there is a strong sense among medical historians that the poliomyelitis epidemics catalyzed the change in care. Why later changes occurred, which would modify the way care was delivered, and why they occurred against understandable objections of new costs and unknown benefit cannot be easily pinpointed. It is likely that sophistication of practice was gradual and stepwise – as it always is – and due to improved surgical techniques, understanding resuscitation of shock, ability to treat infections in a timely fashion with antibiotics, technical advances, and greater availability of positive-pressure mechanical ventilators. The sickest patients would now be admitted to a special ward called the intensive care unit (ICU). The critically ill patient would now have to cared for by newly specialized physicians and greatly specialized nursing staff. (Hilberman, 1975; Grenvik et al., 1981; Calvin et al., 1997; Bryan-Brown, 2007).

In comparison, care of patients with acute brain and spine injury was less developed and incomplete, and sadly initially involved decisions whether the patient was salvageable or not at the time of presentation. Many patients in coma from a massive brain injury inexorably succumbed from hypoxemia and cardiac arrest. It was known to many clinicians that acute brain injury would lead to breathing difficulties and apnea first, and then cardiac arrest. Acutely increased intracranial pressure (for example, from a ruptured cerebral aneurysm) could lead to severe bradycardia or asystole. Once an open airway or ventilatory support could be secured, patients' vital signs stabilized, such that physicians could focus on the

---

*Correspondence to: Eelco F.M. Wijdicks, Department of Neurology, Mayo Clinic, 200 First Street SW, Rochester MN 55905, USA. E-mail: wijde@mayo.edu

treatment of primary and secondary insults to the brain. This fundamental change in care of a severely brain-injured patient prevented patients from rapidly dying, and provided an opportunity to recover, but also maintained some patients in extremis with no realistic chance of improvement. The comprehensive management of acute brain injury came much later, but even then, the involvement of the neurologist would be often little more than to diagnose the acute neurologic disorder and to say whether it is "good or bad."

The care of acutely ill neurologic patients in the USA may have originated in postoperative neurosurgical units, but for many years such patients were also cared for in general, undifferentiated ICUs, next to patients with medical or surgical illnesses. It is still this way today in many hospitals at smaller medical centers and in countries, outside the USA (Bleck and Klawans, 1986; Bleck, 2009).

This chapter is a preliminary and necessarily unfinished attempt at a synthesis. For many decades, epidemics, natural disasters, and mass casualities taught us that the care of an acutely affected population requires both special hospital wards and multidisciplinary interaction. But there was a more profound change in conceptualization of care and we can ask ourselves: what happened in these so-called ICUs (and neuroscience ICUs in particular) and how did models of care evolve? What is it that epitomizes the care of the acutely ill neurologic and neurosurgical patient? What would be needed to maintain expertise and to make progress? Many specialists for many years have cared for critically ill neurologic and neurosurgical patients. The format of the *Handbook of Clinical Neurology* allows us to engage our interest preferentially with the neurologist becoming a neurointensivist. Revisiting some of the earlier landmarks will provide a clearer view of how this specialty came to be and where it could go.

## EARLY BEGINNINGS OF INTENSIVE CARE MEDICINE AND NEUROLOGY

Physicians like to have "fathers" of medicine, but medical historians know better – specialties usually evolve gradually with fits and starts and with contributions of many. History of medicine is not a history of bravura men alone, although several pioneers in critical care medicine must be mentioned (Grenvik et al., 1981; Rosengart, 2006).

The early pioneers of ICUs identified that sick patients needed one-to-one nursing care. In the early 1950s, some hospital staff had the foresight that a specific hospital space would need to be designed to take care of the most critically ill patients, which also would require specifically trained nurses. This model was different from other hospital models. The simple concept

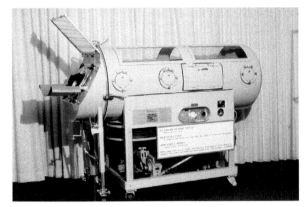

**Fig. 1.1.** Iron lung. Used with the permission of Mayo foundation for Medical Education and Research. All rights reserved.

of having a separate unit for the complicated and unstable patients developed gradually in the USA, but more acutely in Europe after the major poliomyelitis epidemics. Once these epidemics subsided (due to the introduction of Salk's vaccine), hospital administrators, but mostly nursing staff, recognized that these wards could have an important function for future patients.

One can argue that intensive care at the time was defined by the need for mechanical ventilation. In the 1950s, mechanical ventilation was effective with the so-called "iron lung," a tank which incorporated electrically driven blowers and created inspiration with negative pressures and expiration with positive pressures (Fig. 1.1). Within the chamber, sealing the patient at the neck, a negative pressure caused the abdomen and thorax to expand with air flowing into the lungs. A cycle was produced by returning to atmospheric pressure. Depending on the cause of respiratory support, patients could be liberated from the device, or transitioned to a cuirass ventilator. In these early days of mechanical ventilation, hospitals throughout the world would have only a few of these respirators available.

In Europe, intensive care medicine started as an extension of the field of anesthesiology, with Lassen and Ibsen, who handled and organized the care of patients during the major poliomyelitis epidemic in Denmark (Lassen, 1953; Ibsen, 1954). This 1952 outbreak in Denmark resulted in a growing number of admissions of patients with respiratory failure or bulbar weakness who were closing off their airways due to pooling of secretions. Only one iron lung ventilator was available in Blegham hospital, which led to the decision to aggressively treat these patients with an emergency tracheostomy (the technique for emergency tracheostomy had been known for years). Respiratory support was provided with bag ventilation and a soda lime canister to absorb exhaled carbon dioxide (Fig. 1.2). Mortality as

THE LANCET]                                          [JAN. 3, 1953  37

## Special Articles

### A PRELIMINARY REPORT ON
### THE 1952 EPIDEMIC OF POLIOMYELITIS
### IN COPENHAGEN
#### WITH SPECIAL REFERENCE TO THE TREATMENT
#### OF ACUTE RESPIRATORY INSUFFICIENCY

H. C. A. LASSEN

M.D. Copenhagen

PROFESSOR OF EPIDEMIOLOGY IN THE UNIVERSITY OF
COPENHAGEN ; CHIEF PHYSICIAN, DEPARTMENT FOR COM-
MUNICABLE DISEASES, BLEGDAM HOSPITAL, COPENHAGEN

THE 1952 epidemic of poliomyelitis in Greater Copenhagen has been the largest and most severe local epidemic
ever recorded in Denmark.

#### ADMISSIONS

The metropolitan area of Copenhagen has a population
of 1,200,000 people served by a single hospital for
communicable diseases, the Blegdam Hospital. Between
July 24 and Dec. 3 2722 patients with poliomyelitis
were admitted to this hospital—866 with paralysis and
1856 without. In 316 of the 866 paralytic cases we had
to resort to special measures, such as tracheotomy,
artificial respiration, postural drainage, or combinations
of these. The enormous load of severely ill patients is
well illustrated by the fact that in four months we
treated three times as many cases with respiratory
insufficiency, paralysis of the ninth, tenth, and twelfth
cranial nerves, and involvement of the bulbar respiratory
and vasomotor centres as in the preceding ten years.
At times we had 70 patients requiring artificial respiration, and we still have from 50 to 60 requiring it. To
my knowledge nothing comparable has ever been seen
in Europe.

The great number of severely ill patients pouring in
made therapeutic improvisations necessary. During
these months we have in fact been in a state of war,
and at the beginning we were not nearly adequately
equipped to meet an emergency of such vast proportions.

Fig. 1 shows that the epidemic culminated about
Sept. 1. During the week Aug. 28–Sept. 3 our hospital
admitted 335 patients or nearly 50 cases daily. The
descending branch of the epidemic curve is, as usual,
less steep than the ascending branch. At the time of
writing, Dec. 7, the epidemic seems to be nearing its

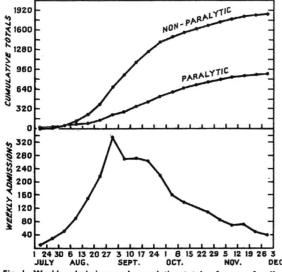

**Fig. I—Weekly admissions and cumulative totals of cases of polio-
myelitis in 1952.**

end. During the last two months the proportion of
paralytic in relation to non-paralytic cases has grown
steadily, but as a whole the ratio is 1 : 2. Naturally the
number of patients admitted with non-paralytic poliomyelitis does not give an accurate picture of the true
incidence of such cases in the epidemic area.

#### TREATMENT OF RESPIRATORY INSUFFICIENCY AND BULBAR DISEASE

In former years our therapeutic results in cases with
respiratory insufficiency and involvement of the lower
cranial nerves and the bulbar centres have always been
very bad.

During the eleven years 1934–44 respirator treatment
was used in 76 cases with a mean mortality-rate of 80%.
Only cuirass respirators were used.

It is generally agreed that respiratory insufficiency of
spinal origin is far easier to treat than respiratory
insufficiency due to the involvement of the lower cranial
nerves and the bulbar centres. Table I shows clearly
the extremely grave prognosis of the pure bulbar and
combined forms of respiratory insufficiency. With very
few exceptions all our patients belonging to these
groups died.

In 1948 we started using tracheotomy in all cases
where it proved impossible to maintain an open airway
because of pooling of secretions and aspiration into the
lungs. In the U.S.A. this procedure seems to have had

TABLE I—RESULTS OF RESPIRATOR TREATMENT OF POLIO-
MYELITIS 1934–44

| Type of disease | No. of cases | No. of deaths |
|---|---|---|
| Respiratory paralysis without bulbar involvement .. .. .. | 17 | 5 (28%) |
| Respiratory paralysis with bulbar involvement .. .. | 51 | 48 (94%) |
| Respiratory paralysis of undetermined type .. .. .. .. | 8 | 8 (100%) |

a beneficial influence on prognosis. In our hands this
has not been so.

Table II shows that all the patients treated by tracheotomy and with respirators died, whereas treatment
with respirators alone had a somewhat better prognosis,
1 man and 4 children surviving. Of these 5 patients
4 had respiratory insufficiency of purely spinal origin, and
1 patient had transient slight impairment of swallowing.

Thus the prognosis of poliomyelitis with respiratory
insufficiency was rather gloomy at the outbreak of the
present epidemic in Copenhagen. At our disposal we
had one tank respirator (Emerson) and six cuirass
respirators. This equipment proved wholly insufficient
when the epidemic developed into a major catastrophe.

Fig. 2 shows the admission dates of the 316 poliomyelitis patients requiring special treatment—i.e.,
tracheotomy, artificial respiration, postural drainage,
and combinations of these forms of treatment. The
chart exclusively comprises patients with respiratory
insufficiency, paralysis of the lower cranial nerves, the
respiratory or vasomotor bulbar centres or combinations of
these forms of paralysis. During the epidemic tracheotomy was performed in about 250 cases. The indication
for this operation was invariably stagnation of secretions
in the upper airway, leading to inadequate ventilation.
By far the greater number of the patients had simultaneously paralysis of the respiratory muscles. The
316 cases did not all come from the metropolitan area,
because in recent years we have done much to centralise
the treatment of such patients. Consequently fig. 2
includes 75 cases brought in from localities outside our
usual area. These admissions account for the three peaks
of the curve.

Until the last week of August we used the therapeutic
methods practised in 1948–50, but during these terrible
weeks the situation became increasingly critical. The

a result of manual ventilation (medical students and staff) dropped from about 80% to 50% with this change (Lassen, 1953). Ibsen was also responsible for better triage of patients after emergency tracheostomy to centers with this capability. Tracheostomy and positive-pressure ventilation made care much easier than care of patients in a tank or shell respirator. These dramatic events led to further innovations in care, and are considered by many practitioners from that era to be "the birth of intensive care" (Ibsen, 1954; Berthelsen and Cronqvist, 2003; Reisner-Senelar, 2011).

In the USA, Max Harry Weil, a physician at the University of Southern California in Los Angeles, developed the Institute of Critical Care Medicine, which eventually moved to Rancho Mirage (Sun and Tang, 2011). Apart from possibly coining the term "critical care" first, he emphasized the need for a specific unit, which was opened with four beds in 1958 and referred to as a "shock ward" – a precursor to the ICU with daily rounding. He was also responsible for the rolling "crash carts," which allowed immediate resuscitation at the bedside; introduced measurement of lactic acid as a marker of organ perfusion; and developed, for the first time, computerized monitoring of critically ill patients (Weil, 1973). Other pioneers were William Schoemaker (a trauma surgeon at Cook Country Hospital in Chicago who advanced optimal treatment of shock) and Peter Safar (an anesthesiologist at the University of Pittsburg who pioneered cardiopulmonary resuscitation) (Safar and Grenvik, 1971; Shoemaker et al., 1984; Safar, 1986). These three physicians from different backgrounds have been identified as the early leaders in critical care medicine and founded the Society of Critical Care Medicine in 1971. The Society eventually further beaconed off its field, welcomed multiple types of specialists, and created training programs and guidelines. Since 1995 the Society has been a professional scientific society. (The European counterpart is the European Society of Intensive Care Medicine (ESICM). The first meeting of the ESICM took place in Geneva in 1981.).

Another notable development in the history of intensive care medicine was the development of methods to predict mortality in more severely affected patients. Knaus and Zimmerman were instrumental in developing the Acute Physiology and Chronic Health Evaluation, better known as the APACHE scale (Knaus et al., 1981, 1985). This system could predict outcome on the basis of physiologic abnormalities, and would substantially improve predictability of outcome, potentially justifying continuation or de-escalation of care. Many variables needed to be tallied, including treatment factors, status before ICU admission, and response to therapies. Glasgow Coma Scale score was incorporated into the APACHE score, and it was not surprising that coma

was an important identifier of outcome (Teres et al., 1982).

The early beginnings of critical care neurology undoubtedly started with the poliomyelitis epidemics, which is where neurologists came in. In the UK, intensive care started with respiratory care units in the late 1950s (Marshall, 1961; Reynolds and Tansey, 2011a, b). Most notable were Batten respiratory care unit and National Hospital for Neurosurgery in London admitting patients with poliomyelitis, myasthenia gravis, and tetanus, among many other patients with more acute and chronic respiratory disease (Bodman et al., 1955; Prys-Roberts et al., 1969). Spalding and Russell (both neurologists) and Crampton Smith (anesthesiologist) were responsible for the respiratory unit of the Churchill hospital in Oxford (Spalding and Crampton, 1963). These units were primarily housed in "Nissen huts," which were temporary, rapidly erected wartime buildings. There were two neurology wards in these "huts," housing about 20 patients in each, and there was an adjoining special ICU with either four or six beds, at least two of which were iron lungs. Russell and Spalding would together develop the Radcliffe ventilator and humidification system (Russell and Schuster, 1953). Many tetanus patients could survive through the combination of mechanical ventilation and pharmacologic neuromuscular paralysis. Russell's work (Fig. 1.3) identified poliomyelitis defined by their respiratory care. He divided cases into cases with difficulty in swallowing with no respiratory weakness, cases involving weakness of respiratory muscles but no oropharyngeal weakness, and combined cases in which there was paralysis of both respiratory muscles and oropharyngeal muscles. He emphasized examination of the respiratory muscles and included the abdominal muscles as playing an important role in coughing up secretions. Inability to count beyond 10 in one breath as a sign of reduced vital capacity is mentioned. Care includes postural drainage to avoid aspiration in patients without respiratory failure and involving inverted V and tilted bed.

In the USA, there were respiratory care units in most academic institutions. Close involvement in direct patient care by neurologists was not often seen in the USA, and neurologists were mostly involved only in the diagnostic evaluation of these patients (Anderson and Ibsen, 1954). Some neurologists were involved in assessment of bulbar dysfunction associated with poliomyelitis requiring emergency tracheostomy and it was combined with a vest-type ventilator to support the respiratory mechanics until positive-pressure respirators were introduced. The most notable exception was the neurologist AB Baker, who reported on the complex care of bulbar poliomyelitis with detailed descriptions of airway management, prevention and treatment of infections, pulmonary edema, gastrointestinal complications, and

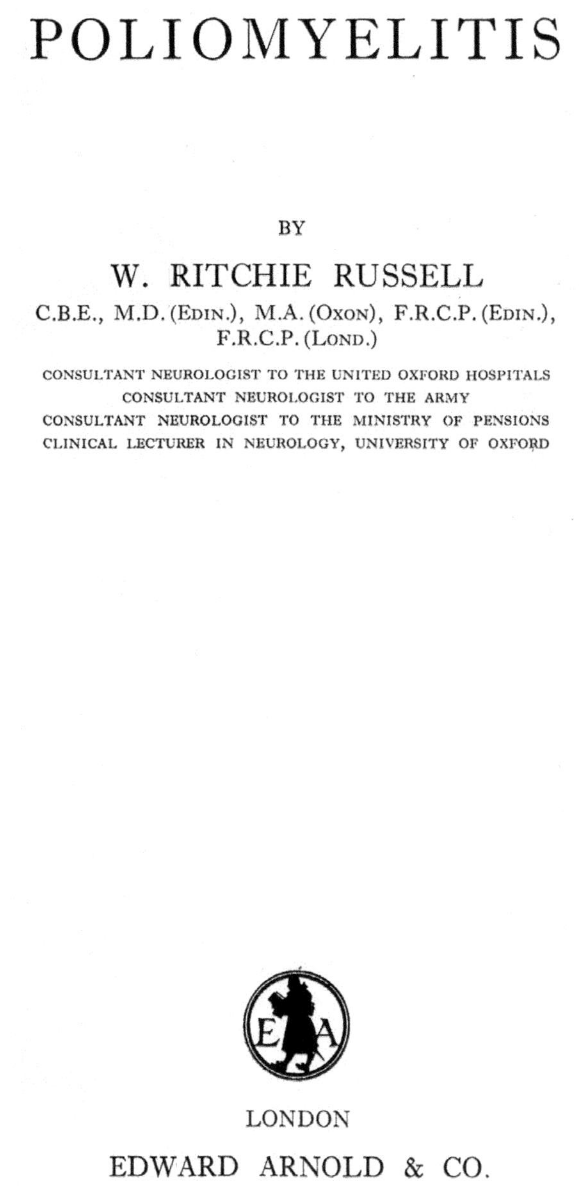

# POLIOMYELITIS

BY

## W. RITCHIE RUSSELL

C.B.E., M.D. (Edin.), M.A. (Oxon), F.R.C.P. (Edin.),
F.R.C.P. (Lond.)

CONSULTANT NEUROLOGIST TO THE UNITED OXFORD HOSPITALS
CONSULTANT NEUROLOGIST TO THE ARMY
CONSULTANT NEUROLOGIST TO THE MINISTRY OF PENSIONS
CLINICAL LECTURER IN NEUROLOGY, UNIVERSITY OF OXFORD

LONDON

EDWARD ARNOLD & CO.

**Fig. 1.3.** W. Ritchie Russell's contribution to the general and respiratory care of poliomyelitis. From Russell and Schuster (1953).

nearly all other aspects of care that concern a modern neurointensivist today (Wijdicks, 2016a, b). This knowledge originated in large part from a 1946 severe poliomyelitis epidemic occurring in Minnesota, with nearly 200 cases admitted to University of Minnesota hospitals. Baker, the chief of neurology, became one of the most experienced US neurologists in the treatment of poliomyelitis and presumably introduced tracheostomy as part of care (Brown and Baker, 1947; Baker, 1954, 1957). Another prominent neurologist was Fred Plum, who developed a respiratory center at Harborview Hospital in Seattle, located between the neurology

and infectious disease ward, that housed patients with acute poliomyelitis. Consequently, he would publish a series of detailed and original papers on the respiratory care of patients with poliomyelitis, and even contributed a detailed chapter to Baker's four-volume book on clinical neurology (Plum and Wolff, 1951; Plum and Dunning, 1956).

More specialized units appeared, with each representing a different path of development. Surgical recovery units became surgical ICUs; patients with treatable cardiac arrhythmias after myocardial infarction were admitted to coronary care units. Any patient with multiorgan trauma ended up in a trauma ICU, coordinated by trauma surgeons and later by surgical intensivists. The ability to place premature newborns in an incubator resulted in the establishment of neonatal ICUs. Similar developments occurred with burn units.

A history of critical care medicine may also be written in terms of improving technology. Advances in mechanical ventilation, reliable venous and arterial access, monitoring of invasive hemodynamics (including the now nearly defunct Swan–Ganz balloon catheter) and noninvasive assessment (ICU sonography) changed practice dramatically.

Besides all that, there was a growing sense that progress in intensive care was not possible without specialized nursing care, with which it is associated. The role of nursing care has often been underappreciated by physicians who have mostly written the histories. Critical care nursing started with the establishment of the American Association of Cardiovascular Nurses in 1969, the name of which was subsequently changed to the American Association of Critical Care Nurses. From the early days to the present, the ingenuity and perseverance of critical care nurses against odds made multidisciplinary care possible. Truth be told, in many ICUs, the daily care and recognition of manifestations of critical illness are in the hands of the nursing staff.

## A NEW PHASE OF CRITICAL CARE NEUROLOGY

After the polio epidemics interest by neurologists in the 1960s was not sustained, and most of the care of acutely ill neurologic patients admitted to ICUs was by intensivists, with neurologists consulting and advising.

It will be difficult to precisely identify pinpoint the beginnings but some of the currently practicing neurointensivists rightfully argue that neurocritical care evolved out of neurosurgery, and thus we have to revisit the first decade of the 20th century starting with neurosurgeon Harvey Cushing. In the words of his biographer Michael Bliss, he decided to open the closed box of the skull, expecting to do more good than harm (Bliss, 2005).

Cushing realized that many of his postoperative patients needed close observation, and in the event of a major postoperative complication, he would not stop until he determined the cause and mechanism. This is best illustrated by his quest to understand postoperative fatality, which in some cases was related to gastric hemorrhages (Wijdicks, 2011).

Neurosurgeon Dandy has been credited by many as having opened one of the first neuroscience ICUs at Johns Hopkins University. In 1932, he refurbished a ward, where he then admitted his sickest postoperative neurosurgical patients. These units were typically used for neurosurgical patients and to allow close monitoring in the postoperative phase. However, the patients were usually managed by anesthesiologist or intensivists if a major systemic complication occurred.

Care of traumatic brain injury became better organized as a result of neurosurgical involvement (most famously the Glasgow neurosurgeons Bryan Jennett and Graham Teasdale). In addition, neurosurgeons were interested in treating increased intracranial pressure after traumatic head injury. When they performed craniotomies for acute subdural hematoma, they sometimes opted for a craniectomy in more severe cases of refractory intracranial hypertension. Almost parallel to care of head injury was better understanding of care of spinal cord injury, which became more organized in the early 1900s, especially after World War I. Two neurosurgeons are responsible for pioneering the care of these devastated patients. One major spinal unit was developed by neurosurgeon Donald Munro (Munro, 1954). He established the first spinal cord unit in the USA at Boston City Hospital in 1936. With his comprehensive approach to care, patients survived more often and with less morbidity. Sir Ludwig Guttmann, a neurologist and neurosurgeon, organized another major spinal cord unit in 1944 at Stoke Mandeville Hospital in Aylesbury, UK. This unit was created in anticipation of casualties of war in the major spring offensive (Guttman, 1967).

The participation of neurologists and neurosurgeons in those years seemed impromptu. Neurosurgical units often had interested neuroanesthesiologists, and this led to specific care protocols and research in traumatic brain injury, not only in the USA and UK, but also in other countries. Care of the majority of patients in these ICUs remained overwhelmingly for neurosurgical trauma and aneurysmal subarachnoid hemorrhage. Guidelines for managing severe traumatic brain injury were first established in 1996 by the Brain Trauma Foundation, and were later accepted by both the American Association of Neurological Surgeons and the World Health Organization Committee in Neurotraumatology (Bullock et al., 1996).

Little is known about the triage of patients with acute neurologic conditions in those days, but neurocritical care in the USA may have emerged from several lineages and has several ancestors. First, in 1985 the American Board of Neurologic Surgeons approved an interspecialty certification for neurosurgical intensive care, but this did not lead to practicing neurosurgical neurointensivists, such that a void remained. Because neurosurgeons performed more extensive surgeries, and needed neurologic coverage of other patients in the unit during these long cases, neurologic services were appreciated. While reconstructing this period, it is clear that the close cooperation between neurology and neurosurgery consultants in the neuroscience ICU was distinctively characteristic. When asked to co-manage these patients, neurologists had to educate themselves to become more knowledgeable, and to become proficient in the treatment of increased intracranial pressure and the management of both neurosurgical and systemic complications. Many of these first units were for either neurosurgical or neurologic patients.

At Mayo Clinic, the first newly built combined neuroscience ICU was at Saint Mary's Hospital (Wijdicks et al., 2011). Patients with meningitis and status epilepticus were admitted there as well. The need for further education also applied to the allied staff. For nursing staff, there was instruction in the basic neurosciences and review of neuroanatomy. Some of the neuroanesthesiologists gave lectures on respiratory care, including safe and effective provision of oxygen. The rehabilitation services were often consulted to assist in use of rocking beds and chest physiotherapy. At that time, use of hypothermia blankets was also common. Teaching of residents in neurosurgery and neurology was done at the bedside during daily attending staff and resident rounds.

It would have to wait until the 1970s for a renewed interest in acute neurology and coma by neurologists. The development of the specialty of critical care and emergency neurology, or neurocritical care, as it is often called, is shown in Table 1.1. The evolution of neurocritical care was possible as a result of energetic, deeply engaged neurologists, and support by departments of neurosurgery and anesthesia, appreciating their added knowledge and expertise in the assessment of acute neurologic illness. Already in the late 1980s neurologists assumed co-director positions in neuroscience ICUs. In the USA, most neurocritical care units matured when combining neurosurgical and neurologic patients. This would seem logical, because acutely ill neurologic patients could need neurosurgical intervention (e.g., cerebral hematoma) and acutely ill neurosurgical patients could benefit from neurologic expertise (e.g., seizure management). Because of the open nature of the neurocritical care unit, physicians from multiple disciplines would closely cooperate in patient management.

*Table 1.1*

**Major landmarks in development of neurocritical care**

| | |
|---|---|
| 1950s | Neurologists interested in acute neurology |
| 1960s | Several papers published on ventilatory care in poliomyelitis by Fred Plum, Richie Russell and A. B. Baker |
| | Publication of *The Diagnosis of Stupor and Coma* by Fred Plum and Jerome Posner (1966) |
| 1970s | Interest and research in treatments of intracranial pressure (ventriculostomy, decompressive craniotomy, barbiturates) |
| 1980s | Research in management of subarachnoid hemorrhage by neurologists (antifibrinolytic treatment for rebleeding, hyponatremia and fluid management) |
| | Neurologists rounding in the neurologic and neurosurgical intensive care |
| | (Allan Ropper at Massachusetts General Hospital, Daniel Hanley at Johns Hopkins, Matthew Fink at Columbia University) |
| | Founding section of critical care and emergency neurology |
| | (American Academy of Neurology) |
| 1990s | Further refinement of the field of critical care neurology (development of best practice) |
| | Start of clinical trials organized by neurointensivists (Factor VII in cerebral hemorrhage, blood pressure management in cerebral hemorrhage, thrombolysis in intraventricular hemorrhage) |
| 2000s | Founding of the Neurocritical Care Society (president Thomas Bleck) |
| | Inaugural issue of *Neurocritical Care* journal |
| | Educational programs (Emergency Neurological Life Support) |
| | Development of fellowship curricula and certification examinations (United Council of Neurologic Specialties) |

A second major development was that neurologists became interested in patients admitted in the ICU, particularly in the USA. In the neurologic literature and textbooks, very little was written on diagnosis of the comatose patient. Before neurologists Plum and Posner would write their original textbook on the diagnosis of stupor and coma, papers on care of the comatose patient were written by other specialists, mostly anesthesiologists. Patient management at the time was directed mostly towards general patient care, with avoidance of hypotension and hypoxemia – the precursors of the "ABC" of resuscitation. Plum and Posner's monograph on stupor and coma, published in 1966, introduced many neurologists to the detailed examination of the comatose patient, including the clinical course of brain herniation. Many neurointensivists from the early beginnings will recall that they became interested in acute neurology after reading this book.

Eventually, neurologists would join intensivists to develop hands-on training, which allowed them to manage these complicated patients (Borel and Hanley, 1985). Management of respiratory failure in acute neuromuscular disorders became better understood, and clinical trials would often admit the severely affected patients to the neurosciences ICU. The first textbook of intensive care neurology grew out of a Harvard-sponsored teaching course, and was edited by Ropper, Kennedy and Zervas (Ropper et al., 1983). Ropper defined neurologic intensive care as primarily concerned with treatment of raised intracranial pressure, care and examination of the comatose patient, treatment of neuromuscular respiratory failure, use of therapies specific for acute stroke, cerebral hemorrhage, aneurysmal subarachnoid hemorrhage, head injury, status epilepticus, among other conditions, and treatment of medical complications typical for acute neurologic illness (Ropper et al., 1983). Recognition of the specifics of deterioration of patients with acute brain injury, Neurologic complications of medical and surgical critical illness, and recognition, treatment, and triage of acute neurology in the emergency department became recognized in the 1990s as important additional areas in the field (Wijdicks, 1995, 1997, 2000).

Neurologists learned their trade "on the go." In the 1990s, there was a marked increment in the number of textbooks and publications, which for the first time refined causes of deterioration in patients with acute brain injury, the treatment and prognostication of coma. A number of important guidelines associated with prognostication and brain death determination followed (Ropper and Davis, 1980; Ropper et al., 1982; Ropper and King, 1984; Ropper and Shafran, 1984; Ropper and Kehne, 1985). In 2004 the Neurocritical Care Society was founded, with Thomas Bleck as the first president, and this also included a founding of a new academic journal (Wijdicks, 2004). In Germany, a neurocritical care society, Deutsche Gesellschaft für Neurointensiv- und Notfallmedizin, was founded in 1983, and is the oldest society, with members from various specialties, including emergency medicine.

More defined practice eventually culminated in certification examinations through the United Council of Neurologic Specialties (UCNS), an administrative body of the American Academy of Neurology. Training involves a 2-year fellowship. The Neurocritical Care Society recognized that, to practice critical care neurology well, training does not consist only of intensive care training after neurology training, as it is in other places in the world. To become knowledgeable and to develop skills in urgent care would require sufficient training in a neurosciences ICU, where patients were admitted and decisions are made. Neurologists and later other specialists could qualify for such a fellowship.

The UCNS provided a template for defining practice, and the body of knowledge that beginning neurointensivists should acquire. It could only come from seeing many patients, with many disorders in all its diverse presentations, who may develop disease-specific complications. Full understanding of electrophysiology and neuroimaging of acute brain disorders was needed, and this would set neurointensivists apart from other intensive care practices. The Society also produced educational material to foster better care. One example is the Emergency Neurological Life Support (ENLS) course, a joint venture between the emergency medicine community and neurointensivists. The purpose was to improve care during the first hour of an acute neurologic emergency (Smith and Weingart, 2012). Consensus meetings on best practice followed and further cemented the major role that the Neurocritical Care Society could play in practice (Diringer et al., 2011).

Currently, most neurointensive care units are combined neurologic and neurosurgical units. With mixing these patients and specialists in neurology and neurosurgery, acutely ill neurosurgical patients could benefit from neurologic expertise, and acutely ill neurologic patients could benefit from neurosurgical expertise or intervention. This markedly improved the care of these patients, and in many centers replaced "open" ICUs, where different physicians and numerous consultants take care of patients, resulting in poor communication and coordination (Mayer et al., 2006a, b; Wijdicks, 2006).

More elaborate monitoring of the patient apart from a comprehensive neurologic examination has become a major new interest. A recent consensus statement concluded that, although several monitoring devices are available which can address several important physiologic parameters, there are a considerable number of shortcomings that perhaps could question the foundation of multimodal monitoring. Some of the monitoring devices have been used predominantly in traumatic brain injury and subarachnoid hemorrhage, and extrapolation to other causes of acute brain injury could not be easily justified. The consensus statement identified that very few studies purport to show that outcome is improved with knowledge of certain physiologic data, and a number of significant flaws were found in a detailed review of published material (Le Roux et al., 2014).

Responsible use of resources and costs remain important considerations (Cullen et al., 1976; Goldstein et al., 1986). The concept of using statistical models to determine if a patient could benefit from intensive care was not immediately and widely accepted. To use a mathematic measure of severity, rather than clinical judgment, was difficult to fathom by many physicians, particularly those with many years of experience. In the early 1980s, care of patients with hopeless neurologic conditions became a topic of considerable interest, although prognosis often was considered an "educated empirical guess." Studies by Bates et al. (1977) and Levy et al. (1981, 1985) identified specific neurologic findings that could predict a poor outcome with a high degree of certainty. These findings in persistently comatose patients included absent pupillary light reflexes and abnormal motor responses, such as pathologic flexion or extension. This was followed by important prediction papers by the Glasgow group, led by Jennett, Teasdale, and Braakman. Neurosurgeon Bryan Jennett initiated an international head injury data bank, which resulted in large data sets using mathematic calculations for predicting outcome (Jennett et al., 1976, 1979, 1980; Jennett and Braakman, 1990). Outcome prediction has improved over time in nontraumatic and traumatic coma, but remains a challenging aspect of daily neurocritical care practice (Wijdicks et al., 2006).

Finally, there have been a substantial number of clinical trials organized by neurointensivists, supported both by industry and the National Institutes of Health (www.braininjuryoutcomes.com).

## A PERSPECTIVE

Although many specialist colleagues thought disparagingly of the "neurointensivist" (and some still do), and territorial disputes were widespread, the care of the critically ill neurologic patient with acute brain, spine, or neuromuscular disorders is widely considered to be a legitimate specialty. The specialty has several names: neurologic intensive care, critical care neurology, and neurocritical care. It has many links to other specialties, but can easily set itself apart as a new specialty (Fig. 1.4) (Lanier, 2012; Mashour, 2012; Kelly et al., 2014).

Certification in the USA is possible through the UCNS. This organization is not recognized by the American Board of Medical Specialties. There is interest in board certification through neurologic societies in Europe. In the UK, progress towards certification is in the early stages, but there is a major demand for training programs to provide an adequate number of opportunities. The majority of case-based teaching for neurocritical care will occur during scheduled rotations in the neurocritical care unit. Simulation of acute neurologic disorders and decision making is increasingly in development. Entrustable professional activities (EPAs) are now used as core assessment tools for neurology trainees,

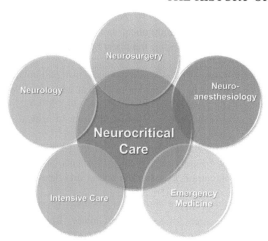

**Fig. 1.4.** Interactions of neurocritical care with other specialties. Used with the permission of Mayo foundation for Medical Education and Research. All rights reserved.

and these EPAs are mapped to milestones within the Accreditation Council for Graduate Medical Education core competencies. Incorporating neurology-specific scenarios into simulation can ensure that specific EPAs are met.

Virtually all of the neuroemergency EPA scenarios are not trained. Some of the most impactful learning experiences occur when physicians faced with neurologic emergencies err. In contrast to the traditional approach, we can reproduce the stress response when faced with an emergency, an unknown clinical situation in flux, a complication of treatment decisions, or an error. Many major academic institutions have centers in place with experienced personnel, and there is major interest to venture into this field. Expertise in neurosimulation requires a new sort of creative teacher with energy and commitment. Some types of acute neurologic illness are more conducive to simulation than others. Scenarios can be built to teach avoidance of errors, course of action, and cerebral resuscitation, but also the difficulties of communicating complex decisions with family members. Using simulation to teach emergency and critical care neurology is a new opportunity (Brydges et al., 2015; Hocker et al., 2015). Exposure should allow the trainee to obtain the knowledge and skills required to manage neurocritical illness.

Care of the patient by the best-qualified specialist should always be emphasized. This also applies to the patient with a major acute brain injury requiring urgent medical and neurologic care. When we look at our times, we need to put a premium of the care of the patient first and leave politics and turf battles behind. Only then can we strive and improve our competency, and gain a better understanding of why patients are not doing so well, and

how to increase the chances of a favorable functional recovery.

The main neurologic ICU models are open, transitional, and closed units. In the closed ICU, one team that is led by neurointensivists cares for all patients, and only neurointensivists or neurosurgeons have admitting privileges. Consultants, fellows, and residents (mostly in final years of training) do provide an integral part of care. Physician assistants in critical care units can also be part of an excellent practice model. Other team members may include nutritional consultants, infectious disease specialists, and medical emergency (acute code) responders. Most studies of ICUs suggest that closed units reduce complications and mortality, but these specific data are not available for neurocritical care (Carson et al., 1996; Multz et al., 1998). The current situation in the USA is a mixed picture, with open ICUs in many major hospitals and relatively few with a strictly closed neurocritical care unit. Neurointensivists often have their own service and are in a co-primary care role with neurosurgeons. Postoperative care typically remains in the hands of the responsible neurosurgeon and neurosurgical trainees, unless a major medical or neurologic complication occurs (i.e., seizures).

It is expected that neurocritical care will branch out into other fields and there is interest in organizing care of pediatric neurocritical conditions (Murphy et al., 2015). It is a truism that the severity of acute brain injury is the main variable for outcome. However, secondary injury remains important, and thus monitoring of these changes and modifying them should remain a priority. There is no question technology could help the field of neurocritical care greatly if studied rigorously and with a healthy dose of skepticism (Le Roux et al., 2014; Bouzat et al., 2015). Ideal setups for multimodal monitoring can be defined, and research may provide valid data. Not all modalities are widely available, nor is there sufficient expertise in interpreting the acquired data. Research collaborations and improvement in standardization are required.

It is not difficult to imagine a patient and computer interface that provides detailed, sophisticated, online information on brain functioning after a major injury that results in secondary neuronal stress. Automatic adjustment of parameters may follow, and digital alerts to smartphones or tablets would inform the nursing staff and neurointensivist. Functional imaging would be commonplace. We will know in the next decades how much this will remain out of reach, or if our means and ways will be completely different. Just as the carefully localizing neurologist may "lose" from magnetic resonance imaging, so it is possible that neurointensivists' clinical assessments in the digital technocracy may "lose" from data recorded by invasive or noninvasive monitoring. Most of us prefer the clinical observation and detailed examination of the neurologic patient. Is it too much to say that the neurology of neurocritical care is such a crucial part of our understanding of pathophysiology and the expected clinical course that it cannot be compromised, or worse, replaced by a device or test (Wijdicks, 2017).

The practice of neurointensivists has evolved and continues to do so. Daily rounding on patients and reviewing of test results, with rapid-fire decisions in acutely evolving conditions, have been commonplace. What sets this specialty apart is dealing with major neurologic morbidity, which affects the mind and physical function. During a normal day, considerable time is spent in communication with family members about the neurologic condition. Neurointensivists see devastating injury in many patients, and this will affect neurointensivists over time. Being frequently involved with neuropalliation creates the potential for burnout and a phenomenon called compassion fatigue, with avoidance behavior, re-experiencing of patients' suffering, emotional exhaustion, a sense of ineffectiveness, and social withdrawal. We do not know how this will affect neurointensivists and other health care professionals who work in neurocritical care units in the long run, and solutions may need to be in place.

Now, in the 21st century, neurocritical care is a well-defined specialty, and neurointensivists are sought after by recruiting chairs of departments. In all modesty, neurointensivists believe they make a difference and improve outcomes of patients.

## REFERENCES

Anderson EW, Ibsen B (1954). The anaesthetic management of patients with poliomyelitis and respiratory paralysis. BMJ 2: 786–788.

Baker AB (1954). Poliomyelitis. XI. Treatment. Neurology 4: 379–392.

Baker AB (1957). Poliomyelitis. 16. A study of pulmonary edema. Neurology 7: 743–751.

Bates D, Caronna JJ, Cartlidge NE et al. (1977). A prospective study of nontraumatic coma: methods and results in 310 patients. Ann Neurol 2: 211–220.

Berthelsen PG, Cronqvist M (2003). The first intensive care unit in the world: Copenhagen 1953. Acta Anaesthesiol Scand 47: 1190–1195.

Bleck TP (2009). Historical aspects of critical care and the nervous system. Crit Care Clin 25: 153–164.

Bleck TP, Klawans HL (1986). Neurologic emergencies. Med Clin North Am 70: 1167–1184.

Bliss M (2005). Harvey Cushing. A life in surgery, Oxford University Press, New York.

Bodman RI, Morton HJ, Thomas ET (1955). Treatment of tetanus with chlorpromazine and nitrous-oxide anaesthesia. Lancet 269: 230–231.

Borel C, Hanley D (1985). Neurologic intensive care unit monitoring. Crit Care Clin 1: 223–239.

Bouzat P, Marques-Vidal P, Zerlauth JB et al. (2015). Accuracy of brain multimodal monitoring to detect cerebral hypoperfusion after traumatic brain injury. Crit Care Med 43: 445–452.

Brown JR, Baker AB (1947). The bulbar form of poliomyelitis; diagnosis and the correlation of clinical with physiologic and pathologic manifestations. JAMA 134: 757–762.

Bryan-Brown CW (2007). My first 50 years of critical care (1956–2006). Am J Crit Care 16: 12–16.

Brydges R, Hatala R, Zendejas B et al. (2015). Linking simulation-based educational assessments and patient-related outcomes: a systematic review and meta-analysis. Acad Med 90: 246–256.

Bullock RM, Chesnut G, Clifton J et al. (1996). Guidelines for the management of severe head injury. Brain Trauma Foundation. Eur J Emerg Med 3: 109–127.

Calvin JE, Habet K, Parrillo JE (1997). Critical care in the United States. Who are we and how did we get here? Crit Care Clin 13: 363–376.

Carson SS, Stocking C, Podsadecki T et al. (1996). Effects of organizational change in the medical intensive care unit of a teaching hospital: a comparison of 'open' and 'closed' formats. JAMA 276: 322–328.

Cullen DJ, Ferrara LC, Briggs BA et al. (1976). Survival, hospitalization charges and follow-up results in critically ill patients. N Engl J Med 294: 982–987.

Diringer MN, Bleck TP, Claude Hemphill 3rd J et al. (2011). Critical care management of patients following aneurysmal subarachnoid hemorrhage: recommendations from the Neurocritical Care Society's Multidisciplinary Consensus Conference. Neurocrit Care 15: 211–240.

Goldstein RL, Campion EW, Thibault GE et al. (1986). Functional outcomes following medical intensive care. Crit Care Med 14: 783–788.

Grenvik A, Leonard JJ, Arens JF et al. (1981). Critical care medicine. Certification as a multidisciplinary subspecialty. Crit Care Med 9: 117–125.

Guttman LI (1967). Organization of spinal units. History of the National Spinal Injuries Centre, Stoke Mandeville Hospital, Aylesbury. Paraplegia 5: 115–126.

Hilberman M (1975). The evolution of intensive care units. Crit Care Med 3: 159–165.

Hocker S, Wijdicks EFM, Feske SK et al. (2015). Use of simulation in acute neurology training: point and counterpoint. Ann Neurol 78: 337–342.

Ibsen B (1954). The anaesthetist's viewpoint on the treatment of respiratory complications in poliomyelitis during the epidemic in Copenhagen, 1952. Proc R Soc Med 47: 72–74.

Jennett B, Braakman R (1990). Severe traumatic brain injury. J Neurosurg 73: 479–480.

Jennett B, Teasdale G, Braakman R et al. (1976). Predicting outcome in individual patients after severe head injury. Lancet 1: 1031–1034.

Jennett B, Teasdale G, Braakman R et al. (1979). Prognosis of patients with severe head injury. Neurosurgery 4: 283–289.

Jennett B, Teasdale G, Braakman R et al. (1980). Treatment for severe head injury. J Neurol Neurosurg Psychiatry 43: 289–295.

Kelly FE, Fong K, Hirsch N et al. (2014). Intensive care medicine is 60 years old: the history and future of the intensive care unit. Clin Med 14: 376–379.

Knaus WA, Zimmerman JE, Wagner DP et al. (1981). APACHE – acute physiology and chronic health evaluation: a physiologically based classification system. Crit Care Med 9: 591–597.

Knaus WA, Draper EA, Wagner DP et al. (1985). APACHE II: a severity of disease classification system. Crit Care Med 13: 818–829.

Lanier WL (2012). The history of neuroanesthesiology: the people, pursuits, and practices. J Neurosurg Anesthesiol 24: 281–299.

Lassen HC (1953). A preliminary report on the 1952 epidemic of poliomyelitis in Copenhagen with special reference to the treatment of acute respiratory insufficiency. Lancet 1: 37–41.

Le Roux P, Menon DK, Citerio G et al. (2014). Consensus Summary Statement of the International Multidisciplinary Consensus Conference on Multimodality Monitoring in Neurocritical Care : A statement for healthcare professionals from the Neurocritical Care Society and the European Society of Intensive Care Medicine. Neurocrit Care 21 (Suppl 2): S1–S26.

Levy DE, Bates D, Caronna JJ et al. (1981). Prognosis in nontraumatic coma. Ann Intern Med 3: 293–301.

Levy DE, Caronna JJ, Singer BH et al. (1985). Predicting outcome from hypoxic-ischemic coma. JAMA 253: 1420–1426.

Marshall J (1961). The work of a respiratory unit in a neurological hospital. Postgrad Med J 37: 26–30.

Mashour GA (2012). Neuroanesthesiology: then and now. Anesth Analg 114: 715–717.

Mayer SA, Coplin WM, Chang C et al. (2006a). Core curriculum and competencies for advanced training in neurological intensive care: United Council for Neurologic Subspecialties guidelines. Neurocrit Care 5: 159–165.

Mayer SA, Coplin WM, Chang C et al. (2006b). Program requirements for fellowship training in neurological intensive care: United Council for Neurologic Subspecialties guidelines. Neurocrit Care 5: 166–171.

Multz AS, Chalfin DB, Samson IM et al. (1998). A "closed" medical intensive care unit (MICU) improves resource utilization when compared with an "open" MICU. Am J Respir Crit Care Med 157: 1468–1473.

Munro D (1954). The rehabilitation of patients totally paralyzed below the waist: with special reference to making them ambulatory and capable of earning their living – an end-result study of 445 cases. N Engl J Med 250: 4–14.

Murphy SA, Bell MJ, Clark ME et al. (2015). Pediatric neurocritical care: a short survey of current perceptions and practices. Neurocrit Care 23: 149–158.

Plum F, Dunning MF (1956). Technics for minimizing trauma to the tracheobronchial tree after tracheotomy. N Engl J Med 254: 193–200.

Plum F, Posner JB (1966). The Diagnosis of Stupor and Coma. F. A. Davis, Philadelphia.

Plum F, Wolff HG (1951). Observations on acute poliomyelitis with respiratory insufficiency. JAMA 146: 442–446.

Prys-Roberts C, Corbett JL, Kerr JH et al. (1969). Treatment of sympathetic overactivity in tetanus. Lancet 1: 542–545.

Reisner-Senelar L (2011). The birth of intensive care medicine: Bjorn Ibsen's records. Intensive Care Med 37: 1084–1086.

Relman AS (1980). Intensive-care units: who needs them? N Engl J Med 302: 965–966.

Reynolds LA, Tansey EM (Eds.), (2011a). Wellcome Witnesses to Twentieth Century Medicine. Queen Mary, University of London, London. No. 42.

Reynolds LA, Tansey EM (Eds.), (2011b). History of British Intensive Care, C.1950–C.2000. Wellcome Witnesses to Twentieth Century Medicine; No. 42, Queen Mary University of London, London.

Ropper AH, Davis KR (1980). Lobar cerebral hemorrhages: acute clinical syndromes in 26 cases. Ann Neurol 8: 141–147.

Ropper AH, Kehne SM (1985). Guillain-Barré syndrome: management of respiratory failure. Neurology 35: 1662–1665.

Ropper AH, King RB (1984). Intracranial pressure monitoring in comatose patients with cerebral hemorrhage. Arch Neurol 41: 725–728.

Ropper AH, Shafran B (1984). Brain edema after stroke. Clinical syndrome and intracranial pressure. Arch Neurol 41: 26–29.

Ropper AH, O'Rourke D, Kennedy SK (1982). Head position, intracranial pressure, and compliance. Neurology 32: 1288–1291.

Ropper AH, Kennedy SF, Zervas NT (1983). Neurological and neurosurgical intensive care, University Park Press, Baltimore.

Rosengart MR (2006). Critical care medicine: landmarks and legends. Surg Clin North Am 86: 1305–1321.

Russell R, Schuster E (1953). Respiratory pump for poliomyelitis. Lancet 1: 707–709.

Safar P (1986). Cerebral resuscitation after cardiac arrest: a review. Circulation 74: IV138–IV153.

Safar P, Grenvik A (1971). Critical care medicine. Organizing and staffing intensive care units. Chest 59: 535–547.

Shoemaker WC, Thomson WL, Holbrook PR (Eds.), (1984). The Society of Critical Care Medicine Textbook of Critical Care, WB Saunders, Philadelphia.

Smith WS, Weingart S (2012). Emergency Neurological Life Support (ENLS): What to do in the first hour of a neurological emergency. Neurocrit Care 17: S1–S3.

Spalding JM, Crampton SA (1963). Clinical Practice and Physiology of Artificial Respiration, Blackwell Scientific Publications, Oxford.

Sun S, Tang W (2011). Max Harry (Hal) Weil, MD, PhD, ScD (hon), MACP Master, FCCP, FACC, FCCM, FAHA 1927 to 2011. J Crit Care 26: 439–440.

Teres D, Brown RB, Lemeshow S (1982). Predicting mortality of intensive care unit patients. The importance of coma. Crit Care Med 10: 86–95.

Weil MH (1973). The Society of Critical Care Medicine, its history and its destiny. Crit Care Med 1: 1–4.

Wijdicks EFM (1995). Neurology of Critical Illness. Contemporary Neurology Series, Philadelphia, FA Davis.

Wijdicks EFM (1997). The Clinical Practice of Critical Care Neurology, Lippincott, Williams and Wilkins, Philadelphia.

Wijdicks EFM (2000). Neurologic Catastrophes in the Emergency Department, Butterworth-Heinemann, Boston.

Wijdicks EFM (2004). A new journal, a new step, a new energy. Neurocrit Care 1: 1–2.

Wijdicks EFM (2006). Neurocritical care; it is what we do and what we do best. Neurocrit Care 5: 81.

Wijdicks EFM (2011). Cushing's ulcer: the eponym and his own. Neurosurgery 68: 1695–1698.

Wijdicks EFM (2016a). Neurology of critical care. Semin Neurol 36: 483–491.

Wijdicks EFM (2016b). W. Ritchie Russell, AB Baker, Fred Plum. Pioneers in respiratory management of poliomyelitis. Neurology 87: 1167–1170.

Wijdicks EFM, Hijdra A, Young GB et al. (2006). Practice parameter: prediction of outcome in comatose survivors after cardiopulmonary resuscitation (an evidence-based review): report of the Quality Standards Subcommittee of the American Academy of Neurology. Neurology 67: 203–210.

Wijdicks EFM, Worden WR, Miers A et al. (2011). The early days of the neurosciences intensive care unit. Mayo Clin Proc 86: 903–906.

*Handbook of Clinical Neurology, Vol. 140 (3rd series)*
*Critical Care Neurology, Part I*
E.F.M. Wijdicks and A.H. Kramer, Editors
http://dx.doi.org/10.1016/B978-0-444-63600-3.00002-7

Chapter 2

# Airway management and mechanical ventilation in acute brain injury

D.B. SEDER[1,2]* AND J. BÖSEL[3]

[1]*Department of Critical Care Services, Maine Medical Center, Portland, ME, USA*

[2]*Tufts University School of Medicine, Boston, MA, USA*

[3]*Department of Neurology, University of Heidelberg, Heidelberg, Germany*

## Abstract

Patients with acute neurologic disease often develop respiratory failure, the management of which profoundly affects brain physiology and long-term functional outcomes. This chapter reviews airway management and mechanical ventilation of patients with acute brain injury, offering practical strategies to optimize treatment of respiratory failure and minimize secondary brain injury. Specific concerns that are addressed include physiologic changes during intubation and ventilation such as the effects on intracranial pressure and brain perfusion; cervical spine management during endotracheal intubation; the role of tracheostomy; and how ventilation and oxygenation are utilized to minimize ischemia-reperfusion injury and cerebral metabolic distress.

## EPIDEMIOLOGY

Respiratory complications are the most important source of secondary morbidity and mortality in the neurocritical care unit. Approximately 10% of stroke patients develop respiratory failure requiring intubation and mechanical ventilation (Grotta et al., 1995; Gujjar et al., 1998), translating to approximately 80 000 patients annually in the USA (Mozaffarian et al., 2016). A large point-prevalence study of international neurocritical care practices showed that 18% of 1545 patients admitted to 143 neurocritical care units in 31 countries were receiving mechanical ventilation (personal communication). Brain-injured patients may develop respiratory complications of their primary illness, such as aspiration pneumonitis, pneumonia, or neurogenic pulmonary edema following a stroke or traumatic brain injury (TBI) (Hannawi et al., 2013). They may also develop primary lung problems, such as acute respiratory distress syndrome (ARDS), in response to inflammation or direct injury (Rincon et al., 2014b), or may have significant underlying lung disease prior to brain injury. Furthermore, because the lungs are an important source of inflammatory mediators that contribute to remote organ injury (Fisher et al., 1999; Kalsotra et al., 2007), respiratory disease should be considered a primary treatment target in patients with brain injury (Holland et al., 2003). Expertise in the nuances of airway management and mechanical ventilation are fundamental to the practice of neurocritical care. Furthermore, airway and ventilation practices are specific to patients with brain injury, whose respiratory management differs fundamentally from the general critical care population (Seder et al., 2015).

Data from the 1980s and 1990s suggest that cerebrovascular and other neurologic patients requiring mechanical ventilation have a poor prognosis, and some authors questioned the usefulness of life support in the neurocritically ill (Steiner et al., 1997; Wijdicks and Scott, 1997; Berrouschot et al., 2000; Mayer et al., 2000), while others demonstrated that even long-term ventilated patients sometimes had good outcomes (Roch et al., 2003; Rabinstein and Wijdicks, 2004). Mechanical ventilation

---

*Correspondence to: David B. Seder, MD, FCCP, FCCM, FNCS, Tufts University School of Medicine, MMC Department of Critical Care Services, Portland ME 04103, USA. Tel: +1-207-662-2179, Fax: +1-207-662-6326, E-mail: sederd@mmc.org

in these early studies was almost invariably an unadjusted indicator of illness severity, and the key elements of its application were rarely described. Today, with increasingly effective medical and surgical therapies for cerebrovascular diseases, improved mechanical ventilation and general intensive care unit (ICU) practices, sophisticated techniques for the detection and prevention of secondary brain injury, and dedicated treatment in specialized neurological ICUs, the published long-term outcomes of mechanically ventilated neurocritical care patients have improved from survival rates of 29–36% (Steiner et al., 1997; Wijdicks and Scott, 1997; Berrouschot et al., 2000; Mayer et al., 2000) to 66% in a recent report (Steffling et al., 2012). Accurate prognostication can usually not be reliably performed in the early hours after presentation to the medical care system, so appropriate airway and respiratory management must be initiated to prevent secondary brain injury during the stabilization phase of care (Souter et al., 2015).

This chapter highlights general principles of airway management and mechanical ventilation in patients with brain injury, and reviews elements of therapy unique to that population.

## RESPIRATORY ANATOMY AND PHYSIOLOGY

### Airway and automaticity

Normal respiration depends not only on an intact respiratory rhythm generator mechanism (Guyenet and Bayliss, 2015), but also intact modulatory impulses from the brainstem and cortical inputs. It requires a normal effector mechanism through the spinal cord and respiratory muscles, and normal chemo-sensing mechanisms in the aortic arch and carotid bodies. A comprehensive review of the neuropathology of breathing is beyond the scope of this review, and readers are referred to the textbook *Neurology of Breathing* (Bolton et al., 2004) for more details.

Brain injuries affect respiration in many overlapping ways, but it is useful to consider the following distinct scenarios. These syndromes reflect different pathophysiologic processes and require an individualized clinical approach, although they may coexist within the same patient:

1. Impaired respiratory automaticity due to low-brainstem injury, in which hypoventilation and even respiratory arrest may occur. The respiratory rhythm generator mechanism in humans is located in the medulla, with critical afferent and efferent connections to pontine nuclei controlling the rate, rise, and depth of ventilation, and many other cortical and subcortical inputs related to volitional and autonomic control of

respiration (Feldman et al., 2013; Guyenet and Bayliss, 2015). Lesions in the brainstem due to infarction, hemorrhage, tumor, vascular malformations, radiation injury, infection, encephalitis, and other processes should immediately trigger an assessment of respiratory stability, and warrant continuous respiratory monitoring, especially during sleep. In particular, care should be taken to identify unstable ventilatory patterns, such as apnea, "ataxic," and "cluster" breathing, which may be signs of impending respiratory arrest (Bolton et al., 2004; Nogués and Benarroch, 2008; Feldman et al., 2013; Guyenet and Bayliss, 2015). Although lesions causing unstable respiratory patterns are typically bilateral in animal models, multiple case reports describe respiratory arrest events in rare patients with unilateral pontine or medullary lesions, such as the lateral medullary syndrome (Hashimoto et al., 1989; Bolton et al., 2004). It should be noted that such injuries in patients with underlying sleep-disordered breathing may have a higher susceptibility to apnea events, as do patients receiving respiratory-suppressant medications like opiates or benzodiazepines (Gross, 2003; Boom et al., 2012). Patients with impaired respiratory automaticity may require continuous long-term ventilation, typically via tracheostomy (Qureshi et al., 2000).

2. Abnormal breathing patterns that are benign, but serve as indicators of other disease processes, include Cheyne–Stokes respirations in heart failure, central hyperventilation in pulmonary embolism or early sepsis, and central hypoventilation due to oversedation. Such patterns should provoke the question, "is there evidence to suggest that the abnormal respiratory pattern is causing secondary neurological injury?" (Carrera et al., 2010; Pynnönen et al., 2011). They should also provoke investigations to diagnose treatable underlying disease states.

3. When a patient has respiratory alkalosis, it is necessary to distinguish between hyperventilation originating from the patient or from the ventilator. When recognized, accidental overventilation should be immediately corrected. When hyperventilation appears to be spontaneous, the clinician should attempt to classify patients according to the following categories:

a. Pathophysiologic central hyperventilation (may worsen brain injury via alkalosis or cerebral vasoconstriction) usually caused by loss of inhibitory input to the respiratory rhythm generator apparatus. This is frequently due to unilateral or bilateral hemispheric lesions

(North and Jennett, 1974), but can be observed in brainstem injury and many other circumstances (Bolton et al., 2004), and is poorly understood. To differentiate appropriate (physiologic) from inappropriate (pathophysiologic) hyperventilation may require cerebral metabolic monitoring. One group showed that spontaneous hyperventilation in patients with severe injury was associated with lower brain tissue oxygen ($Pbto_2$) levels (Carrera et al., 2010), and a second group showed induced hyperventilation was associated with cerebral metabolic distress with elevated tissue lactate and elevated lactate/pyruvate ratios (Marion et al., 2002). In clinical practice, this distinction may be difficult or impossible to make.

b. Physiologic central hyperventilation (physiologically necessary or advantageous hyperventilation), potentially caused by increased intracranial pressure (ICP) or a central acid load requiring respiratory buffering (as discussed above).

4. Impaired airway-protective reflexes, facilitating entry of colonized aerodigestive secretions, gastric acid, or regurgitated stomach contents into the upper and lower airways. Loss of sensory input from the upper aerodigestive tract is common to many stroke subtypes, and clinical impairment is routinely classified by swallowing evaluation utilizing physical examination, video laryngoscopy, and fluoroscopic testing (Flowers et al., 2011; Somasundaram et al., 2014). Lesions of the parabrachial nucleus in the upper pons may additionally inhibit coordination of breathing and swallowing activities in the posterior oropharynx, resulting in aspiration. It is often difficult to be certain when the impairment of swallowing reflexes is so severe as to require placement of an artificial airway.

5. Impaired cough, preventing clearance of secretions that penetrate the glottis, and causing atelectasis (Harraf et al., 2008; Ward et al., 2010).

6. Inability to maintain a patent upper airway for gas exchange purposes. Up to two-thirds of acute ischemic stroke patients suffer from sleep apnea compared to 5–15% in the general population, and sleep apnea is strongly associated with both hypoxia and neurologic deterioration in the first 24 hours after stroke (Iranzo et al., 2002; Malhotra and White, 2002; Bassetti et al., 2006; Herrmann and Bassetti, 2009; Kepplinger et al., 2013). Among critically ill patients with severe stroke, failure to maintain a patent upper airway is both common and potentially catastrophic, as hypoxia, hypercarbia, acidosis, and severe hypertension may follow.

## EFFECTS OF HYPEROXIA AND HYPOXIA ON BRAIN PHYSIOLOGY

Although therapeutic uses of hyperoxia have been described, most notably in TBI (Rangel-Castilla et al., 2010; Vilalta et al., 2011; Rockswold et al., 2013; Taher et al., 2016), many neuroscientists believe that supraphysiologic levels of oxygen provided to acutely ill patients may worsen reperfusion injury and outcomes (Balan et al., 2006; Brucken et al., 2010). Conversely, hypoxia may be an important cause of secondary brain injury (Kilgannon et al., 2011), and the injured and ischemic brain is particularly vulnerable to low oxygen levels. Hyperoxia causes the formation of reactive oxygen species in postischemic tissue beds, impairing mitochondrial function (Davis et al., 2009).

Hyperoxia at a level of $Pao_2 > 300$ mmHg on the first arterial blood gas following resuscitation is independently associated with poor outcomes following TBI (Davis et al., 2009), cardiac arrest (Brucken et al., 2010; Kilgannon et al., 2010, 2011), and stroke (Rincon et al., 2014a), though not all published data support this concern (Rangel-Castilla et al., 2010; Bellomo et al., 2011; Elmer et al., 2015; Taher et al., 2016). Hyperoxia causes the formation of reactive oxygen species, overwhelming antioxidants at sites of tissue injury; directly injures respiratory epithelium and alveoli, inducing inflammation; drives hypercarbia; and leads to reabsorption atelectasis in the lung. In addition to oxidative stress to the brain, it may at least theoretically be associated with hyperoxemia-induced cerebral vasoconstriction (Floyd et al., 2003: Rangel-Castilla et al., 2010; Taher et al., 2016).

It is recommended that 100% oxygen be provided for preoxygenation immediately prior to intubation, but that oxygen be immediately weaned to 50%, or to the lowest $Fio_2$ that will support an oxyhemoglobin saturation of 95–100% following intubation. This normoxic resuscitation strategy is recommended in American Heart Association guidelines for postresuscitation care after cardiac arrest (Callaway et al., 2015) and in Emergency Neurological Life Support (Seder et al., 2015).

## EFFECTS OF $PCO_2$ AND pH ON BRAIN PHYSIOLOGY

When cerebral autoregulation is intact, $PCO_2$ plays a prominent role in determining cerebral blood flow (CBF). Hypoventilation resulting in hypercarbia has the immediate effect of arteriolar vasodilation with increased cerebral blood volume and ICP. Hyperventilation with hypocarbia results in arteriolar constriction, resulting in decreased CBF and cerebral blood volume, and decreased ICP. These processes may be manipulated to physiologic advantage, such as when ICP must urgently be controlled, but may lead to disastrous results when they occur accidentally, as with inadvertent hyperventilation of a patient in the acute phase of ischemic stroke, when excessive ventilation may compromise collateral circulation to an ischemic penumbra, or with hypoventilation of a patient with elevated ICP precipitating a crisis (Seder et al., 2015). Changes in $PCO_2$ have different implications for a patient with aneurysmal subarachnoid hemorrhage, active vasospasm, and cerebral ischemia than a TBI patient with cerebral edema and poor intracranial compliance.

These relationships also highlight how respiratory management differs between the neurocritical care and other critically ill settings. In a general ICU population, permissive hypercarbia is tolerated or encouraged for ventilation of patients with obstructive lung disease (Ijland et al., 2010) or ARDS (The Acute Respiratory Distress Syndrome Network, 2000), but such a strategy after acute brain injury should be approached with great caution, and generally only with ICP monitoring in place (Gopinath et al., 1999). When hyperventilation is used to induce hypocarbia and reduce ICP rapidly, this state of hyperventilation must be quickly weaned as soon as other measures to reduce ICP have started to have an effect, since hyperventilation is associated with higher morbidity and mortality when applied chronically after TBI (Bouma et al., 1991; Muizelaar et al., 1991). The neurointensivist must understand, recognize, and constantly manipulate respiratory parameters to maximal advantage and to minimize secondary brain injury.

## CLINICAL PRESENTATION

Indications for endotracheal intubation of patients with neurologic diseases are failure to oxygenate or ventilate, inability to protect the airway, anticipation of possible neurologic or cardiopulmonary decline, and prevention of ischemia or secondary neurologic injury related to anxiety, pain, work of breathing, or aspiration.

Because of the potential for respiratory arrest, large-volume aspiration, or unsafe hemodynamic fluctuations, intubation and the initiation of mechanical ventilation are critical to protect patients in a period of neurologic decline. In particular, patients who will require transport, neuroimaging, and medical or surgical procedures to ensure clinical stability should be intubated to maintain a stable airway and adequate oxygenation and ventilation. It should be noted that "failure to protect the airway" is a grossly subjective measure, but involves two primary components – adequate airway clearance involving oropharyngeal coordination, cough reflexes and respiratory

muscle strength, and the ability to maintain a patent upper airway. Conversely, many patients in the convalescent or recovery phase following brain injury can be safely extubated despite impaired consciousness, or impaired airway-protective reflexes (Coplin et al., 2000). The assessment for extubation is covered in greater detail in the text to follow.

## Preparation for intubation

Preparation for intubation of the neurologic patient should include a presedation neurologic examination, assessment of factors associated with difficult laryngoscopy and bag-and-mask ventilation, selection of induction agents, as well as consideration of fluids and vasopressors to maintain hemodynamic stability. Anticipatory to intubation, clinicians should assess and consider five categories of risk:

1. Is this a difficult airway or difficult mask ventilation scenario?
2. What medications or maneuvers should be avoided?
3. Is this intubation high-risk due to elevated ICP?
4. Is this intubation high-risk due to threatened cerebral perfusion?
5. Is the cervical spine unstable?

### PREPARATION FOR THE DIFFICULT AIRWAY AND MASK VENTILATION SCENARIOS

Difficult bag-and-mask ventilation is a more dangerous situation than difficult intubation – a sedated or paralyzed patient may sustain a cardiac arrest if s/he cannot be oxygenated or ventilated, while a patient with difficult laryngoscopy and intubation can sometimes be bag-and-mask-ventilated for extended periods of time – long enough for neuromuscular blockade to wear off or help to arrive. The MOANS mnemonic can be used to predict difficulty of bag-and-mask ventilation:

M = mask seal (beard, unusual anatomy)
O = obesity/obstruction
A = age > 55
N = no teeth
S = stiff lungs

The LEMON mnemonic helps to predict the difficult laryngoscopy:

L = look (at the face, mouth, and neck)
E = evaluate the mouth opening and airway position
M = Mallampati score (Mallampati et al., 1985)
O = obstruction
N = neck mobility

The airways of patients with risk factors for either difficult mask ventilation or difficult intubation should be approached with caution. The urgency of the intubation, as well as the skill level of the intubating clinician, must be considered. Because not every difficult intubation can be predicted, clinicians should enter into every situation with a backup plan. Patients anticipated to be difficult to ventilate or intubate should prompt preparation with appropriate backup in terms of skilled individuals (e.g., anesthesiology assistance) and special equipment (Apfelbaum et al., 2013). Adjunct airway devices such as laryngeal mask airways, special blades, video laryngoscopy, intubating stylets, fiberoptic bronchoscopy, and surgical airway equipment should be immediately available. In modern airway management, the availability of basic airway adjunct devices is mandatory.

## CONTRAINDICATIONS TO (ELECTIVE) INTUBATION

Except for a "do not intubate" order, there are no absolute contraindications to endotracheal intubation. Relative contraindications must be weighed against the benefits of intubation for patients in a period of rapid decompensation. Relative contraindications include the need to preserve the neurologic examination without the interfering effects of sedative and analgesic agents; the presence of critical brain ischemia, such as in an acute cerebrovascular flow failure event, in which a large ischemic penumbra is perfused by maximally dilated collateral vasculature (Talke et al., 2014); significant cervical spine instability; and an anticipated difficult airway (such as mechanical upper-airway obstruction) with inadequate resources present. Each of these relative contraindications will be discussed further in this chapter, but clinicians must recognize that these circumstances require special attention, and should not be attempted without a risk–benefit assessment and maximal preparation.

## ALTERNATIVES TO INTUBATION

Intubation and postintubation management often require analgesia and sedation, at times muscle relaxants, and vasoconstrictor agents and/or intravascular fluids to counteract the effects of vasodilating drugs. Intubation is extremely uncomfortable, activates the sympathetic nervous system, and requires frequent analysis of ventilation by arterial blood gas or end-tidal carbon dioxide measurement (Table 2.1). Alternatively, oxygen delivery by a standard or high-flow nasal cannula or face mask device can provide close to 100% inspired oxygen, provide a small amount of positive end-expiratory pressure (PEEP), and may be better tolerated than noninvasive positive-pressure ventilation (NPPV) with a pressure mask.

*Table 2.1*

**Contraindications to noninvasive ventilation**

Cardiac or respiratory arrest
Nonrespiratory organ failure
- Hemodynamic instability or dangerous arrhythmia
- End-organ ischemia with increased work of breathing
- Severe encephalopathy (Glasgow Coma Score < 10)
- Significant upper gastrointestinal bleeding
Facial trauma, surgery, or deformity
Upper-airway obstruction
Inability to cooperate or protect airway
Inability to clear respiratory secretions
High risk for aspiration

Technology to provide NPPV has dramatically improved in recent years, including the development of portable ventilators specifically designed for this purpose that compensate for mask leaks and typically provide excellent patient–ventilator synchrony (Scala and Naldi, 2008; Hess, 2013). Dozens of different interfaces, including hoods, full face masks, oronasal masks, nasal masks, and tight-fitting nasal cannulae make patient comfort during mask ventilation less of an issue than ever before. Using modern equipment, the practical limitations to NPPV are that it provides only partial ventilatory support, offers no lower-airway protection, and does not maintain the upper airway open.

Finally, tracheostomy should be viewed as an alternative to ongoing (prolonged) intubation. Many patients with neurologic disease and especially those with brain injury lack adequate airway-protective reflexes, but are able to ventilate and oxygenate well. In such cases, early tracheostomy provides a reliable and patent upper airway, facilitates suctioning of the lower airways, allows patients to breathe spontaneously, thereby preserving respiratory muscle function, and often eliminates the need for sedating medications that may interfere with neurologic recovery (Seder et al., 2009; Bösel et al., 2013). Tracheostomy will be discussed later in this text.

## PREINTUBATION NEUROLOGIC EVALUATION

Urgent management of the airway should coincide with a rapid but detailed neurologic assessment (Seder et al., 2015). The presedation/intubation neurologic exam is crucial to subsequent triage decisions, and can typically be conducted in a few minutes. It establishes a baseline that is used to assess therapeutic interventions or may identify injuries that are at risk of progressing (e.g., unstable cervical spine fractures). The assessment identifies the most appropriate testing and helps to

*Table 2.2*

Standard elements of the preintubation neurologic evaluation

| |
| --- |
| Level of arousal and orientation, as well as an assessment of cortical functions such as vision, attention, and speech comprehension and fluency |
| Cranial nerve function |
| Motor function of each individual extremity |
| Tone and reflexes |
| Comment on subtle or gross seizure activity |
| Cervical spine tenderness, when appropriate |
| Sensory level in patients with suspected spinal cord injury |

avoid unnecessary and uncomfortable interventions, such as cervical spine immobilization. The preintubation neurologic assessment is the responsibility of the team leader who is coordinating resuscitation efforts; findings should be documented and communicated directly to the treatment team that assumes care of the patient (Table 2.2).

#### REDUCING PERI-INTUBATION RISK

Backup plans for oxygenation and ventilation, and for securing the airway under difficult circumstances, should include airway adjuncts and special equipment, and routine "ramping up" of obese patients prior to administration of muscle relaxants (to optimally align the mouth, pharynx, and larynx) (Lebowitz et al., 2012). Clinicians should use medications best suited to individual patients' pathophysiology, including preemptive intravascular volume expansion, prevention of episodic hypotension with vasopressors and hemodynamically neutral intubating agents, blunting of the ICP response to direct laryngoscopy with analgesics, and minimizing time with the head of the bed flat (McPhee and Seder, 2012) (Fig. 2.1).

## CLINICAL TRIALS AND GUIDELINES

Definitive prospective clinical trials related to airway management and mechanical ventilation of the neurocritically ill have not been performed. However, several important observational studies inform neurocritical care airway and ventilation practices, and form the basis of recommendations in the Emergency Neurological Life Support protocols for airway and ventilation, and the Society for Neuroscience in Anesthesiology and Critical Care consensus statement for anesthetic management of endovascular treatment for acute ischemic stroke (Talke et al., 2014; Seder et al., 2015).

Retrospective data suggest that intubation of patients undergoing endovascular thrombectomy for acute ischemic anterior circulation stroke may be associated with

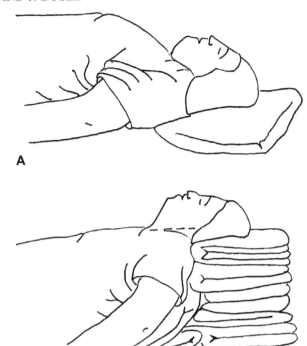

**A**

**B**

**Fig. 2.1.** "Ramping up" an obese patient. (**A**) The usual supine alignment in obesity is shown, creating extremely difficult intubating conditions. (**B**) The patient is "ramped up" with blankets, bringing the external auditory meatus to the level of the sternal notch, and creating a favorable line of sight for direct laryngoscopy. (Adapted from http://www.edexam. com.au/managing-the-obese-difficult-airway.)

worse outcomes than conscious sedation (Brinjikji et al., 2015; Berkhemer et al., 2016). The only randomized trial to address this question prospectively, the single-center SIESTA study, found no differences in short-term early neurologic recovery and most peri-interventional aspects when comparing general anesthesia to conscious sedation (Schönenberger et al., 2016). Nonetheless, there are mechanistic reasons for concern that induction of anesthesia may critically compromise blood flow to the ischemic penumbra, and pre-procedural intubation of patients undergoing endovascular stroke care should be hemodynamically neutral, with preservation of both blood pressure and physiological shunting (Talke et al., 2014).

Many retrospective observational studies suggest that dysventilation and dysoxia, especially in the early hours after acute brain injury, are independently associated with worse outcomes. These data are fairly uniform throughout the literature on cardiac arrest-associated brain injury (Kilgannon et al., 2010; Del Castillo et al., 2012; Schneider et al., 2013) and stroke (Rincon et al., 2014a; Roberts et al., 2015), and have strong preclinical correlates from experimental work in animal models. The role of hyperoxia remains contentious in brain trauma, with conflicting data supporting (Davis et al., 2005, 2006; Dumont et al., 2010) or refuting (Vilalta et al., 2011; Rockswold et al., 2013; Taher et al., 2016) the importance of normoxia in the early period after TBI. Theorized mechanisms of injury include potentiation of ischemia-reperfusion injury by systemic hyperoxia or inadequately buffered acidosis, worsening of ischemic injury by systemic hypoxia, and a critical decrease in CBF related to hyperventilation (Seder et al., 2015; Topjian et al., 2015). For this reason, published guidelines for management of brain trauma, cardiac arrest, and stroke all support immediate normalization of oxygenation and ventilation immediately following resuscitation (Brain Trauma Foundation, 2007; Wijdicks et al., 2014; Callaway et al., 2015).

Although some studies suggest that standard cardiopulmonary weaning criteria fail to predict extubation failure in patients with brain injuries (dos Reis et al., 2013), many patients can be safely extubated (Karanjia et al., 2011). A carefully performed prospective observational study evaluating the safety of extubation of brain-injured patients suggested a benefit to extubation of brain-injured patients that met cardiopulmonary weaning criteria, despite a Glasgow Coma Scale (GCS) < 9. This study compared the outcomes of patients who met standard cardiopulmonary weaning criteria and were extubated despite a low GCS to those who met standard ventilator weaning criteria but were kept intubated because of low GCS. Patients who were extubated seemed to have benefit in terms of length of ICU stay, development of ventilator-associated pneumonia, and mortality, and many patients were safely extubated despite very low GCS (Coplin et al., 2000). These findings, though compelling, have not been replicated, and may be confounded by unrecognized biases, whereby patients who were kept intubated had characteristics associated with worsened outcome. Other studies (Salam et al., 2004; Anderson et al., 2011; Wang et al., 2014) offer alternative predictors of extubation success after brain injury, but suffer from retrospective methodology.

A pilot randomized controlled trial of 60 patients at a single center with severe stroke and respiratory failure compared very early percutaneous tracheostomy performed on or before day 3 to weaning for extubation or delayed tracheostomy performed after day 7. Although the trial showed no difference in the primary endpoint (ICU length of stay), patients receiving early tracheostomy received less sedation and had decreased mortality at 30 days and 6 months following stroke (Bösel et al., 2013). A phase III trial is now under way (Schönenberger et al., 2016b).

## COMPLEX CLINICAL DECISIONS

The approach to a mechanically difficult airway is governed by the urgency of the intubation. In a patient in whom oxygenation cannot be maintained using bag-and-mask ventilation, a mask airway such as a laryngeal mask airway or Combitube should be attempted. If oxygenation and ventilation cannot be adequately achieved using a mask airway, then a true airway emergency exists, and rapid intubation or a surgical airway is required. In such cases, advance preparation, the utilization of an airway algorithm, appropriate airway-adjunct equipment, and the presence of an experienced intubator may be life-saving.

Airway adjuncts can facilitate a difficult intubation, or minimize movement of the cervical spine during intubation. The gum-elastic bougie is a common choice. It is a 60-cm malleable intubating stylet with a 40° angled tip that is placed through the visualized vocal cords. Alternatively, a bougie can be placed blindly through the vocal cords by "feeling" the tracheal rings upon appropriate placement. The endotracheal tube is then advanced and the bougie removed.

Video intubation has revolutionized airway management, in part because there does not need to be a direct line of vision between the eye and the vocal cords – a video camera at the curved tip of an intubating blade allows for an intubating stylet or endotracheal tube to be passed between the vocal cords without a direct line of vision, making difficult anterior airways accessible, and decreasing manipulation of the neck. Flexible bronchoscopy facilitates nasal or oral intubation, though oral intubation is preferred unless absolute spinal neutrality is demanded. Except in unusual circumstances, the video laryngoscope is preferred over the fiberoptic bronchoscope due to its ease of use and utility in anterior displacement of the tongue, improving laryngeal visualization.

When a patient cannot be intubated or ventilated, a surgical airway is necessary. A needle, wire-guided, or surgical cricothyroidotomy should be performed; tracheostomy is a more complex and time-consuming procedure and is typically reserved for nonemergent situations. In a needle cricothyroidotomy, a small catheter over a needle is passed percutaneously in a caudad direction through the cricothyroid membrane. When air bubbles are seen in the syringe, the catheter is advanced over the needle and the syringe and needle are removed. The catheter is then connected to high-pressure oxygen tubing and transtracheal jet ventilation is performed. The guidewire technique is performed similarly, with the exception that a guidewire is placed through the needle and the needle and syringe are removed with only the guidewire left behind. A dilator-airway catheter is passed over the guidewire, the guidewire is removed, and the catheter cuff is inflated.

A surgical airway using a scalpel can be performed quickly, utilizing one of several standard techniques (Scrase and Woollard, 2006).

## Induction medication issues to consider in the neurocritically ill

As a neuromuscular blockade agent, succinylcholine should be withheld in patients with hyperkalemia, as well as those with normal potassium levels but at risk for a surge in serum potassium due to prolonged immobility (Clancy et al., 2001; Martyn and Richtsfeld, 2006). This includes neurologic patients with upper motor neuron lesions.

Ketamine, a dissociative agent that maintains blood pressure, was suspected to increase ICP in older reports, but according to more recent studies is safe if co-administered with a sedative (Cohen et al., 2015). Especially in hypovolemic patients, propofol and opioids may cause excessive vasodilation and blood pressure reductions unless counteracted with vasopressors and fluids.

## Intubation in the setting of elevated intracranial pressure

Patients with cerebral edema are at risk for increased ICP or inadequate cerebral perfusion pressure (CPP) during intubation. Clinicians should pay special attention to the adequacy of sedation and analgesia during laryngoscopy, maintaining head of the bed-up positioning, and adequacy of blood pressure and oxygenation. Direct laryngoscopy causes sympathetic stimulation, potentially triggering tachycardia, hypertension, bronchospasm, and increased ICP (Walls and Murphy, 2008). When preparing for intubation, the head of the bed can be maintained at 30–45°, before briefly bringing it flat during the procedure and then returning it to its original position. If necessary, the patient can be maintained in reverse Trendelenburg positioning throughout the intubation (Seder et al., 2015). Medications that blunt the ICP rise associated with laryngoscopy include intravenous lidocaine (Donegan and Bedford, 1980; Grover et al., 1999; Salhi and Stettner, 2007), analgesics such as fentanyl, and sympatholytics like esmolol. The data to support or refute the routine use of these agents are weak. Hypotension, hypoxemia, and hypercarbia cause vasodilation and an increase in cerebral blood volume, leading to a rise in ICP.

Preoxygenation washes out nitrogen in the lungs and prolongs the time to oxyhemoglobin desaturation. Patients' minute ventilation should be maintained throughout the procedure to avoid $CO_2$ retention, a matter of urgency in the setting of intracranial mass

lesions and elevated ICP. Adequate intravenous access is important to manage hemodynamic changes during intubation, and routine peri-intubation infusion of isotonic crystalloid is suggested. Vasopressors should be readily available in the event of hypotension to maintain adequate CPP.

## Intubation in the setting of impaired cerebral perfusion

In suspected or proven ischemic stroke one should proceed with intubation as with elevated ICP, by avoiding hypotension during induction and postintubation, and taking special precautions to avoid vasodilators, especially in hypotensive patients. When an ischemic stroke is suspected or known to be occurring, or a state of inadequate CBF exists for other reasons, brain ischemia should be presumed.

The cerebrovascular circulation is ordinarily well collateralized, and many patients presenting with stroke symptoms can be seen to have an infarct core and an ischemic penumbra on perfusion computed tomography or magnetic resonance imaging (Campbell et al., 2012). Under these circumstances, the ischemic penumbra may be conceptualized as a region of maximally vasodilated vessels, receiving shunting of the cerebrovascular circulation, yet CBF is severely compromised and at the limits of compensation. Hypertension and tachycardia are physiologic responses to this ischemia and should be allowed to maintain perfusion of the ischemic territory.

Even vasoactive agents that do not drop systemic blood pressure or alter CPP may reverse physiologic shunting of blood to the region of ischemia, and should be avoided in conditions of active ischemia. An episode of relative or actual hypotension, such as would be precipitated by the administration of a sedative medication like propofol to a volume-depleted patient, may worsen infarction size by "stealing" blood flow from maximally dilated watershed territories between vascular territories.

Brain ischemia or infarction can be precipitated by hypotension whenever blood flow is compromised by vasospasm, TBI, intracranial and extracranial cerebrovascular stenosis, intracerebral hemorrhage, and hypoxic-ischemic encephalopathy following resuscitation from cardiac arrest. Strong associations between episodic hypotension in the critical hours following resuscitation and poor neurologic outcome have been noted in TBI and hypoxic-ischemic encephalopathy (Chesnut et al., 1993; Trzeciak et al., 2009). Cerebral and systemic vascular tone must be maintained during airway management. Because of the association between hyperventilation and poor outcome in conditions of brain ischemia, clinicians should maintain normocapnia, and early correlation of an arterial $CO_2$ sample with end-tidal $CO_2$ is suggested, so that continuous capnography can be used to verify normocarbia.

## Intubation of the patient with unstable cervical spine

When spinal column or ligamentous injury to the neck is suspected due to the mechanism of injury, or the cervical spine is known to be unstable, measures must be taken to protect the spinal cord during movements or procedures. Preintubation airway maneuvers that are routinely used in other settings can conceivably injure the spinal cord when cervical instability is present.

Any patient with a confirmed or suspected unstable cervical spine should be immediately placed in a stabilization device. During intubation, manual inline axial stabilization of the head and neck by an assistant is mandatory. Cervical subluxation could occur during chin lift, jaw thrust, bag-and-mask ventilation, and tracheal intubation, as well as maneuvers such as cricoid pressure and head turning; these maneuvers should therefore be minimized. Mask ventilation was found in one study to cause more cervical spine displacement than any method used for tracheal intubation (Hauswald et al., 1991), so extreme caution must be employed through all aspects of the procedure.

Basic principles of cervical spine stabilization have been developed and refined over decades, and the algorithm mapped out by the American College of Surgeons Advanced Trauma Life Support course is recommended. In urgent circumstances in the field, endotracheal intubation is preferred to bag-and-mask ventilation or cricothyrotomy, and should be performed with inline spinal stabilization. Though cricoid pressure is no longer recommended during intubation, it definitely should not be used in patients with cervical spine injury, since it may cause posterior displacement of the cervical spine (Stein et al., 2012).

Hypoxia, hypoventilation, and large-volume aspiration are larger risks to trauma patients than complications of endotracheal intubation; inline spinal stabilization helps ensure safe intubating conditions when direct laryngoscopy is performed and is the standard of care (Grande et al., 1988). A recent systematic review suggested the risk of intubation failure was lower with alternative intubation devices compared with Macintosh laryngoscopy (Suppan et al., 2016), but the minimum amount of anterior–posterior displacement of the cervical spine occurs with flexible fiberoptic intubation, which is preferred when time and circumstances allow, or when known severe instability is present (Brimacombe et al., 2000).

## Problems in ventilation after acute brain injury

Many types of neurologic injury are exacerbated by respiratory compromise. Carbon dioxide and pH are powerful determinants of cerebral vascular tone, and the intended or unintended effects of hyperventilation (decreased CBF, and in turn intracranial blood volume and ICP) should be anticipated, monitored, and manipulated by clinicians. Conversely, hypoventilation and hypercapnia cause cerebral vasodilation and increased ICP. Hyperoxia may exacerbate reperfusion injury, while hypoxia is strongly associated with worse outcomes in stroke, hypoxic-ischemic encephalopathy, and TBI. Finally, when work of breathing is markedly increased, up to 50% of the cardiac output may be diverted to the respiratory muscles, potentially "stealing" blood flow from the ischemic brain or spinal cord. This metabolic stressor can be effectively managed by sedation, intubation, and initiation of full mechanical ventilatory support.

## Effects of hyperventilation and hypoventilation on brain physiology

The relationship between arterial and central pH and $PCO_2$ is complex and incompletely understood. When underlying metabolic acidosis is concurrent with acute brain injury, such as in diabetic ketoacidosis (Wood et al., 1990), it is likely that, because of the blood–brain barrier and central nervous system (CNS) buffering capacity, CNS pH and CBF are often preserved despite a severely acidic systemic pH and very low $PCO_2$.

Alternatively, in patients with chronic respiratory acidosis due to chronic obstructive pulmonary disease, sleep apnea/obesity hypoventilation syndrome, chronic neuromuscular disease, or other etiologies, $CO_2$ responsiveness is typically preserved, but the set point of cerebral $CO_2$ reactivity changes (Van de Ven et al., 2001). It is therefore recommended that mechanical ventilation be adjusted to correct the pH and not the $PCO_2$, or that the estimated "premorbid" $PCO_2$ target be used. This is recommended on both physiologic and practical grounds, since ventilating patients with obstructive lung disease to "normal" $PCO_2$ targets may be difficult. Because a great deal of physiologic uncertainty exists in these cases, CBF and/or metabolic monitoring are helpful, whenever available, to guide the titration of pH and $PCO_2$ targets, with attention to how changes in ventilation affect CBF and metabolism (Carrera et al., 2010; Pynnönen et al., 2011).

Under these circumstances, surrogates for CBF and metabolism may include jugular venous oximetry, direct intracranial monitoring of CBF or brain tissue oxygen tension, or measurement of lactate and pyruvate levels by cerebral microdialysis. These recommendations are based on physiologic knowledge, as well as observational human and experimental animal data, although little prospective experimental human research has been performed in this area (Oddo and Bösel, 2014).

## Acidemic and alkalemic hypocarbia: potential for suppression of spontaneous hyperventilation

Two very different circumstances should be considered in patients with spontaneous hypocarbia: when the response to systemic metabolic acidosis accounts for high ventilatory demand, and when ventilation exceeds systemic metabolic needs.

In patients whose ventilation is driven by metabolic acidosis, suppression of the respiratory drive with sedation or neuromuscular blockade is not recommended, unless direct measurement of brain chemistry suggests that hyperventilation is linked to cerebral metabolic crisis. Under these circumstances, clinicians must find other means to buffer systemic pH.

It has been observed in TBI that, while intubated and mechanically ventilated patients presenting with hypocarbia (due to excessive prehospital ventilation) have worse outcomes compared to those with normocarbia, nonintubated patients presenting with hypocarbia do not, suggesting that such hypocarbia may be a physiologic response and should not be suppressed (Davis et al., 2006).

Alkalemic hypocarbia develops in patients with spontaneous hyperventilation, and its causes and physiologic effects are poorly understood. Theoretically, there are many "physiologic" explanations, more than one of which may be present in an individual patient, including:

- brain tissue acidosis requiring hyperventilation to buffer pH until local bicarbonate-generating mechanisms can compensate
- pain, anxiety, fear, or agitation
- autoregulation of elevated ICP
- irritation of respiratory centers by heme breakdown products
- increased acidity of cerebrospinal fluid in the ventricular system
- mechanical compression of chemoreceptors in the floor of the fourth ventricle
- physiologic dysregulation of the medullary respiratory rhythm generator, due to disrupted afferent inputs from the pons, mesencephalon, and higher cortical centers.

A single trial of patients with severe brain injury showed brain tissue hypoxia to be worsened when end-tidal $CO_2$ values were reduced by spontaneous alkalemic hyperventilation, suggesting possible harm (Carrera et al., 2010). There is a critical deficiency of scientific knowledge in this area, and, since it is rarely known whether alkalemic hypocapnia is a physiologic or pathophysiologic process, suppression of intrinsic respiratory activity is generally not recommended unless there is evidence of hyperventilation causing harm, either by inducing cerebral ischemia or indirectly by increased systemic metabolic demands and work of breathing.

## Purposeful hyperventilation to control elevated ICP

When a patient develops brain herniation with elevated ICP or plateau waves signaling impending herniation, hyperventilation is an appropriate intervention to acutely decrease ICP and prevent widespread infarction of neuronal tissues and death. Maximal cerebral vasoconstriction is usually achieved at a $PCO_2$ of 20 mmHg, so ventilation below this level will be ineffective and may further impede venous return to the heart, decrease blood pressure, and exacerbate cerebral hypoperfusion (Stevens et al., 2015).

During hyperventilation, end-tidal $CO_2$ monitoring (quantitative capnography) is suggested, although this value may be quite discrepant from the actual $PCO_2$ if there is a high dead-space fraction. As soon as other treatments to control ICP are in place (e.g., blood pressure support, osmotherapy, surgical decompression, hypothermia, metabolic therapy), hyperventilation should be rapidly weaned to restore brain perfusion (Oertel et al., 2002).

Hyperventilation for increased ICP is not safe or effective when employed for a prolonged period. Hyperventilation severely reduces CBF, increases the volume of ischemic brain tissue, and, when the patient is weaned off, may result in rebound elevation of ICP (Coles et al., 2002; Diringer et al., 2002). When prolonged (mild) hyperventilation must be employed, it is strongly recommended that both end-tidal $CO_2$ and cerebral metabolic monitoring (jugular oximetry, CBF, brain tissue oxygen, or cerebral microdialysis) be used together with ICP monitoring to verify the adequacy of tissue perfusion.

## Hypoxia and hyperoxia exacerbate primary brain injury

Hypoxia is a major source of secondary brain injury (Helmerhorst et al., 2015), and the injured and ischemic brain is particularly vulnerable to low oxygen levels. Similarly, supraphysiologic levels of oxygen provided to acutely ill patients have the potential to worsen reperfusion injury and outcomes (Balan et al., 2006; Brucken et al., 2010).

An inhaled oxygen fraction of 1.0 is recommended immediately prior to intubation, but oxygen should be weaned immediately following intubation to 0.5, or the lowest $Fio_2$ that will support an oxyhemoglobin saturation of above 95%. This normoxic resuscitation strategy is recommended in the 2015 American Heart Association Guidelines for postresuscitation care after cardiac arrest (Callaway et al., 2015).

One small trial supports the use of hyperoxia to reduce postoperative pneumocephalus (Hong et al., 2015). This technique of facilitating the resorption of nitrogen-containing air should be employed only when the potential harm of hyperoxia is outweighed by the clinical benefit of increased resorption on air. While appropriate after uncomplicated craniotomy, it may not be in a patient with recent ischemic brain injury.

## Acute respiratory distress syndrome

The fundamental principle behind management of ARDS is that patients with injured lungs are susceptible to further injury, due to both the vulnerable, inflamed condition of the lungs, and the high pressures and levels of inhaled oxygen required to achieve adequate oxygenation. Accordingly, lung-protective ventilation must be provided.

Lung-protective ventilation is a strategy of low tidal volumes, low distending pressures, and adequate PEEP to prevent cyclical alveolar collapse, inflammation ("biotrauma"), and excessive inhaled oxygen fraction (>0.6) (The Acute Respiratory Distress Syndrome Network, 2000; Hess, 2014). This combination target can be achieved through a variety of ventilatory modes, but requires close attention and frequent ventilator adjustment. Adjuncts to ventilation, such as prone positioning (Guérin et al., 2013), increased levels of PEEP in patients with more severe lung injury (Santa Cruz et al., 2013), and continuous neuromuscular blockade (Papazian et al., 2010), have resulted in improved outcomes, probably due to their effects on minimizing ventilator-induced lung injury.

Although the landmark study of low-tidal-volume mechanical ventilation (The Acute Respiratory Distress Syndrome Network, 2000) emphasizes permissive hypercarbia; $PCO_2$ is a potent mediator of CBF and ICP, and must be carefully considered in patients with elevated ICP or compromised CBF. Several very small investigations suggest that lung-protective ventilation strategies causing mild hypercarbia in patients with elevated ICP may be well tolerated (Bennett et al., 2007; Petridis et al., 2010; Young and Andrews, 2011), but

more data are needed before this may be considered safe in routine practice. Prone positioning seems to increase ICP (Reinprecht et al., 2003), but the small increase in ICP may be offset by dramatic improvements in oxygenation (Roth et al., 2014). Neurologic patients with ICP elevation or cerebral edema should not be maintained acidemic or in the prone position unless continuous monitoring of ICP and cerebral metabolism is available to verify safety.

## Airway pressure can affect intracranial pressure

When lung compliance is normal, increased intrathoracic pressure may reduce venous return from the brain and increase ICP. Additionally, high PEEP may decrease venous return to the heart, thereby decreasing cardiac output and mean arterial pressure, reducing CPP, and potentially leading indirectly to increased ICP via reflex cerebral vasodilation. However, the individual response to increased PEEP in brain-injured patients varies greatly, probably according to lung, chest wall, and ventricular compliance. Patients with low pulmonary compliance (stiff lungs) usually do not demonstrate PEEP-associated ICP increases (Caricato et al., 2005). In patients with severe stroke, increases in PEEP did not produce a significant increment in ICP, but CPP was reduced (Helbok et al., 2012). In clinical practice, PEEP may be necessary to achieve adequate oxygenation, and clinicians should use physiologic data to weigh the risks and potential benefits of any maneuvers affecting airway and intrathoracic pressures.

## LIBERATING OF THE VENTILATOR

Outcomes of mechanically ventilated stroke patients have improved in recent years, but respiratory failure is strongly associated with greater severity of brain injury, and the high mortality is likely determined more by the brain injury than the respiratory failure. The best approach to predicting respiratory outcomes in patients with concomitant respiratory failure and acute brain injury during their convalescent period is to consider the following questions:

1. Is there compromise of central respiratory rhythm generation? A very small percentage of brain-injured patients have true central apneas and unstable respiratory patterns that could lead to respiratory arrest. In such patients, closely monitored trials of spontaneous ventilation must precede transfer to a lower acuity care unit, and respiratory suppressants like opioids (or even supplemental oxygen, in patients believed to have true hypoxic respiratory drive)

must be minimized or eliminated completely. Patients with impaired central ventilatory drive may require diaphragmatic pacing or permanent mechanical ventilation, often also with placement of a tracheostomy.

2. Is there need for access to the lower airways for suctioning (as in patients with failed secretion management), or to maintain a patent upper airway for gas exchange (as with severe obstructive sleep apnea)? Such patients may recover airway protection mechanisms over a few days or weeks, and many require a temporary tracheostomy. Permanent tracheostomy is required less often.

3. Is mechanical ventilation required, or does the patient simply need airway protection? Tracheostomy for airway protection allows for removal of the endotracheal tube, and often results in rapid discontinuation of sedatives and weaning from mechanical ventilation. A novel score for prediction of the need for tracheostomy in stroke patients with respiratory failure has been proposed and validated (Bösel et al., 2012; Schönenberger et al., 2016b), and a study of early tracheostomy is under way to determine its effect on long-term functional outcome (Schönenberger et al., 2016a).

## Weaning trials

Weaning from mechanical ventilation is a continuous process that should begin as soon as a moderate level of medical and respiratory stability is achieved. While excessive work of breathing should be avoided as a stressor in patients with ongoing neurologic or cardiac ischemia, respiratory work is necessary to prevent muscle atrophy, and increased duration of mechanical ventilation is strongly correlated with the development of ventilator-associated pneumonia and other medical complications (Table 2.3). Ventilator weaning should proceed unless a strong contraindication exists.

Weaning of mechanical ventilation begins with the downward titration of $Fio_2$ and mean airway pressures, such as $Fio_2 \leq 50\%$ and PEEP of $\leq 8$ cm $H_2O$. Compared to gradually reducing the respiratory rate using synchronized mandatory ventilation or the level of pressure support triggered by each breath, the good results can be obtained through the use of spontaneous breathing trials (SBTs), during which most of the work of breathing is performed by the patient. If the SBT is successful, a protocolized assessment is performed to determine suitability for extubation or disconnection from mechanical ventilation. The most common types of SBTs involve placing the patient on continuous positive airway pressure (CPAP) with a low-level pressure

**Table 2.3**

**Contraindications to spontaneous breathing trials in neurological patients**

| |
|---|
| $Fio_2 > 0.6$, PEEP $>10$ cm $H_2O$, or high risk of lung de-recruitment in severe ARDS |
| Deep sedation or paralysis for control of seizures, ICP, or shivering |
| Active neurologic or myocardial ischemia |
| Symptomatic cerebral vasospasm (delayed cerebral ischemia) |
| Inadequate respiratory muscle strength to support even high-pressure support weaning |
| Central apnea |

PEEP, positive end-expiratory pressure; ARDS, acute respiratory distress syndrome; ICP, intracranial pressure.

support sufficient to overcome endotracheal tube resistance; T-piece trials, in which the patient breathes spontaneously for a predetermined duration through the endotracheal tube with oxygen flow-by; or "trach collar" trials. The ability of the patient to tolerate a T-piece or CPAP trial for 30–60 minutes, while maintaining a ratio of respiratory rate (breaths/minute) to tidal volume (liters) less than 105, is a useful predictor of successful extubation, although these parameters were established in medical, rather than neurocritical care, patients (Yang and Tobin, 1991).

In patients with depressed level of consciousness or neuromuscular respiratory weakness, the ability to tolerate a T-piece or CPAP ventilation overnight offers additional reassurance that the patient has adequate stamina to tolerate breathing off the ventilator indefinitely. Indications of tiring during an SBT include an increasing respiratory rate, with decreasing tidal volume, drop in arterial oxygen saturation, diaphoresis, the progressive use of accessory muscles of respiration, or hemodynamic instability. One very small trial showed the feasibility of continuous weaning using an adapted support ventilation mode after stroke (Teismann et al., 2015).

Failure of a weaning trial is a physiologic stressor, and patients with these signs should be returned to mechanical ventilation. Successful SBTs do not predict the ability to protect the airway. A study of systematic daily lightening of sedation in patients with severe brain injury demonstrated dangerous ICP increases, compromised cerebral oxygenation, and release of stress hormones in some patients, suggesting caution is warranted (Helbok et al., 2012).

In patients with tracheostomy or receiving NPPV, detachment from and reconnection to the ventilator is uneventful and easy to perform. Conversely, extubation and reintubation entail risk. Before a planned extubation, the patient's volume status, airway reactivity, secretions, and cardiac function should be optimized. Even with careful patient selection and medical optimization,

10–15% of extubated patients in the neurologic ICU are reintubated within 48 hours (Karanjia et al., 2011; dos Reis et al., 2013). Of all critically ill patients, the extubation success of those with neurologic diseases is the most difficult to predict (Wang et al., 2014).

## Tracheostomy

Percutaneous tracheostomy creates a temporary stoma that is easily and rapidly reversible upon decannulation, while surgical tracheostomy may create a more durable and permanent stoma. Traditionally, tracheostomy is performed for comfort, oral care, secretion management, and to assist in ventilator weaning when mechanical ventilation is required for more than 14 days (Seder and Yahwak, 2012). In comatose patients, or those with profound neuromuscular weakness for whom a prolonged period of ventilator dependence is anticipated, early tracheostomy within 3–5 days of intubation extends these benefits. A recent pilot study of early tracheostomy vs. prolonged endotracheal intubation with

attempted extubation suggested a mortality benefit with early tracheostomy (Bösel et al., 2013), and recent retrospective data support this approach (Villwock et al., 2014). Most patients with significant bulbar dysfunction following an acute brain injury will require tracheostomy for secretion management (Qureshi et al., 2000; Schönenberger et al., 2016b), although they can often be weaned rapidly from mechanical ventilation, and most will be decannulated when cough strength and airway-protective reflexes have recovered. A novel, validated scoring tool can be used to predict the need for tracheostomy after severe stroke, and may be useful to clinicians in determining when and in whom to perform early tracheostomy (Table 2.4) (Schönenberger et al., 2016b).

Although early tracheostomy is a promising tool for accelerating recovery after a severe brain injury, clinicians performing tracheostomy in such patients should be aware of physiologic dangers inherent in the tracheostomy procedure, such as ICP elevation (Kocaeli et al., 2008; Imperiale et al., 2009; Kleffmann et al., 2012; Kuechler et al., 2015) and impaired cerebral perfusion (Stocchetti et al., 2000), and must take steps to minimize those risks.

*Table 2.4*

The SETscore

| Area of assessment | Situation | Points |
|---|---|---|
| Neurologic function | Dysphagia | 4 |
| | Observed aspiration | 3 |
| | Glasgow Coma Scale on admission <10 | 3 |
| Neurologic lesion | Brainstem | 4 |
| | Space-occupying cerebellar | 3 |
| | Ischemic infarct >2/3 middle cerebral artery territory | 4 |
| | Intracerebral hemorrhage volume > 25 cc | 4 |
| | Diffuse lesion | 3 |
| | Hydrocephalus | 4 |
| General organ function/ procedure | (Neuro)surgical intervention | 2 |
| | Additional respiratory disease | 3 |
| | $Pao_2/Fio_2 < 150$ | 2 |
| | APS (of APACHE II) > 20 | 4 |
| | Lung injury score > 1 | 2 |
| | Sepsis | 3 |

Adapted from Schönenberger et al. (2016b).
A SETscore > 10 predicted the need for tracheostomy in patients with severe stroke and respiratory failure with a sensitivity of 64% and specificity of 86%.
APS, acute physiology score; APACHE, Acute Physiology and Chronic Health Evaluation.

## REFERENCES

Apfelbaum JL, Hagberg CA, Caplan RA et al. (2013). Practice guidelines for management of the difficult airway: an updated report by the American Society of Anesthesiologists Task Force on Management of the Difficult Airway. Anesthesiology 118: 251–270.

Anderson CD, Bartscher JF, Scripko PD et al. (2011). Neurologic examination and extubation outcome in the neurocritical care unit. Neurocrit Care 15: 490–497.

Balan IS, Fiskum G, Hazelton J et al. (2006). Oximetry-guided reoxygenation improves neurological outcome after experimental cardiac arrest. Stroke 37: 3008–3013.

Bassetti CL, Milanova M, Gugger M (2006). Sleep-disordered breathing and acute ischemic stroke: diagnosis, risk factors, treatment, evolution, and long-term clinical outcome. Stroke 37: 967–972.

Bellomo R, Bailey M, Eastwood GM et al. (2011). Arterial hyperoxia and in-hospital mortality after resuscitation from cardiac arrest. Crit Care 15: R90.

Bennett SS, Graffagnino C, Borel CO et al. (2007). Use of high frequency oscillatory ventilation (HFOV) in neurocritical care patients. Neurocrit Care 7: 221–226.

Berkhemer OA, van den Berg LA, Fransen PS et al. (2016). The effect of anesthetic management during intra-arterial therapy for acute stroke in MR CLEAN. Neurology 87: 656–664.

Berrouschot J, Rossler A, Koster J et al. (2000). Mechanical ventilation in patients with hemispheric ischemic stroke. Crit Care Med 28: 2956–2961.

Bolton CF, Chen R, Wijdicks EFM et al. (2004). Neurology of Breathing, Butterworth Heinemann, Philadelphia.

Boom M, Niesters M, Sarton E et al. (2012). Non-analgesic effects of opioids: opioid-induced respiratory depression. Curr Pharm Des 18: 5994–6004.

Bösel J, Schiller P, Hacke W et al. (2012). Benefits of early tracheostomy in ventilated stroke patients? Current evidence and study protocol of the randomized pilot trial SETPOINT (Stroke-related Early Tracheostomy vs. Prolonged Orotracheal Intubation in Neurocritical care Trial). Int J Stroke 7: 173–182.

Bösel J, Schiller P, Hook Y et al. (2013). Stroke-related Early Tracheostomy versus Prolonged Orotracheal Intubation in Neurocritical Care Trial (SETPOINT): a randomized pilot trial. Stroke 44: 21–28.

Bouma GJ, Muizelaar JP, Choi SC et al. (1991). Cerebral circulation and metabolism after severe traumatic brain injury: the elusive role of ischemia. J Neurosurg 75: 685–693.

Brain Trauma Foundation (2007). Guidelines for the management of severe traumatic brain injury. XIV. Hyperventilation. J Neurotrauma 24 (Suppl 1): S87–S90.

Brimacombe J, Keller C, Kunzel KH et al. (2000). Cervical spine motion during airway management: a cinefluoroscopic study of the posteriorly destabilized third cervical vertebrae in human cadavers. Anesth Analg 91 (5): 1274–1278.

Brinjikji W, Murad MH, Rabinstein AA et al. (2015). Conscious sedation versus general anesthesia during endovascular acute ischemic stroke treatment: a systematic review and meta-analysis. AJNR Am J Neuroradiol 36: 525–529.

Brucken A, Kaab AB, Kottmann K et al. (2010). Reducing the duration of 100% oxygen ventilation in the early reperfusion period after cardiopulmonary resuscitation decreases striatal brain damage. Resuscitation 81: 1698–1703.

Callaway CW, Donnino MW, Fink EL et al. (2015). Part 8: Post-cardiac arrest care: 2015 American Heart Association guidelines update for cardiopulmonary resuscitation and emergency cardiovascular care. Circulation 132 (18 Suppl 2): S465–S482.

Campbell BC, Christensen S, Levi CR et al. (2012). Comparison of computed tomography perfusion and magnetic resonance imaging perfusion-diffusion mismatch in ischemic stroke. Stroke 43: 2648–2653.

Caricato A, Conti G, Della Corte F et al. (2005). Effects of PEEP on the intracranial system of patients with head injury and subarachnoid hemorrhage: the role of respiratory system compliance. J Trauma 58: 571–576.

Carrera E, Schmidt JM, Fernandez L et al. (2010). Spontaneous hyperventilation and brain tissue hypoxia in patients with severe brain injury. J Neurol Neurosurg Psychiatry 81: 793–797.

Chesnut RM, Marshall SB, Piek J et al. (1993). Early and late systemic hypotension as a frequent and fundamental source of cerebral ischemia following severe brain injury in the Traumatic Coma Data Bank. Acta Neurochir Suppl 59: 121–125.

Clancy M, Halford S, Walls R et al. (2001). In patients with head injuries who undergo rapid sequence intubation using succinylcholine, does pretreatment with a competitive neuromuscular blocking agent improve outcome? A literature review. Emerg Med J 18: 373–375.

Cohen L, Athaide V, Wickham ME et al. (2015). The effect of ketamine on intracranial and cerebral perfusion pressure and health outcomes: a systematic review. Ann Emerg Med 65: 43–51.

Coles JP, Minhas PS, Fryer TD et al. (2002). Effect of hyperventilation on cerebral blood flow in traumatic head injury: clinical relevance and monitoring correlates. Crit Care Med 30: 1950–1959.

Coplin WM, Pierson DJ, Cooley KD et al. (2000). Implications of extubation delay in brain-injured patients meeting standard weaning criteria. Am J Respir Crit Care Med 161: 1530–1536.

Davis DP, Stern J, Sise MJ et al. (2005). A follow-up analysis of factors associated with head-injury mortality after paramedic rapid sequence intubation. J Trauma 59: 486–490.

Davis DP, Idris AH, Sise MJ et al. (2006). Early ventilation and outcome in patients with moderate to severe traumatic brain injury. Crit Care Med 34: 1202–1208.

Davis DP, Meade W, Sise MJ et al. (2009). Both hypoxemia and extreme hyperoxemia may be detrimental in patients with severe traumatic brain injury. J Neurotrauma 26: 2217–2223.

Del Castillo J, Lopez-Herce J, Matamoros M et al. (2012). Hyperoxia, hypocapnia and hypercapnia as outcome factors after cardiac arrest in children. Resuscitation 83: 1456–1461.

Diringer MN, Videen TO, Yundt K et al. (2002). Regional cerebrovascular and metabolic effects of hyperventilation after severe traumatic brain injury. J Neurosurg 96: 103–108.

Donegan MF, Bedford RF (1980). Intravenously administered lidocaine prevents intracranial hypertension during endotracheal suctioning. Anesthesiology 52: 516–518.

dos Reis HF, Almeida ML, da Silva MF et al. (2013). Association between the rapid shallow breathing index and extubation success in patients with traumatic brain injury. Rev Bras Ter Intensiva 25: 212–217.

Dumont TM, Visioni AJ, Rughani AI et al. (2010). Inappropriate prehospital ventilation in severe traumatic brain injury increases in-hospital mortality. J Neurotrauma 27: 1233–1241.

Elmer J, Scutella M, Pullalarevu R et al. (2015). The association between hyperoxia and patient outcomes after cardiac arrest: analysis of a high-resolution database. Intensive Care Med 41: 49–57.

Feldman JL, Del Negro CA, Gray PA (2013). Understanding the rhythm of breathing: so near, yet so far. Annu Rev Physiol 75: 423–452.

Fisher AJ, Donnelly SC, Hirani N et al. (1999). Enhanced pulmonary inflammation in organ donors following fatal non-traumatic brain injury. Lancet 353: 1412–1413.

Flowers HL, Skoretz SA, Streiner DL et al. (2011). MRI-based neuroanatomical predictors of dysphagia after acute ischemic stroke: a systematic review and meta-analysis. Cerebrovasc Dis 32: 1–10.

Floyd TF, Clark JM, Gelfand R et al. (2003). Independent cerebral vasoconstrictive effects of hyperoxia and accompanying arterial hypocapnia at 1 ATA. J Appl Physiol (1985) 95 (6): 2453–2461.

Gopinath SP, Valadka AB, Uzura M et al. (1999). Comparison of jugular venous oxygen saturation and brain tissue Po2 as monitors of cerebral ischemia after head injury. Crit Care Med 27: 2337–2345.

Grande CM, Barton CR, Stene JK (1988). Appropriate techniques for airway management of emergency patients with suspected spinal cord injury. Anesth Analg 67: 714–715.

Gross JB (2003). When you breathe in you inspire, when you don't breathe, you...expire: new insights regarding opioid-induced ventilatory depression. Anesthesiology 99: 767–770.

Grotta J, Pasteur W, Khwaja G et al. (1995). Elective intubation for neurologic deterioration after stroke. Neurology 45: 640–644.

Grover VK, Reddy GM, Kak VK et al. (1999). Intracranial pressure changes with different doses of lignocaine under general anaesthesia. Neurol Ind 47: 118–121.

Guérin C, Reignier J, Richard JC et al. (2013). Prone positioning in severe acute respiratory distress syndrome. N Engl J Med 368: 2159.

Gujjar AR, Deibert E, Manno EM et al. (1998). Mechanical ventilation for ischemic stroke and intracerebral hemorrhage: Indications, timing, and outcome. Neurology 51: 447–451.

Guyenet PG, Bayliss DA (2015). Neural control of breathing and CO2 homeostasis. Neuron 87: 946–961.

Hannawi Y, Hannawi B, Rao CP et al. (2013). Stroke-associated pneumonia: major advances and obstacles. Cerebrovasc Dis 35: 430–443.

Harraf F, Ward K, Man W et al. (2008). Transcranial magnetic stimulation study of expiratory muscle weakness in acute ischemic stroke. Neurology 71: 2000–2007.

Hashimoto Y, Watanabe S, Tanaka F et al. (1989). A case of medullary infarction presented lateral medullary syndrome and respiratory arrest after ataxic respiration. Rinsho Shinkeigako 29: 1017–1022.

Hauswald M, Sklar DP, Tandberg D et al. (1991). Cervical spine movement during airway management: cinefluoroscopic appraisal in human cadavers. Am J Emerg Med 9: 535–538.

Helbok R, Kurtz P, Schmidt MJ et al. (2012). Effects of the neurological wake-up test on clinical examination, intracranial pressure, brain metabolism and brain tissue oxygenation in severely brain-injured patients. Crit Care 16: R226.

Helmerhorst HJ, Roos-Blom MJ, van Westerloo DJ et al. (2015). Association between arterial hyperoxia and outcome in subsets of critical illness: a systematic review, meta-analysis, and meta-regression of cohort studies. Crit Care Med 43: 1508–1519.

Herrmann DM, Bassetti CL (2009). Sleep-related breathing and sleep-wake disturbances in ischemic stroke. Neurology 73: 1313–1322.

Hess DR (2013). Noninvasive ventilation for acute respiratory failure. Respir Care 58: 950–972.

Hess DR (2014). Ventilatory strategies in severe acute respiratory failure. Semin Respir Crit Care Med 35: 418–430.

Holland MC, Mackersie RC, Morabito D et al. (2003). The development of acute lung injury is associated with worse neurologic outcome in patients with severe traumatic brain injury. J Trauma 55: 106–111.

Hong B, Biertz F, Raab P et al. (2015). Normobaric hyperoxia for treatment of pneumocephalus after posterior fossa surgery in the semisitting position: a prospective randomized controlled trial. PLoS One 10 (5): e0125710.

Ijland MM, Heunks LM, van der Hoeven JG (2010). Bench-to-bedside review: hypercapnic acidosis in lung injury – from 'permissive' to 'therapeutic'. Crit Care 14: 237.

Imperiale C, Magni G, Favaro R et al. (2009). Intracranial pressure monitoring during percutaneous tracheostomy "percutwist" in critically ill neurosurgery patients. Anesth Analg 108: 588–592.

Iranzo A, Santamaría J, Berenguer J et al. (2002). Prevalence and clinical importance of sleep apnea in the first night after cerebral infarction. Neurology 58: 911–916.

Kalsotra A, Zhao J, Anakk S et al. (2007). Brain trauma leads to enhanced lung inflammation and injury: evidence for role of P4504Fs in resolution. J Cereb Blood Flow Metab 27: 963–974.

Karanjia N, Nordquist D, Stevens R et al. (2011). A clinical description of extubation failure in patients with primary brain injury. Neurocrit Care 15: 4–12.

Kepplinger J, Barlinn K, Albright KC et al. (2013). Early sleep apnea screening on a stroke unit is feasible in patients with acute cerebral ischemia. J Neurol 260: 1343–1350.

Kleffmann J, Pahl R, Deinsberger W et al. (2012). Effect of percutaneous tracheostomy on intracerebral pressure and perfusion pressure in patients with acute cerebral dysfunction (TIP trial): an observational study. Neurocrit Care 17: 85–89.

Kilgannon JH, Jones AE, Shapiro NI et al. (2010). Association between arterial hyperoxia following resuscitation from cardiac arrest and in-hospital mortality. JAMA 303: 2165–2171.

Kilgannon JH, Jones AE, Parrillo JE et al. (2011). Relationship between supranormal oxygen tension and outcome after resuscitation from cardiac arrest. Circulation 123: 2717–2722.

Kocaeli H, Korfali E, Taşkapilioğlu O et al. (2008). Analysis of intracranial pressure changes during early versus late percutaneous tracheostomy in a neuro-intensive care unit. Acta Neurochir (Wien)150 (12): 1263–1267. discussion 1267. http://dx.doi.org/10.1007/s00701-008-0153-9. Epub 2008 Nov 11.

Kuechler JN, Abusamha A, Ziemann S et al. (2015). Impact of percutaneous dilatational tracheostomy in brain injured patients. Clin Neurol Neurosurg 137: 137–141.

Lebowitz PW, Shay H, Straker T et al. (2012). Shoulder and head elevation improves laryngoscopic view for tracheal intubation in nonobese as well as obese individuals. J Clin Anesth 24: 104–108.

Malhotra A, White D (2002). Obstructive sleep apnea. Lancet 360: 237–245.

Mallampati SR, Gatt SP, Gugino LD et al. (1985). A clinical sign to predict difficult tracheal intubation: a prospective study. Can Anaesth Soc J 32: 429–434.

Marion DW, Puccio A, Wisniewski SR et al. (2002). Effect of hyperventilation on extracellular concentrations of glutamate, lactate, pyruvate, and local cerebral blood flow in patients with severe traumatic brain injury. Crit Care Med 17: 2619–2625.

Martyn JA, Richtsfeld M (2006). Succinylcholine-induced hyperkalemia in acquired pathologic states: etiologic factors and molecular mechanisms. Anesthesiology 104: 158–169.

Mayer SA, Copeland D, Bernardini GL et al. (2000). Cost and outcome of mechanical ventilation for life-threatening stroke. Stroke 31: 2346–2353.

McPhee L, Seder DB (2012). The neurocritical care airway. In: K Lee (Ed.), The Neuro-ICU Book, McGraw Hill, New York, pp. 655–671.

Mozaffarian D, Benjamin EJ, Go AS et al. (2016). Executive summary: heart disease and stroke statistics – 2016 update: a report from the American Heart Association. Circulation 133: 447–454.

Muizelaar JP, Marmarou A, Ward JD et al. (1991). Adverse effects of prolonged hyperventilation in patients with severe head injury: a randomized clinical trial. J Neurosurg 75: 731–739.

Nogués MA, Benarroch E (2008). Abnormalities of respiratory control and the respiratory motor unit. Neurologist 14: 273–288.

North JB, Jennett S (1974). Abnormal breathing patterns associated with acute brain damage. Arch Neurol 31: 338–344.

Oddo M, Bösel J, Participants in the International Multidisciplinary Consensus Conference on Multimodality Monitoring (2014). Monitoring of brain and systemic oxygenation in neurocritical care patients. Neurocrit Care 21: S103–S120.

Oertel M, Kelly DF, Lee JH et al. (2002). Efficacy of hyperventilation, blood pressure elevation, and metabolic suppression therapy in controlling intracranial pressure after head injury. J Neurosurg 97: 1045–1053.

Papazian L, Forel JM, Gacouin A et al. (2010). Neuromuscular blockers in early acute respiratory distress syndrome. N Engl J Med 363: 1107.

Petridis AK, Doukas A, Kienke S et al. (2010). The effect of lung protective permissive hypercapnia in intracerebral pressure in patients with subarachnoid haemorrhage and ARDS. A retrospective study. Acta Neurochir 152: 2143–2145.

Pynnönen L, Falkenbach P, Kämäräinen A et al. (2011). Therapeutic hypothermia after cardiac arrest – cerebral perfusion and metabolism during upper and lower threshold normocapnia. Resuscitation 82: 1174–1179.

Qureshi AI, Suarez JI, Parekh PD et al. (2000). Prediction and timing of tracheostomy in patients with infratentorial lesions requiring mechanical ventilatory support. Crit Care Med 28: 1383–1387.

Rabinstein AA, Wijdicks EF (2004). Outcome of survivors of acute stroke who require prolonged ventilatory assistance and tracheostomy. Cerebrovasc Dis 18: 325–331.

Rangel-Castilla L, Lara LR, Gopinath S et al. (2010). Cerebral hemodynamic effects of acute hyperoxia and hyperventilation after severe traumatic brain injury. J Neurotrauma 27: 1853–1863.

Reinprecht A, Greher M, Wolfsberger S et al. (2003). Prone position in subarachnoid hemorrhage patients with acute respiratory distress syndrome: effects on cerebral tissue oxygenation and intracranial pressure. Crit Care Med 31: 1831–1838.

Rincon F, Kang J, Maltenfort M et al. (2014a). Association between hyperoxia and mortality after stroke: a multicenter cohort study. Crit Care Med 42: 387–396.

Rincon F, Maltenfort M, Dey S et al. (2014b). The prevalence and impact of mortality of the acute respiratory distress syndrome on admissions of patients with ischemic stroke in the United States. J Intensive Care Med 29: 357–364.

Roberts BW, Karagiannis P, Coletta M et al. (2015). Effects of PaCO2 derangements on clinical outcomes after cerebral injury: a systematic review. Resuscitation 91: 32–41.

Roch A, Michelet P, Jullien AC et al. (2003). Long-term outcome in intensive care unit survivors after mechanical ventilation for intracerebral hemorrhage. Crit Care Med 31: 2651–2656.

Rockswold SB, Rockswold GL, Zaun DA et al. (2013). A prospective, randomized Phase II clinical trial to evaluate the effect of combined hyperbaric and normobaric hyperoxia on cerebral metabolism, intracranial pressure, oxygen toxicity, and clinical outcome in severe traumatic brain injury. J Neurosurg 118: 1317–1328.

Roth C, Ferbert A, Deinsberger W et al. (2014). Does prone positioning increase intracranial pressure? A retrospective analysis of patients with acute brain injury and acute respiratory failure. Neurocrit Care 21: 186–191.

Salam A, Tilluckdharry L, Amoateng-Adjepong Y et al. (2004). Neurologic status, cough, secretions and extubation outcomes. Intensive Care Med 30: 1334–1339.

Salhi B, Stettner E (2007). In defense of the use of lidocaine in rapid sequence intubation. Ann Emerg Med 49: 84–86.

Santa Cruz R, Rojas JI, Nervi R et al. (2013). High versus low positive end-expiratory pressure (PEEP) levels for mechanically ventilated adult patients with acute lung injury and acute respiratory distress syndrome. Cochrane Database Syst Rev 6. CD009098.NMB.

Scala R, Naldi M (2008). Ventilators for noninvasive ventilation to treat acute respiratory failure. Respir Care 53: 1054–1080.

Schneider AG, Eastwood GM, Bellomo R et al. (2013). Arterial carbon dioxide tension and outcome in patients admitted to the intensive care unit after cardiac arrest. Resuscitation 84: 927–934.

Schönenberger S, Uhlmann L, Hacke W et al. (2016). Effect of conscious sedation vs general anesthesia on early neurological improvement among patients with ischemic stroke undergoing endovascular thrombectomy: a randomized clinical trial. JAMA 316 (19): 1986–1996.

Schönenberger S, Al-Suwaidan F, Kieser M et al. (2016a). The SETscore to predict tracheostomy need in cerebrovascular neurocritical care patients. Neurocrit Care 25: 94–104.

Schönenberger S, Niesen WD, Fuhrer H et al. (2016b). Early tracheostomy in ventilated stroke patients: study protocol of the international multicentre randomized trial SETPOINT2 (Stroke-related Early Tracheotomy vs. Prolonged Orotracheal Intubation in Neurocritical care Trial 2). Int J Stroke 11: 368–379.

Scrase I, Woollard M (2006). Needle vs surgical cricothyroidotomy: a short cut to effective ventilation. Anaesthesia 61: 962–974.

Seder DB, Yahwak JA (2012). Percutaneous tracheostomy. In: K Lee (Ed.), The Neuro-ICU Book, McGraw Hill, New York, pp. 723–733.

Seder DB, Lee K, Rahman C et al. (2009). Safety and feasibility of percutaneous tracheostomy performed by neurointensivists. Neurocrit Care 10: 264–268.

Seder DB, Jagoda A, Riggs B (2015). Emergency neurological life support: airway, ventilation, and sedation. Neurocrit Care 23 (Suppl. 2): S5–S22.

Somasundaram S, Henke C, Neumann-Haefelin T et al. (2014). Dysphagia risk assessment in acute left-hemispheric middle cerebral artery stroke. Cerebrovasc Dis 37: 217–222.

Souter MJ, Blissitt PA, Blosser S et al. (2015). Recommendations for the critical care management of devastating brain injury: prognostication, psychosocial, and ethical management: a position statement for healthcare professionals from the Neurocritical Care Society. Neurocrit Care 23: 4–13.

Steffling D, Ritzka M, Jakob W et al. (2012). Indications and outcome of ventilated patients treated in a neurological intensive care unit. Nervenarzt 83: 741–750.

Stein DM, Roddy V, Marx J et al. (2012). Emergency neurological life support: traumatic spine injury. Neurocrit Care 17: S102–S111.

Steiner T, Mendoza G, De Georgia M et al. (1997). Prognosis of stroke patients requiring mechanical ventilation in a neurological critical care unit. Stroke 28: 711–715.

Stevens RD, Shoykhet M, Cadena R (2015). Emergency neurological life support: intracranial hypertension and herniation. Neurocrit Care 23: S76–S82.

Stocchetti N, Parma A, Lamperti M et al. (2000). Neurophysiological consequences of three tracheostomy techniques: a randomized study in neurosurgical patients. J Neurosurg Anesthesiol 12: 307–313.

Suppan L, Tramèr MR, Niquille M et al. (2016). Alternative intubation techniques vs Macintosh laryngoscopy in patients with cervical spine immobilization: systematic review and meta-analysis of randomized controlled trials. Br J Anaesth 116: 27–36.

Taher A, Pilehvari Z, Poorolajal J et al. (2016). Effects of normobaric hyperoxia in traumatic brain injury: a randomized controlled clinical trial. Trauma Mon 21 (1): e26772.

Talke PO, Sharma D, Heyer EJ et al. (2014). Society for Neuroscience in Anesthesiology and Critical Care Expert consensus statement: anesthetic management of endovascular treatment for acute ischemic stroke: endorsed by the Society of NeuroInterventional Surgery and the Neurocritical Care Society. J Neurosurg Anesthesiol 26: 95–108.

Teismann IK, Oelschläger C, Werstler N et al. (2015). Discontinuous versus continuous weaning in stroke patients. Cerebrovasc Dis 39: 269–277.

The Acute Respiratory Distress Syndrome Network (2000). Ventilation with lower tidal volumes as compared with traditional tidal volumes for acute lung injury and the acute respiratory distress syndrome. N Engl J Med 342: 1301.

Topjian AA, Berg RA, Taccone FS (2015). Haemodynamic and ventilator management in patients following cardiac arrest. Curr Opin Crit Care 21: 195–201.

Trzeciak S, Jones AE, Kilgannon JH et al. (2009). Significance of arterial hypotension after resuscitation from cardiac arrest. Crit Care Med 37: 2895–2903.

Van de Ven MJ, Colier WN, Van der Sluijs MC et al. (2001). Ventilatory and cerebrovascular responses in normocapnic and hypercapnic COPD patients. Eur Respir J 18: 61–68.

Vilalta A, Sahuquillo J, Merino MA (2011). Normobaric hyperoxia in traumatic brain injury: does brain metabolic state influence the response to hyperoxic challenge? J Neurotrauma 28: 1139–1148.

Villwock JA, Villwock MR, Deshaies EM (2014). Tracheostomy timing affects stroke recovery. J Stroke Cerebrovasc Dis 23: 1069–1072.

Walls RM, Murphy MF (2008). Manual of emergency airway management, 3rd edn. Lippincott Williams & Wilkins, Philadelphia.

Wang S, Zhang L, Huang K et al. (2014). Predictors of extubation failure in neurocritical patients identified by a systematic review and meta-analysis. PLoS One 9 (12): e112198.

Ward K, Seymour J, Steier J et al. (2010). Acute ischaemic hemispheric stroke is associated with impairment of reflex in addition to voluntary cough. Eur Respir J 36: 1383–1390.

Wijdicks EF, Scott JP (1997). Causes and outcome of mechanical ventilation in patients with hemispheric ischemic stroke. Mayo Clin Proc 72: 210–213.

Wijdicks EF, Sheth KN, Carter BS et al. (2014). American Heart Association Stroke Council. Recommendations for the management of cerebral and cerebellar infarction with swelling: a statement for healthcare professionals from the American

Heart Association/American Stroke Association. Stroke 45: 1222–1238.

Wood EG, Go-Wingkun J, Luisiri A et al. (1990). Symptomatic cerebral swelling complicating diabetic ketoacidosis documented by intraventricular pressure monitoring: survival without neurologic sequela. Pediatr Emerg Care 6: 285–288.

Yang KL, Tobin MJ (1991). A prospective study of indexes predicting the outcome of trials of weaning from mechanical ventilation. N Engl J Med 324: 1445–1450.

Young NH, Andrews PJ (2011). High-frequency oscillation as a rescue strategy for brain-injured adult patients with acute lung injury and acute respiratory distress syndrome. Neurocrit Care 15: 623–633.

*Handbook of Clinical Neurology,* Vol. 140 (3rd series)
*Critical Care Neurology, Part I*
E.F.M. Wijdicks and A.H. Kramer, Editors
http://dx.doi.org/10.1016/B978-0-444-63600-3.00003-9

Chapter 3

# Neuropulmonology

A. BALOFSKY[1], J. GEORGE[2], AND P. PAPADAKOS[1,2,3,4]*

[1]*Department of Anesthesiology, University of Rochester Medical Center, Rochester, NY, USA*

[2]*Department of Neurology, University of Rochester Medical Center, Rochester, NY, USA*

[3]*Department of Surgery, University of Rochester Medical Center, Rochester, NY, USA*

[4]*Department of Neurosurgery, University of Rochester Medical Center, Rochester, NY, USA*

## Abstract

Neuropulmonology refers to the complex interconnection between the central nervous system and the respiratory system. Neurologic injury includes traumatic brain injury, hemorrhage, stroke, and seizures, and in each there are far-reaching effects that can result in pulmonary dysfunction. Systemic changes can induce impairment of pulmonary function due to changes in the core structure and function of the lung. The conditions and disorders that often occur in these patients include aspiration pneumonia, neurogenic pulmonary edema, and acute respiratory distress syndrome, but also several abnormal respiratory patterns and sleep-disordered breathing. Lung infections, pulmonary edema – neurogenic or cardiogenic – and pulmonary embolus all are a serious barrier to recovery and can have significant effects on outcomes such as hospital course, prognosis, and mortality. This review presents the spectrum of pulmonary abnormalities seen in neurocritical care.

## INTRODUCTION

Neuropulmonology refers to the complex interactions between the central nervous system and the respiratory system. Neurologic injury occurs due to a variety of mechanisms, including traumatic brain injury (TBI), hemorrhage, stroke, and seizures. While the primary injury occurs in the central nervous system, there are far-reaching systemic effects which often include pulmonary dysfunction. Following the inciting event, systemic and local changes can lead to impairment of pulmonary function due to changes in the core structure and function of the lung. The conditions and disorders that often occur in these patients include pneumonia, neurogenic pulmonary edema (NPE), and acute respiratory distress syndrome (ARDS), as well as the production of abnormal respiratory patterns and sleep-disordered breathing (SDB). These pulmonary complications present a barrier to recovery and treatment, and can have significant effects on outcomes such as hospital course, prognosis, and mortality.

## NEUROCRITICAL DISORDERS ASSOCIATED WITH PULMONARY DISEASE

### Traumatic brain injury

TBI refers to alteration in brain function due to an external force, and it is a severe disabling disorder causing significant morbidity and mortality (Reis et al., 2015). In patients with severe TBI, the most commonly encountered non-neurologic organ dysfunction is respiratory failure, and it is associated with worse outcomes (Zygun et al., 2005). This is not an unexpected result, as it is known that brain injury may increase the vulnerability of lungs to additional mechanical or ischemia-reperfusion injuries (López-Aguilar et al., 2005).

Infectious complications are extremely common following TBI, and pneumonia has been found to occur in 40–65% of patients, most commonly occurring in the first 5 days after severe TBI (Lim and Smith, 2007). Zygun et al. (2006) reported a 45% incidence

*Correspondence to: Peter Papadakos, MD FCCM FAARC, Department of Anesthesiology, University of Rochester Medical Center, 601 Elmwood Ave, Box 604, Rochester NY 14642, USA. Tel: +1-585-273-4750, E-mail: Peter_Papadakos@urmc.rochester.edu

of ventilator-associated pneumonia (VAP) in patients with severe TBI, associated with significant morbidity, including longer duration of mechanical ventilation, more frequent need for tracheostomy, and longer hospital and intensive care unit (ICU) stays, and Hui et al. (2013) found that each additional ventilator day increased the risk of pneumonia by 7%. This is particularly important given that hospital-acquired pneumonia has an independent association with poor outcomes extending 5 years after the occurrence of TBI (Kesinger et al., 2015).

The pathologic changes leading to pulmonary damage and respiratory failure after injury to the brain may occur via a variety of mechanisms. Following head injury, hypoxemia may result due to a failure of mechanisms regulating the ventilation–perfusion balance. This occurs by numerous mechanisms, such as redistribution in regional perfusion, pulmonary microembolism, possibly leading to increased dead-space ventilation, and a depletion of lung surfactant as a result of excessive sympathetic stimulation (Pelosi et al., 2005). Studies have shown that exposure to lethal head injury with stress involving the sympathetic nervous system results in decreased lung compliance and high minimum surface tension of lung wash fluid, possibly mediated in part by changes to alveolar surfactant due to an increase in intra-alveolar cholesterol (Bergren and Beckman, 1975; Sexton and Beckman, 1975; Crittenden and Beckman, 1982). Interestingly, Brueggemann et al. (1976) found that the observed reduction in static compliance only occurs immediately before the time of death. Zhu et al. (2007) found that TBI induces rapid increases of labile zinc and inflammatory mediators in the lung, including tumor necrosis factor-alpha (TNF-$\alpha$) and interleukin-8 (IL-8), and this may further contribute to the development of lung injury. Changes in respiratory dynamics can lead to further pulmonary compromise, and a study of 114 patients post-TBI showed that 79% had a moderate deficit in expiratory reserve volume, with 60% experiencing severe deficits (McHenry, 2001). While severe TBI is known to be associated with acute lung injury (ALI) and pulmonary infectious complications, Vermeij et al. (2013) found that, even with experimentally induced mild TBI in rats, there is observable ALI with protein leakage, lung edema, and an alveolar inflammatory response, as well as systemic immune suppression.

Elevated intracranial pressure (ICP) increases the risk for adverse outcomes in TBI, and while ICP monitoring is routinely performed, there is conflicting evidence regarding its utility, and some studies have demonstrated an association between ICP monitoring and worse outcomes (Haddad and Arabi, 2012). Once these values are known it may lead to treatment, and treatment of intracranial hypertension may itself prove detrimental to the lungs. Hyperventilation is commonly used for the purpose of inducing hypocapnia and reducing ICP, although this may lead to lung injury. Hypocapnia may be injurious to lungs via numerous mechanisms, including potentiation of reperfusion injury, increased lung permeability and edema, decreased compliance, surfactant inhibition, and by potentiating lung inflammation (Curley et al., 2010). Not only is there an increased risk to the pulmonary system, but the risk of brain tissue hypoxia is known to be increased when there is a reduction in end-tidal $CO_2$ (Carrera et al., 2010). While cooling of patients with TBI is an accepted method for treating refractory intracranial hypertension, a study by O'Phelan et al. (2015) found that the use of temperature modulation significantly increased the risk for pulmonary complications, including pneumonia and ARDS.

The impact of TBI on SDB represents another important consideration in this patient population. Almost one-quarter of patients with TBI will experience SDB, including central sleep apnea and obstructive sleep apnea, and it is associated with increased impairment of sustained attention and memory (Vermaelen et al., 2015).

Further understanding of the pathogenesis leading to pulmonary injury will prove useful in developing therapies. Jin et al. (2009) found that, following experimentally induced TBI, mice lacking nuclear factor erythroid 2-related factor 2 (Nrf2) were more susceptible to developing lung injury, evidenced by greater pulmonary capillary permeability and alveolar cell apoptosis, and associated with increased production of pulmonary inflammatory cytokines and decreased pulmonary antioxidant and detoxifying enzymes. Structural changes are known to occur following TBI and are observable in the tracheobronchial epithelia as well as type II pneumocytes, an effect that may be ameliorated through the use of erythropoietin (Yildirim et al., 2004a, b, 2005). This may be in part due to the role erythropoietin plays in inducing an Nrf-2-mediated protective response when administered following TBI (Jin et al., 2011).

Recently there has been a focus on the role of high-mobility group box protein 1 (HMGB1) interaction with the receptor for advanced glycation end products (RAGE) in the pathogenesis of lung dysfunction following TBI. This is particularly important in the setting of lung transplantation, where patients with TBI represent a significant source of organs for transplantation. Weber et al. (2014) found that TBI-induced systemic hypoxia, ALI, pulmonary neutrophilia, and decreased compliance were attenuated in RAGE-deficient mice, and that lungs from RAGE-deficient TBI donors did not develop ALI after transplantation. The neutralization of TBI-induced systemic HMGB1 was found to reverse hypoxia and improve lung compliance. RAGE is also known to be involved in the onset of innate immune inflammatory responses, and is associated with ALI and clinical outcomes in ventilator-induced lung injury (Lopez-Aguilar and Blanch, 2015). While the use of hyperbaric oxygen therapy (HBOT) has been advocated in the treatment of TBI, significant pulmonary compromise has been reported to occur in 13% of patients receiving HBOT, including increased oxygen requirements, infiltrates on chest X-ray, and severe cyanosis and hyperpnea (Bennett et al., 2012). Furthermore, hypoxemia and extreme hyperoxemia are associated with an increase in mortality and a decrease in good outcomes following TBI (Davis et al., 2009).

## Subarachnoid hemorrhage

Pulmonary injury is the most common complication following subarachnoid hemorrhage (SAH), affecting the majority of patients, and includes NPE, ARDS, pneumonia, and pulmonary emboli (Schuiling et al., 2005; Stevens and Nyquist, 2007). Pulmonary complications have been linked to prolonged ICU stay and hospital length of stay, as well as poor functional outcome and mortality (Wartenberg and Mayer, 2010). A large multicenter cooperative aneurysm study found that following aneurysmal SAH, the proportion of deaths from extracerebral complications (23%) equaled the individual proportions of deaths from initial bleeding (19%), rebleeding (22%), and vasopasm (23%), with pulmonary complications being the most common nonneurologic cause of death (Solenski et al., 1995). Twenty-three percent of patients developed pulmonary edema, with 6% experiencing severe pulmonary edema, with the greatest frequency of occurrence being on days 3 through 7. This can have an effect on the neurologic course, as there is an observed higher incidence of symptomatic vasospasm in patients with pulmonary complications after aneurysmal SAH, which may reflect an avoidance of hypervolemic and hyperdynamic therapy due to pulmonary compromise (Friedman et al., 2003).

Bilateral pulmonary infiltrates are a common finding in SAH patients, occurring secondary to NPE, aspiration pneumonia, and cardiogenic pulmonary edema, and are associated with poor neurologic grade on admission and prolonged length of hospital stay (Kramer et al., 2009; Wartenberg and Mayer, 2010). These infiltrates most commonly develop within 3 days of aneurysm rupture, but only infiltrates developing 72 hours after the initial event were predictors for death and poor functional outcome. Pneumonia is a common complication following SAH, and has been reported to occur in 20–49% of patients, with higher incidence in those undergoing mechanical ventilation (Mrozek et al., 2015).

A prospective study (Sarrafzadeh et al., 2011) found pronounced immunodepression in patients following aneurysmal SAH, which was associated with a high incidence of pneumonia. Treatment for SAH may contribute, and hypothermia and barbiturates to reduce ICP may result in immune suppression and decreased leukocyte count, which can predispose to pneumonia (Chen et al., 2014).

Consideration must be given to the numerous pathologic processes occurring after SAH and their role in the development of pulmonary complications. Massive quantities of catecholamines are released following SAH due to hypothalamic stress, particularly in association with posterior-circulation aneurysms, resulting in increased pulmonary vascular permeability and hydrostatic pressure injury to the pulmonary capillaries (Macmillan et al., 2002; Lo et al., 2015).

The incidence of systemic inflammatory response syndrome (SIRS) in SAH patients ranges from 29% to 87% (Chen et al., 2014), and Gruber et al. (1999) suggested that the SIRS following SAH is the primary mechanism for the development of extracerebral organ dysfunction. SAH is known to induce a systemic state of inflammation, during which there is an increase in numerous cytokines, including IL-1, IL-1β, IL-6, and TNF-α. The development and progression of this dysfunction may also be contributed to by a mechanism of central dysregulation, whereby there is direct modulation of the organ function and the predisposition for a systemic inflammatory state, and may be related to hypothalamic and medullary lesions. These lesions can lead to pulmonary dysfunction associated with high pulmonary capillary pressure and increased permeability. The finding that vasospasm after SAH can lead to ischemic neurodegeneration in the dorsal root ganglia of the phrenic nerve causing deterioration of respiratory rhythms provides another explanation for pulmonary dysfunction (Ulvi et al., 2013). SAH leads to structural changes in the lung and Suzuki et al. (2011) found that, in mouse studies, NPE following SAH was associated with pulmonary endothelial cell apoptosis. The location of the aneurysm itself may play a role in the degree of lung dysfunction, and Ochiai et al. (2001) found that the severity of NPE following SAH from vertebral artery aneurysm rupture correlated with deformation of the ventrolateral medulla from the localized hemorrhage. Muroi et al. (2008) found that most patients with NPE following SAH were severely impaired, and all presented with radiologically severe hemorrhage, and that the incidence of NPE was significantly higher when patients presented with posterior-circulation ruptured aneurysms.

Spontaneous hyperventilation is a common finding following SAH, and is associated with worse illness severity and complications like pneumonia and SIRS (Williamson et al., 2015). Further to this point, hypocapnia is a common finding in ventilated patients following SAH, even with minimal ventilator support, and is independently associated with poor functional outcomes (Solaiman and Singh, 2013).

The impaired oxygenation that frequently occurs after SAH is strongly associated with an increased mean length of hospital stay (Vespa and Bleck, 2004).

Laboratory testing may play a role in predicting which patients will go on to develop pulmonary complications after SAH. Early elevation of cerebral lactate following SAH has been found to correlate with the early occurrence of bacterial pneumonia, and may represent a way to predict which patients are at higher risk of developing infections (Radolf et al., 2014). The development of ARDS was found to be correlated with an elevation of troponin I (Naidech et al., 2009), and Chen et al. (2016b) found that electrocardiographic abnormalities, particularly with Q and QS waves and nonspecific ST- or T-wave changes, may predict NPE development within 24 hours following spontaneous SAH. Satoh et al. (2014) found that increased serum lactate, within 1 hour after SAH, was independently associated with early onset of NPE.

## Stroke

Pulmonary dysfunction may occur for multiple reasons after stroke, and these patients are at risk of hypoxia due to respiratory muscle weakness, aspiration, and alterations in the central regulation of respiration (Roffe et al., 2003). Following stroke, patients commonly develop restrictive respiratory patterns (Fugl-Meyer et al., 1983). Ezeugwu et al. (2013) studied stroke survivors to determine lung function when compared to healthy controls. Survivors were observed to have significantly lower values for forced expiratory volume in 1 second, forced vital capacity, peak expiratory flow, and chest excursion. Both ipsilateral and contralateral diaphragmatic paralysis have been reported to occur following stroke (Kumar et al., 2009; Wu et al., 2011; Morís et al., 2012) and Similowski et al. (1996) observed that central corticodiaphragmatic pathways may be involved in the development of diaphragmatic paralysis following stroke. Khedr et al. (2000) studied patients with cortical and subcortical infarction and found there to be abnormal values of cortical latency, central conduction time, amplitude of compound muscle action potentials, and excitability threshold of the affected hemisphere, and a strong association between the site of infarction on computed tomography (CT), diaphragmatic excursion, and degree of respiratory dysfunction. M-mode ultrasonography has been proposed as a noninvasive method that can provide quantitative information regarding diaphragmatic motion that is correlated with pulmonary function (Jung et al., 2014). And while ischemic stroke is known to lead to cardiac complications such as myocardial

stunning, Probasco et al. (2014) found that large-vessel ischemic brainstem stroke was associated with the development of pulmonary edema unrelated to any cardiac dysfunction.

Up to one-third of stroke patients will develop pneumonia, and a prospective cohort study by Sellars et al. (2007) found that pneumonia after stroke is associated with older age, dysarthria or no speech due to aphasia, disability severity, cognitive impairment, and failing the water swallow test. The risk of aspiration pneumonia is increased with vascular bulbar lesions, due to impaired swallow, respiratory abnormalities, reduced vital capacity, and reduction in cough reflex (Howard et al., 2001). Winklewski et al. (2014) proposed a model explaining the increased incidence of pneumonia following ischemic stroke, whereby the intense sympathetic nervous system activation and release of catecholamines following stroke primarily damages the lungs, and the poststroke state of immunosuppression makes them more susceptible to infection.

Breathing after stroke can be disturbed by disruption of central pattern generation and interruption of respiratory pathways with reduced respiratory drive, leading to impairment of both automatic and voluntary ventilatory control (Howard et al., 2001). SDB includes an assortment of conditions, such as central sleep apnea, obstructive sleep apnea (OSA), and sleep-related hypoventilation or hypoxemic syndromes, occurring in as many as 50–70% of patients with stroke, with OSA being the most common (Deak and Kirsch, 2014). Patients with OSA have an increased risk of stroke, and patients with OSA after stroke have a higher mortality and greater disability (Gibson, 2004). SDB improves in the weeks to months following stroke, but remains highly prevalent (Harbison et al., 2002). Bassetti et al. (2006) prospectively studied 152 patients with acute ischemic stroke to investigate the risk factors for SDB. They found that SDB is common in elderly male patients with diabetes, nighttime stroke onset, and macroangiopathy as the cause of stroke. SDB was also found to improve after the acute phase and was associated with increased poststroke mortality.

## Disordered breathing

In order to better understand the effect neurologic injury has on patterns of breathing, the normal control of ventilation must be discussed here. However, the neuronal networks and mechanisms responsible for the neurologic control of ventilation have been intensively studied, yet remain incompletely elucidated.

Recently proposed models regarding the generation of automatic breathing revolve around the concept of a central pattern generator, and have been reviewed in depth (Rybak et al., 2007; Smith et al., 2007; Bianchi and Gestreau, 2009; Garcia et al., 2011; Molkov et al., 2013). These neuronal groups, including the ventral respiratory column in the medulla and the pontine respiratory group, are responsible for production and modulation of the respiratory drive, and control of the three phases of the respiratory cycle – inspiration, postinspiration (or early expiration), and late expiration. The ventral respiratory column is composed of compartments arranged in a rostrocaudal fashion: the Bötzinger complex (BötC), the pre-Bötzinger complex (pre-BötC), and the ventral respiratory group (VRG). The BötC primarily contains expiratory neurons, and the pre-BötC plays an important role in inspiratory rhythmicity. The VRG is further divided into the rostral VRG, containing bulbospinal inspiratory neurons, and the caudal VRG, containing bulbospinal expiratory neurons. The pontine respiratory group includes the parabrachial complex and Kölliker fuse nuclei, responsible for the duration of the respiratory cycle by controlling the transition between inspiration and expiration. Additional important structures include the nucleus tractus solitarii, which acts as the primary site for integrating afferent inputs, and the retrotrapezoid nucleus, medullary raphe nucleus, and the arcuate nucleus, which are involved in chemoreception.

Abnormal breathing patterns are commonly encountered in neurologic diseases, including stroke, but may not be of utility in localizing disease processes (North and Jennett, 1974; Bassetti et al., 1997).

Central sleep apnea refers to a group of periodic breathing disorders in which there is the cessation of air flow without respiratory effort (Malhotra and Owens, 2010), including Cheyne–Stokes respiration, a pattern of periodic breathing with phases of hyperpnea alternating regularly with apnea associated with impairment of the bilateral forebrain and diencephalic function (Posner et al., 2007). Central periodic breathing during wakefulness occurs in up to 53% of patients with acute stroke, is related to large acute cerebral hemispheric lesions with mass effect, and is associated with poor outcome independent of stroke severity (Rowat et al., 2006, 2007). Siccoli et al. (2008) found that patients with extensive unilateral hemispheric brain damage were more prone to develop central apneas and central periodic breathing during sleep. The mechanism by which this abnormal breathing pattern occurs in neurologic disorders is not completely understood, but may be related to delays or interruptions of afferent or efferent neural traffic or the central processing of afferent receptor signals, slowed brain blood flow, or altered chemoresponsiveness (Hudgel et al., 1993). Heightened responsiveness to $CO_2$ (referred to as increased controller gain) and loss of the neurologic protective effect normally preventing apnea from occurring after hyperventilation may also

explain the occurrence of this phenomenon after stroke (Cherniack et al., 2005). Nopmaneejumruslers et al. (2005) found that in patients with stroke, Cheyne–Stokes respiration and central sleep apnea are signs of occult cardiac dysfunction.

Central alveolar hypoventilation syndromes occurring due to the loss of automatic control of ventilation have been reported in a variety of neurologic disorders, including multiple sclerosis, brainstem stroke, congenital brainstem malformations, multiple system atrophies, and encephalitides (Muzumdar and Arens, 2008; Brown, 2010). While the eponymous Ondine's curse usually refers to congenital central hypoventilation syndrome, it is also used for cases of acquired central alveolar hypoventilation due to lesions of ventrolateral medullary chemosensory areas, and bilateral damage to the descending pathways that control automatic respiration in the lateral columns of the spinal cord (Posner et al., 2007). It has been reported to occur following a variety of acquired brainstem disorders, including lateral medullary infarction (Schestatsky and Fernandes, 2004; Planjar-Prvan et al., 2010; Mendoza and Latorre, 2013), transient vertebrobasilar ischemia (Kraus et al., 1999), brainstem glioma (Marin-Sanabria et al., 2006), medullary capillary telangiectasia (Kapnadak et al., 2010), and posterior fossa surgery (Faraji Rad et al., 2015).

Central neurogenic hyperventilation is a syndrome first described by Plum and Swanson (1959) which is characterized by regular, rapid breathing which produces ventilation that ranges from three to six times normal, and continues for hours or days at a time. It occurs with pontine dysfunction, and specifically with damage to the parabrachial nucleus (Posner et al., 2007). It is seen in brainstem infarcts, encephalitis, hypoglycemia, anoxia, sepsis, and hepatic coma (Plum and Brown, 1963) and infiltrative tumors that stimulate the pontine respiratory centers and central chemoreceptors (Tarulli et al., 2005).

Apneusis is a respiratory pause at full inspiration, and apneustic breathing refers to an abnormal pattern of breathing in which each cycle of respiration includes a respiratory pause (Posner et al., 2007). It can be experimentally induced in animals by disruption of the pontine respiratory nuclei (Gromysz and Karczewski, 1980; Wang et al., 1993). Although rare in humans, apneusis has been reported to occur in the setting of hypoxic-ischemic brainstem damage, pontomedullary hemorrhage, pontine infarct, pontine tumor, postmeningitis deafness, cervical cordotomy, achondroplasia, and multiple sclerosis (Saito et al., 1999). The serotonin type 1A receptor agonists buspirone and tandospirone have been used to alleviate apneustic breathing following neurosurgery for an astrocytoma in the pons and medulla, brainstem infarction, hypoxic-ischemic brainstem damage, and in multiple sclerosis (Wilken et al., 1997;

Saito et al., 1999; El-Khatib et al., 2003; O'Sullivan et al., 2008).

Ataxic breathing refers to a variety of abnormal breathings with irregular gasping respiration, indicating damage to the pre-BötC, and is seen with bilateral rostral medullary lesions, while more complete bilateral lesions of the ventrolateral medullary reticular formation cause apnea (Posner et al., 2007).

Biot's breathing is a form of ataxic breathing characterized by breathing that is irregular and rapid, with rhythmic pauses and periods alternating between apnea and tachypnea, and is named for Dr. Camille Biot, who described it in 1876 in a patient with tuberculous meningitis (Wijdicks, 2007).

## Seizures

Seizures can occur in up to 3.3% of critically ill patients with nonneurologic primary pathologies, and nonconvulsive seizures may occur in up to 34% of neurocritically ill patients (Mirski and Varelas, 2008). Primary neurologic disorders such as stroke, hemorrhage, central nervous system infections, and brain tumors all have a high associated incidence of seizures. Seizures can lead to respiratory disturbances that can range from mild to fatal. The occurrence of postictal pulmonary edema appears to be a relatively rare occurrence, with just 42 episodes in 27 patients reported between 1908 and 1982 (Darnell and Jay, 1982).

There is usually a rapid and spontaneous resolution of symptoms, requiring only conservative management with supplemental oxygen (Teplinsky and Hall, 1986). And while usually presenting with an uncomplicated course, gross hemoptysis has been reported to occur (Pacht, 1988). Interestingly, a case of NPE was reported to have occurred following electric shock therapy for depression (Buisseret, 1982).

Ictal respiratory changes and respiratory compromise are known to occur following both tonic-clonic convulsions and partial seizures, where tachypnea occurs following generalized tonic-clonic seizures and hypopnea and apnea with desaturation occur with partial seizures, especially with temporal or orbital-frontal origin (Blum, 2009). Ictal hypoxemia may occur as a result of central apneas and hypopneas, as well as mixed or obstructive apneas during seizures (Bateman et al., 2008). Severe and prolonged increases in end-tidal $CO_2$ have been observed to occur with seizures, which may be due to ventilation–perfusion inequality, resulting from pulmonary shunting or transient NPE (Seyal et al., 2010). Seyal et al. (2012) found that postictal generalized EEG suppression is not associated with central apnea, but is related to the severity of seizure-associated pulmonary dysfunction.

Patients with epilepsy have a risk of sudden death, termed sudden unexpected death in epilepsy (SUDEP) (Devinsky, 2011). Studies have found that the incidence of SUDEP ranges from 0.09/1000 patient-years to as high as 9/1000 patient-years in epilepsy surgery candidates (Tomson et al., 2008), potentially causing as many as 15% of all epilepsy-related deaths (Massey et al., 2014). Massey et al. (2014) proposed a mechanism by which SUDEP occurs. They suggested that seizures lead to activation of neurons projecting to the midbrain and medulla, inhibiting neurons of the ascending arousal system, which then affects the respiratory network in the medulla. This would then lead to inhibition of cardiovascular and respiratory neurons while cortical activity is suppressed. Inhibition of the ascending arousal system would then cause postictal unresponsiveness and postictal generalized EEG suppression. Hypercapnia and hypoxia resulting from hypoventilation during the seizure would then lead to asystole and death.

## Neurogenic pulmonary edema

NPE refers to increased pulmonary and alveolar interstitial fluid that rapidly occurs following a central neurologic insult, initially reported early in the 20th century in relation to epilepsy and head injuries sustained in war. While any cerebral insult can lead to NPE, it has been estimated that 71% of cases of NPE occur following cerebral hemorrhage, 2% following seizure, and 1% with trauma. It may occur in 23% of patients with SAH, 20–50% of patients with head injury, and up to one-third of patients with status epilepticus (Baumann et al., 2007). NPE may present in two forms with differential timing. The early form presents most commonly, developing within minutes to hours following the injury, while the delayed form develops 12–24 hours after injury (Colice et al., 1984).

Patients become acutely dyspneic, tachypneic, and hypoxic, produce a pink frothy sputum, and bilateral rales and crackles are heard on auscultation (Davison et al. (2012b); Busl and Bleck, 2015). Chest radiograph (Fig. 3.1) will show diffuse bilateral infiltrates. Davison et al. (2012b) proposed diagnostic criteria for NPE, as outlined in Table 3.1.

NPE likely develops due to rapid sympathetic discharge, specifically a massive increase in $\alpha$-adrenergic discharge (Busl and Bleck, 2015). There is resultant increased pulmonary capillary hydrostatic pressure, increased endothelial permeability, pulmonary microembolization as a result of intravascular thrombosis and platelet aggregation, and lymphatic obstruction (Malik, 1985). This leads to pulmonary vascular congestion with perivascular edema, along with extravasation and intraalveolar accumulation of protein-rich edema fluid and

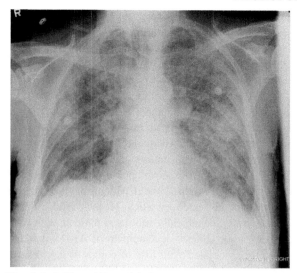

**Fig. 3.1.** Diffuse bilateral infiltrates on X-ray representing pulmonary edema.

*Table 3.1*

**Proposed diagnostic criteria for neurogenic pulmonary edema (Davison et al., 2012b)**

Bilateral infiltrates on imaging
$Pao_2/Fio_2 < 200$
No evidence of left atrial hypertension
Central nervous system injury severe enough to significantly
  increase intracranial pressure
Absence of other common causes of acute respiratory distress
  syndrome

intra-alveolar hemorrhage (Sedý et al., 2008). The medulla and hypothalamus have been implicated as the neuroanatomic locations responsible for the sympathetic nervous system discharge (Malik, 1985). Khademi et al. (2015) found that increased activity of the sympathetic nervous system may also play a role in the development of NPE with cerebral hypoxia in the presence of systemic normoxia. Increased ICP may also play a role in the development of NPE, and Cecchetti et al. (2013) found that in head trauma there is a significant increase in pulmonary permeability when ICP is >15 mmHg, strongly correlated with an increased extravascular lung water index.

Various pharmacologic therapies have been suggested for NPE, including β-blockers to increase lymph flow and reduce pulmonary vascular permeability (Colice et al., 1984), and dobutamine to reduce total peripheral vascular resistance and increase cardiac contractility (Knudsen et al., 1991).

Given that increased sympathetic activity due to excessive α-adrenergic discharge leads to the development of NPE, the use of agents with α-adrenergic blocking activity like chlorpromazine and phentolamine has been recommended for the treatment of NPE (Wohns et al., 1985; Davison et al., 2012a).

## Acute respiratory distress syndrome

The terms ALI and ARDS originally described a continuum of disease with a wide spectrum, characterized by acute-onset nonhydrostatic pulmonary edema, bilateral chest infiltrates on frontal chest radiograph (Fig. 3.2), pulmonary artery wedge pressure <18 mmHg or no clinical evidence of left atrial hypertension, and an abnormal $Pao_2/Fio_2$ ratio (Bernard et al., 1994). While older literature still refers to both ALI and ARDS, this classification has since been supplanted by the Berlin definition, which was shown to have better predictive validity for mortality (ARDS Definition Task Force, 2012). The new definition no longer uses the term ALI, and classifies ARDS as mild, moderate, and severe according to the $Pao_2/Fio_2$ ratio.

ARDS occurs following a variety of neurologic injuries, including brain injury, stroke, and intracranial bleeding. ARDS is reported to occur in 8–31% of patients following isolated TBI (Holland et al., 2003; Rincon et al., 2012), and ARDS following SAH has been reported to occur with an incidence of 18% to as high as 37% (Kahn et al., 2006; Veeravagu et al., 2014). The prevalence of ARDS following acute ischemic stroke increased from 3% in 1994 to 4% in 2008 (Rincon et al., 2014).

The mechanism leading to the development of ARDS in neurologic injury is complex and not completely understood. Theodore and Robin (1976) proposed the "blast theory" of injury for the generation of NPE. An initial massive centrally mediated sympathetic discharge occurs, following which intense vasoconstriction of the

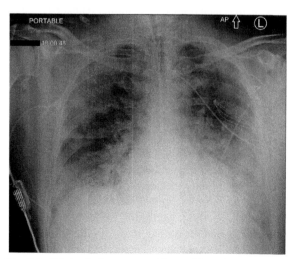

**Fig. 3.2.** Bilateral airspace opacities on X-ray in acute respiratory distress syndrome.

systemic circulation results in fluid shift to the pulmonary circulation. Pulmonary edema then develops due to increased pulmonary vascular pressures and increased volume, resulting in increased hydrostatic pressures, with concurrent alterations in pulmonary capillary permeability.

A systemic inflammatory response is known to occur following head injury, and the associated release of intracranial cytokines has been implicated in the cellular cascade of injury and the pathology of organ dysfunction (Ott et al., 1994). McKeating et al. (1997) found that, following acute brain injury, there is increased intracranial production of cytokines, and particularly IL-6, and Schmidt et al. (2005) found that there is an elevation in cytokines such as TNF, IL-1, and IL-6 which are central mediators of neuroinflammation following head injury. Wu et al. (2006) found that, following experimentally induced intracerebral hemorrhage, there is increased expression of intracellular adhesion molecule-1 (ICAM-1) and tissue factor in both the brain and lung, accompanied by histologic evidence of increased neutrophil infiltration and intra-alveolar structural damage. Kalsotra et al. (2007) found that, following contusion injury to the rat brain, there is a large migration of macrophages and neutrophils in the major airways and alveoli, associated with increased production of leukotriene $B_4$ in the lung.

Given that cytokine-mediated inflammation is known to play an integral role in mediating and perpetuating lung injury, as inflammatory processes contribute to lung dysfunction through injury of epithelial and endothelial cells (Goodman et al., 2003), a "double-hit" model has been proposed to explain the occurrence of extracerebral organ dysfunction following brain injury (Mascia, 2009).

This model proposes that organ dysfunction following TBI occurs in two steps. First, the initial injury leads to the creation of a systemic inflammatory environment. The system is then primed to be further damaged by secondary insults occurring hours and days following the original injury, including infections and mechanical stresses, to which the lungs are particularly susceptible.

Multiple risk factors have been identified for ALI following neurologic injuries. Lou et al. (2013) found that, in patients with isolated severe TBI, increased ICP was associated with an increased risk for developing SIRS and ALI, and that the development of SIRS increased the risk of developing ALI fourfold. Other risk factors independently associated with development of ARDS in severe head injury include the administration of epinephrine and dopamine, as well as a history of drug abuse (Contant et al., 2001). Interestingly, Salim et al. (2008) found that, while the development of ARDS following TBI due to blunt trauma was associated with increased morbidity, and longer ICU and hospital stay when compared to TBI alone, it was not associated with a higher rate of mortality or worse functional capacity at discharge.

Chen et al. (2015) found that administration of TM-1, a thaliporphine derivative, improved ALI and reduced pulmonary edema following TBI. This was theorized to be due in part to the downregulation of the expression of aquaporins, water channel proteins known to be involved in the maintenance of water balance between lung epithelial and microvascular domains.

A prospective multicenter study by Kitamura et al. (2010) found that SIRS developed in 48 of 96 patients following SAH, and that 19 of 26 patients who developed ALI were complicated by SIRS. Hoesch et al. (2012) found that in mechanically ventilated patients with critical neurologic illness, development of ARDS is independently associated with loss of cough or gag reflex, but is not associated with Glasgow Coma Scale (GCS) or the specific etiology of brain injury.

This pulmonary dysfunction may result in further neurologic damage, and it has been found that, when ALI occurs following TBI, it is associated with an increased risk for compromise of brain tissue oxygen tension, independent of concurrent intracerebral and other extracerebral injuries (Oddo et al., 2010).

ARDS is a severe complication following neurologic injury and can play a significant role in patient outcome and survival. Development of ALI following traumatic injury is an independent factor influencing mortality; it is associated with worse neurologic outcomes (Holland et al., 2003; Rincon et al., 2012), and ARDS is common following SAH and is independently associated with worse clinical outcome, although the overall mortality has been decreasing (Kahn et al., 2006; Veeravagu et al., 2014).

While ARDS following acute ischemic stroke is a relatively rare event and associated mortality has decreased over time, ARDS still confers a significantly higher length of stay and risk of death (Rincon et al., 2014). In a study of patients with TBI-induced ARDS, Chen et al. (2016a) found a 40% occurrence of stroke in a 5-year follow-up period and a fourfold increase in the risk of stroke compared to TBI without ARDS, with significantly increased risk of hemorrhagic but not ischemic stroke.

Therapeutic strategies themselves may lead to the development of ARDS. Mascia et al. (2007) found that low $Pao_2/FIo_2$, high tidal volume ventilation, and high respiratory rate are all independent risk factors for ALI in severe brain injury. Given the massive sympathetic activation following brain injury, the use of $\beta$-blockers has been suggested to reduce the associated adverse effects following both SAH and TBI, and while further studies are needed, $\beta$-blockers may also play a role in decreasing lung endothelial damage by reducing pulmonary vascular flow (van der Jagt and Miranda, 2012).

# HOSPITAL COURSE AND MANAGEMENT

The primary goals of management throughout the hospital course for patients who have developed lung dysfunction as a result of a neurologic injury revolve around treating the underlying condition and providing supportive therapy. Mechanical ventilation is often required in the setting of neurologic injury for various indications, including depressed level of consciousness, anticipation of deterioration, brainstem dysfunction, and respiratory dysfunction (Stevens et al., 2008). Given the significant interaction between brain and lung, it is important to consider how both neurologic and pulmonary management affect the disease processes. The complex respiratory mechanics that develop during brain injury must also be taken into account, as brain injury leads to increased flow resistance in the respiratory system, even without respiratory failure, increased respiratory system elastance, and impairment of oxygenation (Koutsoukou et al., 2016). As such, it is important to maintain a coordinated approach to therapy comprised of treatment tailored to the specific ventilatory and fluid requirements of this patient population, in order to both prevent and treat respiratory dysfunction, and improve outcomes. This includes ventilation strategies focused on the prevention of lung collapse and consolidation and maintenance of oxygenation, prevention of pulmonary infection, and therapies to hasten weaning from intensive care requirements (Pelosi et al., 2005).

Management of NPE is primarily focused on treatment of the underlying neurologic insult with the goal of reducing sympathetic discharge that leads to lung injury, and ICP reduction has been shown to improve oxygenation (Davison et al., 2012b), and further therapy consists of supportive treatment of pulmonary edema, volume management, and optimization of oxygenation (Busl and Bleck, 2015).

The Lund concept for the treatment of severe TBI focuses on the regulation of brain volume and perfusion, and includes several methods for lung protection (Koskinen et al., 2014). These include using positive end-expiratory pressure (PEEP) to reduce atelectasis, while avoiding therapies which may potentially worsen pulmonary dysfunction, such as high-dose barbiturates, and restricting use of crystalloids to reduce lung edema.

Most management strategies focus on providing oxygen support to maintain appropriate oxygenation of brain parenchyma (Chang and Nyquist, 2013), but the use of hyperoxia to maintain oxygenation should generally be avoided due to its association with pulmonary injury complications that may impact clinical outcome (Narotam, 2013). Other adjunctive therapies may also lead to deleterious results. The use of hypertonic saline, a common therapy in brain injury, has been shown to increase pulmonary infections in this patient population

(Coritsidis et al., 2015). Fiberoptic bronchoscopy is another important therapy utilized in the care of brain-injured patients, but caution is advised as the procedure may be associated with transient but substantial increases in ICP (Kerwin et al., 2000).

Even mechanical ventilation itself can prove to be injurious, as Quilez et al. (2011) found that in rats it promotes brain activations and leads to an increased occurrence of both systemic and pulmonary inflammation compared to nonventilated controls, and critically ill patients requiring mechanical ventilation and those who survive ARDS show neurologic impairment and cognitive decline (Quílez et al., 2012).

Pelosi et al. (2011) studied 552 neurologic patients (stroke and brain trauma) requiring mechanical ventilation as compared to 4030 patients requiring ventilation for nonneurologic reasons. They found that, while the neurologic patients had fewer complications than their nonneurologic counterparts, they did require mechanical ventilation for longer duration, had higher tracheotomy rates, higher mortality rates, particularly in those with stroke, and the brain trauma patients experienced a higher rate of VAP.

Lung-protective ventilation utilizing low tidal volumes is known to reduce pulmonary complications in ARDS (Neto et al., 2015), and in rats with massive brain damage, low tidal volume ventilation was found to minimize lung morphofunctional changes and inflammation (Krebs et al., 2014).

While PEEP may have varying effects on ICP and cerebral perfusion pressure (CPP) in patients with cerebral injury (Zhang et al., 2011), it can be safely applied along with close monitoring for cerebral and hemodynamic changes (Lou et al., 2012). The application of PEEP in patients with acute stroke is safe as long as mean arterial pressure is maintained in order to maintain CPP (Georgiadis et al., 2001), and a pilot study done by Nemer et al. (2015) found that, in patients with severe TBI and coexisting ARDS, high PEEP successfully improved both brain tissue oxygenation and oxygen saturation without causing increased ICP and decreased CPP.

Lung recruitment techniques are often used in an attempt to improve gas exchange, and while Bein et al. (2002) found that a volume recruitment maneuver led to worsening of cerebral hemodynamics with only minor improvement in oxygenation in patients with brain injury, Nemer et al. (2011) found that the use of a pressure control recruitment maneuver significantly improved oxygenation without affecting ICP and maintained CPP within a safe range in patients who developed ARDS following SAH.

VAP is a serious concern among this patient population. TBI and mechanical ventilation increase the risk of VAP, and as such, it is expected that a reduction in mechanical ventilation will reduce this risk

(Hui et al., 2013). Bilateral dependent consolidation as seen on admission CT is independently associated with the development of VAP following brain injury, and may be helpful in the identification of those patients more likely to experience VAP (Plurad et al., 2013). Jovanovic et al. (2015) found that the development of early VAP following severe brain injury was related to the extent of brain and other organ injury, while late VAP development was related to the extent of brain injury and age; the level of serum procalcitonin has been proposed as a predictive marker for the development of early VAP, and the clinical pulmonary infection score may be helpful in detecting early VAP (Pelosi et al., 2008).

Although chest physiotherapy is commonly employed in the course of therapy following brain injury, compelling evidence is lacking for its utility in preventing or treating VAP, or in reducing the use of mechanical ventilation and ICU stay (Patman et al., 2009; Hellweg, 2012). While further research may yet provide deeper insight into the role of physiotherapy, Olson et al. (2007) did report the case of a patient with a closed head injury and pneumonia, for whom chest physiotherapy provided temporary resolution of high ICP.

Patients with neurologic injury often require prolonged mechanical ventilation and placement of a tracheostomy, the presence of which can reduce peak airway pressures, improve dynamic compliance, and improve PaO2 (Sofi and Wani, 2010). In neurosurgical patients, percutaneous tracheostomy does not lead to significant alterations in ICP, CPP, or GCS (Milanchi et al., 2008), and the timing of the procedure does not appear to have a significant effect on ICP, pneumonia, or mortality (Kocaeli et al., 2008). Decreasing the length of procedure appears to be the most-effective way of avoiding increases in ICP (Kuechler et al., 2015). In patients with brain injury, early placement of tracheostomy has been found to improve mortality (Chintamani et al., 2005), provide better overall clinical outcome (Rizk et al., 2011), shorten length of mechanical ventilation and ICU stay, and decrease antibiotic and sedation needs (Gandía-Martínez et al., 2010; Wang et al., 2012; Alali et al., 2014; Siddiqui et al., 2015).

Other methods of artificial ventilation may be utilized: the use of high-frequency oscillatory ventilation combined with tracheal gas insufflation has been shown to improve gas exchange in ARDS, and can provide another ventilatory strategy in the setting of brain injury (Young and Andrews, 2011; Pelosi and Sutherasan, 2013; Vrettou et al., 2013). In cases of severe lung dysfunction unresponsive to conventional forms of mechanical ventilation following brain injury, extracorporeal membrane oxygenation may be required (Muellenbach et al., 2012). In stroke patients who often develop sleep apnea, noninvasive ventilation is tolerated well and has a low risk of serious complications (Tsivgoulis et al., 2011).

Due to the variety of neurologic insults that lead to the requirement for mechanical ventilation, determining when patients are ready to be liberated from mechanical support can prove to be quite difficult. Numerous factors must thus be taken into account in this decision, including assessment of neurologic status, hemodynamic stability, and respiratory parameters (Lazaridis et al., 2012). Karanjia et al. (2011) found that, in patients with primary brain injury, extubation failure was most often a result of disordered breathing and respiratory distress secondary to altered mental status. A prospective cohort study by Reis et al. (2013) found that, for patients with TBI, failure of extubation was associated with increased hospital stay, requirement for tracheostomy, and pulmonary complications, as well as worse functional outcome and increased hospital mortality.

It may be similarly difficult to ascertain the proper timing of tracheostomy decannulation following TBI. Zanata et al. (2014) proposed a decannulation protocol which takes into account GCS, maintenance of respiration, secretions at the tracheostomy site, as well as evaluations of phonation, swallowing, and coughing.

## CONCLUSIONS

Respiratory failure and the breakdown of normal neuropulmonary interaction are common occurrences in neurocritical illness. Specific disease processes lead to several respiratory dysfunctions but patterns have been recognized and can now be treated.

REFERENCES

Alali AS, Scales DC, Fowler RA et al. (2014). Tracheostomy timing in traumatic brain injury: a propensity-matched cohort study. J Trauma Acute Care Surg 76 (1): 70–76. discussion. 76–78.

ARDS Definition Task Force (2012). Acute respiratory distress syndrome: the Berlin Definition. JAMA 307 (23): 2526–2533.

Bassetti C, Aldrich MS, Quint D (1997). Sleep-disordered breathing in patients with acute supra- and infratentorial strokes. A prospective study of 39 patients. Stroke 28 (9): 1765.

Bassetti CL, Milanova M, Gugger M (2006). Sleep-disordered breathing and acute ischemic stroke: diagnosis, risk factors, treatment, evolution, and long-term clinical outcome. Stroke 37 (4): 967–972.

Bateman LM, Li CS, Seyal M (2008). Ictal hypoxemia in localization-related epilepsy: analysis of incidence, severity and risk factors. Brain 131: 3239–3245.

Baumann A, Audibert G, McDonnell J et al. (2007). Neurogenic pulmonary edema. Acta Anaesthesiol Scand 51 (4): 447–455.

Bein T, Kuhr LP, Bele S et al. (2002). Lung recruitment maneuver in patients with cerebral injury: effects on intracranial pressure and cerebral metabolism. Intensive Care Med 28 (5): 554–558.

Bennett MH, Trytko B, Jonker B (2012). Hyperbaric oxygen therapy for the adjunctive treatment of traumatic brain injury. Cochrane Database Syst Rev 12. CD004609.

Bergren DR, Beckman DL (1975). Pulmonary surface tension and head injury. J Trauma 15 (4): 336–338.

Bernard GR, Artigas A, Brigham KL et al. (1994). The American-European Consensus Conference on ARDS. Definitions, mechanisms, relevant outcomes, and clinical trial coordination. Am J Respir Crit Care Med 149: 818–824.

Bianchi AL, Gestreau C (2009). The brainstem respiratory network: an overview of a half century of research. Respir Physiol Neurobiol 168: 4–12.

Blum AS (2009). Respiratory physiology of seizures. J Clin Neurophysiol 26 (5): 309–315.

Brown LK (2010). Hypoventilation syndromes. Clin Chest Med 31 (2): 249–270.

Brueggemann MW, Loudon RG, McLaurin RL (1976). Pulmonary compliance changes after experimental head injury. J Trauma 16 (1): 16–20.

Buisseret P (1982). Acute pulmonary oedema following grand mal epilepsy and as a complication of electric shock therapy. Br J Dis Chest 76 (2): 194–195.

Busl KM, Bleck TP (2015). Neurogenic Pulmonary Edema. Crit Care Med 43 (8): 1710–1715.

Carrera E, Schmidt JM, Fernandez L et al. (2010). Spontaneous hyperventilation and brain tissue hypoxia in patients with severe brain injury. J Neurol Neurosurg Psychiatry 81 (7): 793–797.

Cecchetti C, Elli M, Stoppa F et al. (2013). Neurogenic pulmonary edema and variations of hemodynamic volumetric parameters in children following head trauma. Minerva Anestesiol 79 (10): 1140–1146.

Chang WT, Nyquist PA (2013). Strategies for the use of mechanical ventilation in the neurologic intensive care unit. Neurosurg Clin N Am 24 (3): 407–416.

Chen S, Li Q, Wu H et al. (2014). The harmful effects of subarachnoid hemorrhage on extracerebral organs. Biomed Res Int 2014: 858496.

Chen GS, Huang KF, Huang CC et al. (2015). Thaliporphine derivative improves acute lung injury after traumatic brain injury. Biomed Res Int 2015: 729831.

Chen GS, Liao KH, Bien MY et al. (2016a). Increased risk of post-trauma stroke following traumatic brain injury-induced acute respiratory distress syndrome. J Neurotrauma 33: 1263–1269.

Chen WL, Huang CH, Chen JH et al. (2016b). Electrocardiographic abnormalities predict neurogenic pulmonary edema in patients with subarachnoid hemorrhage. Am J Emerg Med 34: 79–82.

Cherniack NS, Longobardo G, Evangelista C (2005). Causes of Cheyne–Stokes respiration. Neurocrit Care 3 (3): 271–279.

Chintamani, Khanna J, Singh JP et al. (2005). Early tracheostomy in closed head injuries: experience at a tertiary center in a developing country – a prospective study. BMC Emerg Med 5: 8.

Colice GL, Matthay MA, Bass E et al. (1984). Neurogenic pulmonary edema. Am Rev Respir Dis 130 (5): 941–948.

Contant CF, Valadka AB, Gopinath SP et al. (2001). Adult respiratory distress syndrome: a complication of induced hypertension after severe head injury. J Neurosurg 95 (4): 560–568.

Coritsidis G, Diamond N, Rahman A et al. (2015). Hypertonic saline infusion in traumatic brain injury increases the incidence of pulmonary infection. J Clin Neurosci 22 (8): 1332–1337.

Crittenden DJ, Beckman DL (1982). Traumatic head injury and pulmonary damage. J Trauma 22 (9): 766–769.

Curley G, Kavanagh BP, Laffey JG (2010). Hypocapnia and the injured brain: more harm than benefit. Crit Care Med 38 (5): 1348–1359.

Darnell JC, Jay SJ (1982). Recurrent postictal pulmonary edema: a case report and review of the literature. Epilepsia 23 (1): 71–83.

Davis DP, Meade W, Sise MJ et al. (2009). Both hypoxemia and extreme hyperoxemia may be detrimental in patients with severe traumatic brain injury. J Neurotrauma 26 (12): 2217–2223.

Davison DL, Chawla LS, Selassie L et al. (2012a). Neurogenic pulmonary edema: successful treatment with IV phentolamine. Chest 141 (3): 793–795.

Davison DL, Terek M, Chawla LS (2012b). Neurogenic pulmonary edema. Crit Care 16 (2): 212.

Deak MC, Kirsch DB (2014). Sleep-disordered breathing in neurologic conditions. Clin Chest Med 35 (3): 547–556.

Devinsky O (2011). Sudden, unexpected death in epilepsy. N Engl J Med 365 (19): 1801–1811.

El-Khatib MF, Kiwan RA, Jamaleddine GW (2003). Buspirone treatment for apneustic breathing in brain stem infarct. Respir Care 48 (10): 956–958.

Ezeugwu VE, Olaogun M, Mbada CE et al. (2013). Comparative lung function performance of stroke survivors and age-matched and sex-matched controls. Physiother Res Int 18 (4): 212–219.

Faraji Rad E, Faraji Rad M, Amini S et al. (2015). Sleep apnea syndrome after posterior fossa surgery: a case of acquired Ondine's curse. Iran J Otorhinolaryngol 27 (78): 63–67.

Friedman JA, Pichelmann MA, Piepgras DG et al. (2003). Pulmonary complications of aneurysmal subarachnoid hemorrhage. Neurosurgery 52 (5): 1025–1031.

Fugl-Meyer AR, Linderholm H, Wilson AF (1983). Restrictive ventilatory dysfunction in stroke: its relation to locomotor function. Scand J Rehabil Med Suppl 9: 118–124.

Gandía-Martínez F, Martínez-Gil I, Andaluz-Ojeda D et al. (2010). Analysis of early tracheostomy and its impact on development of pneumonia, use of resources and mortality in neurocritically ill patients. Neurocirugia (Astur) 21 (3): 211–221.

Garcia III AJ, Zanella S, Koch H et al. (2011). (2011). Networks within networks: the neuronal control of breathing. Prog Brain Res 188: 31–50.

Georgiadis D, Schwarz S, Baumgartner RW et al. (2001). Influence of positive end-expiratory pressure on intracranial pressure and cerebral perfusion pressure in patients with acute stroke. Stroke 32 (9): 2088–2092.

Gibson GJ (2004). Sleep disordered breathing and the outcome of stroke. Thorax 59 (5): 361–363.

Goodman RB, Pugin J, Lee JS et al. (2003). Cytokine-mediated inflammation in acute lung injury. Cytokine Growth Factor Rev 14 (6): 523–535.

Gromysz H, Karczewski WA (1980). Generation of respiratory pattern in the rabbit – brainstem transections revisited. Acta Neurobiol Exp (Wars) 40 (6): 985–992.

Gruber A, Reinprecht A, Illievich UM et al. (1999). Extracerebral organ dysfunction and neurologic outcome after aneurysmal subarachnoid hemorrhage. Crit Care Med 27 (3): 505–514.

Haddad SH, Arabi YM (2012). Critical care management of severe traumatic brain injury in adults. Scand J Trauma Resusc Emerg Med 20: 12.

Harbison J, Ford GA, James OF et al. (2002). Sleep-disordered breathing following acute stroke. QJM 95 (11): 741–747.

Hellweg S (2012). Effectiveness of physiotherapy and occupational therapy after traumatic brain injury in the intensive care unit. Crit Care Res Pract 2012: 768456.

Hoesch RE, Lin E, Young M et al. (2012). Acute lung injury in critical neurological illness. Crit Care Med 40 (2): 587–593.

Holland MC, Mackersie RC, Morabito D et al. (2003). The development of acute lung injury is associated with worse neurologic outcome in patients with severe traumatic brain injury. J Trauma 55 (1): 106–111.

Howard RS, Rudd AG, Wolfe CD et al. (2001). Pathophysiological and clinical aspects of breathing after stroke. Postgrad Med J 77 (913): 700–702.

Hudgel DW, Devadatta P, Quadri M et al. (1993). Mechanism of sleep-induced periodic breathing in convalescing stroke patients and healthy elderly subjects. Chest 104 (5): 1503–1510.

Hui X, Haider AH, Hashmi ZG et al. (2013). Increased risk of pneumonia among ventilated patients with traumatic brain injury: every day counts! J Surg Res 184 (1): 438–443.

Jin W, Wang H, Ji Y et al. (2009). Genetic ablation of Nrf2 enhances susceptibility to acute lung injury after traumatic brain injury in mice. Exp Biol Med (Maywood) 234 (2): 181–189.

Jin W, Wu J, Wang H et al. (2011). Erythropoietin administration modulates pulmonary Nrf2 signaling pathway after traumatic brain injury in mice. J Trauma 71 (3): 680–686.

Jovanovic B, Milan Z, Markovic-Denic L et al. (2015). Risk factors for ventilator-associated pneumonia in patients with severe traumatic brain injury in a Serbian trauma centre. Int J Infect Dis 38: 46–51.

Jung KJ, Park JY, Hwang DW et al. (2014). Ultrasonographic diaphragmatic motion analysis and its correlation with pulmonary function in hemiplegic stroke patients. Ann Rehabil Med 38 (1): 29–37.

Kahn JM, Caldwell EC, Deem S et al. (2006). Acute lung injury in patients with subarachnoid hemorrhage: incidence, risk factors, and outcome. Crit Care Med 34 (1): 196–202.

Kalsotra A, Zhao J, Anakk S et al. (2007). Brain trauma leads to enhanced lung inflammation and injury: evidence for role of P4504Fs in resolution. J Cereb Blood Flow Metab 27 (5): 963–974.

Kapnadak SG, Mikolaenko I, Enfield K et al. (2010). Ondine's curse with accompanying trigeminal and glossopharyngeal neuralgia secondary to medullary telangiectasia. Neurocrit Care 12 (3): 395–399.

Karanjia N, Nordquist D, Stevens R et al. (2011). A clinical description of extubation failure in patients with primary brain injury. Neurocrit Care 15 (1): 4–12.

Kerwin AJ, Croce MA, Timmons SD et al. (2000). Effects of fiberoptic bronchoscopy on intracranial pressure in patients with brain injury: a prospective clinical study. J Trauma 48 (5): 878–882. discussion 882–883.

Kesinger MR, Kumar RG, Wagner AK et al. (2015). Hospital-acquired pneumonia is an independent predictor of poor global outcome in severe traumatic brain injury up to 5 years after discharge. J Trauma Acute Care Surg 78 (2): 396–402.

Khademi S, Frye MA, Jeckel KM et al. (2015). Hypoxia mediated pulmonary edema: potential influence of oxidative stress, sympathetic activation and cerebral blood flow. BMC Physiol 15 (1): 4.

Khedr EM, El Shinawy O, Khedr T et al. (2000). Assessment of corticodiaphragmatic pathway and pulmonary function in acute ischemic stroke patients. Eur J Neurol 27 (3): 323–330.

Kitamura Y, Nomura M, Shima H et al. (2010). Acute lung injury associated with systemic inflammatory response syndrome following subarachnoid hemorrhage: a survey by the Shonan Neurosurgical Association. Neurol Med Chir (Tokyo) 50 (6): 456–460.

Knudsen F, Jensen HP, Petersen PL (1991). Neurogenic pulmonary edema: treatment with dobutamine. Neurosurgery 29 (2): 269.

Kocaeli H, Korfali E, Taşkapilioğlu O et al. (2008). Analysis of intracranial pressure changes during early versus late percutaneous tracheostomy in a neuro-intensive care unit. Acta Neurochir (Wien) 150 (12): 1263–1267. discussion 1267.

Koskinen LO, Olivecrona M, Grände PO (2014). Severe traumatic brain injury management and clinical outcome using the Lund concept. Neuroscience 283: 245–255.

Koutsoukou A, Katsiari M, Orfanos SE et al. (2016). Respiratory mechanics in brain injury: a review. World J Crit Care Med 5 (1): 65–73.

Kramer AH, Bleck TP, Dumont AS et al. (2009). Implications of early versus late bilateral pulmonary infiltrates in patients with aneurysmal subarachnoid hemorrhage. Neurocrit Care 10 (1): 20–27.

Kraus J, Heckmann JG, Druschky A et al. (1999). Ondine's curse in association with diabetes insipidus following transient vertebrobasilar ischemia. Clin Neurol Neurosurg 101 (3): 196–198.

Krebs J, Tsagogiorgas C, Pelosi P et al. (2014). Open lung approach with low tidal volume mechanical ventilation attenuates lung injury in rats with massive brain damage. Crit Care 18 (2): R59.

Kuechler JN, Abusamha A, Ziemann S et al. (2015). Impact of percutaneous dilatational tracheostomy in brain injured patients. Clin Neurol Neurosurg 137: 137–141.

Kumar S, Reddy R, Prabhakar S (2009). Contralateral dia-phragmatic palsy in acute stroke: an interesting observa-tion. Indian J Crit Care Med 13: 28–30.

Lazaridis C, DeSantis SM, McLawhorn M et al. (2012). Liberation of neurosurgical patients from mechanical ven-tilation and tracheostomy in neurocritical care. J Crit Care 27 (4): 417.e1–417.e8.

Lim HB, Smith M (2007). Systemic complications after head injury: a clinical review. Anaesthesia 62 (5): 474–482.

Lo BW, Fukuda H, Nishimura Y et al. (2015). Pathophysiologic mechanisms of brain-body associations in ruptured brain aneurysms: a systematic review. Surg Neurol Int 6: 136.

Lopez-Aguilar J, Blanch L (2015). Brain injury requires lung protection. Ann Transl Med 3 (Suppl 1): S5.

López-Aguilar J, Villagrá A, Bernabé F et al. (2005). Massive brain injury enhances lung damage in an isolated lung model of ventilator-induced lung injury. Crit Care Med 33 (5): 1077–1083.

Lou M, Xue F, Chen L et al. (2012). Is high PEEP ventilation strategy safe for acute respiratory distress syndrome after severe traumatic brain injury? Brain Inj 26 (6): 887–890.

Lou M, Chen X, Wang K et al. (2013). Increased intracranial pressure is associated with the development of acute lung injury following severe traumatic brain injury. Clin Neurol Neurosurg 115 (7): 904–908.

Macmillan CS, Grant IS, Andrews PJ (2002). Pulmonary and cardiac sequelae of subarachnoid haemorrhage: time for active management? Intensive Care Med 28 (8): 1012–1023.

Malhotra A, Owens RL (2010). What is central sleep apnea? Respir Care 55 (9): 1168–1178.

Malik AB (1985). Mechanisms of neurogenic pulmonary edema. Circ Res 57 (1): 1–18.

Marin-Sanabria EA, Kobayashi N, Miyake S et al. (2006). Snoring associated with Ondine's curse in a patient with brainstem glioma. J Clin Neurosci 13 (3): 370–373.

Mascia L (2009). Acute lung injury in patients with severe brain injury: a double hit model. Neurocrit Care 11 (3): 417–426.

Mascia L, Zavala E, Bosma K et al. (2007). High tidal volume is associated with the development of acute lung injury after severe brain injury: an international observational study. Crit Care Med 35 (8): 1815–1820.

Massey CA, Sowers LP, Dlouhy BJ et al. (2014). Mechanisms of sudden unexpected death in epilepsy: the pathway to pre-vention. Nat Rev Neurol 10 (5): 271–282.

McHenry MA (2001). Vital capacity following traumatic brain injury. Brain Inj 15 (8): 741–745.

McKeating EG, Andrews PJ, Signorini DF et al. (1997). Transcranial cytokine gradients in patients requiring inten-sive care after acute brain injury. Br J Anaesth 78 (5): 520–523.

Mendoza M, Latorre JG (2013). Pearls and oy-sters: reversible Ondine's curse in a case of lateral medullary infarction. Neurology 80 (2): e13–e16.

Milanchi S, Magner D, Wilson MT et al. (2008). Percutaneous tracheostomy in neurosurgical patients with intracranial pressure monitoring is safe. J Trauma 65 (1): 73–79.

Mirski MA, Varelas PN (2008). Seizures and status epilepticus in the critically ill. Crit Care Clin 24 (1): 115–147.

Molkov YI, Bacak BJ, Dick TE et al. (2013). Control of breath-ing by interacting pontine and pulmonary feedback loops. Front Neural Circuits 7: 16.

Morís G, Arias M, Terrero JM et al. (2012). Ipsilateral revers-ible diaphragmatic paralysis after pons stroke. J Neurol 259 (5): 966–968.

Mrozek S, Constantin JM, Geeraerts T (2015). Brain-lung crosstalk: implications for neurocritical care patients. World J Crit Care Med 4 (3): 163–178.

Muellenbach RM, Kredel M, Kunze E et al. (2012). Prolonged heparin-free extracorporeal membrane oxygenation in multiple injured acute respiratory distress syndrome patients with traumatic brain injury. J Trauma Acute Care Surg 72 (5): 1444–1447.

Muroi C, Keller M, Pangalu A et al. (2008). Neurogenic pul-monary edema in patients with subarachnoid hemorrhage. J Neurosurg Anesthesiol 20 (3): 188–192.

Muzumdar H, Arens R (2008). Central Alveolar Hypoventilation Syndromes. Sleep Med Clin 3 (4): 601–615.

Naidech AM, Bassin SL, Garg RK et al. (2009). Cardiac tro-ponin I and acute lung injury after subarachnoid hemor-rhage. Neurocrit Care 11 (2): 177–182.

Narotam PK (2013). Eubaric hyperoxia: controversies in the management of acute traumatic brain injury. Crit Care 17 (5): 197.

Nemer SN, Caldeira JB, Azeredo LM et al. (2011). Alveolar recruitment maneuver in patients with subarachnoid hem-orrhage and acute respiratory distress syndrome: a compar-ison of 2 approaches. J Crit Care 26 (1): 22–27.

Nemer SN, Caldeira JB, Santos RG et al. (2015). Effects of positive end-expiratory pressure on brain tissue oxygen pressure of severe traumatic brain injury patients with acute respiratory distress syndrome: a pilot study. J Crit Care 30 (6): 1263–1266.

Neto AS, Simonis FD, Barbas CS et al. (2015). Lung-protective ventilation with low tidal volumes and the occur-rence of pulmonary complications in patients without acute respiratory distress syndrome: a systematic review and individual patient data analysis. Crit Care Med 43 (10): 2155–2163.

Nopmaneejumruslers C, Kaneko Y, Hajek V (2005). Cheyne–Stokes respiration in stroke: relationship to hypocapnia and occult cardiac dysfunction. Am J Respir Crit Care Med 171 (9): 1048–1052.

North JB, Jennett S (1974). Abnormal breathing patterns asso-ciated with acute brain damage. Arch Neurol 31 (5): 338.

Ochiai H, Yamakawa Y, Kubota E (2001). Deformation of the ventrolateral medulla oblongata by subarachnoid hemor-rhage from ruptured vertebral artery aneursysms causes neurogenic pulmonary edema. Neurol Med Chir (Tokyo) 41: 529–534.

Oddo M, Nduom E, Frangos S et al. (2010). Acute lung injury is an independent risk factor for brain hypoxia after severe traumatic brain injury. Neurosurgery 67 (2): 338–344.

Olson DM, Thoyre SM, Turner DA et al. (2007). Changes in intracranial pressure associated with chest physiotherapy. Neurocrit Care 6 (2): 100–103.

O'Phelan KH, Merenda A, Denny KG et al. (2015). Therapeutic temperature modulation is associated with pulmonary complications in patients with severe traumatic brain injury. World J Crit Care Med 4 (4): 296–301.

O'Sullivan RJ, Brown IG, Pender MP (2008). Apneusis responding to buspirone in multiple sclerosis. Mult Scler 14 (5): 705–707.

Ott L, McClain CJ, Gillespie M et al. (1994). Cytokines and metabolic dysfunction after severe head injury. J Neurotrauma 11 (5): 447–472.

Pacht ER (1988). Postictal pulmonary edema and hemoptysis. J Natl Med Assoc 80 (3): 337–339. 342.

Patman S, Jenkins S, Stiller K (2009). Physiotherapy does not prevent, or hasten recovery from, ventilator-associated pneumonia in patients with acquired brain injury. Intensive Care Med 35 (2): 258–265.

Pelosi P, Sutherasan Y (2013). High-frequency oscillatory ventilation with tracheal gas insufflation: the rescue strategy for brain-lung interaction. Crit Care 17 (4): R179.

Pelosi P, Severgnini P, Chiaranda M (2005). An integrated approach to prevent and treat respiratory failure in brain-injured patients. Curr Opin Crit Care 11 (1): 37–42.

Pelosi P, Barassi A, Severgnini P et al. (2008). Prognostic role of clinical and laboratory criteria to identify early ventilator-associated pneumonia in brain injury. Chest 134 (1): 101–108.

Pelosi P, Ferguson ND, Frutos-Vivar F et al. (2011). Management and outcome of mechanically ventilated neurologic patients. Crit Care Med 39 (6): 1482–1492.

Planjar-Prvan M, Krmpotić P, Jergović I et al. (2010). Central sleep apnea (Ondine's curse syndrome) in medullary infarction. Acta Med Croatica 64 (4): 29–301.

Plum F, Brown HW (1963). Hypoxic–hypercapnic interaction in subjects with bilateral cerebral dysfunction. J Appl Physiol 18: 1139–1145.

Plum F, Swanson AG (1959). Central neurogenic hyperventilation in man. AMA Arch Neurol Psychiatry 81: 535–549.

Plurad DS, Kim D, Bricker S et al. (2013). Ventilator-associated pneumonia in severe traumatic brain injury: the clinical significance of admission chest computed tomography findings. J Surg Res 183 (1): 371–376.

Posner JB, Saper CB, Schiff ND et al. (2007). Examination of the comatose patient. In: JB Posner, CB Saper, ND Schiff et al. (Eds.), Plum and Posner's Diagnosis of Stupor and Coma, 4th edn. Oxford University Press, New York, pp. 38–87.

Probasco JC, Chang T, Victor D et al. (2014). Isolated pulmonary edema without myocardial stunning in brainstem strokes. J Neurol Transl Neurosci 2 (1): 1040.

Quilez ME, Fuster G, Villar J et al. (2011). Injurious mechanical ventilation affects neuronal activation in ventilated rats. Crit Care 15: R124.

Quílez ME, López-Aguilar J, Blanch L (2012). Organ cross-talk during acute lung injury, acute respiratory distress syndrome, and mechanical ventilation. Curr Opin Crit Care 18 (1): 23–28.

Radolf S, Smoll N, Drenckhahn C et al. (2014). Cerebral lactate correlates with early onset pneumonia after aneurysmal SAH. Transl Stroke Res 5 (2): 278–285.

Reis HF, Almeida ML, Silva MF et al. (2013). Extubation failure influences clinical and functional outcomes in patients with traumatic brain injury. J Bras Pneumol 39 (3): 330–338.

Reis C, Wang Y, Akyol O et al. (2015). What's new in traumatic brain injury: update on tracking, monitoring and treatment. Int J Mol Sci 16 (6): 11903–11965.

Rincon F, Ghosh S, Dey S et al. (2012). Impact of acute lung injury and acute respiratory distress syndrome after traumatic brain injury in the United States. Neurosurgery 71 (4): 795–803.

Rincon F, Maltenfort M, Dey S et al. (2014). The prevalence and impact of mortality of the acute respiratory distress syndrome on admissions of patients with ischemic stroke in the United States. J Intensive Care Med 29 (6): 357–364.

Rizk EB, Patel AS, Stetter CM et al. (2011). Impact of tracheostomy timing on outcome after severe head injury. Neurocrit Care 15 (3): 481–489.

Roffe C, Sills S, Halim M et al. (2003). Unexpected nocturnal hypoxia in patients with acute stroke. Stroke 34 (11): 2641–2645.

Rowat AM, Dennis MS, Wardlaw JM (2006). Central periodic breathing observed on hospital admission is associated with an adverse prognosis in conscious acute stroke patients. Cerebrovasc Dis 21 (5–6): 340–347.

Rowat AM, Wardlaw JM, Dennis MS (2007). Abnormal breathing patterns in stroke: relationship with location of acute stroke lesion and prior cerebrovascular disease. J Neurol Neurosurg Psychiatry 78 (3): 277–279.

Rybak IA, Abdala AP, Markin SN et al. (2007). Spatial organization and state-dependent mechanisms for respiratory rhythm and pattern generation. Prog Brain Res 165: 201–220.

Saito Y, Hashimoto T, Iwata H et al. (1999). Apneustic breathing in children with brainstem damage due to hypoxic-ischemic encephalopathy. Dev Med Child Neurol 41 (8): 560–567.

Salim A, Martin M, Brown C et al. (2008). The presence of the adult respiratory distress syndrome does not worsen mortality or discharge disability in blunt trauma patients with severe traumatic brain injury. Injury 39 (1): 30–35.

Sarrafzadeh A, Schlenk F, Meisel A et al. (2011). Immunodepression after aneurysmal subarachnoid hemorrhage. Stroke 42 (1): 53–58.

Satoh E, Tagami T, Watanabe A et al. (2014). Association between serum lactate levels and early neurogenic pulmonary edema after nontraumatic subarachnoid hemorrhage. J Nippon Med Sch 81 (5): 305–312.

Schestatsky P, Fernandes LN (2004). Acquired Ondine's curse: case report. Arq Neuropsiquiatr 62 (2B): 523–527.

Schmidt OI, Heyde CE, Ertel W et al. (2005). Closed head injury – an inflammatory disease? Brain Res Brain Res Rev 48 (2): 388–399.

Schuiling WJ, Dennesen PJ, Rinkel GJ (2005). Extracerebral organ dysfunction in the acute stage after aneurysmal subarachnoid hemorrhage. Neurocrit Care 3 (1): 1–10.

Sedý J, Zicha J, Kunes J et al. (2008). Mechanisms of neurogenic pulmonary edema development. Physiol Res 57: 499–506.

Sellars C, Bowie L, Bagg J et al. (2007). Risk factors for chest infection in acute stroke: a prospective cohort study. Stroke 38 (8): 2284–2291.

Sexton JD, Beckman DL (1975). Neurogenic influence on pulmonary surface tension and cholesterol in cats. Proc Soc Exp Biol Med 148 (3): 679–681.

Seyal M, Bateman LM, Albertson TE et al. (2010). Respiratory changes with seizures in localization-related epilepsy: analysis of periictal hypercapnia and airflow patterns. Epilepsia 51 (8): 1359–1364.

Seyal M, Hardin KA, Bateman LM (2012). Postictal generalized EEG suppression is linked to seizure-associated respiratory dysfunction but not postictal apnea. Epilepsia 53 (5): 825–831.

Siccoli MM, Valko PO, Hermann DM et al. (2008). Central periodic breathing during sleep in 74 patients with acute ischemic stroke – neurogenic and cardiogenic factors. J Neurol 255 (11): 1687–1692.

Siddiqui UT, Tahir MZ, Shamim MS et al. (2015). Clinical outcome and cost effectiveness of early tracheostomy in isolated severe head injury patients. Surg Neurol Int 6: 65.

Similowski T, Catala M, Rancurel G et al. (1996). Impairment of central motor conduction to the diaphragm in stroke. Am J Respir Crit Care Med 154: 436–441.

Smith JC, Abdala AP, Koizumi H et al. (2007). Spatial and functional architecture of the mammalian brain stem respiratory network: a hierarchy of three oscillatory mechanisms. J Neurophysiol 98 (6): 3370–3387.

Sofi K, Wani T (2010). Effect of tracheostomy on pulmonary mechanics: an observational study. Saudi J Anaesth 4 (1): 2–5.

Solaiman O, Singh JM (2013). Hypocapnia in aneurysmal subarachnoid hemorrhage: incidence and association with poor clinical outcomes. J Neurosurg Anesthesiol 25 (3): 254–261.

Solenski NJ, Haley Jr EC, Kassell NF et al. (1995). Medical complications of aneurysmal subarachnoid hemorrhage: a report of the multicenter, cooperative aneurysm study. Participants of the Multicenter Cooperative Aneurysm Study. Crit Care Med 23 (6): 1007–1017.

Stevens RD, Nyquist PA (2007). The systemic implications of aneurysmal subarachnoid hemorrhage. J Neurol Sci 261 (1–2): 143–156.

Stevens RD, Lazaridis C, Chalela JA (2008). The role of mechanical ventilation in acute brain injury. Neurol Clin 26 (2): 543–563.

Suzuki H, Sozen T, Hasegawa Y et al. (2011). Subarachnoid hemorrhage causes pulmonary endothelial cell apoptosis and neurogenic pulmonary edema in mice. Acta Neurochir Suppl 111: 129–132.

Tarulli AW, Lim C, Bui JD et al. (2005). Central neurogenic hyperventilation: a case report and discussion of pathophysiology. Arch Neurol 62 (10): 1632–1634.

Teplinsky K, Hall J (1986). Postictal pulmonary edema. Report of a case. Arch Intern Med 146 (4): 801–802.

Theodore J, Robin ED (1976). Speculations on neurogenic pulmonary edema (NPE). Am Rev Respir Dis 113 (4): 405–411.

Tomson T, Nashef L, Ryvlin P (2008). Sudden unexpected death in epilepsy: current knowledge and future directions. Lancet Neurol 7 (11): 1021–1031.

Tsivgoulis G, Zhang Y, Alexandrov AW et al. (2011). Safety and tolerability of early noninvasive ventilatory correction using bilevel positive airway pressure in acute ischemic stroke. Stroke 42 (4): 1030–1034.

Ulvi H, Demir R, Aygul R et al. (2013). Effects of ischemic phrenic nerve root ganglion injury on respiratory disturbances in subarachnoid hemorrhage: an experimental study. Arch Med Sci 9 (6): 1125–1131.

van der Jagt M, Miranda DR (2012). Beta-blockers in intensive care medicine: potential benefit in acute brain injury and acute respiratory distress syndrome. Recent Pat Cardiovasc Drug Discov 7 (2): 141–151.

Veeravagu A, Chen YR, Ludwig C et al. (2014). Acute lung injury in patients with subarachnoid hemorrhage: a nationwide inpatient sample study. World Neurosurg 82 (1–2): e235–e241.

Vermaelen J, Greiffenstein P, deBoisblanc BP (2015). Sleep in traumatic brain injury. Crit Care Clin 31 (3): 551–561.

Vermeij JD, Aslami H, Fluiter K et al. (2013). Traumatic brain injury in rats induces lung injury and systemic immune suppression. J Neurotrauma 30 (24): 2073–2079.

Vespa PM, Bleck TP (2004). Neurogenic pulmonary edema and other mechanisms of impaired oxygenation after aneurysmal subarachnoid hemorrhage. Neurocrit Care 1 (2): 157–170.

Vrettou CS, Zakynthinos SG, Malachias S et al. (2013). High-frequency oscillation and tracheal gas insufflation in patients with severe acute respiratory distress syndrome and traumatic brain injury: an interventional physiological study. Crit Care 17 (4): R136.

Wang W, Fung ML, St John WM (1993). Pontile regulation of ventilatory activity in the adult rat. J Appl Physiol (1985) 74 (6): 2801–2811.

Wang HK, Lu K, Liliang PC et al. (2012). The impact of tracheostomy timing in patients with severe head injury: an observational cohort study. Injury 43 (9): 1432–1436.

Wartenberg KE, Mayer SA (2010). Medical complications after subarachnoid hemorrhage. Neurosurg Clin N Am 21 (2): 325–338.

Weber DJ, Gracon AS, Ripsch MS et al. (2014). The HMGB1-RAGE axis mediates traumatic brain injury-induced pulmonary dysfunction in lung transplantation. Sci Transl Med 6 (252): 252ra124.

Wijdicks EF (2007). Biot's breathing. J Neurol Neurosurg Psychiatry 78 (5): 512–513.

Wilken B, Lalley P, Bischoff AM et al. (1997). Treatment of apneustic respiratory disturbance with a serotonin-receptor agonist. J Pediatr 130 (1): 89–94.

Williamson CA, Sheehan KM, Tipirneni R et al. (2015). The association between spontaneous hyperventilation, delayed cerebral ischemia, and poor neurological outcome in patients with subarachnoid hemorrhage. Neurocrit Care 23 (3): 330–338.

Winklewski PJ, Radkowski M, Demkow U (2014). Cross-talk between the inflammatory response, sympathetic activation and pulmonary infection in the ischemic stroke. J Neuroinflammation 11: 213.

Wohns RN, Tamas L, Pierce KR et al. (1985). Chlorpromazine treatment for neurogenic pulmonary edema. Crit Care Med 13 (3): 210–211.

Wu S, Fang CX, Kim J et al. (2006). Enhanced pulmonary inflammation following experimental intracerebral hemorrhage. Exp Neurol 200 (1): 245–249.

Wu MN, Chen PN, Lai CL et al. (2011). Contralateral diaphragmatic palsy after subcortical middle cerebral artery infarction without capsular involvement. Neurol Sci 32: 487–490.

Yildirim E, Kaptanoglu E, Ozisik K et al. (2004a). Ultrastructural changes in pneumocyte type II cells following traumatic brain injury in rats. Eur J Cardiothorac Surg 25 (4): 523–529.

Yildirim E, Solaroglu I, Okutan O et al. (2004b). Ultrastructural changes in tracheobronchial epithelia following experimental traumatic brain injury in rats: protective effect of erythropoietin. J Heart Lung Transplant 23 (12): 1423–1429.

Yildirim E, Ozisik K, Solaroglu I et al. (2005). Protective effect of erythropoietin on type II pneumocyte cells after traumatic brain injury in rats. J Trauma 58 (6): 1252–1258.

Young NH, Andrews PJ (2011). High-frequency oscillation as a rescue strategy for brain-injured adult patients with acute lung injury and acute respiratory distress syndrome. Neurocrit Care 15 (3): 623–633.

Zanata Ide L, Santos RS, Hirata GC (2014). Tracheal decannulation protocol in patients affected by traumatic brain injury. Int Arch Otorhinolaryngol 18 (2): 108–114.

Zhang XY, Yang ZJ, Wang QX et al. (2011). Impact of positive end-expiratory pressure on cerebral injury patients with hypoxemia. Am J Emerg Med 29 (7): 699–703.

Zhu L, Yan W, Qi M et al. (2007). Alterations of pulmonary zinc homeostasis and cytokine production following traumatic brain injury in rats. Ann Clin Lab Sci 37 (4): 356–361.

Zygun DA, Kortbeek JB, Fick GH et al. (2005). Non-neurologic organ dysfunction in severe traumatic brain injury. Crit Care Med 33 (3): 654–660.

Zygun DA, Zuege DJ, Boiteau PJ et al. (2006). Ventilator-associated pneumonia in severe traumatic brain injury. Neurocrit Care 5 (2): 108–114.

*Handbook of Clinical Neurology*, Vol. 140 (3rd series)
*Critical Care Neurology, Part I*
E.F.M. Wijdicks and A.H. Kramer, Editors
http://dx.doi.org/10.1016/B978-0-444-63600-3.00004-0

Chapter 4

# Neurocardiology

N.D. OSTERAAS AND V.H. LEE*

*Section of Cerebrovascular Diseases, Department of Neurological Sciences, Rush University Medical Center, Chicago, IL, USA*

## Abstract

Neurocardiology refers to the interplay between the nervous system and the cardiovascular system. Stress-related cardiomyopathy exemplifies the brain–heart connection and occurs in several conditions with acute brain injury that share oversympathetic activation. The brain's influences on the heart can include elevated cardiac markers, arrhythmias, repolarization abnormalities on electrocardiogram, myocardial necrosis, and autonomic dysfunction. The neurogenic stunned myocardium in aneurysmal subarachnoid hemorrhage represents one end of the spectrum, and is associated with an explosive rise in intracranial pressure that results in excess catecholamine state and possibly CBN. A brain–heart link is more known to cardiologists than neurologists. This chapter provides some insight into the pathophysiology of these pathologic neurocardiac states and their most appropriate management relevant to neurologists.

## INTRODUCTION

The capacity for the brain to injure the heart has been well recognized throughout history, but has only recently gained attention in the field of neurocardiology (van der Wal and Gilst, 2013). The central nervous system (CNS) has an extensive physiologic influence on the cardiovascular system, and the cardiovascular system in turn has both physiologic and, all too frequently, pathologic influences on the CNS (such as cardioembolic stroke and cerebral hypoperfusion). Samuels brought attention to a 1942 article by Cannon on "voodoo death," which studied death from fright, felt to be caused by the sympathetic system (Cannon, 1942; Samuels, 2007a). The emphasis of this chapter will be on the pathologic CNS influences on the cardiovascular system, focusing on the most common vascular pathologies seen in the intensive care setting, specifically, aneurysmal subarachnoid hemorrhage (SAH), ischemic stroke (IS), and intracerebral hemorrhage (ICH), along with a discussion of epilepsy in relationship to sudden unexplained death in epilepsy (SUDEP). Commonly encountered pathologic neurocardiac manifestations in this setting are subendocardial ischemia, repolarization abnormalities, arrhythmias,

autonomic dysfunction, and sudden cardiac death (SCD). In this chapter there is a particular focus on stress-related cardiomyopathy (CMO) syndromes, which include "neurogenic stunned myocardium" and takotsubo CMO.

## BASIC ANATOMY AND PHYSIOLOGY OF NEUROCARDIOLOGY

Although a complete understanding of the anatomy and pathology involved in neurocardiac dysregulation has not yet been achieved, much is known. A brief review of the pertinent anatomy and physiology of the CNS, autonomic nervous system (ANS), and the cardiovascular system is needed prior to a discussion of pathologic processes. Emphasis is placed on the clinically relevant ascending and descending structures in the CNS, peripheral nervous system (PNS), and connections to the cardiovascular system. The ANS has significant influence on the cardiovascular system due to its ability to modulate heart rate and conduction velocity, as well as cardiac contractility. These effects are mediated primarily via parasympathetic and sympathetic nervous system innervation of the sinoatrial (SA) and atrioventricular (AV)

*Correspondence to: Vivien H. Lee, MD, Section of Cerebrovascular Diseases, Department of Neurological Sciences, Rush University Medical Center, 1725 W Harrison St #1121, Chicago IL 60612, USA. Tel: +1-312-942-4500, E-mail: Vivien_lee@rush.edu nodes, and these systems are subject to supratentorial influence as well (Mitchell, 1952). Pathologic disruption at various points in this axis has a variety of clinical manifestations; the general categories are subendocardial ischemia, repolarization abnormalities, arrhythmias, SCD, and cardiovascular autonomic dysfunction; takotsubo CMO and neurogenic stunned myocardium are most commonly described in patients with aneurysmal SAH, but can also occur in patients diagnosed with ICH and IS (Wang et al., 1997; Amaral, 2012).

The cardiovascular system has afferent connections with the CNS which are critical in providing regulatory feedback on cardiac rate and contractility. The afferent system begins with chemoreceptors and baroreceptors (Pereira et al., 2013), with the ascending afferent information transmitted primarily by cranial nerves IX and X. These travel caudally to the nucleus of the solitary tract and dorsal vagal nucleus, and onwards to the parabrachial nucleus. From this nucleus, afferent pathways continue to the central nucleus of the amygdala, hypothalamus, infralimbic cortex (located in the ventromedial prefrontal cortex), as well as ventral basal thalamus. The infralimbic cortex and basal thalamus (specifically, the paraventricular nucleus) have ipsilateral and contralateral afferent connections to the insular cortex. Communication throughout the ascending pathways is mediated by the neurotransmitter $N$-methyl-D-aspartate, along with contributions from alpha-adrenergic and gamma-aminobutyric acid receptors and modulation by multiple peptides (Davis and Natelson, 1993).

In addition to being a prominent endpoint of the ascending afferent system, the insula has significant efferent projections involved in descending autonomic cardiovascular modulation. Efferent pathways from the insula project to the infralimbic cortex, medial dorsal nucleus of the thalamus, nucleus tractus solitarius, and central nucleus of the amygdala, all of which ultimately project to the sympathetic preganglionic neurons in the intermediolateral column of the spinal cord via the ventral lateral medulla (Davis and Natelson, 1993). Efferent projections also exist between the insula and lateral hypothalamus, which descend to synapse in the ventral lateral medulla (Chechetto, 2004).

The descending pathway continues with parasympathetic ganglia and sympathetic pathway afferent signaling through the intermediolateral column of the spinal cord to the cardiac plexus. Cardiac sympathetic innervation consists of superior, middle, and inferior cervical sympathetic cardiac nerves along with innervation from the thoracic sympathetic ganglia. The cardiac plexus, along with the SA node and AV node, are the final targets of the descending autonomic system (Mitchell, 1952). Seven distinct cardiac subplexi have been described which penetrate into the epicardium as well as the myocardium (Pauza et al., 2000).

The parasympathetic branch of the ANS is responsible for slowing heart rate and antagonizing sympathetic input. The sympathetic branch is primarily responsible for the opposite effect, i.e., increasing heart rate and contractility. The actions of the parasympathetic system are mediated via the vagus nerve predominantly using acetylcholine to bind to muscarinic receptors. The sympathetic nervous system, in general, uses norepinephrine as the primary neurotransmitter (Hall, 1990).

The SA and AV nodes, along with the myocardium of the atria, receive extensive innervation from the parasympathetic system; innervation of the ventricular system is much less rich (Kent et al., 1974). The SA node is preferentially innervated by the right vagus nerve, while the AV node receives more of its parasympathetic innervation from the left vagus (Martin, 1977; Yoon et al., 1997). This anatomic asymmetry is an important component in the differing pathophysiologic neurocardiac manifestations of CNS process, and many observational series in humans and animal experiments have frequently demonstrated a component of laterality involved in arrhythmias and repolarization abnormalities as well as with troponin elevations. As examples of lesions having differing effects based on laterality, in the PNS, stellate (sympathetic) blockades on the right in humans have resulted in decreased resting heart rate. This change does not occur when the procedure is performed on the left (Rogers et al., 1978). In the CNS, right insular stimulation in humans has been associated with tachycardia and relative hypotension, while the opposite has been associated with stimulation of the left insula (Oppenheimer et al., 1992) (Fig. 4.1).

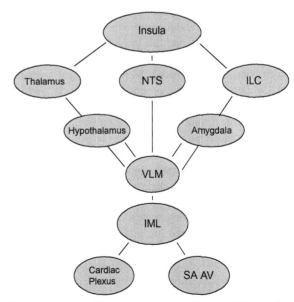

**Fig. 4.1.** Descending sympathetic pathway. NTS, nucleus tractus solitarius; ILC, infralimbic cortex; VLM, ventral lateral medulla; IML, intermediolateral column; SA AV, sinoatrial atrioventricular.

There are proposed mechanisms by which ICH and IS may cause various pathologic neurocardiac findings. It has been hypothesized that damage to the CNS leads to neurocardiac pathology via impairment of regulatory centers of the autonomic nuclei (Barron et al., 1994; Pereira et al., 2013). The insula is a key cortical site of this supratentorial influence (Chechetto, 2004; Christensen et al., 2005; Ay et al., 2006; Oppenheimer, 2006; Nagi et al., 2010). Potential mediating mechanisms include an imbalance between sympathetic and parasympathetic tone as a result of CNS damage to supratentorial modulatory centers, as well as increased production of catecholamines (Lavy et al., 1974, Myers et al., 1981; Lane et al., 1992; Kocan, 1998; Oppenheimer, 2006). It has also been posited that hypoxia associated with neurogenic pulmonary edema, which is common to many acute neurologic pathologies, may contribute to the generation of fatal arrhythmias, although this theory would not account for cases of cerebral arrhythmogenic death without pulmonary involvement (Terrence et al., 1980).

In addition to the associations between neurovascular disease and pathologic dysregulation of the neurocardiac axis, a concurrent catecholamine surge frequently occurs with the neurologic insult and may predispose patients in this population to repolarization abnormalities, as well as premature ventricular beats and other arrhythmias (Myers et al., 1981). These, in turn, could potentially lead to malignant arrhythmias, with SCD as a potential outcome (Myers et al., 1981; Davis and Natelson, 1993; Sörös and Hachinski, 2012).

There is a wealth of support for this hypothesis in the form of animal lesion and cerebral stimulation studies, along with observational studies involving human patients with a variety of neurovascular insults (Oppenheimer et al., 1992). The history of animal experimentation is extensive and cannot be covered in entirety here; it is well summarized by Hoff et al. (1963) with pertinent contemporary research covered extensively by Oppenheimer et al. (1990). Of note, Melville et al. (1969) described a variety of arrhythmias resulting from stimulation of the hypothalamus in monkeys; ectopic beats, heart block, ventricular tachycardia (VT), and unspecified T-wave morphology alterations among others. However, these changes were noted to be similar to those produced by infusion of exogenous catecholamines, making it difficult to attribute the cardiac manifestations solely to a dysregulated neurocardiac axis.

Amygdalar stimulation in animal studies has resulted in heart block and sinus arrhythmia (Reis and Oliphant, 1964). Electric stimulation of the subiculum, cingulate gyrus, and temporal pole in the cortex of cats has resulted in ectopic beats; however, concurrent alterations in blood pressure (out of proportion to the noted increase in heart rate) along with an increase in respiratory rate were also noted. Similar to the hypothalamic stimulation series in monkeys, these alterations in noncardiac parameters raised the possibility that a general sympathetic response may be partially responsible for these autonomic alterations (Oppenheimer et al., 1990).

In order to differentiate between the possibility of insular lesions resulting in a generalized sympathetic response and the possibility of the lesions triggering specific cardiac responses from cortical centers responsible for cardiovascular regulation, Oppenheimer and Cechetto (1990) used a microsimulation technique in a rat model and demonstrated that stimulation of the posterior insula resulted in variation of heart rate without variation in any other measurements, eloquently confirming cortical cardiac chronotropic sites. Subsequent lesion studies by Zhang et al. (1998) located neurons responsible for autonomic baroreceptor reactivity in the right insula of monkeys. In humans, the most dramatic evidence of active, pathologic neurocardiac processes comes from observational studies documenting improvement or even resolution of cardiac abnormalities when the CNS is disconnected from the cardiovascular system, such as in brain death (Dujardin et al., 2001).

Patients with new-onset IS, SAH, and ICH often have elevated systemic levels of epinephrine and norepinephrine independent of any increase in intracranial pressure (ICP) (Myers et al., 1981); this is possibly more often the case when the right insula is involved (Oppenheimer et al., 1992). Strittmatter et al. (2003) demonstrated in a series of 39 patients that patients with right-hemisphere IS have higher levels of norepinephrine and resting heart rate than left-hemisphere infarcts. This may partially account for the high incidence of cardiac arrhythmias and electrocardiogram (ECG) changes seen in these patients (Samuels, 2007b).

Several researchers have demonstrated laterality in many of the neurocardiac sequelae of insular pathology in addition to catecholamine levels. New arrhythmias, presence of elevated cardiac markers in the serum, as well as autonomic dysfunction all have associated research supporting the fact that pathology on one side may be more problematic. One study reviewed cardiac monitor recordings from patients who had been admitted to an inpatient unit and found that, in those patients with tachyarrhythmias, all patients had suffered from IS in the right hemisphere (Lane et al., 1992). In a similar vein, voxel-based analysis of diffusion-weighted magnetic resonance imaging (MRI) images of patients with IS demonstrated that restricted diffusion in the right insula and right inferior parietal lobe have strong correlations with elevations in troponin as well as with significant arrhythmias (Ay et al., 2006; Seifert et al., 2015).

However this laterality has not been consistently replicated in all research (Abdi et al., 2014).

Measurable cardiovascular autonomic dysfunction is a common consequence of IS, and many patients post-IS will demonstrate a decrease in baroreceptor reactivity and alteration in sympathetic tone on formal testing; this autonomic instability may play a pathophysiologic role in clinically significant arrhythmias (Hilz et al., 2011). There is some discrepancy between researchers regarding the culpability of left- versus right-sided insular lesions in cardiovascular dysautonomia, with studies offering conflicting findings. Barron et al. (1994) demonstrated a reduction in beat-to-beat heart rate variability (HRV), a measure of cardiovascular autonomic dysfunction, in patients with both left- and right-sided insular infarcts, but with a greater reduction in HRV associated with infarcts on the right. Tokgözoglu et al. (1999) measured HRV in 62 patients, and demonstrated that rates of autonomic dysfunction were greater in patients with right insular lesions, similar to the findings of Colivicchi et al. (2004) and Meyer et al. (2003). Of the 7 patients who experienced SCD during the study, 5 had right insular lesions. Yoon et al. (1997) measured HRV in patients undergoing sodium amytal injection for preoperative evaluation and noted that sympathovagal balance was significantly altered with left carotid injection, while one research group documented no significant dysautonomia on either side during the same procedure (Reuter et al., 1993).

There is evidence that at least partial recovery of autonomic regulation does take place. One prospective study demonstrated that in patients post IS who initially had impaired cardiac response to three common measures of autonomic regulation (HRV during deep breathing, the Valsalva maneuver. and tilt table testing), these same patients differed from the control group solely on tilt table testing when assessed 6 months later (Korpelainen et al., 1994).

Much of the discussion up to this point has focused on the pathologic action of the sympathetic nervous system in the setting of neurovascular insults and dysautonomic imbalance between the parasympathetic and sympathetic nervous systems and modulated primarily by the right insula. The parasympathetic system is thought to be in general antiarrhythmogenic, although increased activity of the parasympathetic nervous system may result in bradycardia, and, if especially severe, asystole (Bashour et al., 1988). Increased parasympathetic tone may be partially responsible for neurocardiac sequelae that have been described in association with IS in the left insula (Oppenheimer, 2006).

As a critical anatomic structure in the pathophysiology of neurocardiology, the insula is unfortunately a frequent location of pathologic process affecting the CNS. The insula is involved in approximately half of nonlacunar stroke syndromes involving the middle cerebral artery (MCA) territory (Fink et al., 2005). Thus, the insula is a common location for infarction to occur, with the vascular supply predominantly from the "M2" branches of the MCA (Türe et al., 2000). Additionally, mesial temporal-lobe epilepsy is the most common form of epilepsy in adults (Engel, 2001). This close anatomic relationship to the insula may in part explain why some investigators (Oppenheimer et al., 1990) have posited that some cases of sudden death in patients with epilepsy have a cerebroarrhythmogenic origin (Fig. 4.2).

A brief review of cardiac histopathology is in order here. In distinction to infarction-related coagulation necrosis, the classic pathologic myocardial changes in neurogenic stunned myocardium are contraction band

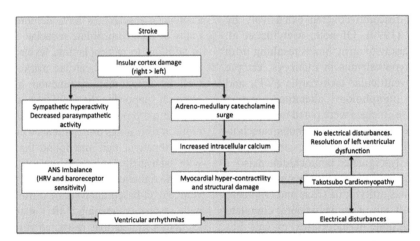

**Fig. 4.2.** Pathophysiology of ventricular arrhythmias after stroke due to autonomic imbalance. ANS, autonomic nervous system; HRV, heart rate variability. (Reproduced from Koppikar et al. (2013) with permission from the publisher. Copyright © 2013 Elsevier.)

necrosis (CBN) changes which have been reproduced in experimental SAH animal models (Sugiura et al., 1985; Elrifai et al., 1996; Parekh et al., 2000; Zaroff et al., 2000b). Myocardial CBN, also known as myocytolysis or myofibrillary degeneration, represents a particular form of myocyte injury characterized by hypercontracted sarcomeres, dense eosinophilic transverse bands, and an interstitial mononuclear inflammatory response (Karch and Billingham, 1986; Elrifai et al., 1996). CBN is most associated with SAH, but the histopathologic changes of CBN occur in an array of conditions, including head trauma, tako-tsubo CMO, pheochromocytoma, near drowning, fatal status asthmaticus, fatal status epilepticus, and violent assault victims in the absence of fatal internal injuries that would explain their death (Doshi and Neil-Dwyer, 1969; Cebelin and Hirsch, 1980; Cruickshank et al., 1987; Drislane et al., 1987; Takeno et al., 2004; Manno et al., 2005; Wittstein et al., 2005). Although these conditions are seemingly unrelated, a pathophysiologic mechanism shared by these conditions is a state of excess sympathetic discharge (Karch and Billingham, 1986).

In addition to associations with SAH, there are associations between CBN and ICH and IS (Kolin and Norris, 1984; Samuels, 2007b). A key differentiating feature between patients with a traditional, purely cardiac etiology and patients who have a neurocardiac etiology responsible for the cardiac injury is that the myofibrillar degeneration occurs specifically in areas of close proximity of the cardiac plexus and nerves (as opposed to the vascular distribution seen in patients with coronary artery disease (CAD)), and CBN is visible on light microscopy (Reichenbach and Benditt, 1970; Samuels, 2007b). As the myofibrillar injury is predominantly subendocardial, it may involve the cardiac conducting system, which in turn could lead to a greater likelihood of cardiac arrhythmias. These lesions are also likely to occur in a background of increased catecholamine release associated with neurovascular diagnosis, which is itself arrhythmogenic, even independent of other structural or cardiac conducting system pathology (Janse et al., 1986).

There are associations between the size of the cerebral lesion and the presence of CBN in both IS and ICH (Kolin and Norris, 1984), with the exception of patients who expired relatively rapidly after the ictus (they did not have detectable CBN). Although the number of cases in this series was low, the pathology was frequently identified. CBN was present in almost 90% of those with SAH, nearly three-quarters of patients with ICH, and approximately half of those with IS.

Animal models that study the effects of elevated ICP on the heart suggest that explosive risk in ICP is likely a mediator of cardiac dysfunction in certain neurologic conditions, most notably aneurysmal SAH (Shivalkar et al., 1993). Brain death is induced in dogs by inflating the same volume of saline into epidural Foley catheters at different rates that cause either an explosive rise in ICP or a gradual rise in ICP (Shivalkar et al., 1993). A sudden rise in ICP yielded a 1000-fold increase in level of epinephrine, whereas a gradual rise in ICP yielded only a 200-fold increase (Shivalkar et al., 1993). Explosive ICP was associated with more area of myocytolysis and necrosis histologically as well, suggesting that an explosive increase in ICP is key to myocardial damage (Shivalkar et al., 1993). Pathology studies in SAH demonstrating hypothalamic lesions, including perivascular hemorrhages, edema, or infarct, suggest a hypothalamic connection to sympathetic activation (Neil-Dwyer et al., 1978).

The baboon animal model of CBN involves inflating an intracranial Foley catheter balloon to produce an increase in ICP, which is associated with clinical signs of brain death and histologic myocardial damage, as well as an immediately high, but transient rise in the levels of circulating catecholamines (Novitzky et al., 1986). Hemodynamic response and CBN pathology were then measured in three groups: group A (control), group B (total denervation of the heart), and group C (incomplete denervation of the heart). The results were similar in the control and incomplete heart denervation group, but the complete heart denervation group showed a modified hemodynamic response and normal myocytes (Novitzky et al., 1986). An intact vagal supply to the heart did not appear to have a role, since CBN still occurs following vagotomy, but can be completely blocked by cardiac sympathectomy or denervation (Novitzky et al., 1986). Since CBN still occurred following bilateral adrenalectomy, circulating catecholamines do not appear to be the crucial mediator of neurogenic cardiac injury, but rather suggest that local release of norepinephrine from myocardial sympathetic nerve terminals is key in the pathogenesis of CBN (Novitzky et al., 1986).

## SPECIFIC CARDIAC DISEASES IN NEUROCRITICALLY ILL PATIENTS

Patients with new neurovascular diagnosis can have concurrent CAD and possibly acute coronary syndrome (ACS) in addition to neurocardiac dysregulation. Compared to patients with SAH, patients who have suffered from IS and ICH are more likely to have comorbid CAD, which can make differentiating between a primarily cardiac versus neurocardiac etiology potentially more of a diagnostic dilemma (Oppenheimer, 2006; Bybee and Prasad, 2008; Koppikar et al., 2013). According to one series, cardiac ischemia in patients with IS of purely cardiac etiology is involved in approximately 3–6% (Jensen et al., 2007; Prosser et al., 2007). Incidence rates are difficult to determine given that many patients with neurovascular pathology will have cardiac enzyme elevations and confirmatory cardiac catheterization is not performed on all patients (Jensen et al., 2007). Myocardial infarction can predate IS; however, meta-analysis by Witt et al. (2006) indicates that for every thousand myocardial infarctions, there are only approximately 14 subsequent incidences of IS.

Many factors further complicate the issue of CAD in this population. Cardiac enzymes are frequently elevated in patients with acute neurovascular illness (Chalela et al., 2004; Ay et al., 2006; Jensen et al., 2007; Abdi et al., 2014; Miller et al., 2015). Echocardiogram findings on occasion demonstrate similar findings to those that occur in ACS in the case of ICH and traumatic brain injury (Dujardin et al., 2001; Chandra et al., 2010). New ST- and T-wave abnormalities have been frequently detected in patients with IS, including those without a cardiac history, ranging from 1 in 10 patients to 1 in 4, depending on the study (Lavy et al., 1974). This can lead to a diagnostic dilemma, as clinical cardiac symptoms in patients with ICH, SAH, and IS may not always be elicited, and changes such as these have a real possibility of indicating myocardial ischemia (Jensen et al., 2009).

Extreme elevation in troponin levels would seem to suggest a cardiac as opposed to neurocardiac etiology; however, there are currently no data to support a cutoff threshold of troponin elevation that is predictive of primarily cardiac etiology (Ay et al., 2006). There are clear differences between CAD and neurocardiac sequelae on histopathology in most cases (Reichenbach and Benditt, 1970; Kolin and Norris, 1984; Samuels, 2007b). However, this information is generally only obtained at autopsy; and in cases of diagnostic uncertainty a cardiac catheterization may be required.

Prognostically, a meta-analysis by Touze et al. (2005) followed nearly 66 000 patients among 39 studies, including patients with diagnosis of transient ischemic attack or IS for a mean period of 3.5 years after discharge, and determined the annual risks at 2.2% for cardiac etiology of adverse outcome, with approximately half of these being fatal. That the deaths occurred months or even years after the acute CNS insult suggests a primarily pure cardiac etiology. However, there is evidence that some autonomic dysfunction and changes on ECG can be persistent (Janse et al., 1986; Korpelainen et al., 1994), theoretically contributing to cardiac death.

Despite the lack of a solid evidence base, basic guidelines do exist. Cardiac enzyme tests, a 12-lead ECG, cardiac monitoring (via telemetry and/or Holter monitoring), in addition to cardiovascular exam by a physician, should be performed in all patients with isolated systolic hypertension, SAH, and ICH (Adams et al., 2007). Supportive

care for patients with myocardial injury following stroke should include beta-blockers, since these agents may reduce sympathetic tone and may prevent further arrhythmias and cardiac damage (although there is currently no evidence that empiric beta blockade alters clinical outcomes (Nagi et al., 2010) and no evidence that empiric magnesium infusions does so either (Koppikar et al., 2013)). A large, blinded, placebo-controlled study using prolonged cardiac monitoring with cardioprotective medications should be conducted in order to establish an evidence base to guide practice (Mikolich et al., 1981; Adams et al., 2007).

Common neurocardiac sequelae of IS, SAH, and ICH include arrhythmias and repolarization abnormalities. Lavy et al. (1974) prospectively followed patients admitted with a new diagnosis of IS and ICH with and without comorbid cardiac disease, and described new-onset sinus bradycardia, nodal bradycardia, supraventricular extrasystolic beats and tachycardia, atrial fibrillation (AF), atrial flutter, and complete AV block. In patients without known cardiac disease, 67% demonstrated changes on ECG or arrhythmias captured on telemetry, while 84% of patients with pre-existing cardiac disease had such findings. Compared to a control population of hospitalized patients, one study demonstrated that patients with a neurovascular diagnosis had an incidence of ST-segment depression and prolonged QTc that occurred at a frequency of 7 and 10 times more often than control patients respectively, with an incidence of T-wave inversion, premature ventricular beats, and conduction abnormalities that was two to four times the rate of control patients (Dimant and Grob, 1977).

Goldstein (1979) reported rates of ECG abnormalities and arrhythmias in stroke patients (IS, ICH, and SAH). ECG abnormalities were detected in approximately three-quarters of the patients; most commonly captured were prolonged QTc, tachycardia, and other arrhythmias, of which AF was the most common among those diagnosed with IS. In patient populations involving multiple CNS pathologies, QTc prolongation is often significant (Perron and Brady, 2000). While not an arrhythmia of itself, QTc prolongation is a significant risk factor for arrhythmia development (Cubeddu, 2003).

Kallmünzer et al. (2012) reported that approximately 25% of patients admitted with diagnosis of acute IS or ICH had an arrhythmia captured on telemetry, most commonly within the first 24 hours of admission. AF was the most prevalent arrhythmia detected in 11% of patients, focal atrial tachycardia in 3%, undetermined supraventricular tachycardia in 2%, type II AV block in 2%, SA block in 2 patients, ventricular ectopy in 1%, nonsustained VT in 1%, atrial flutter in under 1%, and complete AV block in less than 1%. Between 75% and 92% of the patients in this study developed a new ECG abnormality that was not captured on prior ECGs, with the most common being QT prolongation in 45%, followed by ST depression at 45% and U waves in 28%. Similar rates have been reported by Khechinashvili and Asplund (2002). In patients diagnosed with IS, the majority (75% and greater) developed new abnormalities on ECG. The most common abnormality detected was QT prolongation, followed by ST depression. Work by Daniele et al. (2002) involved 450 patients, of which 352 were diagnosed with IS (the remainder diagnosed with ICH) and detected new ECG abnormalities in 75% of patients, with approximately equal rates of arrhythmias in the groups diagnosed with ICH (20.4%) and groups diagnosed with IS (21.9%). However, arrhythmias were more frequently detected in patients with right-sided IS (26.8%) compared to patients with left-sided IS (14.3%). The slightly differing prevalence and incidence rates are likely secondary to differences in methodology between studies. For example, some authors may attempt to account for coexisting CAD while others do not, and only some use Holter data in addition to ECG (Koppikar et al., 2013).

The prognosis in those suffering from acute neurovascular disease has been demonstrated to be significantly worsened by the presence of an arrhythmia. Mortality in all patients was increased by 80% when a "malignant" ventricular arrhythmia was detected (Goldstein, 1979). Prolonged QTc and ventricular extrasystolic beats captured on ECG have also been demonstrated to lead to worse outcomes. Those with a prolonged QTc on ECG (over 440 ms in women, 438 ms in men) were 2½ times more likely to expire within 90 days of admission compared to patients with a normal QTc (Stead et al., 2009). Wong et al. (2003) calculated a relative risk of 2.8 of cardiac mortality when recorded QTc was greater than 480 ms. In one series of patients with ICH, the QTc was significantly increased in patients who expired compared to those who survived (Huang et al., 2004). In another case series, those who expired had approximately twice the rates of ECG evidence of recent myocardial infarction, three times the rate of AF, and five times the rate of conduction deficits (Dimant and Grob, 1977).

As the right insular region has been most closely associated with pathologic neurocardiogenic dysregulation, it may be expected that insular involvement portends a poorer prognosis. A study of over 600 patients demonstrated that there is a hazard ratio of over 3 for fatal cardiac events with both left and right parietal lobe infarctions, whereas insular stroke was not significantly associated with fatal cardiac events when cardiovascular risk factors were statistically controlled for (although there were low numbers of patients with insular lesions in this study) (Rincon et al., 2008). However, another study was able to capture more patients with right insular lesions and demonstrated that patients with right insular lesions have an odds ratio of mortality greater than 6 compared to those without a right insular lesion (Christensen et al., 2005).

Regarding management, little in the way of standardized therapeutic guidelines exists. Electrolytes should be maintained within normal limits, with special attention to magnesium and potassium to minimize potential electrolyte contributions to arrhythmias and repolarization abnormalities of neurocardiac etiology, and detected arrhythmias should be managed appropriately (Fisch, 1973; Adams et al., 2007). Similar to the eventual normalization of abnormalities detected on echocardiogram in myocardial stunning, ECG changes of neurocardiac origin generally persist for 1–2 weeks and subsequently normalize, although they are permanent in a small proportion of patients (Janse et al., 1986).

The most dramatic clinical presentation of neurocardiac dysregulation is SCD (Davis and Natelson, 1993). SCD is defined as either witnessed natural death associated with loss of consciousness or as an unwitnessed, unexpected death with no evidence of a noncardiac cause (Priori et al., 2001). Between 1989 and 1998, SCD was responsible for about half of cardiovascular deaths in the USA, and 74% of cardiac deaths in those between the ages of 35 and 44 (Zheng et al., 2001). Among the general population, approximately 1000 patients who expired secondary to SCD out of 2156 total in the UK had a normal heart on autopsy. Surprisingly, most cases (82%) occurred during sleep, although there are spikes in incidence after significant stress, inducing large-scale events, such as earthquakes (Leor et al., 1996). Associated risk factors in the general population are male gender (Fragkouli and Vougiouklakis, 2010), arrhythmia, prior syncope, family history of sudden death, and epilepsy (Mellor et al., 2014).

The two main categories of arrhythmia that can potentially lead to SCD are tachyarrhythmias and bradyarrhythmias. The tachyarrhythmias associated with SCD include ventricular fibrillation (VF) and VT. The bradyarrhythmias include sinus bradycardia, complete AV block, and sudden asystole (Bashour et al., 1988; Davis and Natelson, 1993; Sörös and Hachinski, 2012). Prolonged QTc is a risk factor for torsades de pointes (Cheung and Hachinski, 2000) and subsequent VF.

SCD is an increasingly recognized consequence of IS (Sörös and Hachinski, 2012). In patients without concurrent CAD, this is most likely mediated by fatal arrhythmias. Among the population with a neurovascular diagnosis, the higher-risk ECG changes for SCD include QTc prolongation, VT, ectopic ventricular beats, and R-on-T phenomenon (Cheung and Hachinski, 2000; Baranchuk et al., 2009). The most common sequence is hypothesized to start with VT, followed by fibrillation and subsequent arrest (Bayés de Luna et al., 1989). Given the association between SCD and agents which prolong the QT interval in combination with the high frequency of QT prolongation present in patients with neurovascular diagnosis (Goldstein, 1979), it is not unreasonable to postulate that prolonged QT leading to torsades de pointes and subsequent cardiac arrest could be a common pathophysiologic sequence leading to SCD as well.

The neurologic condition most classically associated with sudden death is epilepsy (Stecker et al., 2013). SUDEP is defined as an unexpected sudden death (either witnessed or unwitnessed, with or without evidence of a recent seizure) with no evidence of a secondary cause on autopsy (Nashef, 1997). It is the most common cause of death in patients with poorly controlled epilepsy, with incidence ranging from 0.09 per 1000 person-years to 9.3 per 1000 years in the more high-risk patients (Tomson et al., 2008).

Poor seizure control as well as antiepileptic drug use are both associated with increased risk of SUDEP (Tomson et al., 2008; Bardai et al., 2015). Possible mechanisms include sodium channel alterations produced by antiepileptic drug use, along with ion channel abnormalities common in patients with epilepsy (Bardai et al., 2015). Abnormal ion channels may result in abnormalities in both neuronal and cardiac sodium conduction, and they may additionally predispose these patients to more clinically significant cortical spreading depression, resulting in seizure activity that propagates to brain areas critical for maintaining normal cardiovascular function (Aiba and Noebels, 2015). As an argument against the cortical spreading depression hypothesis, despite the well-known association between poor epilepsy control and SUDEP (Tomson et al., 2008), there is some evidence that seizures are not always common occurrences immediately prior to witnessed or unwitnessed death (Stecker et al., 2013).

Fatal cerebrogenic arrhythmias may mediate some causes of sudden death in patients with epilepsy (Oppenheimer et al., 1990). There have been studies demonstrating various cardiac irregularities during seizures captured during concurrent electroencephalogram and ECG monitoring, including tachycardia, ectopic beats, ST- and T-wave changes, along RR variation (Blumhardt et al., 1986). Recent work suggests that there may be some overlap between SCD and SUDEP in the epilepsy population (Lamberts et al., 2015). Although the number of patients with epilepsy in this study was small (18 patients with epilepsy compared to hundreds of controls), the majority of the patients with epilepsy who expired had a cardiac cause (including arrhythmia). These patients would therefore not meet the definition of SUDEP – SCD would be a more appropriate classification, suggesting that in patients with epilepsy there may be

significant overlap between the categories of SUDEP and SCD (Lamberts et al., 2015). Another possibility for sudden death in epilepsy includes stress-related CMO, which has been reported in epilepsy and has been theorized to have a link to SUDEP (Dupuis et al., 2011).

Acute cardiac arrest may occur with aneurysmal rupture and often patients present with asystole or pulseless electric activity arrest. When examined, the acute injury is overwhelmingly severe and a large proportion of patients can be declared brain-dead.

Cardiac enzyme elevations have been well described in association with aneurysmal SAH; however, enzyme elevations occur commonly in the setting of IS and ICH as well (Samuels, 2007b). Prior to widespread use of troponin enzymes in evaluation of cardiac ischemia, Norris et al. (1979) examined cardiac-specific creatine kinase MB fraction (CK-MB) enzyme trends among patients admitted to a stroke intensive care unit. The general trend over days of measurement was a mild and gradual increase in CK-MB levels (as opposed to a rapid rise in cases of ACS), and patients with these elevations were more likely to have detectable arrhythmias and abnormalities on ECG.

Depending on study criteria, elevated cardiac enzymes have been detected in almost none to nearly one-third of patients presenting with IS (Jensen et al., 2007). Troponin is known to be a sensitive marker for cardiac injury (Ross et al., 2000). However troponin elevations have not been shown to be consistently associated with underlying cardiac disease in the acute neurologically ill population. Ay et al. (2006) detected changes on ECG suggestive of cardiac ischemia in only 2 of 10 patients with high troponin levels. One prospective study enrolled 114 patients with IS and found rates of troponin elevation in 17.6%; however, this rate decreased to 5% when including only those patients with normal ECG and creatinine (Abdi et al., 2014). There are significant correlations between troponin elevation and stroke severity as measured by the National Institute of Health Stroke Scale (NIHSS), confirmed by multiple studies (Chalela et al., 2004; Abdi et al., 2014; Miller et al., 2015). However, in the study by Abdi et al. (2014), there was no relationship to the location or laterality of infarct.

Even with comorbid noncardiac medical conditions accounted for, a patient with comorbid cardiac disease is more susceptible to the development of arrhythmias than an otherwise healthy patient (Caplan et al., 1999; Chechetto, 2004). Patients with positive cardiac enzymes are at greater risk for the development of arrhythmias. In one study, approximately 50% of patients admitted with IS and negative cardiac enzymes had detectable cardiac arrhythmias, while those with elevated cardiac enzymes had nearly double this rate, at 92% (Norris et al., 1979).

Troponin elevation in IS has been demonstrated to be a poor prognostic factor in the majority of studies examining the topic (James et al., 2000; Angelantonio et al., 2005; Jensen et al., 2007; Raza et al., 2014). Raza et al. (2014) reviewed 200 patients with IS, elevated troponin levels, and no evidence of ACS on ECG. Elevated troponin was significantly associated with an adverse cardiac outcome. In this same study, troponin elevation was more predictive of a poor outcome than newly diagnosed CMO, which was not associated with a major cardiac event. Death rate post hospitalization in a cohort of patients with a neurovascular diagnosis and elevated troponin was significantly higher when compared to patients with normal troponin levels, with studies calculating a hazard ratio of 2.1 and relative risk at 3.2 (James et al., 2000, Angelantonio et al., 2005).

In patients with ICH, one study involving approximately 100 patients demonstrated no relationship to 30-day mortality and elevated troponin levels (Maramattom et al., 2006). However, a larger study involving more than 200 patients demonstrated a significant increase in hospital mortality among patients with ICH and elevated troponin levels compared to patients without elevated troponin levels (Hays and Diringer, 2006). Garrett et al. (2009) examined several factors involved in mortality in a series of over 100 patients who underwent resection for ICH, and reported that admission troponin and volume of ICH were the only predictors of mortality. Sandhu et al. (2008) compared outcomes and short-term mortality rates in patients with elevated troponin levels in all three major neurovascular diagnoses (aneurysmal SAH, ICH, and IS). Elevated troponin was associated with an equally increased chance of mortality in patients with IS and ICH.

The use of B-type natriuretic peptide (BNP) has been shown to be sensitive, but not specific, in the evaluation of cardiac status in patients with IS, SAH, and ICH (Koenig et al., 2007). Similar to studies examining the relationship between troponin elevation and stroke severity, there are associations between elevation in BNP and stroke severity as measured by NIHSS (Tomita et al., 2007). This same study did not find an association between ICH and BNP elevations. Although BNP lacks specificity in the assessment of cardiac status in patients with IS and ICH, a meta-analysis of almost 3500 patients with IS by García-Berrocoso et al. (2013) demonstrated a relative mortality risk of 2.3 in patients with BNP levels near the upper quartile.

## Cardiac dysfunction and subarachnoid hemorrhage

Stress-related CMO is perhaps most notably illustrated in neurogenic stunned myocardium associated with SAH. Nonspecific and transient ECG abnormalities occur in most SAH patients (50–100%) (Hunt et al., 1969;

Brouwers et al., 1989; Mayer et al., 1995; Yoshikawa et al., 1999; Zaroff et al., 1999). ECG abnormalities are seen near universally in prospective SAH studies with serial monitoring (Brouwers et al., 1989; Mayer et al., 1995). The most common ECG abnormalities reported are sinus bradycardia, ST-segment abnormalities, T-wave abnormalities, and QTc prolongation (Pollick et al., 1988; Brouwers et al., 1989; Mayer et al., 1995). Cardiac arrhythmias are a well-known complication of SAH, with sinus bradycardia and sinus tachycardia being the most commonly associated with SAH, but others include atrial flutter, AF, supraventricular tachycardia, premature ventricular complexes, junctional rhythm, and ventricular arrhythmias (Brouwers et al., 1989; Mayer et al., 1995). The contribution of cardiac arrhythmia to mortality is likely underestimated, especially in the subset of SAH patients who die before reaching medical attention. Sudden death occurs in 12% of SAH patients and, in 92% of these patients, acute pulmonary edema is seen on autopsy (Schievink et al., 1995).

Troponin I is elevated in approximately 20–40% of SAH patients (Parekh et al., 2000; Deibert et al., 2003; Tung et al., 2004; Ramappa et al., 2008). Troponin I is a more sensitive biochemical marker of myocardial injury and left ventricular (LV) dysfunction than CK-MB in the SAH population, and this superiority of troponin I over CK-MB is consistent with the cardiac literature (Luscher et al., 1997; Parekh et al., 2000; Deibert et al., 2003). Elevated troponin I is associated with increased clinical severity of SAH (as measured by Hunt–Hess grade), and typically peaks within 48 hours of ictus, with a subsequent decay thereafter (Parekh et al., 2000; Tung et al., 2004; Naidech et al., 2005; Ramappa et al., 2008; Tanabe et al., 2008). The impact of cardiac injury on functional outcomes in SAH is unclear, with conflicting data. In one study of SAH patients, troponin elevation (categorized into quintiles) in the adjusted analysis was significantly associated with an increased likelihood of poor outcome at discharge, but not at 3 months (Naidech et al., 2005). A meta-analysis suggested that elevated troponin was associated with increased risk of death and poor outcome (van der Bilt et al., 2009).

Although troponin may be associated with worse morbidity, troponin elevation effect on short-term mortality has conflicting reports. Degos et al. (2012) evaluated 526 SAH patients who underwent aneurysm coiling and high troponin was associated with 1-year mortality. Ramappa et al. (2008) reported that peak troponin was an independent predictor of death at discharge in multivariate analysis adjusting for clinical grade in a sample of 250 patients (with 92 troponin levels). However, in other studies, troponin has not been shown to be an independent predictor of in-hospital mortality in SAH after adjusting for clinical severity (Yarlagadda et al., 2006; Gupte et al., 2013).

A characteristic of SAH-induced cardiac dysfunction is severely reduced ejection fraction with large regions of akinesis in the setting of a relatively modest troponin elevation, up to a 10-fold difference from elevations seen with acute myocardial infarction (Bulsara et al., 2003). Transient regional wall motion abnormalities (RWMA) occur in 8% of SAH patients (Mayer et al., 1995), and LV dysfunction on echocardiogram is more commonly seen in SAH patients with elevated cardiac enzymes and BNP, as well as poor neurologic grade (Pollick et al., 1988; Mayer et al., 1999; Parekh et al., 2000; Tung et al., 2004).

Diverse patterns of RWMA in SAH have been described, including LV hypokinesis, which predominantly involves the apex, as well as an apex-sparing pattern (Kono et al., 1994; Mayer et al., 1999; Zaroff et al., 2000a). However, an expected feature of SAH-induced cardiac dysfunction is RWMA extending beyond the territory of a single coronary vessel (Kono et al., 1994; Parekh et al., 2000; Zaroff et al., 2000a). Clinical symptoms of LV dysfunction are more likely in patients with elevated cardiac enzymes, ECG changes, or elevated BNP (Pollick et al., 1988; Mayer et al., 1999; Parekh et al., 2000; Tung et al., 2004). The timing of ejection fraction improvement in SAH-induced LV dysfunction can be variable, with recovery ranging from days to weeks (Mayer et al., 1994; Zaroff et al., 2000a). LV apical thrombus is a rare complication of SAH-induced cardiac dysfunction (Pollick et al., 1988). Depressed cardiac index and pulmonary complications are associated with symptomatic cerebral vasospasm in SAH (Mayer et al., 1994, 1999; Friedman et al., 2003). Rarely, SAH-induced congestive heart failure can be mistakenly triaged as acute myocardial infarction, with delay in the diagnosis of SAH (Handlin et al., 1993). Pulmonary edema occurs in approximately 10% of SAH patients (Friedman et al., 2003), although this can also be due to "neurogenic pulmonary edema," which is the development of lung edema of noncardiogenic origin (i.e., normal pulmonary capillary wedge pressures), possibly due to increased vascular permeability (Mayer et al., 1994; Fontes et al., 2003). Elevated plasma BNP in SAH has been reported to be significantly associated with RWMA and in-hospital mortality (Tung et al., 2005).

## Pathogenesis of SAH neurogenic stunned myocardium

The most widely accepted pathogenesis for SAH-induced neurogenic stunned myocardium is the "catecholamine hypothesis." Other less accepted theories include multivessel coronary artery spasm causing ischemia and microvascular dysfunction. In the cases where coronary angiogram data are available, normal coronary arteries have been documented in the setting of ongoing ST-segment elevation (Yuki et al., 1991; Chang et al., 1998; De Chazal et al., 2005). In the SAH dog model, RWMA in SAH is correlated with angiographic absence of focal coronary spasm (Zaroff et al., 2000b). Given the lack of convincing clinical or animal data supporting the theory of SAH-induced multivessel coronary artery vasospasm, this explanation has mostly been discredited. The alternative theory of myocardial ischemia due to dysfunction on a microvascular level is also unsupported. Microvascular perfusion has been demonstrated to be normal by myocardial contrast echocardiography in the SAH dog model (Zaroff et al., 2000b). Clinical case reports have also failed to demonstrate decreased perfusion in SAH myocardium (Chang et al., 1998). Thus, there is little evidence for decreased perfusion or ischemia on a macro- or microvascular level.

In contrast, the "catecholamine hypothesis" of catecholamine-induced cardiac is supported by robust clinical and animal data. In the SAH dog model, catecholamines increase abruptly 5 minutes after SAH onset (performed by perforating the basilar artery with a microcatheter inserted through the femoral artery) (Masuda et al., 2002). The peak values of cardiac markers (CK-MB and troponin T) correlate with the peak of norepinephrine and epinephrine (Masuda et al., 2002). Arrhythmia scores are greater in SAH animals compared with control sham-operated animals during sympathetic nerve electric stimulation and norepinephrine infusion (Lambert et al., 2002). Experimental SAH animal studies demonstrate immediate excess sympathetic nervous activation, as measured by higher circulating catecholamine levels, as well as increased cardiac sensitivity to sympathetic stimulation, suggesting that elevated sympathetic activity in the acute phase of SAH contributes to the development of cardiac dysfunction (Elrifai et al., 1996; Lambert et al., 2002; Masuda et al., 2002). SAH clinical studies have been in agreement with animal model studies. SAH patients have an increase in plasma norepinephrine within 48 hours after insult compared with control patients, and this increase persists in the first week and normalizes by 6 months (Naredi et al., 2000). In SAH patients, elevated cardiac enzymes are associated with increased concentrations of plasma catecholamines (Kawahara et al., 2003).

## Management of SAH neurogenic stunned myocardium

SAH-induced LV dysfunction is has the potential for recovery, with complete normalization of function expected (Mayer et al., 1994; Zaroff et al., 2000b).

As the condition has the potential for improvement with time, treatment of neurogenic stunned myocardium is mainly supportive. However, the clinician should be vigilant about potential complications that may arise from the combination of reduced LV function in the setting of cerebral vasospasm window, which often requires hemodynamic augmentation with intravenous vasopressors. Treating SAH patients with sympathetic agents such as phenylephrine and norepinephrine to combat hypotensive effects should be considered against, given that catecholamine toxicity is the suspected mechanism causing the original cardiac damage, and inotropic medications may be a better option.

Potential management strategies aimed at reducing the risk of SAH-induced cardiac stunning may include early identification of a high-risk subset and early treatment with alpha/beta blockade, although further investigation is necessary. Pharmacologic alpha or beta blockade has been suggested to prevent myocardial damage in these patients (Cruickshank et al., 1975). In a randomized double-blinded trial of atenolol given for 1 week in 114 acute head injury patients, the atenolol was associated with lower frequency of CK-MB elevation and focal necrosis on pathology. Among SAH patients given propranolol and phentolamine, myocardial lesions on pathology occurred in all 6 placebo patients but in none of the 6 patients in the medication group (Neil-Dwyer et al., 1978).

The explanation of obstructive CAD for cardiac dysfunction is implausible in most SAH patients due to the widespread distribution and reversibility of RWMA already described. However, the clinician should remain vigilant for the rare possibility of previously asymptomatic CAD causing cardiac dysfunction in the SAH population, which can be mistaken for neurogenic stunned myocardium (Hess et al., 2005). However, this should be identifiable by RWMA in a single-vessel territory and comparatively higher elevation of troponin (De Chazal et al., 2005).

## Tako-tsubo cardiomyopathy

Similar to neurogenic stunned myocardium, tako-tsubo CMO is considered to be in the spectrum of stress-related CMO. In the cardiac literature, tako-tsubo CMO is a condition that was originally described in the Japanese population but is now recognized globally and has been designated as a reversible CMO by the American College of Cardiology and American Heart Association (Maron et al., 2006). Tako-tsubo CMO shares similarities with SAH-induced cardiac dysfunction. Also known as apical ballooning syndrome, stress CMO, or "broken heart" syndrome, this syndrome is characterized by transient LV dysfunction.

The clinical presentation of tako-tsubo CMO can mimic acute myocardial infarction. This condition occurs predominantly in postmenopausal women and can be induced by emotional or physical stress. On ventriculogram, the contraction of the heart during systole was felt to resemble a Japanese octopus catcher pot or "tako-tsubo," thus coining its original name (Dote et al., 1994; Tsuchihashi et al., 2001; Abe et al., 2003; Girod et al., 2003; Connelly et al., 2004) (Fig. 4.3).

Patients typically present with ECG abnormalities and minor elevation in cardiac markers in the absence of significant CAD. The diagnostic features of tako-tsubo CMO include reversible RWMA, beyond the territory of a single coronary artery distribution, typically involving the LV apex and mid-ventricle with relative sparing of the basal segment (Dote et al., 1994; Tsuchihashi et al., 2001; Kyuma et al., 2002; Abe et al., 2003; Girod et al., 2003; Bybee et al., 2004a, b; Connelly et al., 2004) (Fig. 4.4). The prognosis tends to be favorable, with spontaneous improvement in LV function expected with supportive care and an in-hospital mortality of less than 1% (Tsuchihashi et al., 2001; Abe et al., 2003; Bybee et al., 2004a, b; Connelly et al., 2004; Wittstein et al., 2005). Rare complications include LV apical thrombus and fatal LV rupture (Akashi et al., 2004; Takaki et al., 2004).

The most widely accepted hypothesis for pathogenesis in tako-tsubo CMO is the catecholamine hypothesis. A cardiac MRI study of tako-tsubo CMO showed no evidence of myocardial necrosis on contrast-enhanced imaging in patients with endomyocardial biopsy demonstrating CBN and lymphocytic infiltrate, and elevated plasma catecholamine levels compared to controls (with myocardial infarction (Wittstein et al., 2005). Other studies have not been able to demonstrate plasma catecholamine levels or 24-hour urine catecholamine levels beyond the normal range (Madhavan et al., 2009).

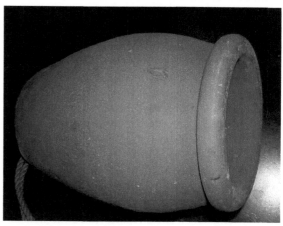

**Fig. 4.3.** Japanese octopus catcher pot, "tako-tsubo."

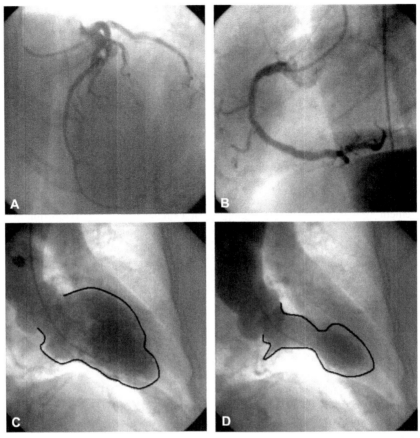

**Fig. 4.4.** (**A, B**) Coronary angiogram demonstrates normal coronary arteries. (**C, D**) Left ventriculogram demonstrates apical and mid-ventricular wall motion abnormalities characteristic of tako-tsubo cardiomyopathy. (Reproduced from Chen et al., 2006.)

However, in contrast to ST-elevated myocardial infarction patients, patients with tako-tsubo CMO have a higher elevation in BNP (three- to fourfold greater) (Madhavan et al., 2009).

Animal models give us insight into the striking female predominance (over 90%) (Kawai et al., 2000; Tsuchihashi et al., 2001; Abe et al., 2003; Wittstein et al., 2005). The rat model of tako-tsubo CMO uses immobilization stress to reproduce the ECG and ventriculogram changes of apical ballooning (Ueyama, 2004). Cardiac dysfunction is prevented by pretreatment with combined alpha- and beta-blockers, but not by calcium channel blockers or nitroglycerin. Furthermore, an increase of serum estrogen partially attenuated these cardiac changes, suggesting that the postmenopausal female predominance may be related to a relative state of estrogen depletion (Ueyama, 2004).

Capture myopathy (CM) is an intriguing condition observed in wild animals that have been captured, and may represent a wildlife model that may explain the evolutionary origins of stress-related CMO in humans. A recent study reconstructed the evolution of CM in ungulates and found that CM was an adaptation associated with faster running speed, greater group size, greater brain mass, and greater longevity (Blumstein et al., 2015). These results suggest that CM developed as an evolutionary response to threat (i.e., increased running speed requires an explosive sympathetic response), and CM can be understood to be an unavoidable consequence to predator risk.

Until recently, tako-tsubo and neurogenic stunned myocardium were considered unrelated conditions. Most series on tako-tsubo specifically excluded SAH patients, and the proposed Mayo diagnostic criteria for apical ballooning syndrome require the exclusion of head trauma and intracranial bleeding (Bybee et al., 2004b). The ventriculogram pattern of apical ballooning has been seen in SAH patients as well, although other patterns of RWMA can also be seen (Lee et al., 2006). The overlap between tako-tsubo CMO and neurogenic stunned myocardium due to SAH is considerable and includes similar population (both conditions predominate in postmenopausal females), shared hypothesis (excess catecholamine state), evidence of exaggerated sympathetic activation (elevated plasma catecholamine levels), absence of coronary artery spasm or obstruction, and shared cardiac histopathology (CBN). The consensus opinion currently is that tako-tsubo CMO and SAH-induced cardiac dysfunction are likely on a continuum of the same pathophysiology, with SAH-induced cardiac dysfunction being on the more severe end of the spectrum (Ako et al., 2003).

## REFERENCES

Abdi S, Oveis-Gharan O, Sinaei F et al. (2014). Elevated troponin T after acute ischemic stroke: association with severity and location of infarction. Iran J Neurol 14: 35–40.

Abe Y, Kondo M, Matsuoka R et al. (2003). Assessment of clinical features in transient left ventricular apical ballooning. J Am Coll Cardiol 41: 737–742.

Adams HP, Del Zoppo G, Alberts MJ et al. (2007). Guidelines for the early management of adults with ischemic stroke: a guideline from the American Heart Association/American Stroke Association Stroke Council, Clinical Cardiology Council, Cardiovascular Radiology and Intervention Council, and the Atherosclerotic Peripheral Vascular Disease and Quality of Care Outcomes in Research Interdisciplinary Working Groups. Circulation 115: 478–534.

Aiba I, Noebels JL (2015). Spreading depolarization in the brainstem mediates sudden cardiorespiratory arrest in mouse SUDEP models. Sci Transl Med 282: FS14.

Akashi YJ, Tejima T, Sakurada H et al. (2004). Left ventricular rupture associated with takotsubo cardiomyopathy. Mayo Clin Proc 79: 821–824.

Ako J, Honda Y, Fitzgerald PJ (2003). Tako-tsubo-like left ventricular dysfunction. Circulation 108: e158.

Amaral S (2012). Takotsubo cardiomyopathy and acute ischemic stroke. JMC 3: 347–351.

Angelantonio DI, Fiorelli M, Toni D et al. (2005). Prognostic significance of admission levels of troponin I in patients with acute ischaemic stroke. J Neurol Neurosurg Psychiatry 76: 76–81.

Ay H, Koroshetz WJ, Benner T et al. (2006). Neuroanatomic correlates of stroke-related myocardial injury. Neurology 66: 1325–1329.

Baranchuk A, Nault MA, Morillo CA (2009). The central nervous system and sudden cardiac death: what should we know? Cardiol J 16: 105–112.

Bardai A, Bom MT, van Noord C et al. (2015). Sudden cardiac death is associated both with epilepsy and with the use of antiepileptic medications. Heart 101: 17–22.

Barron SA, Rogoviski Z, Hemli J (1994). Autonomic consequences of cerebral hemisphere infarction. Stroke 25: 113–116.

Bashour TT, Cohen MS, Ryan C et al. (1988). Sinus node suppression in acute strokes-case reports. Angiology 39: 1048–1055.

Bayés de Luna A, Coumel P, Leclercq JF (1989). Ambulatory sudden cardiac death: mechanisms of production of fatal arrhythmia on the basis of data from 157 cases. Am Heart J 117: 151–159.

Blumhardt LD, Smith PEM, Owen L (1986). Electrocardiographic accompaniments of temporal lobe epileptic seizures. Lancet 2: 1052–1055.

Blumstein DT, Buckner J, Shah S et al. (2015). The evolution of capture myopathy in hooved mammals: a model for human stress cardiomyopathy? Evol Med Public Health: 195–203.

Brouwers PJ, Wijdicks EF, Hasan D et al. (1989). Serial electrocardiographic recording in aneurysmal subarachnoid hemorrhage. Stroke 20: 1162–1167.

Bulsara KR, McGirt MJ, Liao L et al. (2003). Use of the peak troponin value to differentiate myocardial infarction from reversible neurogenic left ventricular dysfunction associated with aneurysmal subarachnoid hemorrhage. J Neurosurg 98: 524–528.

Bybee KA, Prasad A (2008). Stress related cardiomyopathy syndromes. Circulation 118: 397–409.

Bybee KA, Prasad A, Barsness GW et al. (2004a). Clinical characteristics and thrombolysis in myocardial infarction frame counts in women with transient left ventricular apical ballooning syndrome. Am J Cardiol 94: 343–346.

Bybee KA, Kara T, Prasad A et al. (2004b). Systemic review: transient left ventricular apical ballooning: a syndrome that mimics ST-segment elevation myocardial Infarction. Ann Intern Med 141: 858–865.

Cannon WB (1942). "Voodoo" death. Am Anthropol 44: 169–181.

Caplan LR, Hurst JW, Chimowitz MI (1999). Cardiac and cardiovascular findings in patients with nervous system disease. In: SZ Goldhaber, H Bounnameaux (Eds.), Clinical Neurocardiology, Marcel Dekker, New York, pp. 298–435.

Cebelin MS, Hirsch CS (1980). Human stress cardiomyopathy. Myocardial lesions in victims of homicidal assaults without internal injuries. Hum Pathol 11: 123–132.

Chalela JA, Ezzeddine MA, Davis L et al. (2004). Myocardial injury in acute stroke: a troponin I study. Neurocrit Care 1: 343–346.

Chandra S, Sign V, Nehra M et al. (2010). ST-segment elevation in non-atherosclerotic coronaries: a brief overview. Intern Emerg Med 6: 129–139.

Chang PC, Lee SH, Hung HF et al. (1998). Transient ST elevation and left ventricular asynergy associated with normal coronary artery and Tc-99 m PYP myocardial infarct scan in subarachnoid hemorrhage. Int J Cardiol 63: 189–192.

Chechetto DF (2004). Forebrain control of healthy and diseased hearts. In: JA Amor, JL Ardell (Eds.), Basic and Clinical Neurocardiology. Oxford Press, New York, pp. 220–251.

Chen Y-L, Yu T-H, Fu M (2006). Takotsubo cardiomyopathy – transient left ventricular apical ballooning mimicking acute myocardial infarction. J Formos Med Assoc 105: 839–843.

Cheung RTF, Hachinski V (2000). The insula and cerebrogenic sudden death. Arch Neurol 57: 1685–1688.

Christensen H, Boysen G, Christensen AF et al. (2005). Insular lesions, ECG abnormalities, and outcome in acute stroke. J Neurol Neurosurg Psychiatry 76: 269–271.

Colivicchi F, Bassi A, Santini M et al. (2004). Cardiac autonomic derangement and arrhythmias in right-sided stroke with insular involvement. Stroke 35: 2094–2098.

Connelly KA, MacIsaac AI, Jelinek VM (2004). Stress, myocardial infarction, and the "tako-tsubo" phenomenon. Heart 90: e52.

Cruickshank JM, Neil-Dwyer G, Lane J (1975). The effect of oral propranolol upon the ECG changes occurring in subarachnoid haemorrhage. Cardiovasc Res 9: 236–245.

Cruickshank JM, Neil-Dwyer G, Degaute JP et al. (1987). Reduction of stress/catecholamine-induced cardiac necrosis by beta 1-selective blockade. Lancet 2: 585–589.

Cubeddu LX (2003). QT prolongation and fatal arrhythmias: a review of clinical implications and effects of drugs. Am J Ther 10: 452–457.

Daniele O, Caravaglios G, Fierro B et al. (2002). Stroke and cardiac arrhythmias. J Stroke Cerebrovasc Dis 11: 28–33.

Davis AM, Natelson B (1993). Brain–heart interactions. The neurocardiology of arrhythmia and sudden cardiac death. Tex Heart Inst J 20: 158–169.

De Chazal I, Parham WM, Liopyris P et al. (2005). Delayed cardiogenic shock and acute lung injury after aneurysmal subarachnoid hemorrhage. Anesth Analg 100: 1147–1149.

Degos V, Apfel CC, Sanchez P et al. (2012). An admission bioclinical score to predict 1 year outcomes in patients undergoing aneurysm coiling. Stroke 43: 1253–1259.

Deibert E, Barzilai B, Braverman AC et al. (2003). Clinical significance of elevated troponin I levels in patients with nontraumatic subarachnoid hemorrhage. J Neurosurg 98: 741–746.

Dimant J, Grob D (1977). Electrocardiographic changes and myocardial damage in patients with acute cerebrovascular accidents. Stroke 8: 448–455.

Doshi R, Neil-Dwyer G (1969). A clinicopathological study of patients following a subarachnoid hemorrhage. Am Heart J 77: 479–488.

Dote K, Sato H, Tateishi H et al. (1994). Myocardial stunning due to simultaneous multivessel coronary spasms: a review of 5 cases. J Cardiol 21: 203–214.

Drislane FW, Samuels MA, Kozakewich H et al. (1987). Myocardial contraction band lesions in patients with fatal asthma: possible neurocardiologic mechanism. Am Rev Respir Dis 135: 498–501.

Dujardin KS, McCully RB, Wijdicks EF et al. (2001). Myocardial dysfunction associated with brain death: clinical, echocardiographic, and pathologic features. J Heart Lung Transplant 20: 350–357.

Dupuis M, van Rijckevorsel K, Evrard F et al. (2011). Takotsubo syndrome (TKS): a possible mechanism of sudden unexplained death in epilepsy (SUDEP). Seizure 21: 51–54.

Elrifai AM, Bailes JE, Shih SR et al. (1996). Characterization of the cardiac effects of acute subarachnoid hemorrhage in dogs. Stroke 27: 737–741.

Engel J (2001). Mesial temporal lobe epilepsy, what have we learned? Neuroscientist 7: 340–352.

Fink JN, Selim MHS, Kumar S et al. (2005). Insular cortex infarction in acute middle cerebral artery territory stroke. Predictor of stroke severity and vascular lesion. Arch Neurol 62: 1081–1085.

Fisch C (1973). Relation of electrolyte disturbances to cardiac arrhythmias. Circulation 47: 408–419.

Fontes RB, Aguiar PH, Zanetti MV et al. (2003). Acute neurogenic pulmonary edema: case reports and literature review. J Neurosurg Anesthesiol 15: 144–150.

Fragkouli K, Vougiouklakis T (2010). Sudden cardiac death: an 11-year postmortem analysis in the region of Epirus, Greece. Pathol Res Pract 206: 690–694.

Friedman JA, Pichelmann MA, Piepgras DG et al. (2003). Pulmonary complications of aneurysmal subarachnoid hemorrhage. Neurosurgery 52: 1025–1031.

García-Berrocoso T, Giralt D, Bustamante A et al. (2013). B-type natriuretic peptides and mortality after stroke: a systematic review and meta-analysis. Neurology 81: 1976–1985.

Garrett M, Komotar R, Starke R et al. (2009). Elevated troponin levels are predictive of mortality in surgical intracerebral hemorrhage patients. Neurocrit Care 12: 199–203.

Girod JP, Messerli AW, Zidar F et al. (2003). Tako-tsubo-like transient left ventricular dysfunction. Circulation 107: e120–e121.

Goldstein DS (1979). The electrocardiogram in stroke: relationship to pathophysiological type and comparison with prior tracings. Stroke 10: 253–259.

Gupte M, John S, Prabhakaran S et al. (2013). Troponin elevation in subarachnoid hemorrhage does not impact in-hospital mortality. Neurocrit Care 18: 368–373.

Hall DW (1990). An overview of the autonomic nervous system. In: HD Walker, DW Hall, JW Just (Eds.), Clinical Methods: The History, Physical, and Laboratory Examinations, 3rd edn. Butterworth Publishers, Boston. chapter 75.

Handlin LR, Kindred LH, Beauchamp GD et al. (1993). Reversible left ventricular dysfunction after subarachnoid hemorrhage. Am Heart J 126: 235–240.

Hays A, Diringer MN (2006). Elevated troponin levels are associated with higher mortality following intracerebral hemorrhage. Neurology 66: 1330–1334.

Hess EP, Boie ET, White RD (2005). Survival of a neurologically intact patient with subarachnoid hemorrhage and cardiopulmonary arrest. Mayo Clin Proc 80: 1073–1076.

Hilz MJ, Moeller S, Akhundova A et al. (2011). High NISS values predict impairment of cardiovascular autonomic control. Stroke 42: 1528–1533.

Hoff EC, Kell JF, Carroll MN (1963). Effects of cortical stimulation and lesions on cardiovascular function. Physiol Rev 43: 68–114.

Huang CH, Chen WJ, Chang WT et al. (2004). QTc dispersion as a prognostic factor in intracerebral hemorrhage. Am J Emerg Med 22: 141–144.

Hunt D, McRae C, Zapf P (1969). Electrocardiographic and serum enzyme changes in subarachnoid hemorrhage. Am Heart J 77: 479–488.

James P, Ellis CJ, Whitlock RM et al. (2000). Relation between troponin T Concentration and mortality in patients presenting with an acute stroke: observational study. BMJ 320: 1502–1504.

Janse MJ, Kleber AG, Cappuci A et al. (1986). Electrophysiological basis for arrhythmias caused by acute ischemia: role of the subendocardium. J Mol Cell Cardio 19: 339–355.

Jensen JK, Kristensen SR, Bak S et al. (2007). Frequency and significance of troponin T elevation in acute ischemic stroke. Am J Cardiol 99: 108–112.

Jensen JK, Mickley H, Bak S et al. (2009). Electrocardiographic ST-T changes during acute ischemic stroke. Int J Cardiol 133: 398.

Kallmünzer B, Breuer L, Kahl N (2012). Serious cardiac arrhythmias after stroke: incidence, time course, and predictors – a systematic, prospective analysis. Stroke 43: 2892–2897.

Karch SB, Billingham ME (1986). Myocardial contraction bands revisited. Hum Pathol 17: 9–13.

Kawahara E, Ikeda S, Miyahara Y et al. (2003). Role of autonomic nervous dysfunction in electrocardiographic abnormalities and cardiac injury in patients with acute subarachnoid hemorrhage. Circ J 67: 753–756.

Kawai S, Suzuki H, Yamaguchi H et al. (2000). R. Ampulla cardiomyopathy ('takotsubo' cardiomyopathy) – reversible left ventricular dysfunction: with ST segment elevation. Jpn Circ J 64: 156–159.

Kent KM, Epstein SE, Copper T et al. (1974). Cholinergic innervation of the canine and human ventricular conducting system. Anatomic and electrophysiologic correlations. Circulation 50: 948–955.

Khechinashvili G, Asplund K (2002). Electrocardiographic changes in patients with acute stroke: a systematic review. J Cerebrovasc Dis 13: 67–76.

Kocan MJ (1998). The brain–heart connection: cardiac effects of acute ischemic stroke. J Cardiovasc Nurs 13: 57–68.

Koenig MA, Puttgen HA, Prabhakaran V et al. (2007). B-type natriuretic peptide as a marker of heart failure in patients with acute stroke. J Intensive Care Med 33: 1587–1593.

Kolin A, Norris JW (1984). Myocardial damage from acute cerebral lesions. Stroke 15: 990–993.

Kono T, Morita H, Kuroiwa T et al. (1994). Left ventricular wall motion abnormalities in patients with subarachnoid hemorrhage: neurogenic stunned myocardium. J Am Coll Cardiol 24: 636–640.

Koppikar S, Baranchuk A, Guzman JC et al. (2013). Stroke and ventricular arrhythmias. Int J Cardio 168: 653–659.

Korpelainen JT, Sotaneieme KA, Suominen K et al. (1994). Cardiovascular autonomic reflexes in brain infarction. Stroke 25: 787–792.

Kyuma M, Tsuchihashi K, Shinshi Y et al. (2002). Effect of intravenous propranolol on left ventricular apical ballooning without coronary artery stenosis (ampulla cardiomyopathy): three cases. Circ J 66: 1181–1184.

Lambert E, Du XJ, Percy E et al. (2002). Cardiac response to norepinephrine and sympathetic nerve stimulation following experimental subarachnoid hemorrhage. J Neurol Sci 198: 43–50.

Lamberts RJ, Blom MT, Wassenaar M et al. (2015). Sudden cardiac arrest in people with epilepsy in the community. Circumstances and risk factors. Neurology 85: 212–218.

Lane RD, Wallace JD, Petrosky PP et al. (1992). Supraventricular tachycardia in patients with right hemisphere strokes. Stroke 23: 362–366.

Lavy SL, Yaar I, Melamed E et al. (1974). The effect of acute stroke on cardiac functions as observed in an intensive stroke care unit. Stroke 5: 775–780.

Lee VH, Connolly HM, Fulgham JR et al. (2006). Tako-tsubo cardiomyopathy in aneurismal subarachnoid hemorrhage: an under-appreciated ventricular dysfunction. J Neurosurg 105: 1–7.

Leor J, Poole WK, Kloner RA (1996). Sudden cardiac death triggered by an earthquake. N Engl J Med 334: 413–419.

Luscher MS, Thygesen K, Ravkilde J et al. (1997). Applicability of cardiac troponin T and I for early risk stratification in unstable coronary artery disease. TRIM Study Group. Thrombin inhibition in myocardial ischemia. Circulation 96: 2578–2585.

Madhavan M, Borlaug BA, Lerman A et al. (2009). Stress hormone and circulating biomarker profile of apical ballooning syndrome (takotsubo cardiomyopathy): insights into the clinical significance of B-type natriuretic peptide and troponin levels. Heart 95: 1436–1441.

Manno EM, Pfeifer EA, Cascino GD et al. (2005). Cardiac pathology in status epilepticus. Ann Neurol 58: 954–957.

Maramattom BV, Manno EM, Fulgham JR et al. (2006). Clinical importance of cardiac troponin release and cardiac abnormalities in patients with supratentorial cerebral hemorrhages. Mayo Clin Proc 81: 192–196.

Maron BJ, Towbin JA, Thiene G et al. (2006). American Heart Association contemporary definitions and classification of the cardiomyopathies: American Heart Association scientific statement from the Council on Clinical Cardiology, Heart Failure and Transplantation Committee; Quality of Care and Outcomes Research and Functional Genomics and Translational Biology Interdisciplinary Working Groups; and Council on Epidemiology and Prevention. Circulation 113: 1807–1816.

Martin P (1977). The influence of the parasypathetic nervous system on atrioventricular conduction. Circ Res 41: 593–599.

Masuda T, Sato K, Yamamoto S et al. (2002). Sympathetic nervous activity and myocardial damage immediately after subarachnoid hemorrhage in a unique animal model. Stroke 33: 1671–1676.

Mayer SA, Fink ME, Homma S et al. (1994). Cardiac injury associated with neurogenic pulmonary edema following subarachnoid hemorrhage. Neurology 44: 815–820.

Mayer SA, LiMandri G, Sherman D et al. (1995). Electrocardiographic markers of abnormal left ventricular wall motion in acute subarachnoid hemorrhage. J Neurosurg 83: 889–896.

Mayer SA, Lin J, Homma S et al. (1999). Myocardial injury and left ventricular performance after subarachnoid hemorrhage. Stroke 30: 780–786.

Mellor G, Raju H, Noronha S et al. (2014). Clinical characteristics and circumstances of death in the sudden arrhythmic death syndrome. Cir Arrhythm Electrophsyiol 7: 1078–1083.

Melville KI, Garvey HL, Shister HE et al. (1969). Central nervous system stimulation and cardiac ischemic changes in monkeys. Ann N Y Acad Sci 156: 241–260.

Meyer S, Stittmatter M, Fischer C et al. (2003). Lateralization in autonomic dysfunction in ischemic stroke involving the insular cortex. NeuroReport 15: 357–361.

Mikolich JR, Jacobs CW, Fletcher GF (1981). Cardiac arrhythmias in patients with acute cerebrovascular accidents. JAMA 246: 1314–1417.

Miller BR, Alkachroum AM, Chami T et al. (2015). Troponin elevations in ischemic stroke are associated with stroke severity and advanced age. Circulation 132: A19723.

Mitchell GAG (1952). The innervation of the heart. Br Heart J 15: 159–171.

Myers MG, Norris JW, Hachinski VC et al. (1981). Plasma norepinephrine in stroke. Stroke 12: 200–204.

Nagi M, Hoshide S, Kario K (2010). The insular cortex and cardiovascular system: a new insight into the brain–heart axis. J Am Soc Hypertens 4: 174–182.

Naidech AM, Kreiter KT, Janjua N et al. (2005). Cardiac troponin elevation, cardiovascular morbidity, and outcome after subarachnoid hemorrhage. Circulation 112: 2851–2856.

Naredi S, Lambert G, Eden E et al. (2000). Increased sympathetic nervous activity in patients with nontraumatic subarachnoid hemorrhage. Stroke 31: 901–906.

Nashef L (1997). Sudden unexpected death in epilepsy: terminology and definitions. Epilepsia 38: S6–S8.

Neil-Dwyer G, Walter P, Cruickshank JM et al. (1978). Effect of propranolol and phentolamine on myocardial necrosis after subarachnoid haemorrhage. Br Med J 2: 990–992.

Norris JW, Hachinski VC, Myers MG et al. (1979). Serum cardiac enzymes in stroke. Stroke 10: 548–553.

Novitzky D, Wicomb WN, Cooper KC et al. (1986). Prevention of myocardial injury during brain death by total cardiac sympathectomy in the chacma baboon. Ann Thorac Surg 41: 520–524.

Oppenheimer SM (2006). Cerebrogenic cardiac arrhythmias: cortical lateralization and clinical significance. Clin Auton Res 16: 6–11.

Oppenheimer SM, Cechetto DF (1990). Cardiac chronotropic organization of the rat insular cortex. Brain Res 533: 66–72.

Oppenheimer SM, Cechetto DF, Hacinski VC (1990). Cerebrogenic cardiac arrhythmias. Cerebral electrocardiographic influences and their role in sudden death. Arch Neurol 47: 513–519.

Oppenheimer SM, Gelb AW, Girvin JP et al. (1992). Cardiovascular effects of human insular stimulation. Neurology 42: 1727–1732.

Parekh N, Venkatesh B, Cross D et al. (2000). Cardiac troponin I predicts myocardial dysfunction in aneurysmal subarachnoid hemorrhage. J Am Coll Cardiol 36: 1328–1335.

Pauza DH, Skripka V, Pauziene N et al. (2000). Morphology, distribution, variability of the epicardiac neural ganglionated subplexuses of in the human heart. Anat Rec 259: 353–382.

Pereira VH, Cerqueira JJ, Palha JA et al. (2013). Stressed brain, diseased heart: a review on the pathophysiologic mechanisms of neurocardiology. Int J Cardio 166: 30–37.

Perron AD, Brady WJ (2000). Electrocardiographic manifestations of CNS events. Am J Emerg Med 18: 715–720.

Pollick C, Cujec B, Parker S et al. (1988). Left ventricular wall motion abnormalities in subarachnoid hemorrhage: an echocardiographic study. J Am Coll Cardiol 12: 600–605.

Priori SG, Aliot E, Blomstrom-Lundqvist C et al. (2001). Task Force on Sudden Cardiac Death of the European Society of Cardiology. Eur Heart J 22: 1374–1450.

Prosser J, MacGregor L, Lees KR et al. (2007). Predictors of early cardiac morbidity and mortality after ischemic stroke. Stroke 38: 2295–2302.

Ramappa P, Thatai D, Coplin W et al. (2008). Cardiac troponin-I: a predictor of prognosis in subarachnoid hemorrhage. Neurocrit Care 8: 398–403.

Raza F, Alkouli M, Sandhu P et al. (2014). Elevated cardiac troponin in acute stroke without acute coronary syndrome predicts long-term adverse cardiovascular outcomes. Stroke Res Treat. 6 pages.

Reichenbach DD, Benditt EP (1970). Catecholamines and cardiomyopathy: the pathogenesis and potential importance of myofibrillar degeneration. Hum Pathol 1: 125–150.

Reis DJ, Oliphant MC (1964). Bradycardia and tachycardia following electrical stimulation of the amygdaloid region in monkey. J Neurophysio 27: 893–912.

Reuter BM, Kuthen M, Linke DM (1993). Does lateralized hemispheric control of cardiovascular activity exist? A Wada test study. Z Exp Angew Psychol 40: 267–278.

Rincon F, Dhamoon M, Moon Y et al. (2008). Stroke location and association with fatal cardiac outcomes. Northern Manhattan Study. Stroke 39: 2425–2431.

Rogers MC, Battit G, McPeek B et al. (1978). Lateralization of sympathetic control of the human sinus node: ECG changes of stellate ganglion block. Anesthesiology 48: 139–141.

Ross G, Bever FN, Uddin Z et al. (2000). Troponin I sensitivity and specificity for the diagnosis of acute myocardial infarction. J Am Osteopath Assoc 100: 29–32.

Samuels MA (2007a). "Voodoo" death revisited. The modern lesions of neurocardiology. CCJM 74: s8–s16.

Samuels MA (2007b). The brain–heart connection. Circulation 116: 77–84.

Sandhu R, Aronow WS, Radjdev A et al. (2008). Relation of cardiac troponin I levels with in-hospital mortality in patients with ischemic stroke, intracerebral hemorrhage, and subarachnoid hemorrhage. Am J Cardiol 102: 632–634.

Schievink WI, Wijdicks EF, Parisi JE et al. (1995). Sudden death from aneurysmal subarachnoid hemorrhage. Neurology 45: 871–874.

Seifert F, Kallmünzer B, Gutjahr I et al. (2015). Neuroanatomical correlates of severe cardiac arrhythmias in acute ischemic stroke. J Neurol 5: 1182–1190.

Shivalkar B, Van Loon J, Wieland W et al. (1993). Increase intracranial pressure on myocardial structure and function. Circulation 87: 230–239.

Sörös P, Hachinski V (2012). Cardiovascular and neurological causes of sudden death after ischaemic stroke. Lancet Neurol 11: 179–188.

Stead LG, Gilmore RM, Bellolio MF et al. (2009). Prolonged QTc as a predictor of mortality in acute ischemic stroke. J Stroke Cerebrovasc Dis 18: 469–474.

Stecker EC, Reinier K, Uy-Evandado A et al. (2013). Relationship between seizure episode and sudden cardiac arrest in patients with epilepsy: a community-based study. Circ Arrhythm Electrophysiol 6: 912–916.

Strittmatter M, Meyer S, Fischer C et al. (2003). Location-dependent patterns in cardio-autonomic dysfunction in ischaemic stroke. Eur Neurol 50: 30–38.

Sugiura M, Yozawa Y, Kubo O et al. (1985). Myocardial damage (myocytolysis) caused by subarachnoid hemorrhage. No to Shinkei - Brain & Nerve 37: 1155–1161.

Takaki A, Ogawa H, Wakeyama T et al. (2004). Ampulla cardiomyopathy with left ventricular apical mural thrombi resolved by anticoagulant therapy without systemic complication: a case report. J Cardiol 44: 243–250.

Takeno Y, Eno S, Hondo T et al. (2004). Pheochromocytoma with reversal of tako-tsubo-like transient left ventricular dysfunction: a case report. J Cardiol 43: 281–287.

Tanabe M, Crago EA, Suffoletto MS et al. (2008). Relation of elevation in cardiac troponin I to clinical severity, cardiac dysfunction, and pulmonary congestion in patients with subarachnoid hemorrhage. Am J Cardiol 102: 1545–1550.

Terrence CF, Rao GR, Perper JA (1980). Neurogenic pulmonary edema in unexpected, unexplained death of epileptic patients. Ann Neurol 9: 458–464.

Tokgözoglu S, Batur MK, Topçuoglu MA et al. (1999). Effects of stroke localization on cardiac autonomic balance and sudden death. Stroke 30: 1307–1311.

Tomita H, Metoki N, Saitoh G et al. (2007). Elevated plasma brain natriuretic peptide levels independent of heart disease in acute ischemic stroke: correlation with stroke severity. Hypertens Res 31: 1695–1702.

Tomson T, Nashef L, Ryvlin P (2008). Sudden unexpected death in epilepsy: current knowledge and future directions. Lancet Neurol 7: 1021–1031.

Touze E, Varenne O, Chatellier G et al. (2005). Risk of myocardial infarction and vascular death after transient ischemic attack and ischemic stroke: a systematic review and meta-analysis. Stroke 36: 2748–2755.

Tsuchihashi K, Ueshima K, Uchida T et al. (2001). Angina pectoris-myocardial infarction Investigations in Japan. Transient left-ventricular apical ballooning without coronary artery stenosis: a novel heart syndrome mimicking acute myocardial infarction. J Am Coll Cardiol 38: 11–18.

Tung P, Kopelnik A, Banki N et al. (2004). Predictors of neurocardiogenic injury after subarachnoid hemorrhage. Stroke 35: 548–551.

Tung PP, Olmsted E, Kopelnik A et al. (2005). Plasma B-type natriuretic peptide levels are associated with early cardiac dysfunction after subarachnoid hemorrhage. Stroke 36: 1567–1571.

Türe U, Yaşargil MG, Al-Mefty O (2000). Arteries of the Insula. J Neurosurg 92: 676–687.

Ueyama T (2004). Emotional stress-induced tako-tsubo cardiomyopathy: animal model and molecular mechanism. Ann N Y Acad Sci 1018: 437–444.

van der Bilt IAC, Hasan D, Vandertop WP et al. (2009). Impact of cardiac complication's on outcome after aneurysmal subarachnoid hemorrhage a meta-analysis. Neurology 72: 635–642.

van der Wal EE, Gilst WH (2013). Neurocardiology: close interaction between heart and brain. Neth Heart J 21: 51–52.

Wang TD, Wu CC, Lee YT (1997). Myocardial stunning after cerebral infarction. Int J Cardiol 58: 308–311.

Witt BJ, Ballman KV, Brown RD et al. (2006). The incidence of stroke after myocardial infarction: a meta-analysis. Am J Med 119: 354.e1–354.e9.

Wittstein IS, Thierman DR, Lima JA et al. (2005). Neurohumoral features of myocardial stunning due to sudden emotional stress. N Engl J Med 352: 539–548.

Wong KY, Mac Walter RS, Douglas D et al. (2003). Long QTc predicts future cardiac death in stroke survivors. Heart 89: 377–381.

Yarlagadda S, Rajendran P, Miss JC et al. (2006). Cardiovascular predictors of in-patient mortality after subarachnoid hemorrhage. Neurocrit Care 5: 102–107.

Yoon BW, Morillo CA, Cechetto DF et al. (1997). Cerebral hemispheric lateralization in cardiac autonomic control. Arch Neurol 54: 741–744.

Yoshikawa D, Hara T, Takahasi K et al. (1999). An association between QTc prolongation and left ventricular hypokinesis during sequential episodes of subarachnoid hemorrhage. Anesth Analg 89: 962–964.

Yuki K, Kodama Y, Onda J et al. (1991). Coronary vasospasm following subarachnoid hemorrhage as a cause of stunned myocardium. J Neurosurg 75: 308–311.

Zaroff JG, Rordorf GA, Newell JB et al. (1999). Cardiac outcome in patients with subarachnoid hemorrhage and electrocardiographic abnormalities. Neurosurgery 44: 34–39. discussion 39–40.

Zaroff JG, Rordorf GA, Ogilvy CS et al. (2000a). Regional patterns of left ventricular systolic dysfunction after subarachnoid hemorrhage: evidence for neurally mediated cardiac injury. J Am Soc Echocardiogr 13: 774–779.

Zaroff JG, Rordorf GA, Titus JS et al. (2000b). Regional myocardial perfusion after experimental subarachnoid hemorrhage. Stroke 31: 1136–1143.

Zhang ZH, Dougherty PM, Oppenheimer SM (1998). Characterization of baroreceptor-related neurons in the monkey insular cortex. Brain Res 796: 303–306.

Zheng Z, Croft J, Giles WH et al. (2001). Sudden cardiac death in the United States. Circulation 104: 2158–2163.

*Handbook of Clinical Neurology, Vol. 140 (3rd series)*
*Critical Care Neurology, Part I*
E.F.M. Wijdicks and A.H. Kramer, Editors
http://dx.doi.org/10.1016/B978-0-444-63600-3.00005-2

Chapter 5

# Principles of intracranial pressure monitoring and treatment

M. CZOSNYKA[1]*, J.D. PICKARD[1], AND L.A. STEINER[2]

[1]*Department of Clinical Neurosciences, University of Cambridge, Cambridge, UK*

[2]*Department for Anesthesia, Surgical Intensive Care, Prehospital Emergency Medicine and Pain Therapy, University Hospital of Basel, Basel, Switzerland*

## Abstract

Intracranial pressure (ICP) is governed by volumes of intracranial blood, cerebrospinal fluid, and brain tissue. Expansion of any of these volumes will trigger compensatory changes in the other compartments, resulting in initially limited change in ICP. Due to the rigid skull, once compensatory mechanisms are exhausted, ICP rises very rapidly. Intracranial hypertension is associated with unfavorable outcome in brain-injured patients. This chapter discusses the pathophysiology of raised ICP, as well as typical waveforms, monitoring techniques, and clinical management. The dynamics of ICP are more important than the absolute value at any given time point, but mean ICP exceeding 20–25 mmHg is usually treated aggressively. Algorithms based on data from patients with traumatic brain injury are applied also in other conditions. However, an understanding of the underlying pathophysiology allows adaptation of therapies to other pathologies. Typically, a three-staged approach is used, starting with restoration of systemic physiology, sedation, and analgesia. If these measures are insufficient, surgical options, such as drainage of cerebrospinal fluid or evacuation of mass lesions, are considered. In the absence of surgical options, stage 2 treatments are initiated, consisting of either mannitol or hypertonic saline. If these measures are insufficient, stage 3 therapies include hypothermia, metabolic suppression, or craniectomy.

## NEUROPATHOLOGY AND PATHOPHYSIOLOGY OF INTRACRANIAL HYPERTENSION:

### Essential principles and semiquantitative relationships

In most organs, perfusion pressure equals the difference between inlet (arterial) and outlet (venous) pressures. Intracranial outlet pressure differs in this respect from central venous pressure or cerebral venous sinus pressure, as the brain is surrounded by a rigid skull. Intracranial venous pressure is coupled to intracranial pressure (ICP). Therefore, cerebral perfusion pressure (CPP) is defined as follows (Miller et al., 1972):

$$\text{Mean CPP} = \text{mean arterial pressure} - \text{mean ICP}$$

One might expect that a rise in ICP would impede blood flow and cause ischemia. However, this is not the case, assuming autoregulation of cerebral blood flow (CBF) works correctly.

ICP is a complex modality derived from volumetric changes of intracranial blood, cerebrospinal fluid (CSF), brain parenchyma plus, in pathologic states, space-occupying lesions. Classically, the Monro–Kellie doctrine states that the sum of all intracranial volumes must remain constant. This is probably not 100% accurate, as the volume of the dural sac in the lumbar channel may expand slightly against internal vertebral venous plexuses.

ICP has dynamic (changing in time) and static (which may also change over time, but at a much slower rate) components. Both fast and slow changes in ICP are

*Correspondence to: Marek Czosnyka, PhD, Professor of Brain Physics, Department of Clinical Neurosciences, University of Cambridge, UK. Tel: +44-1223-336946, E-mail: mc141@medschl.cam.ac.uk

associated with a change of volume of arterial and venous blood, CSF, and brain tissue (edema formation) or other volume/space-occupying lesions (e.g., hematomas, tumors, or abscesses). It is important to distinguish between different components of ICP, as optimal clinical strategies to combat intracranial hypertension depend on which component is elevated. For example, arterial blood volume may raise ICP to very high levels in a matter of minutes and these elevations are known as plateau waves, which are secondary to massive, intrinsic arterial dilatation. Rapid, short-term hyperventilation usually reduces ICP in such cases. The CSF-circulatory component may elevate ICP in a scenario of acute hydrocephalus. In such cases, extraventricular drainage is particularly helpful. Venous outflow obstruction may also elevate ICP, and proper head positioning or investigation of possible venous thrombosis may be crucial. Finally, if ICP is elevated due to brain edema or a space-occupying lesion, osmotherapy or surgical intervention (including decompressive craniectomy) may be especially beneficial.

Dynamic components of ICP are mainly derived from the circulation of cerebral blood and CSF (the mathematic operator in the formula below should not be represented by a simple sum, therefore the generic symbol # is used):

$$\mathrm{ICP} = \mathrm{ICP_{vascular}} \, \# \, \mathrm{ICP_{CSF}}$$

The vascular component is difficult to express quantitatively. It is probably derived from the pulsation of the cerebral blood volume (CBV) detected and averaged by nonlinear mechanisms of regulation of cerebral blood and CSF volumes. More generally, multiple variables such as the arterial pressure, state of autoregulation, and cerebral venous outflow all contribute to the vascular component.

The CSF-circulatory component may be expressed using Davson's equation (Davson et al., 1970):

$$\mathrm{ICP_{CSF}} = (\text{resistance to CSF outflow}) * (\text{CSF formation}) + (\text{pressure in sagittal sinus})$$

Any factor which, under physiologic (e.g., compression of jugular veins) or pathologic conditions (e.g., brain swelling, space-occupying lesion, or obstruction of CSF absorption) disturbs CSF circulation, may provoke an increase in ICP according to this formula.

## Cerebral autoregulation and pressure-volume compensation

Autoregulation concerns the relationship between CPP and cerebrovascular resistance. It is difficult to express quantitatively; therefore, only a pictorial representation is offered. Normally, resistive small arteries and arterioles dilate when CPP decreases. This helps to stabilize CBF within a wide range of CPP. This range is limited by maximal dilatation in the lower range of CPP and maximal vasoconstriction in the upper range (Lassen, 1964). These critical levels of CPP are respectively termed the lower and upper range of autoregulation. Thus, the relationship between CBF and CPP is nonlinear (Fig. 5.1). As CPP represents the pressure gradient

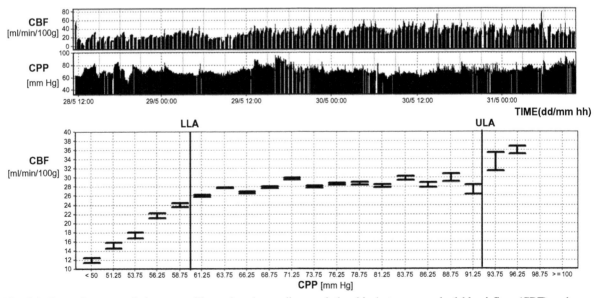

**Fig. 5.1.** Lassen's autoregulation curve illustrating the nonlinear relationship between cerebral blood flow (CBF) and cerebral perfusion pressure (CPP). CBF (using thermodilution probe; gaps in monitoring are related to periodic self-calibration cycles of the CBF monitor) and CPP (mean arterial blood pressure minus mean intracranial pressure) were monitored continuously over 3.5 days in a patient after severe traumatic brain injury. Values of CBF averaged within 2.5-mmHg intervals of CPP from 50 to 100 mmHg and 2 standard error bars were plotted. LLA, lower limit of autoregulation; ULA, upper limit of autoregulation.

acting along the cerebrovascular bed, it is an important factor in the regulation of CBF. Sufficient CPP is required to maintain stable CBF. The autoregulatory reserve is interpreted as the difference between the current mean CPP and the lower limit of autoregulation. Low CPP (beyond a threshold of 40–60 mmHg) may result in exhaustion of the autoregulatory reserve. However, this lower threshold may vary within broader limits, as much as 40–90 mmHg between individual patients. Policies to therapeutically maintain a high CPP are controversial. If the cerebral vessels are nonreactive, an increase in CPP may result in hyperemia, worsening of vasogenic edema, and a secondary increment in ICP. It is also probable that patient- and time-dependent variations in the level of CPP at which autoregulation functions properly may be considerable. Therefore, the threshold between adequate and inadequate CPP should be assessed individually and frequently, as it may change over time (Steiner et al., 2002).

Secondary to cerebral autoregulation is control of cerebral arterial blood volume. Increases or decreases in cerebrovascular resistance lead to its square-root-proportional rise or fall in blood volume in resistive arterioles; the volume of conductive arteries is thought to be more stable. This, in turn, may produce exponential changes in ICP due to the shape of the intracranial pressure–volume curve (Marmarou et al., 1978). It is a relationship between changes of net intracerebral volume and ICP (Fig. 5.2, left).

There is no consensus about which volume should be represented along the x-axis of this model of intracranial compliance. CSF volume can be changed using bolus or constant-rate injection, and can be investigated during diagnostic tests of hydrocephalus patients. When the volume of extra- or subdural balloons is studied experimentally, a linear relationship between volume and mean ICP is observed at low pressures. Above a certain ICP threshold (usually still within the range of normal ICP values), an exponential relationship exists:

$$p = (p_b - p_o) \cdot e^{E\Delta V} + p_o$$

where $p_b$ is baseline pressure and $\Delta V$ is an increase in volume; $E$ is elasticity of the system; and $p_o$ is an elusive reference pressure (some researchers consider it to be zero). This curve may also have an upper deflection point, seen when so-called critical ICP is exceeded (Löfgren et al., 1973). This curve may explain the relationship between the pulse amplitude of ICP and mean ICP. For ICP below the linear-exponential breakpoint on the pressure–volume curve, the pulse amplitude does not depend on ICP. The amplitude increases with ICP within the limits of the exponential portion of the pressure–volume curve. Above a critical pressure, it starts to decrease with further increments in ICP (Fig. 5.2, right).

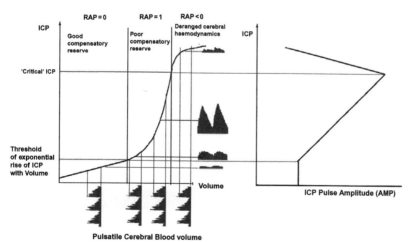

**Fig. 5.2.** Intracranial pressure–volume curve (left) and relationship between mean intracranial pressure (ICP) and amplitude of pulsatile component of ICP waveform (right). The pressure–volume curve has three zones (along the volume axis): first, ICP changes proportionally to changes of intracranial volume (good compensatory reserve). Then ICP increases exponentially with further rise in volume (poor compensatory reserve). Above certain critical ICPs, the pressure–volume curve deflects to the right, probably due to collapse of the cerebral arteriole bed. Accordingly (right panel), pulse amplitude of ICP is not dependent on mean ICP within the range of good compensatory reserve. Then it increases proportionately with increase in mean ICP. Above critical ICP, amplitude decreases when ICP rises further. RAP is the correlation coefficient between changes in pulse amplitude and mean ICP, and is a useful parameter for continuous monitoring of cerebral compensatory reserve.

## CLINICAL PRESENTATION AND NEURODIAGNOSTICS

### Methods of measurement

An intraventricular drain connected to an external pressure transducer is still considered to be the "gold-standard" method (Guillaume and Janny, 1951). ICP is measured as a fluid pressure and can be lowered by CSF drainage. ICP values monitored with an open drain are invalid in most cases. The transducer may be zeroed externally as often as necessary. However, with increasing duration of monitoring, particularly beyond 5 days, the risk of infection starts to increase, with an overall risk estimated to be about 5%. Insertion of the ventricular catheter may be difficult or impossible in cases of advanced brain swelling with compression of the lateral ventricles.

Modern intraparenchymal microtransducers (the most popular types include Camino, Codman, Raumedic, and Pressio-Sophysa) have lower infection rates than ventricular drains. The risk of clinically significant hemorrhage is less than 1% (Koskinen et al., 2013). These monitors have excellent metrologic properties, as revealed during bench tests (i.e., bandwidth and linearity). However, there is a drawback: uniformly distributed ICP can probably only be seen when CSF circulates freely between all its natural fluid pools, equilibrating pressure everywhere according to Pascal's law. With little or no CSF volume left due to brain swelling, the assumption of one uniform value of ICP is questionable. With the most common intraparenchymal probes, measured pressure may be compartmentalized, and not necessarily representative of equally distributed ICP. Moreover, brain tissue microtransducers do not actually directly measure a pressure, but rather a tensor of force (strain) within a tissue. Measurements may be dampened by a direction of this strain that is not necessarily perpendicular to the pressure-sensitive element. In addition, microtransducers can generally not be re-zeroed after insertion, and considerable zero drift may occur during long-term monitoring.

Contemporary epidural sensors are much more reliable than 10 years ago. But the question as to whether epidural pressure can express ICP with confidence and under all circumstances remains unanswered.

Lumbar CSF pressure is seldom measured in neurointensive care, although it could have a role in monitoring of spinal cord perfusion. This form of assessment of craniospinal dynamics is more often used in management of hydrocephalus and idiopathic intracranial hypertension. It is important to emphasize that reliable monitoring over at least a half-hour period, with recording of pressure and pulse amplitude, should be required in making clinical decisions. Instant, manometric assessment by measuring the height of the CSF column (as during a lumbar puncture) may be misleading, since CSF pressure may vary considerably over time (Fig. 5.3).

### Attempts to measure ICP and CPP noninvasively

It would be very helpful to measure ICP and CPP without invasive transducers. A number of techniques are available, but are still in a phase of technical or clinical

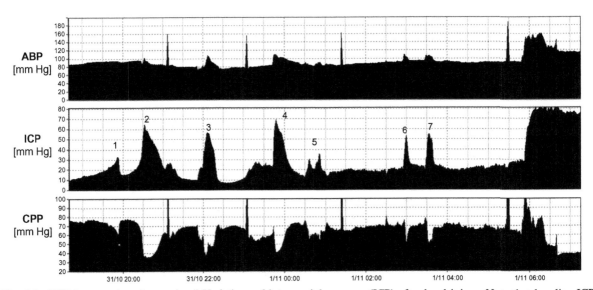

**Fig. 5.3.** "ICP is more than the number." Variations of intracranial pressure (ICP) after head injury. Note that baseline ICP was < 20 mmHg. ICP plateau waves are present with ICP > 60 mmHg. After seven spontaneous plateau waves, the eighth was sustained, with ICP > 70 mmHg and cerebral perfusion pressure (CPP) < 40 mmHg preceding the patient's death. ABP, arterial blood pressure.

evaluation (Robba et al., 2016). Aaslid's description of transcranial Doppler (TCD) sonography in 1982 permitted noninvasive, repeated (or even continuous) monitoring of one index of CBF (Aaslid et al., 1982). TCD measures flow velocity in branches of the circle of Willis, most commonly the middle cerebral artery (MCA). The compliant walls of this large artery can be compared to two physiologic pressure transducers. The pattern of flow within the MCA is modulated by transmural pressure (i.e., CPP), vascular tone affecting arterial compliance, and distal vascular resistance (which is also modulated by CPP). The trouble, as we remain ignorant about the calibration factor, is how stable it is over time, and how we should compensate for unknown nonlinear distortions.

There is a reasonable correlation between the pulsatility index of the MCA velocity and CPP after head injury, but absolute measurements of CPP cannot be done with an accuracy better than 30–35 mmHg. Others have suggested that critical closing pressure derived from flow velocity and arterial pressure waveform approximates ICP (Dewey et al., 1974). This is not accurate, as critical closing pressure is a sum of ICP and arterial wall tension. In a state of intracranial normotension (ICP less than 15 mmHg), wall tension on average amounts to 70–80% of a value of critical closing pressure.

Aaslid et al. (1986) suggested that an index of CPP could be derived from the ratio of the amplitudes of the first harmonics of the arterial blood pressure (ABP) and the TCD MCA multiplied by mean flow velocity. More recently, a method for the noninvasive assessment of CPP has been reported, derived from mean arterial pressure multiplied by the ratio of diastolic to mean flow velocity (Schmidt et al., 2001). This estimator can predict real CPP with an error of less than 10 mmHg for more than 80% of measurements.

A more complex method aimed at the noninvasive assessment of ICP has been introduced and tested by Schmidt et al. (1997). The method is based on the presumed linear transformation between arterial pressure and ICP waveforms. Coefficients of this transformation are derived from a database of real ABP and ICP recordings. A similar linear transformation is built, using the same database, between flow velocity and arterial pressure. Then, the model assumes a linear relationship between arterial pressure and flow velocity and between arterial pressure and ICP. Multiple regression coefficients are calculated. Finally, for each prospective study, ICP is calculated using an ABP to ICP transformation, formed by an ABP to flow velocity transformation and transposed using precalculated regression coefficients.

Comparison of the intraocular and intracranial portions of the ophthalmic artery TCD pulse waveform allows detection when intraocular pressure equilibrates ICP. With external compression of eyeball, such a measurement was demonstrated to be accurate (absolute accuracy ±5 mmHg). A prototype of this promising device is now under test in clinical practice (Ragauskas et al., 2012).

## Typical waves and trends observed in ICP monitoring

It is difficult to establish a universal "normal value" for ICP, as it depends on age, body posture, clinical conditions, and many other factors. In the horizontal position, the normal ICP in a healthy adult subject is estimated to be within the range of 7–15 mmHg. In the vertical body position, it is zero or slightly negative, but not lower than –8 mmHg (based on our own experience in patients suffering from hydrocephalus).

The definition of raised ICP depends on the specific pathology. In hydrocephalus, a pressure above 15 mmHg can be regarded as elevated. Following traumatic brain injury (TBI), anything above 20 mmHg is abnormal, and aggressive treatment usually starts above 25 mmHg. However, recent studies in TBI may justify individualization of elevated ICP, with a proposed definition being the level above which autoregulation of CBF starts to be affected (Lazaridis et al., 2014), which may vary from 15 to 40 mmHg.

It is important to recognize that ICP is "more than a number," and in most cases is time-varying. Averaging for at least 30 minutes is needed to calculate mean ICP. Instant values of ICP read at a once-per-hour interval are not accurate.

The ICP waveform consists of three components, which overlap in the time domain, but can be separated in the frequency domain (Fig. 5.4). The pulse waveform has fundamental and several higher harmonic components. The fundamental component has a frequency equal to the heart rate. The amplitude of this component is very useful for the evaluation of intracranial physiology. The respiratory waveform is related to the frequency of the respiratory rate (8–20 breaths/minute). "Slow waves" are not as precisely defined as in the original Lundberg thesis (Lundberg, 1960). All components that have a spectral representation within the frequency limits of 20 seconds to a 3-minute period can be classified as slow waves. The magnitude of these waves can be calculated as the square root of the power of the signal at the output of the digital filter.

In time domain, ICP pulse waveform usually presents three peaks: P1, P2, and P3 (Cardoso et al., 1983). The earliest peak, P1, called the percussion peak, is probably related to the immediate distension of arterial walls when arterial pressure pulse waveform reaches its systolic maximum. The two delayed peaks, P2 and P3, are probably related to an arterial blood volume increase, and

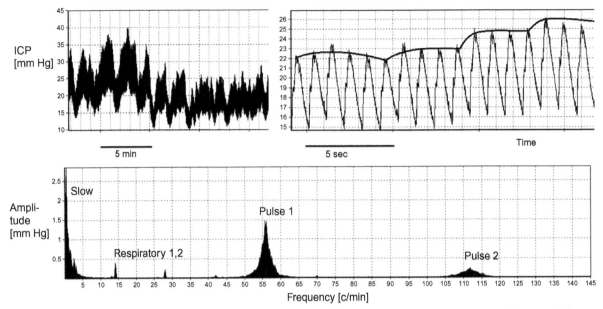

**Fig. 5.4.** Components of intracranial pressure (ICP) observed in the time domain (top) and frequency domain (bottom). Left upper panel illustrates slow vasogenic waves (0.005–0.05 Hz) associated with continuous vasomotor activity, controlling cerebrovascular resistance, cerebral blood flow, and cerebral blood volume. Right upper panel shows pulse waveform of ICP and slower wave. All these components are well separated in the frequency domain: the power spectrum of ICP signal shows slow, respiratory, and pulse waves (fundamentals and higher harmonics).

transport from conductive large cerebral arteries to resistive arterioles, influenced also by intracranial compliance, as described by the pressure–volume curve. Some investigators associate peak P3 with the dicrotic notch and second peak of ABP, which in turn may be attributable to closure of the aortic valve (Fig. 5.5).

There is much more information contained in the ICP waveform than only a time-averaged mean value. Computer-supported displays, with multiscale averaging, show a complexity of different ICP waveform components. When monitored continuously in the acute state (e.g., TBI, poor-grade subarachnoid hemorrhage (SAH), intracerebral hemorrhage), ICP waveforms may show specific fluctuations. They may have the character of repetitive waves or irregular transients. Already mentioned, "slow waves" (also referred to as "B waves," according to the Lundberg nomenclature) have a repetitive character. In the frequency domain, they fall into the bandwidth of 0.005–0.05 Hz. They are coherent with fluctuation of arterial blood volume assessed with near-infrared spectroscopy (NIRS) (Fig. 5.6). Sometimes they are synchronized with fluctuations of ABP. They are thought to be related to cerebral vasocycling, secondary to multiple mechanisms of CBF control, working together and sometimes synchronizing at these specific frequencies. Within faster spectra (around 0.1 Hz for a 10-second period), regular B waves may have a character of Mayer waves, initiated by fluctuations of arterial pressure brought about by oscillations in baroreceptor and

chemoreceptor control systems. These waves produce autoregulatory-induced changes in CBV and are phase-shifted compared to responses seen in ICP. Both Mayer waves and classic B waves are important. In clinical practice, they may be used for monitoring a state of cerebral autoregulation (see below).

Lundberg A waves or plateau waves usually have a dramatic appearance. They produce increases of ICP up to 100 mmHg, lasting from minutes to hours, associated with an increase in ICP, loss of autoregulation, and reduction in CPP, CBF, and brain tissue oxygen tension ($P_{bti}O_2$) (Dias et al., 2014) (Fig. 5.7). A waves may be observed as one-off transients or occur in a cyclic manner (e.g., once every hour or every few hours). The mechanism of plateau waves has been explained elegantly by Rosner and Becker (1984) as a "vasodilatatory cascade." This vasodilatory cascade involves a "vicious cycle" or "positive-feedback loop" that is initiated by cerebral vasodilatation, which increases CBV and ICP, and decreases CPP, which in turn produces further cerebral vasodilation, eventually resulting in a crisis. This occurs especially when autoregulation is working and the pressure–volume curve is steep. A "vasoconstriction cascade" works under the same principle, but in the opposite direction, leading to termination of plateau waves. Although they usually terminate spontaneously after a few minutes, every plateau wave constitutes a potential ischemic insult. Plateau waves are relatively common, occurring in approximately 40% of TBI patients, and their appearance is not categorically

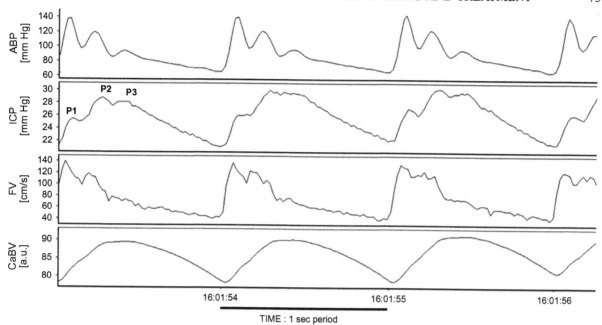

**Fig. 5.5.** P1, P2, and P3 are peaks of the intracranial pulse waveform. P1 is undoubtedly associated with systole of arterial blood pressure waveform. Flow velocity (FV) and cerebral arterial blood volume (CaBV) show recorded parameters of blood FV and CaBV using middle cerebral artery transcranial Doppler tracing. Peaks P2 and P3 are usually associated with peaks seen on CaBV – they are related to blood volume rise and its transmission through the linear pressure–volume curve (Fig. 5.2). ABP, arterial blood pressure; ICP, intracranial pressure.

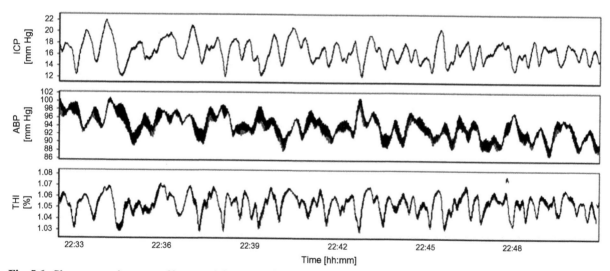

**Fig. 5.6.** Slow vasogenic waves of intracranial pressure (ICP) seem to be ideally synchronized with slow fluctuations of the total hemoglobin index (THI), recorded using near-infrared spectroscopy, which may be treated as surrogate index of changing (fluctuating) cerebral blood volume. ABP, arterial blood pressure.

associated with poor outcomes. However, longer duration of plateau waves, especially when exceeding 30 minutes, has been correlated with worse outcomes (Castellani et al., 2009). At the bedside, any intervention that induces cerebral vasoconstriction, such as transient hyperventilation or a bolus of hypertonic saline, may be sufficient to terminate longer plateau waves.

Low and stable ICP, with low waveform amplitude can be observed in TBI just after admission. More frequently, we see elevated and stable ICP (>20 mmHg). Many ICP waves and transients are related to changes in arterial pressure. If changes in ABP are deep and very fast, ICP usually changes in the same direction (Fig. 5.8A). If changes in ABP are slower, the direction

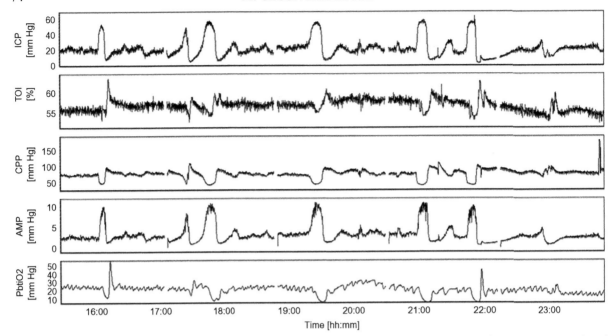

**Fig. 5.7.** Plateau waves of intracranial pressure (ICP) in multimodal monitoring (brain tissue oxygenation ($P_{bti}O_2$), near-infrared spectroscopy-derived tissue oxygenation index (TOI), cerebral perfusion pressure (CPP), and pulse amplitude of ICP tracing (AMP)). During each plateau wave, CPP, $P_{bti}O_2$, and TOI decrease. Cerebral blood flow (not monitored in this segment) also decreases and amplitude increases. Specific periods of hyperemia can be seen in $P_{bti}O_2$ and TOI after each plateau wave.

of changes in ICP depends on cerebrovascular reactivity. With reactive vessels, ICP changes in the opposite direction to changes in ABP. With nonreactive vessels the change is in the same direction (Fig. 5.8B). Elevations of ICP can be also seen during hyperemia. In this case, changes in ICP are in the same direction as changes in CBF or $P_{bti}O_2$, due to an increase in CBV (Fig. 5.8C). Episodes of refractory intracranial hypertension are sometimes accompanied by the characteristic upper breakpoint in the relationship between ICP pulse amplitude and mean ICP level (Fig. 5.8D).

## Cerebrovascular pressure reactivity and autoregulation

A useful ICP-derived modality is the pressure–reactivity index (PRx), which incorporates the philosophy of assessing cerebrovascular reactions by observing the response of ICP to slow spontaneous changes in ABP (Czosnyka et al., 1997). When the cerebrovascular bed is reactive, any change in ABP produces an inverse change in CBV and hence ICP. When reactivity is disturbed, changes in ABP are passively transmitted to ICP. Using computational methods, PRx is determined by calculating the correlation coefficient between 30 consecutive, 10-second time-averaged data points of ICP and ABP. A positive PRx signifies a positive gradient of the regression line between the slow components of ABP and ICP, which we hypothesize to be associated

with passive behavior of a nonreactive vascular bed. A negative value of PRx reflects a normally reactive vascular bed, as ABP waves provoke inversely correlated waves in ICP.

PRx is strongly dependent on CPP. It increases with decreasing CPP, when the lower limit of cerebral autoregulation is breached (Brady et al., 2008). In clinical practice (TBI patients), PRx correlates well with indices of autoregulation based on TCD ultrasonography. It has been positively verified against the static rate of autoregulation with positron emission tomography-mapped CBF (Steiner et al., 2003). It can also be used to illustrate changes in cerebrovascular reactivity during phenomena containing a strong vascular component (e.g., loss of reactivity during plateau waves of ICP (Fig. 5.9A) or during refractory intracranial hypertension (Fig. 5.9B).

Averaged PRx is, besides age, Glasgow Coma Scale, and mean ICP, an independent predictor of outcome after TBI. A critical value of PRx, associated with increased mortality, is approximately +0.25. The prognostic implications of average value from +0.25 to 0 are uncertain, while an average PRx < 0 is associated with favorable outcome (Sorrentino et al., 2012).

## Optimal CPP and critical ICP

PRx plotted against CPP often shows a U-shaped curve (Steiner et al., 2003). The minimum of this curve theoretically indicates the midpoint between the lower and

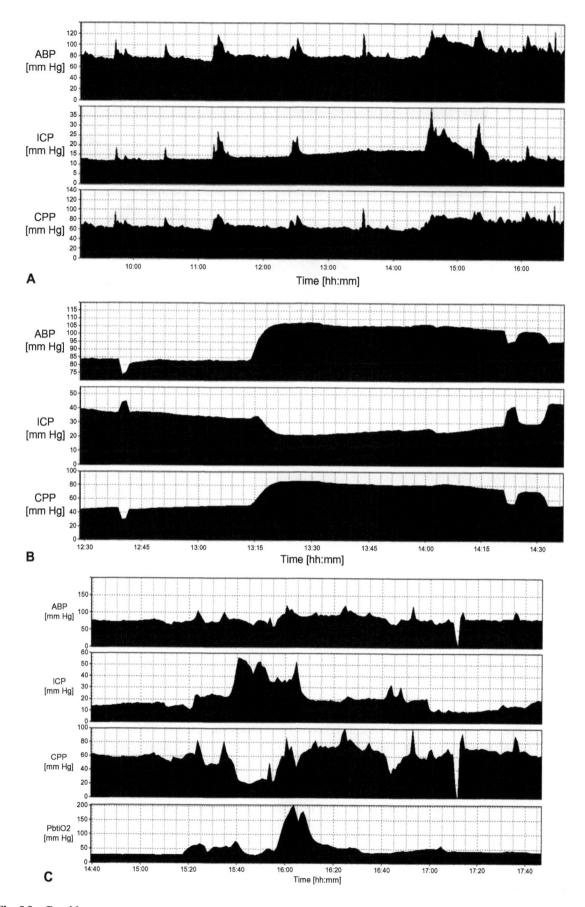

**Fig. 5.8—Cont'd**

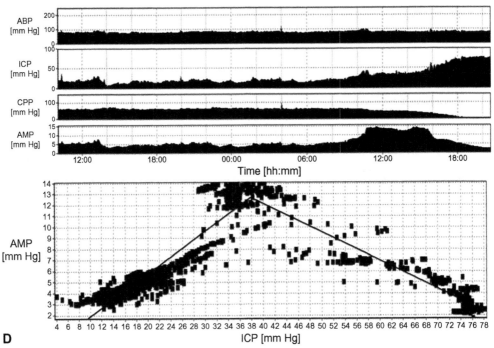

**D**

**Fig. 5.8—Cont'd** Typical intracranial pressure (ICP) patterns, seen in continuous monitoring. (**A**) ICP-arterial blood pressure (ABP) fast waves. Fast changes in ABP (faster than 0.1 mmHg/second, experimental data; Barzó et al., 1993) are always transmitted to ICP, regardless of the state of cerebral autoregulation. (**B**) ICP-ABP responses during slower transients in ABP. Association may be positive (disturbed autoregulation) or negative (functional autoregulation). In this case autoregulation was intact. (**C**) Hyperemic waves. Increases in ICP secondary to increase in cerebral blood flow. $P_{bti}O_2$ also increases with CBF and after the wave- reacting with temporary deep hyperaemia. (**D**) Refractory rise in ICP, related to uncontrollable increase in brain swelling, increasing ICP > 50 mmHg. Note the behavior of ICP pulse amplitude and an amplitude (AMP)–pressure line, presenting upper breakpoint associated with "critical ICP" at 36 mmHg. CPP, cerebral perfusion pressure.

upper breakpoint of the autoregulatory curve (Fig. 5.1). PRx increases below the lower limit of autoregulation (ischemia) and above the upper limit (hyperemia). This optimal CPP can be clinically estimated in real time by plotting and analyzing PRx–CPP curves in sequential 4-hour time windows (Fig. 5.10A). It has been demonstrated in retrospective studies that a greater discrepancy between the actual and optimal CPP is associated with worse outcomes in TBI patients (Steiner et al., 2002; Aries et al., 2012). This potentially useful methodology attempts to refine and individualize CPP-oriented therapy. Both too low (ischemia) and too high CPP (hyperemia and secondary increase in ICP) are detrimental. In one study, ischemia was associated with increased mortality, while hyperemia was associated with an increased rate of severe disability (Aries et al., 2012). Hence, it has been suggested that CPP should be optimized to maintain cerebral perfusion in the globally most favorable state. However, this concept still awaits multicenter prospective study. Retrospective analysis shows that optimal CPP may vary individually (from 60 to 100 mmHg) and may differ dramatically from guideline-fixed thresholds. Moreover, optimal CPP

may vary over the course of postinjury intensive care. This same concept is probably valid in patients after poor-grade SAH (Bijlenga et al., 2010).

Several related methods have been suggested to detect and monitor optimal CPP with 1-minute averaged ICP and ABP values to calculate a so-called "long-PRx" (Santos et al., 2011) and using varying time windows for tracing an optimal CPP using the long-PRx versus CPP U-shaped curve (Depreitere et al., 2014).

PRx and the optimal CPP U-shape curve are only valid if pressure–volume compensatory reserve is normal or low. In patients with increased reserve (e.g., following decompressive craniectomy), detection is problematic. In such cases, instead of using PRx, the PAx index may be helpful (correlation between pulse amplitude of ICP and mean ABP: Radolovich et al., 2011). In addition, NIRS-based indices of cerebrovascular reactivity (see further remarks) have some potential value (Brady et al., 2008).

Per analogy to the U-shaped PRx–CPP curve, the relationship between PRx and ICP can be observed. Usually, PRx monotonically increases with rising ICP. The value

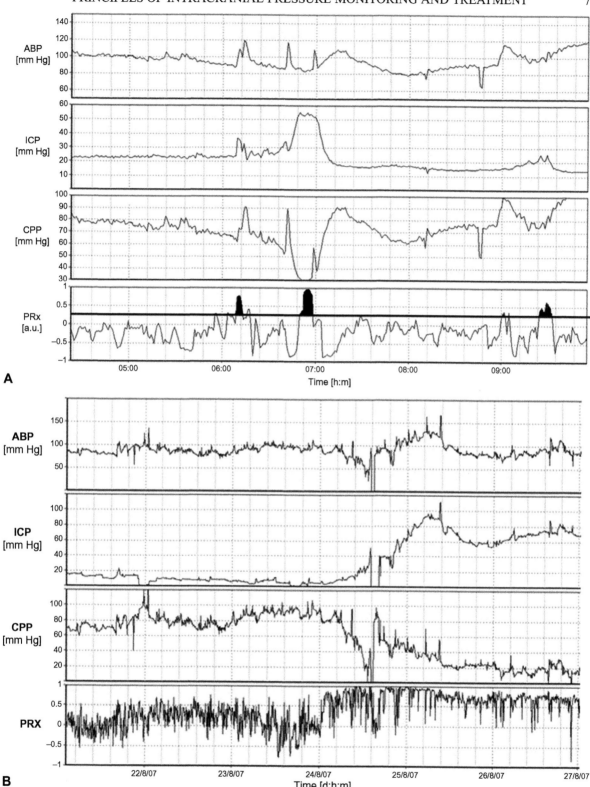

**Fig. 5.9.** Variability in pressure–reactivity index (PRx). (**A**) During plateau wave, PRx increased to nearly +1. (**B**) During refractory intracranial hypertension, PRx increased above 0.3, 12 hours before ICP increased above 20 mmHg, initiating a positive-feedback loop leading to final transtentorial herniation. ABP, arterial blood pressure; ICP, intracranial pressure; CPP, cerebral perfusion pressure.

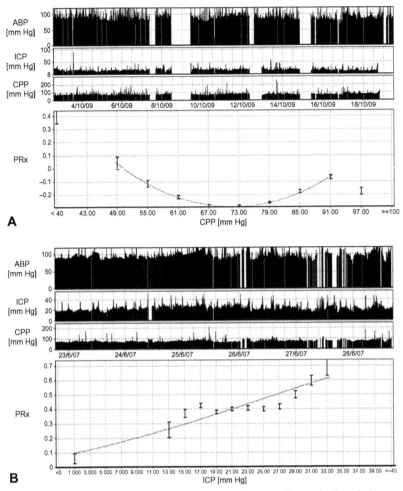

**Fig. 5.10.** It is not true that "one shoe number suits everyone." Therapeutic targets for cerebral perfusion pressure (CPP) and intracranial pressure (ICP) can be assessed individually. (**A**) Pressure–reactivity index (PRx) plotted against CPP, often usually a U-shaped curve. Minimum of this curve indicates midpoint between lower limit of autoregulation and upper limit of autoregulation (compare with Fig. 5.1). This is a hypothetic "optimal" value of CPP, which may substantially vary from patient to patient. (**B**) PRx plotted against ICP usually shows monotonically rising level. Value of ICP for which PRx increases above 0.3 is postulated as therapeutic threshold for elevated ICP. ABP, arterial blood pressure.

of ICP above which vascular reactivity is disturbed (PRx > 0.25) has been postulated as the individual critical ICP level (Fig. 5.10B). In a group of more than 300 patients after TBI, the critical threshold of ICP varied from 15 to 40 mmHg (mean 24 mmHg) (Lazaridis et al., 2014). Time with ICP greater than this individual critical ICP correlated with worse outcome, stronger than mean ICP, or fixed-threshold time integral of ICP.

## Pressure–volume compensatory reserve

Theoretically, compensatory reserve can be studied through the relationship between ICP and changes in volume of the intracranial space, known as the pressure–volume curve. The index RAP (correlation coefficient ($R$) between amplitude ($A$) and mean ICP ($P$)) can be derived by calculating the linear correlation between consecutive, time-averaged data points of amplitude and ICP (usually 30 averages are used) acquired over a reasonably long period to average respiratory and pulse waves (usually 10-second periods) (Czosnyka et al., 1994).

An RAP coefficient close to 0 indicates a lack of synchronization between changes in amplitude and average ICP. This denotes favorable pressure–volume compensatory reserve at low ICP (Fig. 5.2), where a change in intracranial volume produces little change of ICP. When RAP rises to +1, amplitude varies directly with ICP, indicating that the working point of the intracranial space shifts towards the right to the steep part of the pressure–volume curve, where compensatory reserve is low. Therefore, any further rise in volume may produce a rapid increase in ICP. Following TBI and subsequent brain swelling, RAP is usually close to +1. With any further increase in ICP, amplitude decreases and RAP values fall below zero. This occurs when the cerebral autoregulatory capacity is exhausted and the pressure–volume curve bends sharply to the right as the capacity of cerebral arterioles to dilate further in response to a CPP decrement has reached its limit, and the arterioles tend to collapse passively (Fig. 5.2). This indicates terminal cerebrovascular derangement with a decrease in pulse pressure transmission from the arterial bed to the intracranial compartment. Monitoring of RAP in time after head injury may be helpful in understanding phenomena related to increase or decrease of brain edema, or when ICP level reaches the critical threshold for the integrity of CBF (Fig. 5.11).

## Other methods of ICP analysis

There are numerous controversies about how to best utilize and characterize the ICP signal. Even how to perform time averaging, is a source of disagreement. With its various waves and transients, ICP is "more than a number"; information about changes over time contains potentially useful clinical information. Averaging over the whole monitoring period gives us a single number, which is associated with outcome after TBI. The "dose of ICP" above a certain predefined threshold (Vik et al., 2008) produces a number with apparently stronger outcome association. Cumulative time above an individual threshold of

critical ICP, above which pressure reactivity of cerebral vessels is impaired has been advocated as an even stronger outcome predictor (Lazaridis et al., 2014).

Another high priority in brain monitoring would be to develop a technique that helps predict decompensation or herniation. Rises of ICP can be anticipated within a 10–30-minute time horizon using sophisticated data analysis methods and machine-learning algorithms (Güiza et al., 2013).

Brain compliance monitoring (Piper et al., 1993), integrated into the so-called Spiegelberg monitor, was an interesting concept. It was based on direct measurement of the rise of ICP to repetitive expansion of a balloon placed in the intracranial space. Initial results were promising, but wider use was hampered by the invasive nature of the method.

Analysis of the pulse waveform of ICP, known as the high-frequency centroid, was based on evaluation of the power spectrum of a single-pulse ICP waveform and calculation of its power-weighted average frequency within the range of 5–15 Hz. The high-frequency centroid was demonstrated to decrease with increasing ICP. The centroid increases in the state of refractory intracranial hypertension where the blood flow regulation mechanism fails (Robertson et al., 1989).

Pulse transmission between arterial pressure and mean ICP has been investigated by various groups

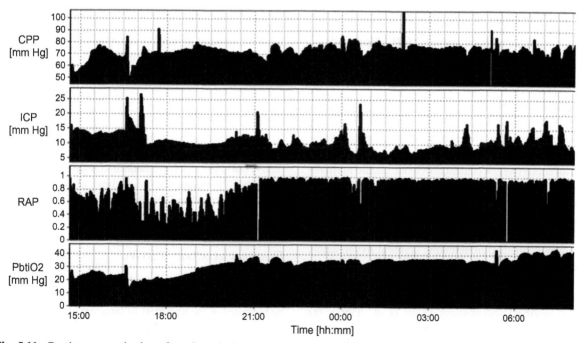

**Fig. 5.11.** Continuous monitoring of cerebrospinal compensatory reserve. Patient with traumatic brain injury monitored over first day after head injury. Compensatory reserve was good during initial period (RAP around 0.4) with gradual depletion of the reserve (RAP close to +1) later, due to brain swelling. Note that this is not automatically associated with a rise in mean intracranial pressure (ICP). CPP, cerebral perfusion pressure; RAP, correlation coefficient ($R$) between amplitude ($A$) and mean intracranial pressure ($P$).

(Piper et al., 1990). The utility of this approach depends upon assumptions about the linearity of the transmission model. Such assumptions are probably unrealistic, particularly in pathologic circumstances.

Morphologic analysis of pulse ICP waveform, with a sophisticated method of detection of peaks P1, P2, P3, and delineation of different curvatures and proportions between peaks and valleys (Hu et al., 2010), was proposed to detect ischemic brain insults, prediction of intracranial hypertensive episodes, and state of vascular wall tension.

Recently, the power of slow waves of ICP was reported to be predictive of outcome in patients suffering from intracranial hypertension following TBI. A low proportion of slow waves in the overall ICP dynamics was associated with a fatal outcome (Balestreri et al., 2005), highlighting a possible link of these events with cerebral autoregulation. Also, the complexity of long-term monitored ICP signals after TBI showed promising clinical correlation (Lu et al., 2012). Multiscale entropy measured as a global index was decreased in patients with worse outcome.

No matter how sophisticated new variables or outcome-predicting models become, perhaps the most useful tool at the bedside is a computerized display that presents the trends of multiple parameters over time. This gives an opportunity to react to a crisis situation, understand cerebral dynamics in multiple dimensions, and predict an optimal strategy for individual patients' care.

## Consequences of raised ICP observed with multimodal brain monitoring

### Cerebral oxygenation

Jugular venous bulb oxygen saturation ($S_jO_2$) may be monitored, preferably continuously, with an indwelling catheter. Single measurements of $S_jO_2$ are of little value given the many fluctuations during the day. The cerebral arteriovenous oxygen content difference should normally be 5–7 mL/dL. Values below 4 mL/dL may indicate cerebral hyperemia, whereas values above 9 mL/dL suggest global cerebral ischemia.

Transcutaneous, transcranial NIRS is a completely noninvasive method of assessing cerebral oxygenation. NIRS is a promising technique, but the scope for technologic refinement is still very large. While contamination of extracranial blood has been largely eliminated with spatial resolved spectroscopy (Lam et al., 1997), the unknown sample volume still poses problems. Moreover, fractioning between arterial, capillary, and venous blood sampling remains unknown. The cerebral oxygenation index is not always well correlated with $S_jO_2$. However, changes in NIRS-derived tissue oxygenation index, and slow waves of blood pressure or CPP have

great potential to monitor cerebrovascular reactivity or cerebral autoregulation. Moreover, these data are useful to evaluate optimal CPP or optimal ABP in pediatric patients (Brady et al., 2009), neonates (da Costa et al., 2015), and adults (Zweifel et al., 2010).

Oxygen content of cerebral tissue is reactive to high ICP. However, $P_{bti}O_2$ may be provoked by other factors, such as hyperventilation, low ABP, microvascular problems, and mitochondrial dysfunction. Therefore, the specificity of the method is low. Moreover, the measurement covers only a limited area of the brain. Changes in cerebral oxygenation reactive to changes in ICP can be observed in multimodal monitoring of the injured brain (Fig. 5.7).

### Cerebral biochemistry/microdialysis

Limitations specific for brain oxygenation parenchymal probes can also be raised in the case of microdialysis. Measurement is extremely local and invasive, and the sampling rate is low (classically one per hour, although prototypes of fast microdialysis machines are now available). Measurement of the lactate/pyruvate ratio is an accepted marker of brain ischemia, with a proven correlation with outcome and cerebrovascular pressure reactivity (Timofeev et al., 2011). However, a high lactate/pyruvate ratio may also occur in the absence of ischemia, referred to as metabolic distress. Glutamate is an excitatory neurotransmitter that may rise in the extracellular space because of excessive release from neurons or impaired cellular uptake. Glycerol is a marker of membrane degradation. Each of these markers may have a patient-specific interaction with raised ICP.

### Cerebral blood flow

CBF can be monitored clinically using TCD (more global but nonquantitative) or a thermal diffusion method (quantitative but regional). Increments in ICP that lead to reductions in CPP below the lower limit of autoregulation produce a decrease in CBF. Both modalities are extremely useful for direct monitoring of cerebral autoregulation.

### Cerebral electric activity

The compressed electroencephalogram (EEG) is helpful in deciding whether cerebral metabolic depressants may be indicated in the treatment of intracranial hypertension. Such therapy will be less helpful if EEG activity is already markedly suppressed. During seizures, ICP is often transiently elevated due to increase in CBV (Vespa et al., 2007). Changes in ICP during cortical spreading depolarization are less specific, and either an increase or decrease in ICP may be observed (Rogatsky et al., 2003).

# HOSPITAL COURSE AND MANAGEMENT

## Treatment of raised intracranial pressure

Due to the many interactions between intracranial pathophysiology and extracranial variables, intensive care treatment of raised ICP is complex. Guidelines that classify the current evidence and make recommendations for a systematic approach are only available for TBI (Bratton et al., 2007a) and to a lesser extent for stroke (Broderick et al., 1999; Adams et al., 2003). However, depending on the dominant mechanism leading to intracranial hypertension, these algorithms may be adapted to suit the needs of patients with other forms of brain injury. Management algorithms usually intensify treatment in a stepwise fashion based on the results of neuromonitoring (Table 5.1). As clinical signs, particularly in unconscious patients on a ventilator, are not reliable, ICP should be monitored when intracranial hypertension is expected or when active treatment is started in unconscious patients. For TBI patients, there are guidelines for when monitoring of ICP is appropriate (Bratton et al., 2007b). For all other patients, the decision to insert monitors must be based on the computed tomography (CT) scan and the clinical presentation.

### TREATMENT THRESHOLDS

Based on data from TBI patients showing worse outcome in patients with ICP above 20–25 mmHg, current guidelines recommend treating ICP if it exceeds 22 mmHg (Brain Trauma Foundation, 2016; Bratton et al., 2007c). Such a fixed threshold has been recently challenged, with many clinicians and researchers believing that ICP thresholds should instead be individualized (Lazaridis et al., 2014). Moreover, ICP therapy has side-effects and needs to be selectively targeted if it is not to be counterproductive.

### FIRST LEVEL OF TREATMENT INTENSITY: PREVENTION OF INTRACRANIAL HYPERTENSION

This section lists simple general medical and nursing care preventive measures and interventions that should be used in all patients who are either at risk of developing intracranial hypertension or are documented to have raised ICP. A summary of relevant factors that may increase ICP is shown in Table 5.2.

The position of the patient's head should minimize any obstruction of cerebral venous drainage. It is standard practice to raise the head of the bed to improve venous drainage from the brain. Direct measurement of global CBF and CPP suggests that elevation to 30° is safe, but CPP needs to be monitored carefully in individual patients. It is recommended to zero blood pressure transducers to the ear, which roughly corresponds to

*Table 5.1*

Generic treatment algorithm for raised intracranial pressure (ICP)

---

**First level of treatment intensity: correct factors that may increase ICP**
- Head-up positioning (maximum 30°)
- Maintain cerebral perfusion pressure 50–70 mmHg
- $Pa_{O_2} > 8$ kPa (60 mmHg), preferably > 10 (75 mmHg) or even 12 kPa (90 mmHg)
- Keep $Pa_{CO_2}$ normal (4.5–5.0 kPa; 34–38 mmHg)
- Sedation (propofol, fentanyl, neuromuscular blockers where required)
- Temperature: normothermia (36–37.5°C)

If ICP >20 mmHg, perform computed tomography scan and check for surgical treatment options (new or increasing space-occupying lesions that require surgical treatment or drainage of cerebrospinal fluid).

If there are no surgical options go to second level.

**Second level of treatment intensity: increased intensity of medical treatment**
- Mannitol 20% (e.g., 2 mL/kg up to three doses; caution if osmolality > or 320 mosmol/L)
- Hypertonic saline (e.g., 5% NaCl 2 ml/kg (do not repeat if Na >155 mmol/L)
- Consider reducing $Pa_{CO_2}$ (3.5–4.5 kPa; 30–34 mmHg) and establishing ischemia monitoring ($P_{bti}O_2$ or $S_jO_2$)
- Consider electroencephalogram and anticonvulsants if indicated
- Consider lowering body temperature to 35°C

If ICP > 20–25 mmHg despite these measures, go to third level.

**Third level of treatment intensity: therapies with controversial impact on outcome**
- Consider deeper hypothermia (target 33–34°C)
- Consider barbiturate coma (maintain cerebral perfusion pressure)
- Consider craniectomy

---

adapted from Patel HC, Menon DK, Tebbs S, Hawker R, Hutchinson PJ, Kirkpatrick PJ (2002). Specialist neurocritical care and outcome from head injury. Intensive Care Med 28 (5): 547–553. Epub 2002 Feb 14. PubMed PMID: 12029400.

the foramen of Monro, rather than to the heart level. Relevant obstruction to venous outflow can also be caused by lateral head tilt, tight cervical collars, bands used for fixation of endotracheal tubes, thrombosis of the internal jugular vein, or inappropriately high levels of positive end-expiratory pressure (PEEP).

Maintaining adequate CPP is critical, and ICP treatment must consider CPP, as the two parameters are often closely linked. Low CPP will lead to ischemia, which may increase cytotoxic edema and, in turn, ICP. Moderately low CPP may also increase ICP due to cerebrovascular autoregulation. In patients with intact autoregulation, decreases in CPP will lead to vasodilatation, which may lead to an

*Table 5.2*

**Potential problems exacerbating raised intracranial pressure**

Technical problems
- Incorrect calibration of intracranial pressure and arterial blood pressure transducers and monitors
- Dysfunction/obstruction of external ventricular drainage

Obstruction of venous drainage from the head
- Inappropriate position of head and neck
- Constricting tape/tube fixations around neck
- Thrombosis of internal jugular vein

Cardiovascular problems
- Inadequate cerebral perfusion pressure
- Cerebral vasodilating drugs

Respiratory problems
- Hypercapnia
- Hypoxia
- Inappropriately high positive end-expiratory pressure
- Secretions, bronchospasm, coughing

Metabolic problems
- Fever
- Infusion of hypo-osmotic fluids

Intensive care unit management
- Insufficient sedation and/or analgesia
- Inappropriate muscle activity (e.g., shivering, straining)

Seizures

Developing or new intracerebral space-occupying lesions

---

increase in ICP, particularly in patients with low intracranial compliance. In patients with impaired autoregulation, increases in CPP will be mirrored by increments in ICP. Excessively high CPP will increase vasogenic edema. There is no consensus as to the level of CPP that is appropriate in an individual patient. The current guidelines of the Brain Trauma Foundation recommend a CPP target range of 60–70 mmHg (Brain Trauma Foundation, 2016; Bratton et al., 2007d). Other studies suggest that the best, or optimal CPP level, should be individually set at the pressure where cerebral autoregulation works best (Steiner et al., 2002; Aries et al., 2012). Clinical proof of this concept is still awaiting appropriate prospective trials. Consideration must also be given to the effects of aggressive blood pressure augmentation on hemodynamics and gas exchange.

For pediatric TBI, specific guidelines with age-dependent thresholds are available (Adelson et al., 2003a, b). If CPP is too high and the decision is made to decrease blood pressure (e.g., in patients with hemorrhagic stroke or untreated ruptured subarachnoid aneurysms), it is important to use a drug that has no vasodilating effect on the cerebral vasculature.

Adequate ventilation is critical. There is no role for prophylactic hyperventilation in brain-injured patients, and the arterial partial pressure of $CO_2$ ($Pa_{CO_2}$) should initially be kept in the low normal range (4.5–5.0 kPa; 34–38 mmHg) (Bratton et al., 2007f). Hypoxia must be avoided, as it is one of the most important secondary insults to the injured brain. On the other hand, short-term hypocapnia can be safely used for terminating sudden increases in ICP during plateau waves. Waves longer than 30 minutes (with ICP > 40 mmHg) are detrimental and are clearly associated with poor outcome (Castellani et al., 2009). An arterial partial pressure of oxygen ($Pa_{O_2}$) below 8 kPa (60 mmHg) lowers arterial oxygen content enough to cause vasodilatation, and treatment algorithms for brain-injured patients typically aim for 10 kPa (75 mmHg) or more of $Pa_{O_2}$. There is a certain reluctance to use PEEP > 5 cmH$_2$O in brain-injured patients, as the associated increase in intrathoracic pressure may impede venous drainage from the brain and raise ICP. However, in many patients with raised ICP, the gradient governing cerebral venous drainage is not the difference between arterial and central venous pressure, but the difference between arterial pressure and ICP. Accordingly, ICP will often not rise if PEEP remains lower than ICP. Nevertheless, this will have to be tested in an individual patient. Management must be adapted to optimize the effects of PEEP on ICP and $Pa_{O_2}$. The effects of supranormal levels of $Pa_{O_2}$ on the brain are controversial; this is an area of active investigation.

Fever not only increases cerebral metabolism and, hence, CBV, but also cerebral edema. Patients should be kept normothermic, by administration of acetaminophen, nonsteroidal anti-inflammatory drugs, provided there are no concerns regarding their effects on platelet function, active cooling, or a combination of these. With active cooling, attempts should be made to avoid shivering, as it may have deleterious effects on brain oxygenation and metabolism. Brain temperature is usually about 0.5°C higher than core temperature, although this may vary from one patient to another.

Severe hyperglycemia should be treated aggressively. There is considerable evidence that cerebral ischemia and infarction are made worse by hyperglycemia, and the use of glucose solutions is contraindicated unless there is significant evidence of benefit in a particular metabolic encephalopathy. Target values for serum glucose are typically in the range of 6–10 mmol/L (Oddo et al., 2008). Lower blood glucose values have been associated with insufficient glucose supply to the injured brain. If glucose-containing solutions are used, they should be administered as a solution with normal osmolality. Because of concerns about worsening cerebral edema by infusing fluids with low osmolarity, many units also avoid Ringer's lactate or similar balanced solutions in brain-injured patients, and instead use normal saline as the preferred maintenance fluid.

Adequate sedation and analgesia are important components of initial management, even in comatose patients, and are essential to control ICP. Coughing, straining, and "fighting the ventilator" all lead to considerable increases in ICP. Sedation not only alleviates stress, but also suppresses cerebral metabolism, thereby improving the supply–demand balance. Propofol is widely used because of its cerebral vasoconstrictor effect and its relatively short duration of action, but care has to be taken to avoid hypotension, which is likely to occur in hypovolemic patients. Due to the possibility of the "propofol infusion syndrome," propofol is not commonly used for sedation in children. However, the syndrome has also been documented in adults, especially with prolonged usage (Kam and Cardone, 2007). Short-acting benzodiazepines, such as midazolam or lorazepam, may also be used for sedation. More recently, dexmedetomidine has been suggested as a useful sedative drug. However, at present there are insufficient data with regard to sedation of brain-injured patients (Grof and Bledsoe, 2010; Erdman et al., 2014).

Seizures have long been known to increase ICP, and have the potential to induce cerebral ischemia, due to an increment in cerebral electric activity and oxidative metabolism. Up to 25% of patients have been shown to have seizures in the first 7 days after TBI, and it has been estimated that more than 10% have nonconvulsive seizures that may only be detectable with continuous EEG monitoring (Varelas et al., 2013). Seizures must be treated aggressively, but may be difficult to recognize when patients are pharmacologically paralyzed. Some units use continuous EEG monitoring to detect occult seizures. Prophylactic administration of anticonvulsants has been advocated for cortical tumors, head-injured patients with acute subdural hematomas (evacuated and nonevacuated), depressed skull fractures, and penetrating missile injuries. Phenytoin can be administered intravenously, and is widely used, despite lingering concerns about potential long-term neuropsychologic effects. It is unknown whether modern antiepileptic drugs such as levetiracetam would be preferable. Many antibiotics, including carbapenems, fluoroquinolones, and metronidazole, are known to have proconvulsant properties.

Glucocorticoids such as dexamethasone are effective at reducing vasogenic edema around focal, relatively chronic, cerebral lesions. Patients deteriorating with a cerebral tumor or an abscess rapidly improve within as little as 24 hours of administration. However, steroids are harmful and should not be used in the management of raised ICP in patients with TBI (Roberts et al., 2004).

## SECOND LEVEL OF TREATMENT INTENSITY

If, despite these measures, ICP exceeds 20 mmHg, more invasive treatments must be considered. If no CT scan has been performed recently, repeat imaging is advisable to exclude conditions that are amenable to surgical interventions. Apart from evacuation of expanding intracranial hematomas or other mass lesions, external ventricular drainage of CSF is a rapid procedure to reduce raised ICP. CSF should generally be removed gradually against a positive pressure of 15–25 cmH$_2$O to avoid unrestrained drainage. In patients with diffuse brain swelling, the ventricles are small and not always easy to cannulate. Even when cannulation is successful, catheters in very tight ventricles may easily become blocked. CSF drainage is the optimal method of controlling intracranial hypertension in patients with SAH where the predominant cause is often a disturbance of CSF circulation. Biventricular drainage may be required for third ventricular lesions, which occlude both foramina of Munro. In the case of posterior fossa tumors, upward herniation may be precipitated if the supratentorial ventricles are drained too rapidly. In patients with a hemispheric mass lesion causing midline shift and contralateral hydrocephalus, drainage of that ventricle may make the shift worse. In certain patients, particularly those with communicating hydrocephalus, lumbar drainage of CSF may be an option (Munch et al., 2001).

## HYPEROSMOLAR TREATMENT: MANNITOL AND HYPERTONIC SALINE

On the second level of treatment, hyperosmolar therapy with mannitol or hypertonic saline is usually the first step. Intravenous mannitol is invaluable as a first-aid measure in a patient with brain herniation as a result of raised ICP (Wakai et al., 2013). In practice, mannitol tends to be given as an intermittent bolus (2 mL/kg of a 20% solution over 15–20 minutes) whenever individual patients' ICP rises significantly above the threshold of 20–25 mmHg. Effects of mannitol last for up to 4 hours. Since osmotic diuresis may lead to hypovolemia, it is crucial to avoid volume depletion and latent hypotension, with careful attention to fluid balance. Mannitol has traditionally not been recommended once the plasma osmolality exceeds 320 mosmol/L, although this opinion is not based on high-quality data. Repeated doses of mannitol should generally not be given unless ICP is monitored.

Hypertonic saline solutions ranging from 1.6 to 29.2% have been used. Commonly recommended regimens include 2 mL/kg 5% NaCl, 250 mL of 7.5% NaCl, or 30–60 mL of 23.4% NaCl. The action of hypertonic saline may be augmented if colloids are administered at the same time. A duration of action of approximately 2 hours has been reported (Lazaridis et al., 2013). There is more than one mechanism of action. Hypertonic saline has an osmotic effect, which leads to removal of water from the interstitial and intracellular compartment in areas with intact blood–brain barrier. In addition, there is an increase in regional CBF, most likely caused by a reduction in size of swollen endothelial cells. Hypertonic saline should generally no longer be used once plasma Na has reached 155 mmol/L. It is preferred that it be given through a central venous line due to its high osmolarity.

## HYPERVENTILATION

Hyperventilation reduces ICP via a reduction of CBV. Unfortunately, hyperventilation also causes a reduction in CBF and, therefore, the main concern when patients are hyperventilated is the possibility of inducing cerebral ischemia. Prophylactic hyperventilation of TBI patients to a $Pa_{CO_2}$ of 3.4 kPa (26 mmHg) has been shown to be detrimental to outcome and aggressive hyperventilation to below a $Pa_{CO_2}$ of 3.5 kPa is therefore not recommended. There is an ongoing controversy about the risk of moderate hyperventilation ($Pa_{CO_2}$ 4.5–3.5 kPa; 34–26 mmHg) to cause ischemia in brain injury. Nevertheless, it is recommended to monitor cerebral oxygenation if moderate hyperventilation is used. Our means of monitoring critical reductions of CBF during hyperventilation are very limited. $S_{jv}O_2$ or $P_{bti}O_2$ monitors are frequently used to avoid overaggressive hyperventilation (Bratton et al., 2007e). There is growing awareness that hyperventilation should be used sparingly, primarily to treat ICP plateau waves and herniation. For TBI patients, the Brain Trauma Foundation guidelines recommend moderate hyperventilation as a short-term measure only, except when other forms of medical ICP treatment have failed (Bratton et al., 2007f).

## THIRD LEVEL OF TREATMENT INTENSITY – THERAPIES WITH CONTROVERSIAL IMPACT ON OUTCOME

If the second-level measures are inadequate to control ICP, therapy will again be intensified. The three options are hypothermia, barbiturate coma, and craniectomy. All these treatment options have relevant side-effects, and there is no clear evidence that they improve patient outcome.

## HYPOTHERMIA

Hypothermia exerts many theoretic beneficial effects on the injured brain and can be used to lower ICP (Polderman, 2004a). In contrast to sedation, which only reduces electric activity, hypothermia also reduces the metabolic demand caused by the processes needed to uphold structural integrity. Typically, temperature is not reduced beyond 33–35°C. Hypothermia can be achieved by surface cooling or with various forms of heat

exchangers that are inserted into a large vein, possibly combined with initial rapid infusion of cold fluids. Patients may shiver when cooled, and may require neuromuscular blockade.

The Eurotherm trial recently demonstrated that earlier use of hypothermia (administered as a second-level therapy prior to consideration of osmotic agents) to a target temperature of 32–35°C is harmful, even if it did reduce the need for other third-level therapies (Andrews et al., 2015). As such, hypothermia should not be applied prophylactically, and should only be used as a rescue therapy when other treatments have been ineffective. The safety of maintaining temperature below 35°C has been questioned by these results.

When it is used, the question of how long hypothermia should be maintained has not been answered definitively. One approach is to cool the patient until ICP is consistently less than 20 mmHg and then to increase temperature slightly (e.g. 0.1°C/hour) and observe the response of ICP. Too rapid rewarming may be detrimental to an injured brain. For SAH, a trial to prove the efficacy of intraoperative hypothermia (IHAST) was also negative. Hypothermia has relevant side-effects: a significantly higher rate of pneumonia, electrolyte abnormalities, and thrombocytopenia when compared to normothermic patients (Polderman, 2004b).

## METABOLIC SUPPRESSION – BARBITURATE COMA

Hypnotic agents such as propofol or barbiturates depress cerebral oxidative metabolism and, hence, lower CBF, CBV, and ICP. Barbiturates are commonly used for this purpose. Cerebral electric activity and normal coupling mechanisms between metabolism and flow must be present if barbiturates are to lower ICP. Flow metabolism coupling mechanisms may be assessed by the cerebrovascular response to carbon dioxide, and barbiturates are only effective if some $CO_2$ reactivity is retained. For thiopental, repeated boluses of 250 mg (up to 3–5 grams) are recommended, followed by an infusion of 4–8 mg/kg/h. Pentobarbital is initiated with a loading dose of 10 mg/kg, possibly followed by 5 m/kg/h for 1–3 hours, and then an infusion of 1–5 mg/kg/h. Barbiturate therapy should be targeted to a predefined EEG burst suppression ratio. Unfortunately, all agents that depress cerebral metabolism have adverse effects. For propofol and barbiturates, the most relevant effect is systemic hypotension, which is often exacerbated by hypovolemia. Synergy with even moderate hypothermia may be helpful, provided mean arterial pressure is maintained. After initial reports of the effectiveness of short-acting barbiturates in lowering ICP after head injury, several trials have failed to show any significant improvement in outcome, or reduction in the number of patients dying with intracranial hypertension (Roberts and Sydenham 2012). Elimination of barbiturates takes several days, and an unconfounded neurologic assessment will not be possible during this time.

## DECOMPRESSIVE CRANIECTOMY

Decompressive craniectomy (i.e., removal of a bone flap) has become more popular as a treatment for refractory intracranial hypertension. Although there is a place for decompressive craniotomy following head injury, there is also the potential to do harm. Hemicraniectomy is effective in the treatment of large ischemic strokes in the region of the MCA (Vahedi et al., 2007). In selected patients with raised ICP following aneurysmal SAH, a benefit of craniectomy has also been suggested (Holsgrove et al., 2014). In patients with TBI, the data are unclear, as it has not been possible to show that craniectomies improve outcomes (Cooper et al., 2011; Hutchinson et al., 2016). Due to the insufficient evidence, craniectomy is often only performed when medical treatment, including hypothermia and/or barbiturate coma, has failed.

## TREATMENT OF ACUTE EXACERBATIONS OF INTRACRANIAL PRESSURE

Patients who are rapidly deteriorating or are unconscious require immediate resuscitation followed by a diagnostic CT scan. As initial treatment goals before invasive monitoring are established, a systolic blood pressure of more than 90 mmHg and a peripheral arterial oxygen saturation >90% are required. Patients with a Glasgow Coma Scale score ≤8 need to be intubated and ventilated to protect their airway prior to scanning. In this particular circumstance, hyperventilation may be used as a temporizing measure. An intravenous bolus of mannitol 20% (2–5 mL/kg over 15 minutes) may be required if there is evidence of transtentorial herniation, such as unilateral pupillary dilatation. Ventricular dilatation necessitates immediate ventricular drainage, sometimes bilateral if the lesion is midline. Significant space-occupying lesions require surgical intervention. If an intracranial tumor or abscess is identified as the cause of intracranial hypertension, dexamethasone (initial dose 10 mg IV bolus) should be given.

## IS ICP MONITORING USEFUL?

The continuous measurement of ICP is an essential modality in most brain monitoring systems. After decades of enthusiastic attempts to introduce new modalities for brain monitoring (e.g., $P_{bti}O_2$, microdialysis, CBF, TCD, $S_jO_2$), it is obvious that ICP measurement is robust, only moderately invasive, and can be realistically conducted in regional hospitals.

Clearly, the treatment of raised ICP has side-effects. It has never been shown conclusively that monitoring ICP and using treatment protocols such as the one discussed above, based on monitoring, improve outcome. Indeed, the recent publication of the BEST TRIP trial (Chesnut et al., 2012) has fueled further controversy regarding the usefulness of monitoring of ICP and its treatment in head-injured patients. To put the results of this important trial into perspective, a consensus statement of 23 clinically active, international opinion leaders in TBI management has been published (Chesnut et al., 2015). It was concluded that the BEST TRIP trial: 1) studied protocols, not ICP-monitoring *per se*; 2) applies only to those protocols and specific study groups and should not be generalized to other treatment approaches or patient groups; 3) strongly calls for further research on ICP interpretation and use; 4) should be applied cautiously to regions with much different treatment milieu; 5) did not investigate the utility of treating monitored ICP in the specific patient group with established intracranial hypertension; 6) should not change the practice of those currently monitoring ICP; and 7) provided a protocol, used in non-monitored study patients, that should be considered when treating without ICP monitoring.

In addition to these statements, we would re-emphasize that "ICP is more than a number," and end-hour instant values of ICP read from the bedside monitor are not an efficient modality to manage intracranial hypertension.

A previously published audit (Patel et al., 2005) showed substantially lower mortality in neurosurgical centers where ICP is usually monitored versus general intensive care units where it is not monitored. However, the availability of ICP monitoring is not the only difference between neurosurgical and general intensive care units that might explain the difference in mortality after head injury.

The ICP waveform contains valuable information about the nature of cerebrospinal pathophysiology. Autoregulation of CBF and compliance of cerebrospinal system are both expressed in ICP. Methods of waveform analysis are useful both to derive this information and to guide the management of patients.

The value of ICP in acute states such as TBI, poorgrade SAH, and intracerebral hematoma depends on a close link between monitoring and therapy. CPP-oriented protocols, osmotherapy, and the Lund protocol cannot be conducted correctly without ICP guidance. A decision about decompressive craniectomy is often supported by the close inspection of the trend of ICP

*Table 5.3*

**Summary of management of raised intracranial pressure (ICP) in patients other than those suffering from traumatic brain injury**

Conscious patient
- Diagnosis based on suspicious history (new headaches, nausea, vomiting, visual blurring/obscurations, diplopia) with or without papilledema on examination

Any patient with drowsiness or fluctuation in level of consciousness merits emergency referral to neurosurgery
- Definitive investigation by CT scan combined with general medical assessment

Never perform a lumbar puncture in a patient with suspected raised ICP, even if papilledema is absent, until a CT scan has shown no evidence of either a mass lesion or diffuse brain swelling
- Management depends on the presumptive diagnosis after CT and proceeds in consultation with neurosurgery:
  - Tumors: dexamethasone, tissue diagnosis and excision, radiotherapy, chemotherapy, as appropriate
  - Abscess: aspiration/excision
  - Hydrocephalus: CSF shunt with or without prior ICP monitoring and CSF infusion studies
  - Idiopathic intracranial hypertension: referral to combined neurosurgery/neuro-ophthalmology service for CSF monitoring, diuretics/steroids/diet for mild cases. Venous stenting in case of active stenosis (Higgins et al., 2002), CSF shunt/optic nerve sheath fenestration for severe/refractory cases

**Unconscious patient**
Emergency resuscitation for patients no longer obeying commands
- Intubation and ventilation
- Intravenous mannitol (2 mL/kg) if signs of herniation present
- Definitive investigation:
  - CT scan in combination with general medical assessment
- Consider ICP monitoring

Management of raised ICP
- Institute specific treatment for etiology
- Mass lesions: surgical evacuation
- Hydrocephalus: external ventricular drainage
- Cerebral edema and brain swelling:
  Dexamethasone for tumors only, not for trauma, consider for abscesses
- Use generic algorithm (Table 5.1) where and as applicable

CT, computed tomography; CSF, cerebrospinal fluid.

and, preferably, by information derived from its waveform. In encephalitis, acute liver failure, and cerebral infarction after stroke, ICP monitoring is used less commonly. However, an increasing number of reports highlight its importance, including noninvasive ICP monitoring methodology.

In summary, despite a lack of clear evidence, the recommendation to treat raised ICP > 20–25 mmHg is standard practice. However, it is important to realize that treatment of raised ICP is associated with a multitude of potential complications, and stringent clinical judgment is required, particularly when guidelines that are based on data from TBI are adapted for patients with other forms of brain injury. A possible approach to the patient suffering from disease other than TBI is shown in Table 5.3.

## REFERENCES

Aaslid R, Markwalder TM, Nornes H (1982). Noninvasive transcranial Doppler ultrasound recording of flow velocity in basal cerebral arteries. J Neurosurg 57: 769–774.

Aaslid R, Lundar T, Lindegaard K-F et al. (1986). Estimation of cerebral perfusion pressure from arterial blood pressure and transcranial Doppler recordings. In: JD Miller, GM Teasdale, JO Rowan et al. (Eds.), Intracranial pressure VI. Springer Verlag, Berlin, pp. 229–231.

Adams Jr HP, Adams RJ, Brott T et al. (2003). Guidelines for the early management of patients with ischemic stroke: a scientific statement from the Stroke Council of the American Stroke Association. Stroke 34: 1056–1083.

Adelson PD, Bratton SL, Carney NA et al. (2003a). Guidelines for the acute medical management of severe traumatic brain injury in infants, children, and adolescents. Chapter 6. Threshold for treatment of intracranial hypertension. Pediatr Crit Care Med 4: S25–S27.

Adelson PD, Bratton SL, Carney NA et al. (2003b). Guidelines for the acute medical management of severe traumatic brain injury in infants, children, and adolescents. Chapter 8. Cerebral perfusion pressure. Pediatr Crit Care Med 4: S31–S33.

Andrews PJ, Sinclair HL, Rodriguez A et al. (2015). Eurotherm3235 Trial Collaborators. Hypothermia for Intracranial Hypertension after Traumatic Brain Injury. N Engl J Med 373 (25): 2403–2412. http://dx.doi.org/10.1056/NEJMoa1507581. Epub 2015 Oct 7. PubMed PMID: 26444221.

Aries MJ, Czosnyka M, Budohoski KP et al. (2012). Continuous determination of optimal cerebral perfusion pressure in traumatic brain injury. Crit Care Med 40: 2456–2463.

Balestreri M, Czosnyka M, Steiner LA et al. (2005). Association between outcome, cerebral pressure reactivity and slow ICP waves following head injury. Acta Neurochir Suppl 95: 25–28.

Barzó P, Bari F, Dóczi T et al. (1993). Significance of the rate of systemic change in blood pressure on the short-term autoregulatory response in normotensive and spontaneously hypertensive rats. Neurosurgery 32 (4): 611–618.

Bijlenga P, Czosnyka M, Budohoski KP et al. (2010). "Optimal cerebral perfusion pressure" in poor grade patients after subarachnoid hemorrhage. Neurocrit Care 13: 17–23.

Brady KM, Lee JK, Kibler KK et al. (2008). Continuous measurement of autoregulation by spontaneous fluctuations in cerebral perfusion pressure: comparison of 3 methods. Stroke 39: 2531–2537.

Brady KM, Shaffner DH, Lee JK et al. (2009). Continuous monitoring of cerebrovascular pressure reactivity after traumatic brain injury in children. Pediatrics 124: e1205–e1212.

Brain Trauma Foundation (2016). Guidelines for the management of severe traumatic brain injury.

Bratton SL, Chestnut RM, Ghajar J et al. (2007a). Guidelines for the management of severe traumatic brain injury. J Neurotrauma 24 (Suppl 1): S1–S106.

Bratton SL, Chestnut RM, Ghajar J et al. (2007b). Guidelines for the management of severe traumatic brain injury. VI. Indications for intracranial pressure monitoring. J Neurotrauma 24 (Suppl 1): S37–S44.

Bratton SL, Chestnut RM, Ghajar J et al. (2007c). Guidelines for the management of severe traumatic brain injury. VIII. Intracranial pressure thresholds. J Neurotrauma 24 (Suppl 1): S55–S58.

Bratton SL, Chestnut RM, Ghajar J et al. (2007d). Guidelines for the management of severe traumatic brain injury. IX. Cerebral perfusion thresholds. J Neurotrauma 24 (Suppl 1): S59–S64.

Bratton SL, Chestnut RM, Ghajar J et al. (2007e). Guidelines for the management of severe traumatic brain injury. X. Brain oxygen monitoring and thresholds. J Neurotrauma 24 (Suppl 1): S65–S70.

Bratton SL, Chestnut RM, Ghajar J et al. (2007f). Guidelines for the management of severe traumatic brain injury. XIV. Hyperventilation. J Neurotrauma 24 (Suppl 1): S87–S90.

Broderick JP, Adams Jr HP, Barsan W et al. (1999). Guidelines for the management of spontaneous intracerebral hemorrhage: a statement for healthcare professionals from a special writing group of the Stroke Council, American Heart Association. Stroke 30: 905–915.

Cardoso ER, Rowan JO, Galbraith S (1983). Analysis of the cerebrospinal fluid pulse wave in intracranial pressure. J Neurosurg 59: 817–821.

Castellani G, Zweifel C, Kim DJ et al. (2009). Plateau waves in head injured patients requiring neurocritical care. Neurocrit Care 11: 143–150.

Chesnut RM, Temkin N, Carney N et al. (2012). A trial of intracranial-pressure monitoring in traumatic brain injury. N Engl J Med 367: 2471–2481.

Chesnut RM, Bleck TP, Citerio G et al. (2015). A consensus-based interpretation of the benchmark evidence from South American trials: Treatment of Intracranial Pressure Trial. J Neurotrauma 32: 1722–1724.

Cooper DJ, Rosenfeld JV, Murray L et al. (2011). Decompressive craniectomy in diffuse traumatic brain injury. N Engl J Med 364: 1493–1502.

Czosnyka M, Price DJ, Williamson M (1994). Monitoring of cerebrospinal dynamics using continuous analysis of intracranial pressure and cerebral perfusion pressure in head injury. Acta Neurochir (Wien) 126 (2–4): 113–119.

Czosnyka M, Smielewski P, Kirkpatrick P et al. (1997). Continuous assessment of the cerebral vasomotor reactivity in head injury. Neurosurgery 41 (1): 11–17.

da Costa CS, Czosnyka M, Smielewski P et al. (2015). Monitoring of cerebrovascular reactivity for determination of optimal blood pressure in preterm infants. J Pediatr 167: 86–91.

Davson H, Hollingsworth G, Segal MB (1970). The mechanism of drainage of the cerebrospinal fluid. Brain 93: 665–678.

Depreitere B, Güiza F, Van den Berghe G et al. (2014). Pressure autoregulation monitoring and cerebral perfusion pressure target recommendation in patients with severe traumatic brain injury based on minute-by-minute monitoring data. J Neurosurg 120: 1451–1457.

Dewey RC, Pieper HP, Hunt WE (1974). Experimental cerebral hemodynamics. Vasomotor tone, critical closing pressure, and vascular bed resistance. Neurosurgery 41: 597–606.

Dias C, Maia I, Cerejo A et al. (2014). Pressures, flow, and brain oxygenation during plateau waves of intracranial pressure. Neurocrit Care 21: 124–132.

Erdman MJ, Doepker BA, Gerlach AT et al. (2014). A comparison of severe hemodynamic disturbances between dexmedetomidine and propofol for sedation in neurocritical care patients. Crit Care Med 42: 1696–1702.

Grof TM, Bledsoe KA (2010). Evaluating the use of dexmedetomidine in neurocritical care patients. Neurocrit Care 12: 356–361.

Guillaume J, Janny P (1951). Manometrie intracranienne continué interest de la methode et premiers resultants. Rev Neurol 84: 131–142.

Güiza F, Depreitere B, Piper I et al. (2013). Novel methods to predict increased intracranial pressure during intensive care and long-term neurologic outcome after traumatic brain injury: development and validation in a multicenter dataset. Crit Care Med 41: 554–564.

Higgins JN, Owler BK, Cousins C et al. (2002). Venous sinus stenting for refractory benign intracranial hypertension. Lancet 359 (9302): 228–230.

Holsgrove DT, Kitchen WJ, Dulhanty L et al. (2014). Intracranial hypertension in subarachnoid hemorrhage: outcome after decompressive craniectomy. Acta Neurochir Suppl 119: 53–55.

Hu X, Glenn T, Scalzo F et al. (2010). Intracranial pressure pulse morphological features improved detection of decreased cerebral blood flow. Physiol Meas 31: 679–695.

Hutchinson PJ, Kolias AG, Timofeev IS et al. (2016). Trial of decompressive craniectomy for traumatic intracranial hypertension. N Engl J Med 375: 1119–1139.

Kam PC, Cardone D (2007). Propofol infusion syndrome. Anaesthesia 62: 690–701.

Koskinen LO, Grayson D, Olivecrona M (2013). The complications and the position of the Codman MicroSensor™ ICP device: an analysis of 549 patients and 650 sensors. Acta Neurochir (Wien) 155: 2141–2148.

Lam JM, Smielewski P, al-Rawi P et al. (1997). Internal and external carotid contributions to near-infrared spectroscopy during carotid endarterectomy. Stroke 28: 906–911.

Lassen NA (1964). Autoregulation of cerebral blood flow. Circ Res 1964 (15 Suppl): 201–204.

Lazaridis C, Neyens R, Bodle J et al. (2013). High-osmolarity saline in neurocritical care: systematic review and meta-analysis. Crit Care Med 41: 1353–1360.

Lazaridis C, DeSantis SM, Smielewski P et al. (2014). Patient-specific thresholds of intracranial pressure in severe traumatic brain injury. J Neurosurg 120: 893–900.

Löfgren J, von Essen C, Zwetnow NN (1973). The pressure–volume curve of the cerebrospinal fluid space in dogs. Acta Neurol Scand 49: 557–574.

Lu CW, Czosnyka M, Shieh JS et al. (2012). Complexity of intracranial pressure correlates with outcome after traumatic brain injury. Brain 135: 2399–2408.

Lundberg N (1960). Continuous recording and control of ventricular fluid pressure in neurosurgical practice. Acta Psych Neurol Scand 36 (Suppl 149): 1–193.

Marmarou A, Shulman K, Rosende RM (1978). A nonlinear analysis of the cerebrospinal fluid system and intracranial pressure dynamics. J Neurosurg 48: 332–344.

Miller JD, Stanek A, Langfitt TW (1972). Concepts of cerebral perfusion pressure and vascular compression during intracranial hypertension. Prog Brain Res 35: 411–432.

Munch EC, Bauhuf C, Horn P et al. (2001). Therapy of malignant intracranial hypertension by controlled lumbar cerebrospinal fluid drainage. Crit Care Med 29: 976–981.

Oddo M, Schmidt JM, Mayer SA et al. (2008). Glucose control after severe brain injury. Curr Opin Clin Nutr Metab Care 11: 134–139.

Patel HC, Bouamra O, Woodford M et al. (2005). Trends in head injury outcome from 1989 to 2003 and the effect of neurosurgical care: an observational study. Lancet 366: 1538–1544.

Piper IR, Miller JD, Dearden NM et al. (1990). Systems analysis of cerebrovascular pressure transmission: an observational study in head-injured patients. J Neurosurg 73: 871–880.

Piper IR, Chan KH, Whittle IR et al. (1993). An experimental study of cerebrovascular resistance, pressure transmission, and craniospinal compliance. Neurosurgery 32: 805–815.

Polderman KH (2004a). Application of therapeutic hypothermia in the ICU: opportunities and pitfalls of a promising treatment modality. Part 1: Indications and evidence. Intensive Care Med 30: 556–575.

Polderman KH (2004b). Application of therapeutic hypothermia in the intensive care unit. Opportunities and pitfalls of a promising treatment modality. Part 2: Practical aspects and side effects. Intensive Care Med 30: 757–769.

Radolovich DK, Aries MJ, Castellani G et al. (2011). Pulsatile intracranial pressure and cerebral autoregulation after traumatic brain injury. Neurocrit Care 15: 379–386.

Ragauskas A, Matijosaitis V, Zakelis R et al. (2012). Clinical assessment of noninvasive intracranial pressure absolute value measurement method. Neurology 78: 1684–1691.

Robba C, Bacigaluppi S, Cardim D et al. (2016). Non-invasive assessment of intracranial pressure. Acta Neurol Scand 134: 4–21.

Roberts I, Yates D, Sandercock P et al. (2004). Effect of intravenous corticosteroids on death within 14 days in 10008 adults with clinically significant head injury (MRC CRASH trial): randomised placebo-controlled trial. Lancet 364: 1321–1328.

Roberts I, Sydenham E (2012). Barbiturates for acute traumatic brain injury. Cochrane Database Syst Rev 12. CD000033. PMID: 23235573.

Robertson CS, Narayan RK, Contant CF et al. (1989). Clinical experience with a continuous monitor of intracranial compliance. J Neurosurg 71: 673–680.

Rogatsky GG, Sonn J, Kamenir Y et al. (2003). Relationship between intracranial pressure and cortical spreading depression following fluid percussion brain injury in rats. J Neurotrauma 20 (12): 1315–1325. PubMed PMID: 14748980.

Rosner MJ, Becker DP (1984). Origin and evolution of plateau waves. Experimental observations and a theoretical model. J Neurosurg 60: 312–324.

Santos E, Diedler J, Sykora M et al. (2011). Low-frequency sampling for PRx calculation does not reduce prognostication and produces similar CPPopt in intracerebral haemorrhage patients. Acta Neurochir (Wien) 153: 2189–2195.

Schmidt B, Klingelhofer J, Schwarze JJ et al. (1997). Noninvasive prediction of intracranial pressure curves using transcranial Doppler ultrasonography and blood pressure curves. Stroke 28: 2465–2472.

Schmidt EA, Czosnyka M, Gooskens I et al. (2001). Preliminary experience of the estimation of cerebral perfusion pressure using transcranial Doppler ultrasonography. J Neurol Neurosurg Psychiatry 70: 198–204.

Sorrentino E, Diedler J, Kasprowicz M et al. (2012). Critical thresholds for cerebrovascular reactivity after traumatic brain injury. Neurocrit Care 16: 258–266.

Steiner LA, Czosnyka M, Piechnik SK et al. (2002). Continuous monitoring of cerebrovascular pressure reactivity allows determination of optimal cerebral perfusion pressure in patients with traumatic brain injury. Crit Care Med 30: 733–738.

Steiner LA, Coles JP, Johnston AJ et al. (2003). Assessment of cerebrovascular autoregulation in head-injured patients: a validation study. Stroke 34: 2404–2409.

Timofeev I, Carpenter KL, Nortje J et al. (2011). Cerebral extracellular chemistry and outcome following traumatic brain injury: a microdialysis study of 223 patients. Brain 134: 484–494.

Vahedi K, Vicaut E, Mateo J et al. (2007). Sequential-design, multicenter, randomized, controlled trial of early decompressive craniectomy in malignant middle cerebral artery infarction (DECIMAL Trial). Stroke 38: 2506–2517.

Varelas PN, Spanaki MV, Mirski MA (2013). Seizures and the neurosurgical intensive care unit. Neurosurg Clin N Am 24: 393–406.

Vespa PM, Miller C, McArthur D et al. (2007). Nonconvulsive electrographic seizures after traumatic brain injury result in a delayed, prolonged increase in intracranial pressure andmetabolic crisis. Crit Care Med 35 (12): 2830–2836. PubMed PMID: 18074483; PubMed Central PMCID: PMC4347945.

Vik A, Nag T, Fredriksli OA et al. (2008). Relationship of "dose" of intracranial hypertension to outcome in severe traumatic brain injury. J Neurosurg 109: 678–684.

Wakai A, McCabe A, Roberts I et al. (2013). Mannitol for acute traumatic brain injury. Cochrane Database Syst Rev 8. CD001049.

Zweifel C, Castellani G, Czosnyka M et al. (2010). Noninvasive monitoring of cerebrovascular reactivity with near infrared spectroscopy in head-injured patients. J Neurotrauma 27: 1951–1958.

*Handbook of Clinical Neurology*, Vol. 140 (3rd series)
*Critical Care Neurology, Part I*
E.F.M. Wijdicks and A.H. Kramer, Editors
http://dx.doi.org/10.1016/B978-0-444-63600-3.00006-4

Chapter 6

# Multimodal neurologic monitoring

G. KORBAKIS[1] AND P.M. VESPA[1,2]*

[1]*Department of Neurosurgery, UCLA David Geffen School of Medicine, Los Angeles, CA, USA*

[2]*Department of Neurology, UCLA David Geffen School of Medicine, Los Angeles, CA, USA*

## Abstract

Neurocritical care has two main objectives. Initially, the emphasis is on treatment of patients with acute damage to the central nervous system whether through infection, trauma, or hemorrhagic or ischemic stroke. Thereafter, attention shifts to the identification of secondary processes that may lead to further brain injury, including fever, seizures, and ischemia, among others. Multimodal monitoring is the concept of using various tools and data integration to understand brain physiology and guide therapeutic interventions to prevent secondary brain injury. This chapter will review the use of electroencephalography, intracranial pressure monitoring, brain tissue oxygenation, cerebral microdialysis and neurochemistry, near-infrared spectroscopy, and transcranial Doppler sonography as they relate to neuromonitoring in the critically ill. The concepts and design of each monitor, in addition to the patient population that may most benefit from each modality, will be discussed, along with the various tools that can be used together to guide individualized patient treatment options. Major clinical trials, observational studies, and their effect on clinical outcomes will be reviewed. The future of multimodal monitoring in the field of bioinformatics, clinical research, and device development will conclude the chapter.

## INTRODUCTION

The term multimodal monitoring (MMM) describes the many tools being used for neurologic monitoring of the brain-injured patient. Traditionally, vigilant monitoring with serial bedside neurologic examinations has been the mainstay for determining changes in brain function; however, changes in neurologic examination may lag behind alterations in cerebral physiology and can sometimes only be detected once catastrophic damage has already occurred. The main goal of MMM is to identify these fluctuations prior to any major changes and intervene in a timely fashion in order to prevent secondary brain injury. This secondary injury can come in the form of seizures, inflammation, edema, or ischemia, and numerous devices are available to identify and examine these changes.

This chapter will explore the various resources available to monitor brain injury and examine the concepts behind their use in the neurocritical care setting. Electroencephalography (EEG) as a tool for diagnosis of seizures, as well as for prognostication based on quantitative measures, will be surveyed, followed by evaluation of various methods of intracranial pressure (ICP) and cerebral perfusion pressure (CPP) monitoring. More advanced techniques evaluating brain tissue oxygenation with noninvasive near-infrared spectroscopy (NIRS) and more invasive intraparenchymal probes or jugular venous oxygen saturation ($S_{jv}O_2$) are discussed. A review of cerebral microdialysis and energy metabolism, including nonischemic causes of metabolic crisis, follows. Lastly, cerebral blood flow (CBF) is examined, primarily through the use of noninvasive transcranial Doppler (TCD) sonography, but also with a brief review of newer intracranial probes. The conclusion will focus on the future of MMM and the field of bioinformatics.

The findings and recommendations of the Neurocritical Care Society consensus conference regarding MMM

*Correspondence to: Paul M. Vespa, MD, FCCM, FAAN, FANA, FNCS, UCLA David Geffen School of Medicine, 757 Westwood Blvd, RR UCLA # 6236A, Los Angeles CA 90095, USA. Tel: +1-310-267-9448, E-mail: Pvespa@mednet.ucla.edu

*Table 6.1*

Monitoring modalities, specific indications for clinical use, strength of recommendations, and quality of evidence based on selected recommendations from the 2014 Consensus Summary Statement of the International Multidisciplinary Consensus Conference on Multimodality Monitoring in Neurocritical Care (LeRoux et al., 2014)

| Modality | Indication | Recommendation | Quality of evidence |
|---|---|---|---|
| EEG | All patients with unexplained and persistent altered consciousness | Strong | Low |
| EEG | Convulsive SE that does not return to baseline within 60 minutes of seizure medication | Strong | Low |
| EEG | Refractory SE | Strong | Low |
| EEG | During therapeutic hypothermia and within 24 hours of rewarming in all comatose patients after cardiac arrest | Strong | Low |
| EEG | Detecting DCI in comatose SAH patients | Weak | Low |
| ICP/CPP | High risk for high ICP based on clinical exam and/or imaging | Strong | Moderate |
| ICP/CPP | Guiding medical and surgical interventions for life-threatening, imminent herniation | Strong | High |
| ICP | ICP should not be used in isolation as a prognostic marker | Strong | High |
| Pressure reactivity | Monitoring of autoregulation should be considered for targeting CPP goals and prognostication | Weak | Moderate |
| Brain oxygen monitoring | Monitoring in patients with or at risk for cerebral ischemia and/or hypoxia | Strong | Low |
| Brain oxygen monitoring | Assist titration of medical and surgical therapies to guide ICP/CPP therapy and help manage DCI | Weak | Low |
| Cerebral MD | Monitoring in patients with or at risk of ischemia, hypoxia, energy failure, and glucose deprivation | Strong | Low |
| Cerebral MD | Used in combination with other monitoring modalities for prognostication | Strong | Low |
| Cerebral MD | Titrating systemic glucose control and treatment of DCI | Weak | Moderate |
| TCDs | Predicting angiographic vasospasm after aneurysmal SAH | Strong | High |

EEG, electroencephalogram; SE, status epilepticus; DCI, delayed cerebral ischemia; SAH, subarachnoid hemorrhage; ICP, intracranial pressure; CPP, cerebral perfusion pressure; MD, microdialysis; TCD, transcranial Doppler.

are summarized in Table 6.1. A summary of treatment thresholds for various monitoring modalities is provided in Table 6.2. Figures 6.1 and 6.2 show images of patients receiving MMM, while Figure 6.3 shows a representative example of the type of data generated.

## ELECTROENCEPHALOGRAPHY

One of the most widely used noninvasive monitoring tools is the EEG. An increasing number of studies have demonstrated that seizures are relatively common in critically ill patients. One of the earlier studies to identify seizures using continuous EEG (cEEG) found a rate of 22% in moderate to severe traumatic brain injury (TBI) patients, where half were nonconvulsive or clinically silent, and nearly one-third were defined as status epilepticus (Vespa et al., 1999). Both focal and generalized seizures were observed. While there was no significant difference in poor outcomes between the seizure and nonseizure group, all patients with status epilepticus died. Similarly, in another study using cEEG in spontaneous intracerebral hemorrhage (ICH) patients, seizures were observed in 31% of patients, and again over half were purely electrographic (Claassen et al., 2007). Seizures were associated with hematoma expansion and poor outcomes. There has also been a high rate of seizures identified in subarachnoid hemorrhage (SAH) patients, with one study finding nonconvulsive seizures or status epilepticus in one-fourth of patients monitored with cEEG (Claassen et al., 2006). Epileptiform discharges and status epilepticus were associated with poor outcomes, even after adjusting for clinical and radiographic findings. Finally, in the postcardiac arrest period, a high rate of seizures has again been identified. In one study involving patients treated with therapeutic hypothermia, an incidence of 15% was reported. A larger proportion of patients with seizures (82%) died during the hospitalization compared to nonseizure patients (50%)

*Table 6.2*

**Commonly used normal values for various monitors and clinical conditions in which they have been evaluated**

| Modality | Lower limit | Upper limit | Clinical application |
|---|---|---|---|
| EEG: PAV | 0.2 | | TBI – prognosis |
| ICP | | 20–25 mmHg | TBI, SAH, hepatic failure, encephalitis/meningitis – prognosis and mortality |
| $S_{jv}O_2$ | 55% | 75% | TBI, SAH – ischemia vs. hyperemia, no data on outcomes |
| $P_{bt}O_2$ | 20 mmHg | | TBI, SAH – prognosis and mortality |
| MD: glucose | 0.2 mmol/L | | TBI, SAH – detection of ischemia, prognosis |
| MD: LPR | | 25–40 | TBI, SAH – detection of ischemia, prognosis |
| NIRS | 60% | 75% | TBI, SAH, ischemic stroke – no studies for isolated use |
| TCDs | | | SAH – DCI detection |
| MCA flow velocity | | 120–200 cm/s | |
| Lindegaard ratio | | 3–6 | |

EEG, electroencephalogram; PAV, percent alpha variability; TBI, traumatic brain injury; ICP, intracranial pressure; SAH, subarachnoid hemorrhage; MD, microdialysis; LPR, lactate/pyruvate ratio; NIRS, near-infrared spectroscopy; TCD, transcranial Doppler; MCA, middle cerebral artery; DCI, delayed cerebral ischemia.

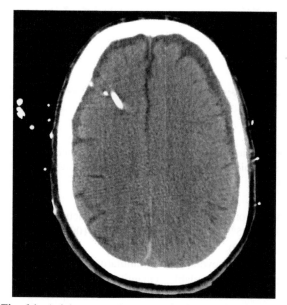

**Fig. 6.1.** Axial computed tomography image of patient with severe traumatic brain injury with right frontal external ventriculostomy drain, brain tissue oxygen, and microdialysis probes.

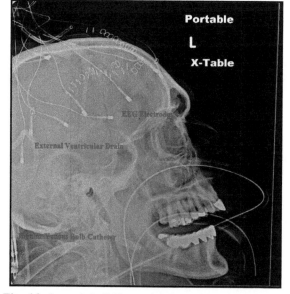

**Fig. 6.2.** Lateral skull X-ray of patient with traumatic brain injury showing jugular venous bulb catheter, external ventricular drain, and electroencephalogram (EEG) electrodes.

(Knight et al., 2013). Recognizing seizures that occur after acute brain injury is important for diagnosis, treatment, and prognostication.

Seizures are a consequence of brain injury, but may also lead to long-term neurologic damage. Vespa et al. (1999) found electrographic seizures in 28% of ICH patients, and seizures were associated with increasing midline shift ($p < 0.03$). Another study observed higher ICP and findings of metabolic distress based on cerebral microdialysis in TBI patients with seizures (Vespa et al.,

2007). Seizures are more common in ICH than with ischemic stroke (Szaflarski et al., 2008), which may be due to the toxic and proconvulsant effects of iron in the brain. *In vivo* models in animals have demonstrated that cortical injection of ferrous chloride causes recurrent focal epileptiform discharges and convulsions (Willmore et al., 1978). Additionally, seizures in the acute phase following brain injury are thought to be due to a cascade of metabolic and chemical events that are potentially epileptogenic, including elevations in excitatory amino

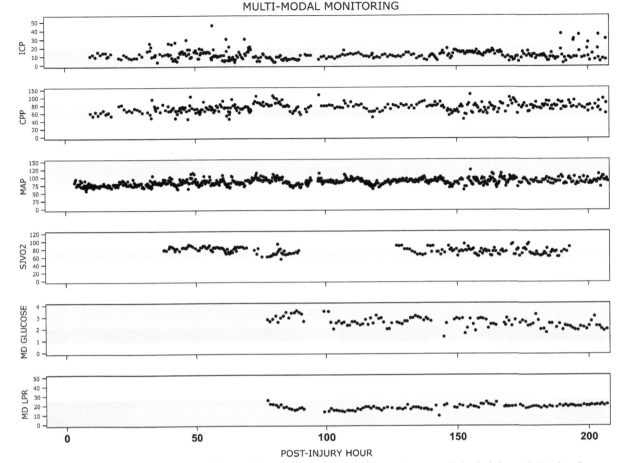

**Fig. 6.3.** Time-synchronized data of multiple variables collected from a patient with traumatic brain injury admitted to the neurointensive care unit; shaded blue area indicates normal ranges. ICP, intracranial pressure; CPP, cerebral perfusion pressure; MAP, mean arterial pressure; MD, microdialysis; LPR, lactate/pyruvate ratio.

acids and neurotransmitters (Bullock et al., 1995), and hyperglycolysis (Bergsneider et al., 1997). Seizures can cause long-term damage, including cell death, particularly in the hippocampus (Vespa et al., 2010). Early detection and treatment of seizures are therefore crucial in preventing these detrimental changes.

EEG is not only used for seizure detection, but also for prognostication. Lack of sleep architecture has been associated with poor prognosis in high-grade SAH patients (Claassen et al., 2006). A quantitative EEG element, percent alpha variability, has been assessed in TBI patients, and impairment has been associated with thalamic injury and poor long-term outcomes (Hebb et al., 2007). Additionally, EEG reactivity was found to be a good predictor of recovery of consciousness in a group of acutely brain-injured patients, including those with TBI, cerebrovascular disease, or anoxia (Logi et al., 2011). For postcardiac arrest patients, one study showed a nonreactive or discontinuous EEG background to be strongly associated with unfavorable outcomes; 34 comatose patients underwent cEEG during hypothermia and none of the survivors had a nonreactive EEG (positive predictive value of 100%, 95% confidence interval 74–100%) (Rossetti et al., 2010).

In the last several years, quantitative EEG has become more widely available. Quantitative EEG transforms EEG waves into numeric values that are compressed over a large period of time to form visual graphs, allowing the reader to compare one cerebral hemisphere to the other and visualize bursts in power frequencies. This was first noted in the 1970s during carotid endarterectomy procedures, when changes in CBF were noted to correlate with EEG changes, specifically a replacement of faster alpha-range frequencies for slower theta- and delta-range components (Sharbrough et al., 1973). These changes are reversible and this concept is now applied to detection of delayed cerebral ischemia (DCI) in SAH patients. A decrease in the alpha–delta ratio or in the percent alpha variability occurs up to 3 days prior to any clinical or radiographic evidence of DCI (Vespa et al., 1997; Gollwitzer et al., 2015; Rots et al., 2016). Detection of these changes on quantitative EEG could potentially allow for treatment of DCI prior to the manifestation of clinical symptoms.

There are important limitations to the use of cEEG monitoring in the intensive care unit. These include availability of technicians to apply and maintain electrodes, significant artifact in the intensive care unit setting, and ability of physicians to interpret the EEG in a sufficiently timely fashion (Gavvala et al., 2014). Additionally, there is an inherent degree of variability and subjectivity between EEG interpretation depending on the reader's exposure and experience, although recent studies suggest that interrater agreement is quite high, particularly when readers have been trained in use of standardized nomenclature (Gaspard et al., 2014). Newer technologies are available for automated seizure detection and remote access for EEG viewing, which may aid centers that currently lack the resources or expertise to monitor and interpret cEEG data (Claassen and Mayer, 2002).

Invasive cEEG monitoring is also available for identifying seizures that are not visible using scalp electrodes. These devices come in the form of subdural strip electrodes or intracortical depth electrodes, which can be placed at the bedside (Claassen and Vespa, 2014). A study of continuous intracortical EEG compared to scalp EEG in 14 patients with acute brain injury found that 10 of those with depth electrode placement had electrographic seizures and 6 of these had no corresponding ictal activity on the scalp EEG (Waziri et al., 2009). Moreover, in a study of 48 comatose SAH patients, intracortical seizures were seen in 38% of patients and only 8% had seizures detected by scalp electrodes (Claassen et al., 2013). Use of intracranial EEG monitoring may provide a higher sensitivity for detecting seizures and improve signal-to-noise ratio when compared to surface electric activity.

## INTRACRANIAL PRESSURE MONITORING

ICP monitoring is the foundation of neuromonitoring in the injured brain. ICP has long been recognized as an important factor affecting brain function and outcomes. Since 1965, when Nils Lundberg published his landmark study on continuous ICP monitoring using ventricular cannula in brain-injured patients (Lundberg et al., 1965), ICP monitoring has evolved and is used in the evaluation and treatment of hydrocephalus, central nervous system infection, and hepatic failure, but is best studied in TBI. It has long been recognized that elevated ICP is associated with a worse prognosis (Miller et al., 1977). The current Brain Trauma Foundation (BTF) guidelines recommend ICP monitoring for patients with a Glasgow Coma Scale (GCS) score of 8 or less with an abnormal head computed tomography (CT) (level II) or severe TBI with a normal head CT and two or more of the following: age greater than 40 years, motor posturing, or systolic blood pressure less than 90 mmHg (level III) (Bratton et al., 2007a). Generally, patients are initially treated for an ICP greater than 20 mmHg (Marmarou et al., 1991). However, refractory ICP and response to treatment for intracranial hypertension may be better predictors of outcome than absolute ICP values (Treggiari et al., 2007).

Despite these guidelines, there is still controversy regarding the use of ICP monitors in TBI. In many studies, the rate of ICP monitor usage for severe TBI is less than 50%; however, some studies suggest improved survival when these monitors are utilized (Talving et al., 2013; Dawes et al., 2015; MacLaughlin et al., 2015). For example, in one study of 844 severe TBI patients, ICP monitors were placed in 46% of patients, and positively associated with younger age and CT findings of mass lesion or mass effect. ICP monitor placement reduced the risk-adjusted mortality rate by more than 8% (Dawes et al., 2015). Others have reported opposite findings. In another study, 194 patients with severe TBI underwent ICP monitoring analysis and patients without monitors were 20% more likely to survive compared to the patients who did have ICP monitoring (Tang et al., 2015). It should be noted, however, that in the ICP monitored group, compliance with the BTF guidelines for ICP was poor. While adherence to the guidelines and management of ICP are quite variable, intracranial monitors remain the standard of care and recommended for severe TBI.

The value of ICP monitoring was further questioned by the results of the BEST-TRIP trial. This study was a randomized multicenter study where 324 patients with severe TBI (GCS 3–8) were assigned to two groups (Chesnut et al., 2012). The first had intraparenchymal monitors placed and were treated to maintain an ICP of less than 20 mmHg. The other group was treated for high ICP based on imaging findings and clinical examination with a standardized protocol of hyperosmolar therapy, mild hyperventilation and, if persistent, barbiturates. Primary outcome was a composite of several measures assessed at 6 months. There was no significant difference between the two groups and 6-month mortality was 39% in the ICP monitoring group and 41% in the imaging-clinical examination group ($p = 0.60$). A recent consensus interpretation has been published emphasizing that the BEST-TRIP trial compares two ICP treatment protocols and is not a study of the efficacy of ICP monitoring (Chesnut et al., 2015). Additionally, the study further demands ongoing research on the interpretation of ICP, and expert opinion maintains that the results of this trial should not alter the practice for those currently monitoring ICP.

CPP is another target for patients with severe brain injury. The mean arterial pressure minus the ICP equals CPP, and if this value reaches a critical low, cerebral ischemia may occur. Additionally, very high CPP values are also associated with a lower probability of favorable outcome (Balestreri et al., 2006). The BTF currently recommends a target CPP of 50–70 mmHg, with the upper limit largely because a previous clinical trial suggested that aggressive attempts to maintain CPP above 70 mmHg resulted in a higher incidence of pulmonary complications (Robertson et al., 1999; Bratton et al., 2007b). However, some research has suggested that the ischemia threshold for CPP may vary over time, and should be individualized. The pressure–reactivity index (PRx) has been proposed to assess autoregulation, and is calculated as the moving correlation coefficient between consecutive samples of ICP and arterial blood pressure averaged over time. PRx has been correlated with fluctuations in mean middle cerebral artery flow velocity, as based on TCD ultrasonography (Czosnyka et al., 1997). A negative value suggests intact autoregulation (a change in blood pressure triggers an inverse change in blood volume to maintain a stable CPP), whereas a positive PRx implies impairment of autoregulation. A positive value has been associated with higher mortality rate in severe TBI (Zweifel et al., 2008). When the PRx is plotted against CPP, a U-shaped curve is seen in some patients, and the point where PRx is minimal has been suggested as the "optimal" CPP. In patients where the mean CPP was close to the calculated optimal CPP, outcomes were more favorable. However, the optimal CPP could only be identified in 60% of patients (Steiner et al., 2002). The concept of "optimal" CPP is still debated and research in this area is ongoing.

## BRAIN TISSUE OXYGENATION

Systemic oxygenation is crucial to critical care and likewise maintenance of cerebral oxygenation is imperative for the neurocritical care patient. Cerebral hypoxia may result from several mechanisms, including reduced CBF (for example, from hypotension or vasospasm), perivascular edema, or blood–brain barrier breakdown, which disrupt oxygen diffusion and extraction, and anemia. If severe enough, cerebral hypoxia may lead to ischemia and cell death. Ischemia has long been identified as a major component of secondary damage following acute brain injury, particularly in TBI and SAH. Autopsy studies have demonstrated ischemic changes in about 90% of fatal TBI cases (Graham et al., 1989). Similarly, antemortem studies using positron emission tomography (PET) scanning measuring CBF, cerebral oxygen metabolism, and oxygen extraction fraction have found a moderate volume of

brain ischemia in head injury patients when compared to controls, and this has been associated with poor outcomes at 6 months after injury (Coles et al., 2004). In addition to ischemia, hyperemia also occurs following brain injury. The ability to assess and recognize these changes is fundamental for the neurointensivist to prevent further irreversible damage. Unfortunately, there is no current continuous imaging method to measure the above variables but two modes exist for bedside monitoring of cerebral oxygenation and will be discussed below.

### Jugular venous bulb oximetry

Jugular venous bulb oximetry is a global measure of cerebral oxygenation and is determined by oxygen delivery to the brain minus the cerebral metabolic rate of oxygen, and reported as the jugular venous saturation ($S_{jv}O_2$). The catheter should be placed in the dominant internal jugular vein and a lateral skull X-ray is recommended to confirm placement, ideally at the level of the first cervical vertebra (Fig. 6.2). Normal $S_{jv}O_2$ values are 55–75%. Complication rates are low, with the most common being nonocclusive jugular vein thrombosis (Coplin et al., 1997). $S_{jv}O_2$ elevation is associated with either reduced cerebral metabolic rate or hyperemia with impaired autoregulation (Fortune et al., 1994). One study of 450 severe TBI patients found a high $S_{jv}O_2$ (75% or greater) in almost 20% of patients, which was not consistently related to CBF or CPP; this group had a worse outcome compared to the normal $S_{jv}O_2$ group, with nearly 75% of patients dying or surviving with severe disability (Cormio et al., 1999). Low $S_{jv}O_2$ indicates ischemia, which can be treated by augmenting the CPP with volume and/or vasopressors, or perhaps transfusing with red blood cells or allowing the $P_{CO_2}$ to rise slightly (Vigué et al., 1999). Elevations in ICP can also cause desaturations in $S_{jv}O_2$. Treatment of ICP with hyperosmolar therapy or CSF drainage via ventriculostomy can raise $S_{jv}O_2$ values, but the responses are inconsistent (Fortune et al., 1995). Though mainly studied in TBI patients, one small study of SAH patients found that a significant rise in cerebral oxygen extraction, as measured by jugular bulb oximetry, was seen 1 day prior to the onset of neurologic deficits caused by vasospasm (Heran et al., 2004). The cerebral oxygen extraction and clinical symptoms improved with hypertensive treatment.

One key use of jugular bulb oximetry is guiding hyperventilation therapy for management of high ICP. Using oxidative PET, Coles et al. (2002) showed that the volume of hypoperfused brain is significantly increased during hyperventilation when $Pa_{CO_2}$ is lowered from 36 to 29 mmHg despite increases in CPP and reductions in ICP. This was not associated with global ischemia based on a conventional $S_{jv}O_2$ definition (<50%). In a subsequent study, hyperventilation was associated with higher ischemic brain volume, which was undetected by jugular bulb monitoring (Coles et al., 2007). Regardless of the beneficial effects of hyperventilation, it can potentially lead to ischemia and permanent tissue damage. Assessing brain oxygenation and making adjustments to mechanical ventilation and blood pressure are helpful to avoid further brain injury. However, $S_{jv}O_2$ may underestimate the degree of regional brain ischemia. Clinicians should likely be concerned about ischemia at levels below 60%.

## Intraparenchymal cerebral oxygen monitoring

Contrary to jugular venous bulb oximetry for the assessment of global cerebral oxygenation, intraparenchymal monitors are available to assess regional changes in brain tissue oxygen tension ($P_{bt}O_2$). The $P_{bt}O_2$ value is thought to signify the partial pressure of oxygen in the brain and represents the balance between oxygen delivery and utilization. The probe is easily inserted at the bedside and ideally resides within a border zone region of white matter between the middle and anterior cerebral arteries. Additionally, the probe should be placed in normal-appearing brain to provide a better reflection of global brain oxygenation and should avoid contusions or perilesional edema, as this can affect the recorded values (Ponce et al., 2012). These catheters have been found to be safe and reliable (Dings et al., 1998). Normal $P_{bt}O_2$ values range from 20 to 40 mmHg. Brain ischemia typically develops when values drop below 15 mmHg. Treatments for low $P_{bt}O_2$ include increasing supplemental oxygen, blood transfusion, sedation, raising blood pressure, and permitting mild to moderate hypercapnia. The $P_{bt}O_2$ can be used to target a CPP that balances oxygen supply and demand. For example, one prospective study of severely head-injured patients found that a CPP > 70 mmHg reduced the percentage of hypoxic $P_{bt}O_2$ (≤15 mmHg) to 10% from 50% when CPP was below 60 mmHg (Marín-Caballos et al., 2005). While this is higher than the generally recommended CPP threshold of 60 mmHg, this study illustrates the importance of monitoring brain tissue oxygenation, and tailoring therapies for each patient.

The BOOST 2 trial was a phase II randomized clinical trial assessing the safety and efficacy of brain tissue oxygen monitoring in the management of severe TBI (Diaz-Arrastia, 2014). A total of 110 patients were randomized to treatment based on ICP monitoring alone versus treatment based on ICP and $P_{bt}O_2$ monitoring with a goal ICP < 20 mmHg and $P_{bt}O_2$ > 20 mmHg using a specific tiered protocol. The primary outcome was the proportion of time that $P_{bt}O_2$ was < 20 mmHg; this was markedly reduced in the brain tissue monitoring group. There was no significant difference in adverse events. A phase III trial is being planned.

Several studies have shown an association between low $P_{bt}O_2$ and worse outcomes. The majority of data come from severe TBI patients showing lower mortality and better functional outcomes among those with higher $P_{bt}O_2$ values (Narotam et al., 2009; Spiotta et al., 2010; Eriksson et al., 2012; Lin et al., 2015). Brain hypoxia is also a predictor of poor outcome independent of elevated ICP and low CPP (Oddo et al., 2011). Two studies of severe TBI patients managed with ICP and $P_{bt}O_2$ monitoring were compared to historic controls managed solely by ICP/CPP monitoring, and both studies found higher $P_{bt}O_2$ values in survivors (Spiotta et al., 2010). One also found improved Glasgow Outcome Scale score at 6 months in the $P_{bt}O_2$ monitored group (Narotam et al., 2009).

Cerebral oxygenation monitoring is also used in the evaluation of patients with SAH. Lower $P_{bt}O_2$ is seen in nonsurvivors (Ramakrishna et al., 2008). SAH patients are particularly vulnerable to ischemia due to vasospasm and other potential mechanisms (Dhar and Dringer, 2015), including disruptions in autoregulation. Much like PRx, the brain tissue oxygen pressure–reactivity index (ORx) may provide useful information on cererbrovascular autoregulation. ORx is calculated as the moving correlation coefficient between CPP and $P_{bt}O_2$, and was found to correlate significantly with PRx in TBI patients (Jaeger et al., 2006). ORx was calculated in 67 severe SAH patients, was found to be significantly higher (indicating impaired autoregulation) in those who developed cerebral infarction, and is suggested as a prognostic indicator of DCI (Jaeger et al., 2007). Interestingly, changes in $P_{bt}O_2$ alone were not predictive of cerebral infarction.

## Near-infrared spectroscopy

NIRS is a noninvasive monitor of cerebral oxygenation. It was initially used to monitor for cerebral ischemia during carotid and cardiovascular surgery. The device is applied across the forehead and measures the transmission and absorption of light in the near-infrared spectrum as it passes through tissue. It is an indirect measure of the relative oxygenation of blood in cerebral tissue (Ghosh et al., 2012). Normal values are between 60 and 75%, but trends in values are considered more important than the absolute number (Highton et al., 2010). NIRS has been used to assess CBF autoregulation in TBI (Zweifel et al., 2010a) and SAH (Zweifel et al., 2010b), with some promise. More recently, it has been used to predict outcomes during endovascular treatment for acute ischemic stroke (Hametner et al., 2015). NIRS has been suggested as a monitor for vasospasm in comatose SAH patients, though sufficient data are lacking. One study showed an ipsilateral drop in cerebral oxygen saturation during angiographic vasospasm, and the degree of vasospasm was associated with a greater drop in NIRS signal (Bhatia et al., 2007). On the other hand, another study found no correlation between vasospasm, either angiographic or clinical (Naidech et al., 2008). NIRS is currently not recommended for routine monitoring of adult neurocritical care patients based on the International Multidisciplinary Consensus Conference on Multimodality Monitoring (Oddo et al., 2014).

## BRAIN METABOLISM AND CEREBRAL MICRODIALYSIS

Cerebral microdialysis is a method for continuous bedside monitoring of brain metabolism. It was first introduced in the early 1990s as a method of monitoring neurochemical markers in acutely brain-injured patients (Persson and Hillered, 1992). The device continues to be used for research and clinical purposes, mostly in TBI and SAH patients. Microdialysis catheters can be placed at the bedside and are inserted through a burrhole or a bolt system, typically about 1.5–2 cm below the skin. They are tunneled beneath the scalp and loosely sutured to the skin to allow flow of perfusate and dialysate, then covered with a sterile dressing. The catheter is attached to a perfusion pump and normal saline or other isotonic fluid is perfused through the catheter at a constant flow rate. Molecules within the interstitial fluid of the brain then diffuse across the semipermeable membrane at the tip of the probe and the dialysate is collected for analysis in small vials at 60-minute time intervals. The concentration of molecules in the dialysate is believed to be proportional to the concentration in the interstitial fluid (Tisdall and Smith, 2006). The first sample is usually not analyzed, as the probe needs time to stabilize and equilibrate. A CT scan is obtained to confirm correct placement. Insertion of the probe is considered to be safe, based on the experience of large cohort studies (Hutchinson et al., 2015). Microdialysis is used to monitor for changes in energy metabolism and brain ischemia and has enhanced our understanding of the pathophysiology of brain injury.

Standard metabolites to be measured include lactate, glucose, and pyruvate. Glucose is the main energy substrate for the brain and understanding glucose delivery and utilization is critical for the brain-injured patient. Under normal conditions, glucose is metabolized to pyruvate, which then is converted to acetyl-CoA and enters mitochondria to participate in the Krebs cycle. A series of redox reactions occurs, producing NADH, which then is used in the electron transport chain to generate adenosine triphosphate through the process of oxidative phosphorylation. When ischemia or hypoxia occurs, the lack of oxygen delivery to the mitochondria results in a shift from aerobic to anaerobic metabolism, and NADH is instead used to convert pyruvate to lactate. Thus, measuring the interstitial levels of glucose, lactate, and pyruvate provides information on the extent of anaerobic glycolysis. In particular, the lactate/pyruvate ratio (LPR) is a reflection of the intracellular redox state of the cell and is a measurement of mitochondrial function. A low interstitial glucose level indicates a lack of glucose delivery (Hillered et al., 2005). The LPR has been found to be a more specific measure of cerebral ischemia compared to lactate alone (Enblad et al., 1996).

Other markers studied using cerebral microdialysis include glutamate and glycerol. Glutamate is the main excitatory amino acid in the brain. Its accumulation leads to calcium influx and secondary brain injury (Hillered et al., 2005). Elevated levels of glutamate have been found in both TBI (Zauner et al., 1996; Chamoun et al., 2010) and SAH (Nilsson et al., 1999), and are correlated with cerebral ischemia and poor outcome. However, the theory of high interstitial glutamate as an indicator of excitotoxicity has been challenged, since the measured glutamate in interstitial fluid by microdialysis is not necessarily a reflection of the concentration of glutamate at the synaptic cleft, and levels of glutamate necessary to produce depolarization and cell death are not attained in acute brain injury (Obrenovitch, 1999). Elevated microdialysis glutamate levels are seen in association with seizures (Vespa et al., 1998) and, more recently, have been connected to spreading depolarizations following TBI (Hinzman et al., 2015). Similarly, elevations in glycerol are also seen following brain injury. Glycerol is thought to be a degradation product from cell membrane phospholipid breakdown following acute brain injury and may be triggered by calcium influx and reactive oxygen species (Hillered et al., 2005). Elevated glycerol levels have also been found to be associated with ischemia and poor outcomes in TBI (Hillered et al., 1998; Paraforou et al., 2011) and SAH (Nilsson et al., 1999; Schulz et al., 2000) patients. Higher-molecular-weight molecules, such as cytokines, can be measured using specialized catheters.

Cerebral microdialysis can be used for prognostication in neurocritical care patients. Multiple studies using cerebral microdialysis, typically in conjunction with other monitoring techniques, have shown poor outcome in TBI patients with abnormal glucose and lactate values (Zauner et al., 1997; Goodman et al., 1999; Timofeev et al., 2011; Stein et al., 2012). In one study of 223 TBI patients, independent positive predictors of mortality included low microdialysate glucose, elevated LPR, as well as increasing age, ICP, and PRx. Those patients with a favorable outcome at 6 months postinjury had significantly lower median LPR and lactate levels (Timofeev et al., 2011). In another study of TBI patients, low glucose and elevated LPR were again associated with poor outcome at 6 months despite adequate resuscitation and controlled ICP (Stein et al., 2012). Elevated LPR after TBI has also been associated with frontal-lobe atrophy on magnetic resonance imaging at 6 months postinjury (Marcoux et al., 2008). Similarly, in SAH patients, high LPR is more common in poor-grade patients and associated with worse neurologic outcomes (Kett-White et al., 2002; Sarrafzadeh et al., 2004). Conversely, elevated lactate levels in SAH may be a predictor of good outcomes. One study of 31 poor-grade SAH patients undergoing concurrent cerebral microdialysis and brain tissue oxygenation monitoring were classified into two patterns of elevated brain lactate: hypoxic (low $P_{bt}O_2$) or nonhypoxic; and hyperglycolytic (elevated pyruvate) or nonhyperglycolytic. Mortality was associated with hypoxic elevated brain lactate but good recovery at 6 months was associated with hyperglycolysis and elevated brain lactate (Oddo et al., 2012). The authors postulate that elevated lactate due to increased aerobic glycolysis in astrocytes is used as an alternative fuel in neurons, leading to improved survival. Other studies have shown that lactate can indeed act as an energy source via the Krebs cycle in humans with TBI (Gallagher et al., 2009). While infrequently studied in this patient population, low LPR has also been associated with favorable outcomes at 6 months in patients with spontaneous ICH (Nikaina et al., 2012).

Cerebral microdialysis can also be used to predict secondary brain injury. Several studies have shown an ischemic pattern on microdialysis that precedes the onset of symptomatic vasospasm in SAH (Sarrafzadeh et al., 2002; Skjøth-Rasmussen et al., 2004). One study of aneurysmal SAH patients found an increase in the lactate/glucose ratio and LPR in 17 out of 18 patients who experienced delayed ischemic neurologic deficits, and this preceded the development of symptoms by a mean of 11 hours (Skjøth-Rasmussen et al., 2004). Another study found that microdialysis has a higher specificity over TCD or angiography for confirming vasospasm in asymptomatic SAH patients (Unterberg et al., 2001). Additionally, changes in cerebral microdialysis may precede elevations in ICP in severe TBI patients (Belli et al., 2008).

Glucose delivery and utilization play major roles in acute brain injury and monitoring brain chemistry can guide systemic glucose control. Hyperglycemia is a well-established poor prognostic indicator for aneurysmal SAH (Kruyt et al., 2009). However, low cerebral glucose is also associated with poor outcomes in SAH and is not necessarily related to blood glucose levels (Schlenk et al., 2008a). Additionally, variations in systemic glucose levels are also associated with higher mortality rates and cerebral metabolic distress in SAH (Kurtz et al., 2014). Initiation of insulin therapy to control hyperglycemia is necessary, but insulin can reduce cerebral glucose levels as well, and microdialysis may play an important role in monitoring cerebral metabolism during treatment with insulin to avoid further brain injury and metabolic crisis (Schlenk et al., 2008b). Cerebral microdialysis can also be used to monitor cerebral glucose levels during initiation of enteral nutrition (Kinoshita et al., 2010), and may be important in the future for optimizing enteral feedings in brain-injured patients. Similarly, optimal glucose control has not been defined in TBI. Low interstitial glucose has also been associated with poor outcomes in TBI patients, and not necessarily related to cerebral ischemia (Vespa et al., 2003). Furthermore, tight blood glucose control (80–120 mg/dL) was associated with reduced cerebral glucose, metabolic crisis with elevated LPR, and increased mortality in a study of 20 patients with severe brain injury (Oddo et al., 2008). Intensive insulin therapy in another study of TBI patients also found lower microdialysis glucose concentrations and markers of cellular distress, including elevated glutamate and LPR (Vespa et al., 2006). However, in this study, mortality and 6-month outcomes were the same when compared to patients treated with a loose insulin protocol. Further research is necessary to determine optimal therapies and targets for glucose control and maintenance of stable cerebral metabolism.

Cerebral microdialysis is a unique tool to assess brain metabolism and has potential benefits. The Consensus Statement from the 2014 International Microdialysis Forum described cerebral microdialysis to be a reliable and safe technique for the clinical management of severe TBI or SAH patients (Hutchinson et al., 2015). It includes reference values for commonly measured substrates and ranks them based on quantity and usefulness of clinical data, with glucose and LPR being at the top, followed by glutamate and then glycerol. When using cerebral microdialysis, one must always be aware of the location of the catheter (pericontusional versus normal brain), as results vary widely (Engström et al., 2005). In one study, use of microdialysis probes was associated with lower mortality in TBI and SAH patients when used in conjunction with ICP data, compared to patients managed with a CPP strategy alone; it is not entirely clear how microdialysis modified treatment in this study (Dizdarevic et al., 2012). When used, cerebral microdialysis should always be combined with other monitoring modalities for accurate interpretation of the data. Potential additional uses of the cerebral microdialysis probe include identification of ischemic stroke progression in patients with hemispheric infarcts (Woitzik et al., 2014), discovery of new biomarkers (Lööv et al., 2015), and measurement of drug levels (particularly antibiotics and anticonvulsants) for pharmacokinetic studies (Shannon et al., 2013).

## TRANSCRANIAL DOPPLER ULTRASONOGRAPHY

TCD ultrasound is a noninvasive tool for assessing cerebral hemodynamics. A probe is used to insonate the major cerebral arteries and peak systolic, end-diastolic, and mean flow velocities, as well as the pulsatility index, are recorded (Springborg et al., 2005). An inverse relationship between blood vessel diameter based on cerebral angiogram and TCD flow velocities has been demonstrated (Aaslid et al., 1984). Generally a mean flow velocity greater than 120 cm/second is indicative of vasospasm in the anterior circulation. A hemispheric index has also been proposed by Lindegaard et al. (1988), and this divides the middle cerebral artery flow velocity by the ipsilateral extracranial internal carotid artery flow velocity to adjust for variations in total blood flow, which will impact TCD velocity even when vascular caliber remains constant. A hemispheric index greater than 3 suggests vasospasm. The TCD flow velocity trend has also been examined, with a rapid increase of 50 cm/second or more during a 24-hour period used to predict vasospasm (Ekelund et al., 1996). TCD seems reliable and is strongly recommended by the International Multidisciplinary Consensus Conference of MMM in Neurocritical Care for prediction of angiographic vasospasm after aneurysmal SAH (LeRoux et al., 2014), although there is some literature to suggest that there is poor sensitivity (e.g., 63% in one study of 441 aneurysmal SAH patients), such that alternative methods of identifying DCI and vasospasm are necessary (Carrera et al., 2009). When TCD values are combined with clinical factors and measures of CBF, a vasospasm probability index with more than 80% sensitivity has been described (Gonzalez et al., 2007).

Vasospasm is primarily a phenomenon following aneurysmal SAH, but can also occur in other disease states, particularly TBI. One study of 299 patients found an incidence of posttraumatic vasospasm of 45% (Oertel et al., 2005), highlighting another potentially important role for TCD in neurocritical care. While TCDs are mostly used in SAH patients for the detection of vasospasm, the calculated pulsatility index (peak systolic velocity – end-diastolic velocity/mean flow velocity) can also be utilized as a noninvasive estimate of ICP (Bellner et al., 2004). Akin to other monitoring methods,

TCD values need to be combined with other variables and the clinical examination to integrate information and assess the need for therapeutic intervention.

## CEREBRAL BLOOD FLOW

There are several imaging modalities in use to measure CBF, including PET, magnetic resonance, or CT perfusion and xenon-CT. While these are valuable in determining areas of ischemia, they are limited by the need to transfer the patient and lack of continuous imaging, in that they only provide data for one point in time during the hospital course. TCD studies, as described previously, are used to estimate CBF in large areas of the brain, but are also limited by operator variability. CBF can be monitored with invasive probes, but these are limited to small regions of the brain. Laser Doppler flowmetry is a method that assesses the microcirculatory flux (a measure of red blood cell concentration and velocity) and has been used to continuously monitor CBF in TBI patients (Kirkpatrick et al., 1994), and, when correlated with CPP and arterial blood pressure, has been applied to determine disruptions in autoregulation, which may have prognostic significance (Lam et al., 1997). A thermal diffusion microprobe has also been designed for the continuous evaluation of CBF. The catheter contains two thermistors. The distal one is heated, and heat transfer through brain tissue is measured at the proximal end, which is ultimately correlated with CBF (Vajkoczy et al., 2000). The probe has been used safely in patients with TBI and allows for assessment of autoregulation (Rosenthal et al., 2011). While measures of CBF and determination of an optimal CPP are important, there are also nonischemic mechanisms of cellular damage in brain-injured patients (Vespa et al., 2005), and emphasis is optimally placed on integrating data collected from MMM in a comprehensive manner.

## BIOINFORMATICS AND THE FUTURE OF MMM

Over the last 20 years, there has been an exponential increase in the use of various monitoring devices in neurocritical care. There are huge amounts of physiologic data collected, but systematic approaches to documenting and interpreting the data are lacking. A critically ill patient may have dozens of continuously collected variables between hemodynamic recordings, laboratory values, and neuromonitoring-derived data (ICP, CPP, $P_{bt}O_2$, microdialysis values, TCD flow velocities, etc.). Processing this information manually is nearly impossible and subject to human error. The integration of all these variables to identify trends, and aid in clinical decision making, is part of the growing field of bioinformatics (De Turck et al., 2007). Future studies will likely use analytic software such as multivariate analysis (Sorani et al., 2007) or symbolic regression (Narotam et al., 2014) to identify trends and patterns in patients' pathophysiologic variables, in addition to the creation of electronic interfaces to better understand the complex interactions following brain injury, thereby allowing therapies to be tailored to individual patients. Currently, there is a large amount of data available but the ability to better analyze it in real time will be the next step in neurocritical bioinformatics.

The future will also envision new devices or new applications of currently existing devices. For example, combining various monitoring methods into a single probe for simultaneous data measurements (Li et al., 2012) or creating portable devices for bedside assessment would be significant advances. One example of such technology is a near-infrared-based device that has been shown to reliably detect ICH of greater than 3.5 cc (Robertson et al., 2010). Lastly, new technologies for noninvasive ICP measurement, including ocular ultrasound for detection of optic nerve sheath diameter (Cammarata et al., 2011) and pupillometry (Chen et al., 2011), may be beneficial in selected cases or as triaging tools.

Studies assessing the impact of brain monitors on clinical outcomes are needed. However, randomized clinical trials, the gold standard of evidence-based medicine, have found few interventions in critical care to be efficacious. This may largely be due to the heterogeneity of patient subjects, particularly in TBI and SAH, and lack of generalizability of protocols used in clinical trials, thereby leading to practice misalignment (Deans et al., 2010). The future of neurocritical care will likely increasingly involve large, international databases of standardized, prospectively collected data that focus on observational cohorts and comparative effectiveness research (Maas et al., 2012). Examination of not just neuromonitors, but also how management strategies using data collected from the monitors guide individual care, will open the door to new therapeutic interventions.

## CONCLUSION

Neurocritical care has focused on the identification and prevention of secondary brain injury. While the neurologic examination is still essential, more advanced monitoring of patients while in coma or under sedation is necessary, as the physical examination is limited in these situations. This chapter has reviewed the major cerebral monitoring modalities and what information has been gained with these monitors to help enhance our understanding of brain pathophysiology. No single value or device can provide all the information about the status of brain function and thus MMM and integration of

various variables, in addition to imaging studies, provide a more thorough view of the complex patient and allow the clinician to make individualized decisions. This will be enhanced in the future with modern technologies for device development and the growing field of bioinformatics.

## REFERENCES

Aaslid R, Huber P, Nornes H (1984). Evaluation of cerebrovascular spasm with transcranial Doppler ultrasound. J Neurosurg 60 (1): 37–41.

Balestreri M, Czosnyka M, Hutchinson P et al. (2006). Impact of intracranial pressure and cerebral perfusion pressure on severe disability and mortality after head injury. Neurocrit Care 4 (1): 8–13.

Belli A, Sen J, Petzold A et al. (2008). Metabolic failure precedes intracranial pressure rises in traumatic brain injury: a microdialysis study. Acta Neurochir (Wien) 150 (5): 461–469.

Bellner J, Romner B, Reinstrup P et al. (2004). Transcranial Doppler sonography pulsatility index (PI) reflects intracranial pressure (ICP). Surg Neurol 62 (1): 45–51.

Bergsneider M, Hovda DA, Shalmon E et al. (1997). Cerebral hyperglycolysis following severe traumatic brain injury in humans: a positron emission tomography study. J Neurosurg 86 (2): 241–251.

Bhatia R, Hampton T, Malde S et al. (2007). The application of near-infrared oximetry to cerebral monitoring during aneurysm embolization: a comparison with intraprocedural angiography. J Neurosurg Anesthesiol 19 (2): 97–104.

Bratton SL, Bullock R, Carney N et al. (2007a). Guidelines for the management of severe brain injury. VIII Intracranial pressure thresholds. J Neurotrauma 24 (Suppl 1): S55–S58.

Bratton SL, Chesnut RM, Ghajar J et al. (2007b). Guidelines for the management of severe traumatic brain injury. IX Cerebral perfusion thresholds. J Neurotrauma 24 (Suppl 1): S59–S64.

Bullock R, Zauner A, Myseros JS et al. (1995). Evidence for prolonged release of excitatory amino acids in severe human head trauma. Relationship to clinical events. Ann N Y Acad Sci 765: 290–297.

Cammarata G, Ristagno G, Cammarata A et al. (2011). Ocular ultrasound to detect intracranial hypertension in trauma patients. J Trauma 71 (3): 779–781.

Carrera E, Schmidt JM, Oddo M et al. (2009). Transcranial Doppler for predicting delayed cerebral ischemia after subarachnoid hemorrhage. Neurosurgery 65 (2): 316–323.

Chamoun R, Suki D, Gopinath SP et al. (2010). Role of extracellular glutamate measured by cerebral microdialysis in severe traumatic brain injury. J Neurosurg 113 (3): 564–570.

Chen JW, Gombart ZJ, Rogers S et al. (2011). Pupillary reactivity as an early indicator of increased intracranial pressure: the introduction of the Neurological Pupil Index. Surg Neurol Int 2: 82.

Chesnut RM, Temkin N, Carney N et al. (2012). A trial of intracranial-pressure monitoring in traumatic brain injury. N Engl J Med 367 (26): 2471–2481.

Chesnut RM, Bleck TP, Citerio G et al. (2015). A consensus-based interpretation of the BEST TRIP ICP trial. J Neurotrauma 32 (22): 1722–1724.

Claassen J, Mayer SA (2002). Continuous electroencephalographic monitoring in neurocritical care. Curr Neurol Neurosci Rep 2 (6): 534–540.

Claassen J, Vespa P (2014). Electrophysiologic monitoring in acute brain injury. Neurocrit Care 21: S129–S147.

Claassen J, Hirsch LJ, Frontera JA et al. (2006). Prognostic significance of continuous EEG monitoring in patients with poor-grade subarachnoid hemorrhage. Neurocrit Care 4 (2): 103–112.

Claassen J, Jetté N, Chum F et al. (2007). Electrographic seizures and periodic discharges after intracerebral hemorrhage. Neurology 69 (13): 1356–1365.

Claassen J, Perotte A, Albers D et al. (2013). Nonconvulsive seizures after subarachnoid hemorrhage: multimodal detection and outcomes. Ann Neurol 74 (1): 53–64.

Coles JP, Minhas PS, Fryer TD et al. (2002). Effect of hyperventilation on cerebral blood flow in traumatic head injury: clinical relevance and monitoring correlates. Crit Care Med 30 (9): 1950–1959.

Coles JP, Fryer TD, Smielewski P et al. (2004). Incidence and mechanisms of cerebral ischemia in early clinical head injury. J Cereb Blood Flow Metab 24 (2): 202–211.

Coles JP, Fryer TD, Coleman MR et al. (2007). Hyperventilation following head injury: effect on ischemic burden and cerebral oxidative metabolism. Crit Care Med 35 (2): 568–578.

Coplin WM, O'Keefe GE, Grady MS et al. (1997). Thrombotic, infectious and procedural complications of the jugular bulb catheter in the intensive care unit. Neurosurgery 41 (1): 101–107.

Cormio M, Valadka AB, Robertson CS (1999). Elevated jugular venous oxygen saturation after severe head injury. J Neurosurg 90 (1): 9–15.

Czosnyka M, Smielewski P, Kirkpatrick P et al. (1997). Continuous assessment of the cerebral vasomotor reactivity in head injury. Neurosurgery 41 (1): 11–17.

Dawes AJ, Sacks GD, Cryer HG et al. (2015). Intracranial pressure monitoring and inpatient mortality in severe traumatic brain injury: a propensity score-matched analysis. J Trauma Acute Care Surg 78 (3): 492–501.

De Turck F, Decruyenaere J, Thysebaert P et al. (2007). Design of a flexible platform for execution of medical decision support agents in the intensive care unit. Comput Biol Med 37 (1): 97–112.

Deans KJ, Minneci PC, Danner RL et al. (2010). Practice misalignments in randomized controlled trials: identification, impact and potential solutions. Anesth Analg 111 (2): 444–450.

Dhar R, Diringer MN (2015). Relationship between angiographic vasospasm, cerebral blood flow, and cerebral infarction after subarachnoid hemorrhage. Acta Neurochir Suppl 120: 161–165.

Diaz-Arrastia R (2014). Brain tissue oxygen monitoring in traumatic brain injury (TBI) (BOOST 2). In: Presented at the 12th Annual Neurocritical Care Society Meeting; 2014 Sept 11–14, Seattle, WA.

Dings J, Meixensberger J, Jäger A et al. (1998). Clinical experience with 118 brain tissue oxygen partial pressure catheter probes. Neurosurgery 43 (5): 1082–1095.

Dizdarevic K, Hamdan A, Omerhodzic I et al. (2012). Modified Lund concept versus cerebral perfusion pressure-targeted therapy: a randomized controlled study in patients with secondary brain ischaemia. Clin Neurol Neurosurg 114 (2): 142–148.

Ekelund A, Säveland H, Romner B et al. (1996). Is transcranial Doppler sonography useful in detecting late cerebral ischaemia after aneurysmal subarachnoid haemorrhage? Br J Neurosurg 10 (1): 19–25.

Enblad P, Valtysson J, Andersson J et al. (1996). Simultaneous intracerebral microdialysis and positron emission tomography in the detection of ischemia in patients with subarachnoid hemorrhage. J Cereb Blood Flow Metab 16 (14): 637–644.

Engström M, Polito A, Reinstrup P et al. (2005). Intracerebral microdialysis in severe brain trauma: the importance of catheter location. J Neurosurg 102 (3): 460–469.

Eriksson EA, Barletta JF, Figueroa BE et al. (2012). The first 72 hours of brain tissue oxygenation predicts patient survival with traumatic brain injury. J Trauma Acute Care Surg 72 (5): 1345–1349.

Fortune JB, Feustel PJ, Weigle CG et al. (1994). Continuous measurement of jugular venous oxygen saturation in response to transient elevations of blood pressure in head-injured patients. J Neurosurg 80 (3): 461–468.

Fortune JB, Feustel PJ, Graca L et al. (1995). Effect of hyperventilation, mannitol, and ventriculostomy drainage on cerebral blood flow after head injury. J Trauma 39 (6): 1091–1097.

Gallagher CN, Carpenter KL, Grice P et al. (2009). The human brain utilizes lactate via the tricarboxylic acid cycle: a 13C-labelled microdialysis and high-resolution nuclear magnetic resonance study. Brain 132: 2839–2849.

Gaspard N, Hirsch LJ, LaRoche SM et al. (2014). Interrater agreement for critical care EEG terminology. Epilepsia 55 (9): 1366–1373.

Gavvala J, Abedn N, LaRoche S et al. (2014). Continuous EEG monitoring: a survey of neurophysiologists and neurointensivists. Epilepsia 55 (11): 1864–1871.

Ghosh A, Elwell C, Smith M (2012). Cerebral near-infrared spectroscopy in adults: a work in progress. Anesth Analg 115: 1373–1383.

Gollwitzer S, Groemer T, Rampp S et al. (2015). Early prediction of delayed cerebral ischemia in subarachnoid hemorrhage base on quantitative EEG: a prospective study in adults. Clin Neurophysiol 126 (8): 1514–1523.

Gonzalez NR, Boscardin WJ, Glenn T et al. (2007). Vasospasm probability index: a combination of transcranial Doppler velocities, cerebral blood flow and clinical risk factors to predict cerebral vasospasm after aneurysmal subarachnoid hemorrhage. J Neurosurg 107 (6): 1101–1112.

Goodman JC, Valadka AB, Gopinath SP et al. (1999). Extracellular lactate and glucose alterations in the brain after head injury measured by microdialysis. Crit Care Med 27 (9): 1965–1973.

Graham DI, Ford I, Adams JH et al. (1989). Ischaemic brain damage is still common in fatal non-missile head injury. J Neurol Neurosurg Psychiatry 52 (3): 346–350.

Hametner C, Stanarcevic P, Stampfl S et al. (2015). Noninvasive cerebral oximetry during endovascular therapy for acute ischemic stroke: an observational study. J Cereb Blood Flow Metab 35 (11): 1722–1728.

Hebb MO, McArthur DL, Alger J et al. (2007). Impaired percent alpha variability on continuous electroencephalography is associated with thalamic injury and predicts poor long-term outcome after human traumatic brain injury. J Neurotrauma 24 (4): 579–590.

Heran NS, Hentschel SJ, Toyota BD (2004). Jugular bulb oximetry for prediction of vasospasm following subarachnoid hemorrhage. Can J Neurol Sci 31 (1): 80–86.

Highton D, Elwell C, Smith M (2010). Noninvasive cerebral oximetry: is there light at the end of the tunnel? Curr Opin Anaesthesiol 23: 576–581.

Hillered L, Valtysson J, Enblad P et al. (1998). Interstitial glycerol as a marker for membrane phospholipid degradation in the acutely injured human brain. J Neurol Neurosurg Psychiatry 64 (4): 486–491.

Hillered L, Vespa PM, Hovda DA (2005). Translational neurochemical research in acute human brain injury: the current status and potential future for cerebral microdialysis. J Neurotrauma 22 (1): 3–41.

Hinzman J, Wilson JA, Mazzeo AT et al. (2015). Excitotoxicity and metabolic crisis are associated with spreading depolarizations in severe traumatic brain injury patients. J Neurotrauma [Epub ahead of print].

Hutchinson PJ, Jalloh I, Helmy A et al. (2015). Consensus statement from the 2014 International Microdialysis Forum. Intensive Care Med 41 (9): 1517–1528.

Jaeger M, Schuhmann MU, Soehle M et al. (2006). Continuous assessment of cerebrovascular autoregulation after traumatic brain injury using brain tissue oxygen pressure reactivity. Crit Care Med 34: 1783–1788.

Jaeger M, Schuhmann MU, Soehle M et al. (2007). Continuous monitoring of cerebrovascular autoregulation after subarachnoid hemorrhage by brain tissue oxygen pressure reactivity and its relation to delayed cerebral infarction. Stroke 38 (3): 981–986.

Kett-White R, Hutchinson PJ, Al-Rawi PG et al. (2002). Adverse cerebral events detected after subarachnoid hemorrhage using brain oxygen and microdialysis probes. Neurosurgery 50 (6): 1213–1221.

Kinoshita K, Moriya T, Utagawa A et al. (2010). Change in brain glucose after enteral nutrition in subarachnoid hemorrhage. J Surg Res 162 (2): 221–224.

Kirkpatrick PJ, Smielewski P, Czosnyka M et al. (1994). Continuous monitoring of cortical perfusion by laser Doppler flowmetry in ventilated patients with head injury. J Neurol Neurosurg Psychiatry 57 (11): 1382–1388.

Knight WA, Hart KW, Adeoye OM et al. (2013). The incidence of seizures in patients undergoing therapeutic hypotehmia after resuscitation from cardiac arrest. Epilepsy Res 106 (3): 396–402.

Kruyt ND, Biessels GJ, de Haan RJ et al. (2009). Hyperglycemia and clinical outcome in aneurysmal subarachnoid hemorrhage: a meta-analysis. Stroke 40 (6): e424–e430.

Kurtz P, Claassen J, Helbok R et al. (2014). Systemic glucose variability predicts cerebral metabolic distress and mortality after subarachnoid hemorrhage: a retrospective observational study. Crit Care 18 (3): R89.

Lam JM, Hsiang JN, Poon WS (1997). Monitoring of autoregulation using laser Doppler flowmetry in patients with head injury. J Neurosurg 86 (3): 438–445.

LeRoux P, Menon DK, Citerio G et al. (2014). The International Multidisciplinary Consensus Conference on Multimodality Monitoring in Neurocritical Care: a statement for healthcare professionals from the Neurocritical Care Society and the European Society of Intensive Care Medicine. Neurocrit Care 21 (Suppl2): S1–S26.

Li C, Wu PM, Hartings JA et al. (2012). Micromachined lab-on-a-tube sensors for simultaneous brain temperature and cerebral blood flow measurements. Biomed Microdevices 14 (4): 759–768.

Lin CM, Lin MC, Huang SJ et al. (2015). A prospective randomized study of brain tissue oxygen pressure-guided management in moderate and severe traumatic brain injury patients. Biomed Res Int 2015: 529580.

Lindegaard KF, Nornes H, Bakke SJ et al. (1988). Cerebral vasospasm after subarachnoid haemorrhage investigated by means of transcranial Doppler ultrasound. Acta Neurochir Suppl (Wien) 42: 81–84.

Logi F, Pasqualetti P, Tomaiuolo F (2011). Predict recovery of consciousness in post-acute severe brain injury: the role of EEG reactivity. Brain Inj 25 (10): 972–979.

Lööv C, Nadadhur AG, Hillered L et al. (2015). Extracellular ezrin: a novel biomarker for traumatic brain injury. J Neurotrauma 32 (4): 244–251.

Lundberg N, Troupp H, Lorin H (1965). Continuous recording of the ventricular-fluid pressure in patients with severe acute traumatic brain injury: a preliminary report. J Neurosurg 22: 581–590.

Maas A, Menon DK, Lingsma HF et al. (2012). Re-orientation of clinical research in traumatic brain injury: report of an international workshop of comparative effectiveness research. J Neurotrauma 29 (1): 32–46.

MacLaughlin BW, Plurad DS, Sheppard W et al. (2015). The impact of intracranial pressure monitoring on mortality after severe traumatic brain injury. Am J Surg 210: 1082–1086.

Marcoux J, McArthur DA, Miller C et al. (2008). Persistent metabolic crisis as measured by elevated cerebral microdialysis lactate-pyruvate ratio predicts chronic frontal lobe brain atrophy after traumatic brain injury. Crit Care Med 36 (10): 2871–2877.

Marín-Caballos AJ, Murillo-Cabezas F, Cayuela-Domínguez A et al. (2005). Cerebral perfusion pressure and risk of brain hypoxia in severe head injury: a prospective observational study. Crit Care 9 (6): R670–R676.

Marmarou A, Anderson RL, Ward JD et al. (1991). Impact of ICP instability and hypotension on outcome in patients with severe head trauma. J Neurosurg 75: S159–S166.

Miller JD, Becker DP, Ward JD et al. (1977). Significance of intracranial hypertension in severe head injury. J Neurosurg 47 (4): 503–516.

Naidech AM, Bendok BR, Ault ML et al. (2008). Monitoring with the Somanetics INVOS 5100C after aneurysmal subarachnoid hemorrhage. Neurocrit Care 9 (3): 326–331.

Narotam PK, Morrison JF, Nathoo N (2009). Brain tissue oxygen monitoring in traumatic brain injury and major trauma: outcome analysis of a brain tissue oxygen-directed therapy. J Neurosurg 111 (4): 672–682.

Narotam PK, Morrison JF, Schmidt MD et al. (2014). Physiological complexity of acute traumatic brain injury in patients treated with a brain oxygen protocol: utility of symbolic regression in predictive modeling of a dynamical system. J Neurotrauma 31 (7): 630–641.

Nikaina I, Paterakis K, Paraforos G et al. (2012). Cerebral perfusion pressure, microdialysis biochemistry, and clinical outcome in patients with spontaneous intracerebral hematomas. J Crit Care 27 (1): 83–88.

Nilsson OG, Brandt L, Ungerstedt U et al. (1999). Bedside detection of brain ischemia using intracerebral microdialysis: subarachnoid hemorrhage and delayed ischemic deterioration. Neurosurgery 45 (5): 1176–1184.

Obrenovitch TP (1999). High extracellular glutamate and neuronal death in neurological disorders. Cause, contribution or consequence? Ann N Y Acad Sci 890: 273–286.

Oddo M, Schmidt JM, Carrera E et al. (2008). Impact of tight glycemic control on cerebral glucose metabolism after severe brain injury: a microdialysis study. Crit Care Med 36 (12): 3233–3238.

Oddo M, Levine JM, Mackenzie L et al. (2011). Brain hypoxia is associated with short-term outcome after severe traumatic brain injury independently of intracranial hypertension and low cerebral perfusion pressure. Neurosurgery 69 (5): 1037–1045.

Oddo M, Levine JM, Frangos S et al. (2012). Brain lactate metabolism in humans with subarachnoid hemorrhage. Stroke 43: 1418–1421.

Oddo M, Bösel J et al. (2014). Monitoring of brain and systemic oxygenation in neurocritical care patients. Neurocrit Care Suppl 2: S103–S120.

Oertel M, Boscardin WJ, Obrist WD et al. (2005). Posttraumatic vasospasm: the epidemiology, severity, and time course of an underestimated phenomenon: a prospective study performed in 299 patients. J Neurosurg 103 (5): 812–824.

Paraforou T, Paterakis K, Fountas K et al. (2011). Cerebral perfusion pressure, microdialysis biochemistry and clinical outcome in patients with traumatic brain injury. BMC Res Notes 4: 540.

Persson L, Hillered L (1992). Chemical monitoring of neurosurgical intensive care patients using intracerebral microdialysis. J Neurosurg 76 (1): 72–80.

Ponce LL, Pillai S, Cruz J et al. (2012). Position of probe determines prognostic information of brain tissue PO2 in severe traumatic brain injury. Neurosurgery 70 (6): 1492–1502.

Ramakrishna R, Stiefel M, Udoetuk J et al. (2008). Brain oxygen tension and outcome in patients with aneurysmal subarachnoid hemorrhage. J Neurosurg 109 (6): 1075–1082.

Robertson CS, Valadka AB, Hannay HJ et al. (1999). Prevention of secondary ischemic insults after severe head injury. Crit Care Med 27 (10): 2086–2095.

Robertson CS, Zager EL, Narayan RK et al. (2010). Clinical evaluation of a portable near-infrared device for detection of traumatic intracranial hematomas. J Neurotrauma 27 (9): 1597–1604.

Rosenthal G, Sanchez-Mejia RO, Phan N et al. (2011). Incorporating a parenchymal thermal diffusion cerebral blood flow probe in bedside assessment of cerebral autoregulation and vasoreactivity in patients with severe traumatic brain injury. J Neurosurg 114 (1): 62–70.

Rossetti AO, Urbano LA, Delodder F et al. (2010). Prognositc value of continuous EEG monitoring during therapeutic hypothermia after cardiac arrest. Crit Care 14 (5): R173.

Rots ML, van Putten MJ, Hoedemaekers CW et al. (2016). Continuous EEG monitoring for early detection of delayed cerebral ischemia in subarachnoid hemorrhage: a pilot study. Neurocrit Care 24: 207–216.

Sarrafzadeh AS, Sakowitz OW, Kiening KL et al. (2002). Bedside microdialysis: a tool to monitor cerebral metabolism in subarachnoid hemorrhage patients? Crit Care Med 30: 1062–1070.

Sarrafzadeh A, Haux D, Küchler I et al. (2004). Poor-grade aneurysmal subarachnoid hemorrhage: relationship of cerebral metabolism to outcome. J Neurosurg 100 (3): 400–406.

Schlenk F, Nagel A, Graetz D et al. (2008a). Hyperglycemia and cerebral glucose in aneurysmal subarachnoid hemorrhage. Intensive Care Med 34 (7): 1200–1207.

Schlenk F, Graetz D, Nagel A et al. (2008b). Insulin-related decrease in cerebral glucose despite normoglycemia in aneurysmal subarachnoid hemorrhage. Crit Care 12 (1): R9.

Schulz MK, Wang LP, Tange M, Bjerre P (2000). Cerebral microdialysis monitoring: determination of normal and ischemic cerebral metabolisms in patients with aneurysmal subarachnoid hemorrhage. J Neurosurg 93 (5): 808–814.

Shannon RJ, Carpenter KL, Guilfoyle MR et al. (2013). Cerebral microdialysis in clinical studies of drugs: pharmacokinetic applications. J Pharmacokinet Pharmacodyn 40 (3): 343–358.

Sharbrough FW, Messick JM, Sundt TM (1973). Correlation of continuous electroencephalograms with cerebral blood flow measurements during carotid endarterectomy. Stroke 4: 674–683.

Skjøth-Rasmussen J, Schulz M, Kristensen SR et al. (2004). Delayed neurological deficits detected by an ischemic pattern in the extracellular cerebral metabolites in patients with aneurysmal subarachnoid hemorrhage. J Neurosurg 100 (1): 8–15.

Sorani MD, Hemphill JC, Morabito D et al. (2007). New approaches to physiological informatics in neurocritical care. Neurocrit Care 7 (1): 45–52.

Spiotta AM, Stiefel MF, Gracias VH et al. (2010). Brain tissue oxygen-directed management and outcome in patients with severe traumatic brain injury. J Neurosurg 113 (3): 571–580.

Springborg JB, Frederiksen HJ, Eskesen V et al. (2005). Trends in monitoring patients with aneurysmal subarachnoid haemorrhage. Br J Anaesth 94 (3): 259–270.

Stein NR, McArthur DL, Etchepare M et al. (2012). Early cerebral metabolic crisis after TBI influences outcome despite adequate hemodynamic resuscitation. Neurocrit Care 17 (1): 49–57.

Steiner LA, Czosnyka M, Piechnik SK et al. (2002). Continuous monitoring of cerebrovascular pressure reactivity allows determination of optimal cerebral perfusion pressure in patients with traumatic brain injury. Crit Care Med 30 (4): 733–738.

Szaflarski JP, Rackley AY, Kleindorfer DO et al. (2008). Incidence of seizures in the acute phase of stroke: a population-based study. Epilepsia 49 (6): 974–981.

Talving P, Karamanos E, Teixeira PG et al. (2013). Intracranial pressure monitoring in severe head injury: compliance with Brain Trauma Foundation guidelines and effect on outcomes: a prospective study. J Neurosurg 119 (5): 1248–1254.

Tang A, Pandit V, Fennell V et al. (2015). Intracranial pressure monitor in patients with traumatic brain injury. J Surg Res 194 (2): 565–570.

Timofeev I, Carpenter KLH, Nortje J et al. (2011). Cerebral extracellular chemistry and outcome following traumatic brain injury: a microdialysis study of 223 patients. Brain 134: 484–494.

Tisdall MM, Smith M (2006). Cerebral microdialysis: research technique or clinical tool. Br J Anaesth 97 (1): 18–25.

Treggiari MM, Schutz N, Yanez ND et al. (2007). Role of intracranial pressure values and patterns in predicting outcome in traumatic brain injury: a systematic review. Neurocrit Care 6 (2): 104–112.

Unterberg AW, Sakowitz OW, Sarrafzadeh AS et al. (2001). Role of bedside microdialysis in the diagnosis of cerebral vasospasm following aneurysmal subarachnoid hemorrhage. J Neurosurg 94 (5): 740–749.

Vajkoczy P, Roth H, Horn P et al. (2000). Continuous monitoring of regional cerebral blood flow: experimental and clinical validation of a novel thermal diffusion microprobe. J Neurosurg 93 (2): 265–274.

Vespa PM, Nuwer MR, Juhász C et al. (1997). Early detection of vasospasm after acute subarachnoid hemorrhage using continuous EEG ICU monitoring. Electroencephalogr Clin Neurophysiol 103 (6): 607–615.

Vespa P, Prins M, Ronne-Engstrom E et al. (1998). Increase in extracellular glutamate caused by reduced cerebral perfusion pressure and seizures after human traumatic brain injury: a microdialysis study. J Neurosurg 89 (6): 971–982.

Vespa PM, Nuwer MR, Nenov V et al. (1999). Increased incidence and impact of nonconvulsive and convulsive seizures after traumatic brain injury as detected by continuous electroencephalographic monitoring. J Neurosurg 91 (5): 750–760.

Vespa PM, McArthur D, O'Phelan K et al. (2003). Persistently low extracellular glucose correlates with poor outcome 6 months after human traumatic brain injury despite a lack of increased lactate: a microdialysis study. J Cereb Blood Flow Metab 23: 865–877.

Vespa P, Bergsneider M, Hattori N et al. (2005). Metabolic crisis without brain ischemia is common after traumatic brain injury: a combined microdialysis and positron emission tomography study. J Cereb Blood Flow Metab 25 (6): 763–774.

Vespa P, Boonyaputthikul R, McArthur DL et al. (2006). Intensive insulin therapy reduces microdialysis glucose values without altering glucose utilization or improving the lactate/pyruvate ratio after traumatic brain injury. Crit Care Med 34 (3): 850–856.

Vespa PM, Miller C, McArthur D et al. (2007). Nonconvulsive electrographic seizures after traumatic brain injury result in intracranial pressure and metabolic crisis. Crit Care Med 35 (12): 2830–2836.

Vespa PM, McArthur DL, Xu Y et al. (2010). Nonconvulsive seizures after traumatic brain injury are associated with hippocampal atrophy. Neurology 75 (9): 792–798.

Vigué B, Ract C, Benayed M et al. (1999). Early SjvO2 monitoring in patients with severe brain trauma. Intensive Care Med 25 (5): 445–451.

Waziri A, Claassen J, Stuart RM et al. (2009). Intracortical electroencephalography in acute brain injury. Ann Neurol 66 (3): 366–377.

Willmore LJ, Sypert GW, Munson JV et al. (1978). Chronic focal epileptiform discharges induced by injection of iron into rat and cat cortex. Science 200 (4349): 1501–1503.

Woitzik J, Pinczolits A, Hecht N et al. (2014). Excitotoxicity and metabolic changes in association with infarct progression. Stroke 45 (4): 1183–1185.

Zauner A, Bullock R, Kuta AJ et al. (1996). Glutamate release and cerebral blood flow after severe human head injury. Acta Neurochir Suppl 67: 40–44.

Zauner A, Doppenberg E, Woodward JJ et al. (1997). Multiparametric continuous monitoring of brain metabolism and substrate delivery in neurosurgical patients. Neurol Res 19 (3): 265–273.

Zweifel C, Lavinio A, Steiner LA et al. (2008). Continuous monitoring of cerebrovascular pressure reactivity in patients with head injury. Neurosurg Focus 25 (4): E2.

Zweifel C, Castellani G, Czosnyka M et al. (2010a). Noninvasive monitoring of cerebrovascular reactivity with near infrared spectroscopy in head-injured patients. J Neurotrauma 27 (11): 1951–1958.

Zweifel C, Castellani G, Czosnyka M et al. (2010b). Continuous assessment of cerebral autoregulation with near-infrared spectroscopy in adults after subarachnoid hemorrhage. Stroke 41 (9): 1963–1968.

*Handbook of Clinical Neurology*, Vol. 140 (3rd series)
*Critical Care Neurology, Part I*
E.F.M. Wijdicks and A.H. Kramer, Editors
http://dx.doi.org/10.1016/B978-0-444-63600-3.00007-6

Chapter 7

# Continuous EEG monitoring in the intensive care unit

G.B. YOUNG[1]* AND J. MANTIA[2]

[1]*Departments of Clinical Neurological Sciences and Medicine (Critical Care), Western University, London, Ontario, Canada*

[2]*Clinical Neurophysiology Unit, Sunnybrook Health Sciences Centre, Toronto, Ontario, Canada*

## Abstract

The purpose and indications for continuous electroencephalography monitoring (CEEG) in intensive care unit (ICU) patients include seizure detection, monitoring the effects of treatment (including depth of sedation), grading and classification of EEG abnormalities, ischemia detection and prognostication. Practical considerations of ICU CEEG include: choice of montages (patterns of electrode placement and connections), EEG electrodes, recognition of artifacts, and the use of automated or computerized analysis. These aspects are reviewed, along with an identifcation of current advances and challenges for the future of CEEG in the ICU.

Continuous electroencephalography (CEEG) in the intensive care unit (ICU) with scalp electrodes allows for "real-time" assessment of cerebral cortical function. It is sensitive to subcortical activity only insofar as such activity projected from the thalamus affects cortical rhythms or from the "disconnecting" effect of lesions in the cerebral white matter. In the clinically unresponsive, immobile patient, the EEG provides a window to cortical activity that is otherwise inaccessible at the bedside. Discontinuous or "routine" 20–30-minute recordings certainly have a place, especially for prognostication, but the trending of EEG over at least 24–48 hours can give a much clearer picture of how the brain is doing over time.

Some of the indications for CEEG monitoring include: (1) detection of seizures and monitoring the effects of seizure therapy; (2) clarifying the nature of abnormal movements; (3) monitoring the depth of sedation; (4) grading the severity of encephalopathy; and (5) prognostication, especially in anoxic-ischemic encephalopathy. Each of these indications will be discussed, followed by a review of practical issues of CEEG.

## DETECTION AND MANAGEMENT OF SEIZURES:

Claassen and colleagues (2004) have shown that most (approaching 90%) seizures in comatose ICU patients are nonconvulsive and would not be detectable without EEG. A single 20–30-minute EEG will capture about 15% of recurring seizures captured by CEEG over the first 48 hours of ICU admission (Figs 7.1 and 7.2) (Claassen et al., 2004).

With the exception of absence status epilepticus, there is abundant evidence that nonconvulsive seizures (NCS), especially nonconvulsive status epilepticus (NCSE), can contribute to brain damage and prolong ICU stay and ventilator dependency, with associated morbidity (e.g., infections and ICU-acquired weakness) and mortality (Trieman et al., 1981; Lothman, 1990; Bogousslavsky et al., 1992; Wasterlain et al., 1993; Krumholz et al., 1995; DeGiorgio et al., 1996; Scholtes et al., 1996; Young and Jordan, 1998; Vespa et al., 2010).

The incidence of NCS/NCSE varies with the population studied. In general ICUs, the incidence is 8–20%, while over 20% of ICU patients with head injury have

*Correspondence to: G. Bryan Young, MD, FRCPC, Emeritus Professor, Departments of Clinical Neurological Sciences and Medicine (Critical Care), Western University, London, Ontario, Canada. Tel: +1-519-371-5809, Fax: +1-519-371-0404, E-mail: bryan.young@lhsc.on.ca

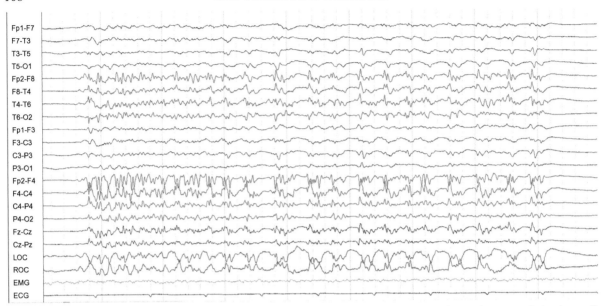

**Fig. 7.1.** A focal seizure from the right hemisphere (channels 1–4 and 13–16) is captured. Note the continuous evolution in amplitude, frequency, and morphology and the abrupt cessation. LOC and ROC, eye movement monitors; EMG, electromyogram (recording over limb muscle); ECG, electrocardiogram.

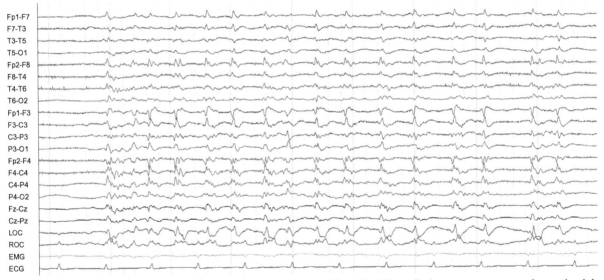

**Fig. 7.2.** A generalized seizure occurs while on a midazolam infusion. The epileptiform discharges are more complex on the right side (channels 1–4 and 13–16). LOC and ROC, eye movement monitors; EMG, electromyogram (recording over limb muscle); ECG, electrocardiogram.

NCS, and almost half of patients who fail to recover consciousness after having convulsive seizures have NCS/NCSE (Table 7.1) (DeLorenzo et al., 1998; Vespa et al., 1999; Towne et al., 2000; Young and Doig, 2005; Alroughani et al., 2009). The literature is somewhat imprecise because of varied definitions of NCSE: do the seizure discharges have to be continuous for at least 30 minutes or are they just frequently recurring? There is a need for more precision – perhaps the concept

of "seizure density," namely the amount of time spent/ unit time (e.g., hour or day) in seizure activity, would be more useful.

It seems axiomatic that the detection of seizures and proving that they have stopped will produce benefit. Demonstrating the success of pharmacologic therapy in controlling NCS and NCSE requires CEEG. Monitoring also enables clinicians to gauge the degree of central nervous system suppression by anesthetic agents. Most

*Table 7.1*

**Incidence of nonconvulsive status epilepticus in comatose patients**

|  | Towne et al. (2000) | Young and Doig (2005) | Alroughani et al. (2009) | Vespa et al. (2010) | DeLorenzo et al. (1998) |
|---|---|---|---|---|---|
| Number of patients | 236 | 55 | 451 | 94 | 164 |
| Patient population | General ICU | General ICU | General ICU | TBI patients | Coma after convulsive seizures |
| % with NCS or NCSE | 8% | 20% | 9% | 22% | 47% |

ICU, intensive care unit; TBI, traumatic brain injury; NCS, nonconvulsive seizures; NCSE, nonconvulsive status epilepticus.
Note that, in the series of Young and Doig, NCS occurred in 10/31 (33%) of those with acute structural brain lesions, and in only 4/24 (17%) of those with metabolic/septic etiologies.

clinicians aim for a burst suppression pattern in controlling refractory status epilepticus. There is controversy, however, as to whether this is sufficient to really stop the seizures and to prevent brain damage, especially when within the bursts there is continuous/ongoing seizure activity. Complete suppression for a period of time might be a better target, but the profound suppression with anesthetic agents has potential complications, including hypotension, sepsis, and ileus (Perks et al., 2012). Unfortunately, there are no trials to show which target, burst suppression vs. complete suppression, is more effective. Since seizure activity can persist within bursts of EEG activity, the concept of "seizure density" (Sarkela, unpublished) or the amount of seizure activity over time might be worth considering.

Claassen and others performed multimodality studies on critically ill patients with aneurysmal subarachnoid hemorrhage and traumatic brain injury (Claassen et al., 2013; Vespa et al., 2016). They found generalized hemodynamic and profound local metabolic changes sometimes accompanied NCS captured on intracortical depth recordings that were not seen on surface EEG. Furthermore, outcomes were worse in such patients than if seizures reached surface electrodes. It remains controversial, however, as to whether depth-only seizures represent additional damage done by the seizures or whether such seizures just reflect more severe brain damage and disconnection of cortical structures. It is also unclear whether vigorous antiseizure treatment is indicated for such seizures. These important preliminary studies clearly require further research, including therapeutic trials.

## CLARIFYING THE NATURE OF MOVEMENTS

Various movements, such as myoclonus, posturing, sustained head or eye deviation, or even pupillary hippus, may raise concern about underlying seizures. The application of video-EEG can be invaluable in such cases in helping to address these concerns, since the association between the movements and the corresponding EEG tracing can be made. In some cases, where muscle activity obscures the EEG tracing, judicious use of a short-acting neuromuscular blocker will allow the underlying EEG to be more clearly seen. This can be done safely in the intubated, ventilated comatose patient.

## MONITORING DEPTH OF SEDATION

CEEG provides a useful method of titrating the degree of cortical suppression with anesthesia in the control of NCS/NCSE. In the ventilated patient receiving pharmacologic paralysis, quantitative EEG (QEEG) is a helpful method of assuring that the patient is sufficiently anesthetized to not be conscious. QEEG can occasionally also be used to guide sedation in awake, quadriplegic patients. For example, we have utilized QEEG in patients with severe Guillain–Barré syndrome, some of whom had lost even pupillary reactivity from their disease, in monitoring sedation (Savard et al., 2009; Claasssen et al., 2013). For example, one can aim for "delta coma" using the QEEG spectral edge frequency (SEF). The SEF-95 represents the frequency under which 95% of the EEG power is contained (Fig. 7.3).

## GRADING SEVERITY OF ENCEPHALOPATHY

We have studied patients with various degrees of sepsis-associated encephalopathy (Young et al., 1992; Vespa et al., 2016). The EEG showed a series of changes that correlated with various indices of multiorgan failure. The earliest changes consisted of mild slowing in the theta (>4 but <8 Hz) frequency range. This was followed by delta (4 Hz or less), at first intermittent and rhythmic and later continuous and more arrhythmic, then by triphasic waves, and finally a burst suppression pattern (Figs 7.4–7.7). There was a strong, almost linear, correlation between worsening of the EEG pattern and increasing mortality (Table 7.2). Patients died from multiorgan failure rather than from their encephalopathy.

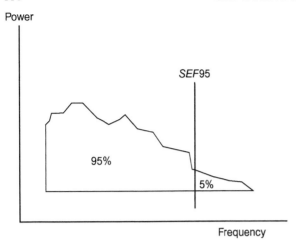

Fig. 7.3. The concept of spectral edge frequency (SEF95) or the frequency (on *x*-axis) containing 95% of the power (*y*-axis) in an electroencephalogram that has been subjected to Fourier transformation.

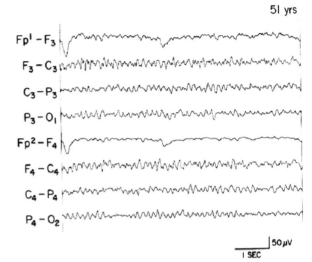

Fig. 7.4. Generalized slowing in the theta range (<8 but > 4 Hz) in a patient with mild confusion.

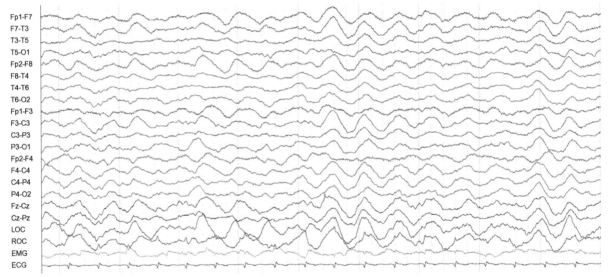

Fig. 7.5. Generalized slowing in the delta range in a comatose patient. LOC and ROC, eye movement monitors; EMG, electromyogram (recording over limb muscle); ECG, electrocardiogram.

This is quite different from the mortality seen with anoxic-ischemic encephalopathy (see below). The EEG should never be used in isolation in making decisions regarding withdrawal of life-sustaining therapy in septic patients. Serial EEG or CEEG could also be applied in examining the course and effect of therapy in other encephalopathies in ICU patients.

## PROGNOSTICATION

Standard EEG, CEEG and evoked responses, especially somatosensory evoked potentials (SSEPs), should be used to assess prognosis only in those conditions causing permanent/irreversible damage to neurons or their connections. These include especially anoxic-ischemic encephalopathy, usually from cardiac arrest, ischemic or hemorrhagic stroke, and traumatic brain injury. This is still a "work in progress" and the definitive role for EEG in prognosis needs be better defined. At best, EEG provides part of the picture, and should not be used as the sole prognostic test.

In anoxic-ischemic encephalopathy, the following patterns have a strong association with very poor outcome, with patients not recovering awareness (i.e., remaining in a vegetative state or dying without recovering consciousness): complete suppression, a burst suppression pattern with generalized epileptiform activity within the bursts, or generalized periodic epileptiform discharges

Triphasic Waves

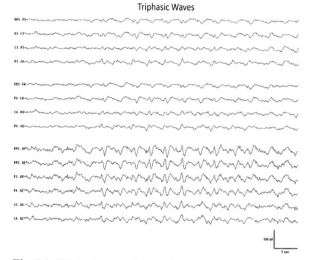

**Fig. 7.6.** Triphasic waves begin after the first 3 seconds of the recording. The triphasic complexes are best seen on the bottom six channels (referred to the ipsilateral ear) compared to the bipolar arrangement in the top eight channels, in which electrodes are compared to adjacent scalp electrodes.

*Table 7.2*

**Graded mortality with electroencephalogram (EEG) classification in sepsis-associated encephalopathy**

| EEG grade | Percentage mortality |
| --- | --- |
| Theta | 40 |
| Delta | 48 |
| Triphasic waves | 53 |
| Burst suppression | 70 |

on an otherwise flat background (Fig. 7.8) (Young, 2000; Savard et al., 2009).

Lack of EEG reactivity to stimulation (a change in amplitude or frequency after the application of stimulus) also has prognostic value in anoxic-ischemic encephalopathy (Fig. 7.9). The lack of reactivity is an unfavorable feature that is associated with mortality or severe disability in most cases; conversely, the presence of reactivity conveys a better chance for

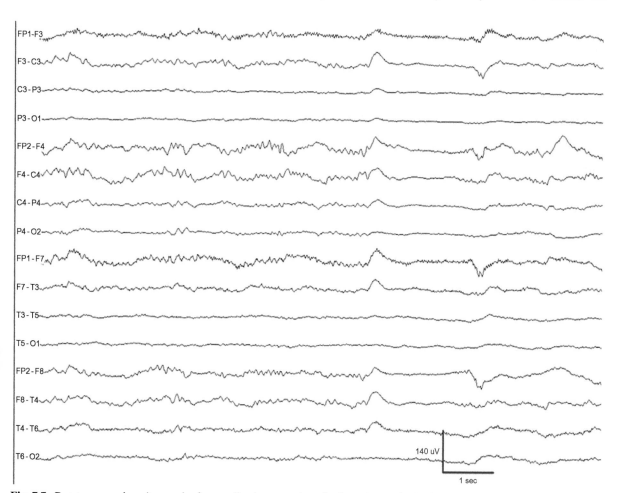

**Fig. 7.7.** Burst suppression: An epoch of generalized suppression of voltage is seen in the last one-third of the tracing. The faster activity is drug-induced.

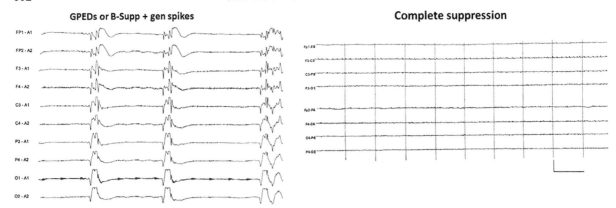

**Fig. 7.8.** Electroencephalograms (EEGs) associated with a poor prognosis in patients with anoxic-ischemic encephalopathy. The left figure shows a burst suppression pattern with epileptiform activity within the bursts (alternatively called generalized periodic complexes). The right figure illustrates complete suppression of cortical activity as recorded by scalp EEG. B-supp, burst suppression; Gen, generalized; GPEDs, generalized periodic epileptiform discharges.

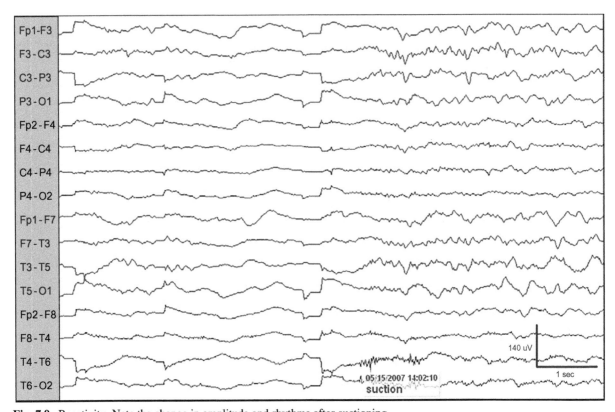

**Fig. 7.9.** Reactivity. Note the change in amplitude and rhythms after suctioning.

recovery of awareness (Young et al., 1992; Young, 2000; Al Thenayan et al., 2010; Rossetti et al., 2010). Again, reactivity should not be considered as the sole prognostic test, but can be considered together with other factors in estimating the likelihood of a favorable or poor outcome. Multiple types of stimuli should be applied, as patients may respond more to some than others. Traditionally, loud sounds, calling the patient's name, passive eye opening, and painful somatosensory stimuli are used (Young et al., in preparation).

SSEPs can be thought of as a "computerized EEG" in which the technique of computerized averaging is used to extract cortical and subcortical signals that are time-locked to the stimulus (most often an electric stimulus applied to the median nerve at the wrist). This allows for assessment of conduction along the sensory pathway (Fig. 7.10).

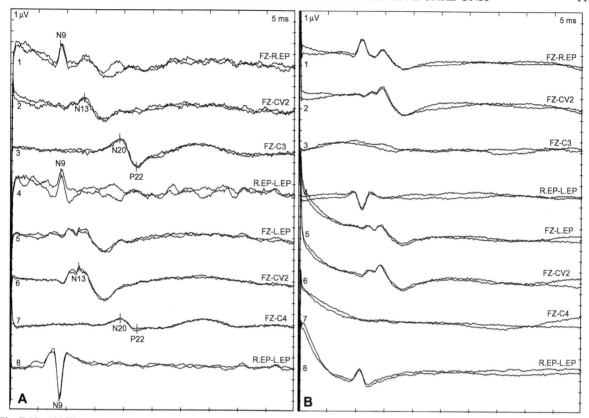

**Fig. 7.10.** (**A**) The waves are a series of averaged evoked responses along the sensory pathway after stimulation of the contralateral median nerve at the wrist. The N9 potential is generated from the brachial plexus; the N13 is from the high cervical spinal cord and the N20 is generated from the primary somatosensory cortex. (**B**) The N9 and N13 are present, but the N20 is absent, indicative of an intracranial interruption of the sensory pathway – this is usually due to cerebral cortical damage.

When only the cortical potential is lost, it can be assumed that the problem lies inside the brain. Assessment of SSEPs is the most definitive electrophysiologic test for prognosis after cardiac arrest, with specificity for poor outcome of nearly 100% with bilateral absence of the cortical N20 responses. They are not as sensitive to poor outcome, however, in that even when they are present, patients still do poorly nearly half the time (Zandbergen et al., 2006; Rossetti et al., 2010). SSEPs have also been shown to be helpful in the prognosis of trauma and in stroke (Tzvetanov et al., 2005; Zandbergen et al., 2006; Al Thenayan et al., 2010; Houlden et al., 2010), but further research is needed to more specifically define their role in conjunction with other clinical factors.

## TECHNICAL AND LOGISTIC CONSIDERATIONS

The ICU poses a number of challenges for the recording and interpretation of CEEG. Consideration will be given to the following: selection of the pattern of electrode placement or montages, selection of types of electrodes, artifacts, and the choice of raw EEG versus quantitative displays.

## EEG montages

It is sometimes not feasible to use the full 10-20 system of EEG electrode placement (Jasper, 1958; Houlden et al., 2010), due to unavailability of EEG technologists, or when it is not possible to place electrodes on the scalp (e.g., recent neurosurgical operations, scalp infections, or burns). Some centers, including ours, have used recordings below the hairline (subhairline EEG) in such situations (Tzvetanov et al., 2005; Young et al., 2009). These can be readily applied by nontechnologists (e.g., housestaff or nurses), usually using adhesive (e.g., electrocardiographaphy) electrodes to nonhairy skin over the forehead, anterior to the ear and over the mastoids. By gently scraping the skin to lower impedance and then applying the electrodes, one can obtain technically good recordings for at least 24 hours. In a study using the 10-20 system as the gold standard, about 70% of seizures, usually nonconvulsive, were captured using a subhairline montage (Jasper, 1958; Young et al., 2006).

A disadvantage of some of the EEG modules provided with bedside ICU monitors is that the sampling rate is below recommended standards (often about 100 Hz rather than the recommendation of >200 Hz). This creates difficulty in differentiating electrocardiographic and electromyographic artifact from EEG spikes or epileptiform discharges. However, seizures can still be detected by recognizing their evolutionary pattern (continual changes in amplitude, frequency, and morphology), and their spread to adjacent electrodes. Subhairline EEG can also play a role in titrating the depth of anesthesia.

In general it is recommended that both bipolar and referential montages be used. Bipolar montages, in which each EEG channel displays the two adjacent electrodes, are best for localizing discharges of focal slowing. Referential recordings (in which each electrode is connected to common electrode or to several electrodes together) are better suited to assess widespread phenomena, such as triphasic waves, generalized epileptiform discharges, or rhythmic delta activity.

## Electrodes

Standard collodion-applied, 1-cm disk electrodes filled with conducting jelly begin to fail after an average of about 6 hours in the ICU, and are often worse in this regard than the adhesive electrodes discussed above. In contrast, we have found that subdermal wire electrodes secured by collodion or other sealant can provide very suitable, artifact-free recordings for several days (Jasper, 1958; Stewart et al., 2010a).

## Raw EEG vs. quantitative displays

Continuous EEG monitoring in ICUs is very labor-intensive. By reducing the amount of data and indicating frequency and amplitude changes that may represent seizures, automated EEG has greatly facilitated seizure detection at the bedside in ICU. The interpretation of the raw or unprocessed EEG requires training and experience. If one does not have this background, it is helpful to have an automated display. This is especially useful for the nurse who is always at the bedside. Automated displays commonly use a fast Fourier transformation to break the EEG signal into various frequencies and, at the same time, display changes in voltage (usually voltage-squared or power). The techniques most commonly used are color density spectral array (CDSA) and amplitude-integrated EEG (Young et al., 2009). These techniques compress the EEG such that epochs of time appear on the same screen and it is easier to trend the changes. Seizures are typically detected by abrupt changes in EEG power that can be readily seen on the display, perhaps best with CDSA (Fig. 7.11). Using commercially available EEG machines with CDSA, the sensitivity for seizure detection is over 80% (Stewart et al., 2010b). More sophisticated techniques provide a sensitivity for seizure detection of over 90% (Tzallas et al., 2007; Ocak, 2009;

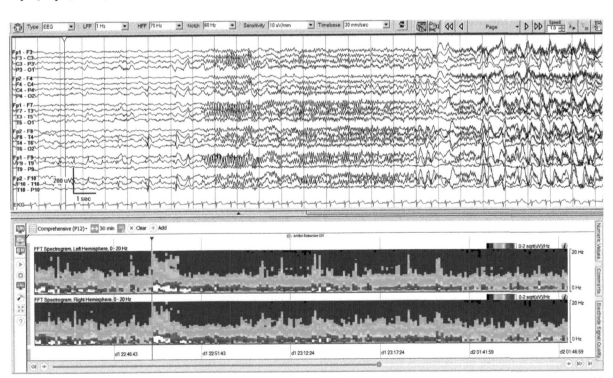

**Fig. 7.11.** The top panel shows a raw electroencephalogram (EEG) with a recorded seizure. Note the evolutionary changes with initially an abrupt high-frequency discharge followed by slower, high-frequency, sharply contoured waves. The lower panel is a color density spectral array (CDSA) with time on the x-axis. Voltage is on the y-axis and the color coding represents voltage divided by frequency: higher-frequency, higher-voltage discharges are green, while lower frequencies are red. The spikes in voltage on CDSA represent seizures as confirmed by the associated raw EEG. (Courtesy of Dr. Peter Tai.)

Sackellares et al., 2011). False detection, e.g., mistaking artifact for seizures, is still a problem but can be reduced using improved algorithms.

It is essential to not rely on the quantitative EEG alone, but to also provide confirmation with examination of the raw EEG. Seizures are usually stereotyped within the same patient, and once one has been confirmed, subsequent recognition is easier.

## Artifacts

The ICU is a much more hostile environment for EEG than the EEG laboratory or an epilepsy monitoring unit. An EEG technologist or electroencephalographer is infrequently at the bedside to check for sources of artifact. Electrode artifacts can be both biologic and external to the person. Commonly encountered biologic artifacts include those due to patient movement, muscle activity, pulsations from blood vessels (i.e., electrode overlying a scalp artery), electrocardiogram, displacement with each heart beat (ballistocardiographic), salt bridging between electrodes from perspiration, and those due to respiration. Artifacts attributable to external factors include electrode artifact, 60 Hz (North America) or 50 Hz (Europe) line artifact, ventilator activity, ventilator tubing (due to condensation of water and its displacement with each ventilation), physiotherapy, displacement of the bed, external perfusion machines (e.g., continuous renal replacement therapy), and pacemakers (Young and Campbell, 1999).

## CONTROVERSIES AND FUTURE ENDEAVORS

There are still a number of unresolved issues surrounding EEG monitoring in the ICU. Some are being addressed through standardization of terminology and technical aspects of recording and data management, advances in technology, further prospective observational studies, multicentered collaboration, meetings, reviews, and debates.

## Standardization

The American Clinical Neurophysiology Society (ACNS) has been instrumental in developing standardized terminology for ICU EEG recordings (Hirsch et al., 2013). This has helped in identifying various phenonema and providing unambiguous definitions. Many of the epileptiform entities fit into the "ictal–interictal continuum": lateralized periodic discharges (LPDs – formerly periorodic lateralized epileptiform discharges or PLEDs), LPDs +, stimulus-induced evolving patterns (Chong and Hirsch, 2005; Claassen, 2009). Challenges remain in exploring the underlying pathophysiology of these entities. The collaboration of basic science with clinical neurophysiology

and ICU neurology may be fruitful in clarifying their significance and rationale for therapy.

The ACNS has also been helpful in the standardization of some aspects of recording, including sampling rates for recording, montages, and displays (ACNS, 2016). Further collaboration under such organizations will improve the quality of research in CEEG in the ICU.

## CONCLUSIONS

CEEG is very demanding of human and technical resources, yet it can be very helpful if there is clarity about its purpose. It is too simplistic to demand that CEEG be justified in terms of improved outcomes in critically ill patients. This will be difficult/impossible to accomplish, given the numerous variables and difficulties with study design. For example, for NCS in the ICU, how can one detect seizures if monitoring is not done? Is it ethically justifiable not to treat seizures when they occur? It makes more sense to approach the issues depending on the purpose we are asking of such monitoring. Is it primarily for detection of seizures and/or ischemia? Is it for following the course of an encephalopathy? Is it for sedation monitoring? Is it for prognosis? Often multiple issues are addressed when a patient is recorded. It is clear that EEG yields information that we did not have before and this information can only help in patient management.

## REFERENCES

ACNS (June 7, 2016). Guidelines and Consensus Statements.

Al Thenayan E, Savard M, Sharpe MD et al. (2010). Electroencephalogram for prognosis after cardiac arrest. J Crit Care 25 (2): 300–304.

Alroughani R, Javidan M, Qasem A et al. (2009). Nonconvulsive status epilepticus; the rate of occurrence in a general hospital. Seizure 18 (1): 38–42.

Bogousslavsky J, Martin R, Regli F et al. (1992). Persistent worsening of stroke sequelae after delayed seizures. Arch Neurol 39: 385–388.

Chong DJ, Hirsch LJ (2005). Which EEG patterns warrant treatment in the critically ill? Reviewing the evidence for treatment of periodic epileptiform discharges and related patterns. J Clin Neurolphysiol 22: 79–91.

Claassen J (2009). How I, treat patients with EEG patterns on the ictal-interictal continuum in the neuro-ICU. Neurocrit Care 11: 437–444.

Claassen J, Mayer SA, Kowalski RG et al. (2004). Detection of electrographic seizures with continuous EEG monitoring in critically ill patients. Neurology 62: 1743–1748.

Claassen J, Perotte A, Albers D et al. (2013). Nonconvulsive seizures after subarachnoid hemorrhage: multifocal detection and outcomes. Ann Neurol 74: 53–64.

DeGiorgio CM, Gott PS, Rabinowicz AL et al. (1996). Neuro-specific enolase, a marker for acute neuronal injury, is increased in complex partial status epilepticus. Epilepsia 37: 606–609.

DeLorenzo RJ, Waterhouse EJ, Towne AR et al. (1998). Persistent nonconvulsive status epilepticus after the control of convulsive status epilepticus. Epilepsia 39 (8): 833–840.

Hirsch LJ, LaRoche SM, Gaspard N et al. (2013). American Clinical Neurophysiology Society's standardized critical care EEG terminology: 2012 version. J Clin Neurophysiol 30: 1–27.

Houlden DA, Taylor AB, Feinstein A et al. (2010). Early somatosensory evoked potential grades in comatose traumatic brain injury patients predict cognitive and functional outcome. Crit Care Med 38 (1): 167–174.

Jasper HH (1958). The 10-20 electrode system of the International Federation. Electroenceph Clin Neurophysiol 10: 371–375.

Krumholz A, Sung GY, Fisher RS et al. (1995). Complex partial status epilepticus accompanied by serious mortality and morbidity. Neurology 145: 1499–1504.

Lothman EW (1990). The biochemical basis and pathophysiology of status epilepticus. Neurology 40 (Suppl 2): 13–23.

Ocak H (2009). Automatic detection of epileptic seizures in EEG using discrete wavelet transform and approximate entropy. Expert Syst Appl 36: 2027–2036.

Perks A, Cheema S, Mohanraj R (2012). Anaesthesia and epilepsy. Br J Anaesth 108 (4): 562–571.

Rossetti A, Oddo M, Logroscino G et al. (2010). Prognositication after cardiac arrest: a prospective study. Ann Neurol 67 (3): 301–307.

Sackellares JC, Shiau DS, Halford JJ et al. (2011). Quantitative EEG analysis for automated detection of nonconvulsive seizures in intensive care units. Epilepsy Behav 22 (Suppl 1): S69–S73.

Savard M, Al Thenayan E, Sharpe MD et al. (2009). Continuous EEG monitoring in severe Guillain-Barré syndrome patients. J Clin Neurophysiol 26: 21–33.

Scholtes FB, Renier WO, Meinardi H (1996). Nonconvulsive status epilepticus: causes, treatment and outcome in 65 patients. J Neurol Neurosurg Psychiatry 61: 93–95.

Stewart CP, Otsubo H, Ochi A et al. (2010a). Seizure identification in the ICU using quantitative EEG displays. Neurology 75: 1501–1508.

Stewart CP, Otsubo H, Ochi A et al. (2010b). Seizure identification in the ICU using quantitative EEG displays. Neurology 75 (17): 1501–1508.

Towne AR, Waterhouse EJ, Boggs JG et al. (2000). Prevalence of nonconvulsive status epilepticus in comatose patients. Neurology 54: 340–345.

Trieman DM, Degado-Escueta AV, Clark MA (1981). Impairment of memory following complex partial status epilepticus. Neurology 31: 109.

Tzallas AT, Tsipouras MG, Fotadis DI (2007). Automatic seizure detetion based on time-frequency analysis and artificial neural networks. Comput Intell Neuroscidec 5. http://dx.doi.org/10.1155/2007/80510.

Tzvetanov P, Rousseff RT, Atanassova P (2005). Prognostic value of median and tibial somatosensory evoked potentials in acute stroke. Neurosci Lett 380 (1–2): 99–104.

Vespa PM, Nuwer MR, Nenov V et al. (1999). Increased incidence and impact of nonconvulsive and convulsive status epilepticus after traumatic brain injury as detected by continuous electroencephalographic monitoring. J Neurosurg 91 (5): 750–760.

Vespa PM, McArthur DL, Xu Y et al. (2010). Nonconvulsive seizures after traumatic brain injury are associated with hippocampal atrophy. Neurology 75 (9): 792–798.

Vespa P, Tubi M, Claassen J et al. (2016). Metabolic crisis occurs with seizures and periodic diseharges after brain trauma. Ann Neurol 79: 579–590.

Wasterlain CG, Fujikawa DG, Penix L et al. (1993). Pathophysiological mechanisms of brain damage from status epilepticus. Epilepsia 34 (Suppl 1): 37–53.

Young GB (2000). The EEG, in coma. J Clin Neurophysiol 17: 473–485.

Young GB, Campbell VC (1999). EEG monitoring in the ICU: pitfalls and caveats. J Clin Neurophysiol 16: 40–45.

Young GB, Doig GS (2005). Continuous EEG monitoring in comatose intensive care patients: epileptiform activity in etiologically distinct groups. Neurocrit Care 2: 5–10.

Young GB, Jordan KG (1998). Do nonconvulsive seizures damage the brain? Yes. Arch Neurol 55: 117–119.

Young GB, Bolton CF, Austin TW et al. (1992). The electroencephalogram in sepsis-associated encephalopathy. J Clin Neurophysiol 9: 145–152.

Young GB, Ives JR, Chapman MG et al. (2006). A comparison of subdermal wire electrodes with collodion-applied disk electrodes in long-term EEG recordings in ICU. Clin Neurophysiol 117: 1376–1379.

Young GB, Sharpe MD, Savard M et al. (2009). Seizure detection with a commercially available bedside EEG monitor and the subhairline montage. Neurocrit Care 11: 411–416.

Zandbergen EG, Koelman JH, de Haan RJ et al. (2006). SSEPS and prognosis in postanoxic coma: only short and also long latency responses? Neurology 22 (4): 583–586. 67.

*Handbook of Clinical Neurology*, Vol. 140 (3rd series)
*Critical Care Neurology, Part I*
E.F.M. Wijdicks and A.H. Kramer, Editors
http://dx.doi.org/10.1016/B978-0-444-63600-3.00008-8

Chapter 8

# Management of the comatose patient

E.F.M. WIJDICKS*

*Division of Critical Care Neurology, Mayo Clinic and Neurosciences Intensive Care Unit, Mayo Clinic Campus, Saint Marys Hospital, Rochester, MN, USA*

## Abstract

Coma has many causes but there are a few urgent ones in clinical practice. Management must start with establishing the cause and an attempt to reverse or attenuate some of the damage. This may include early neurosurgical intervention, efforts to reduce brain tissue shift and raised intracranial pressure, correction of markedly abnormal laboratory abnormalities, and administration of available antidotes. Supporting the patient's vital signs, susceptible to major fluctuations in a changing situation, remains the most crucial aspect of management.

Management of the comatose patient is in an intensive care unit and neurointensivists are very often involved. This chapter summarizes the principles of caring for the comatose patient and everything a neurologist would need to know. The basic principles of neurologic assessment of the comatose patient have not changed, but better organization can be achieved by grouping comatose patients according to specific circumstances and findings on neuroimaging. Ongoing supportive care involves especially aggressive prevention of medical complications associated with mechanical ventilation and prolonged immobility. Waiting for recovery—and many do- is often all that is left. Neurorehabilitation of the comatose patient is underdeveloped and may not be effective. There are, as of yet, few proven options for neurostimulation in comatose patients.

## INTRODUCTION

Management of the comatose patient is divided into two major priorities. First, the cause should be elucidated, so that attempts can be made to reverse it. Second, these extremely vulnerable patients should be protected in every possible way. This includes appropriate airway management, adequate oxygenation, and possibly mechanical ventilation. Other abnormal vital signs should also be corrected, such as blood pressure and temperature. Each of these simple mundane tasks is essential in the initial hours of care. In patients brought to the emergency department, coma can be due to traumatic brain injury, cerebral or cerebellar hemorrhage, acute basilar artery embolus, anoxic-ischemic brain injury after cardiopulmonary resuscitation, and drug overdose. Once the cause of coma is established, management should proceed quickly. This is most pertinent in patients with an expanding mass lesion causing shift of the thalamus or brainstem, acute obstructive hydrocephalus, and central nervous system (CNS) infection (Wijdicks, 2010, 2014; Salottolo et al., 2016). Any acute metabolic arrangement requires correction, albeit slowly in some situations (i.e., acute hyponatremia). Seizures and nonconvulsive status epilepticus need urgent treatment. The evaluation of the comatose patient usually runs through a logical sequence, starting with initial medical support, detailed examination of the patient, finding the cause of coma, and treatment. Using a combination of neurologic findings and neuroimaging, clinicians can elucidate the cause of coma. Because of its specialization, there are good reasons to involve a neurologist in the assessment of coma in patients admitted to general intensive care units (Wijdicks, 2016).

The management of the comatose patient is multidisciplinary from the onset, with many specialties and allied

---

*Correspondence to: Eelco F.M. Wijdicks, Department of Neurology, Mayo Clinic, 200 First Street SW, Rochester MN 55905, USA. E-mail: wijde@mayo.edu

healthcare workers involved. This chapter provides the main essentials for care and treatment, not only in the acute stage, but also in the weeks and sadly sometimes months or years ahead.

## CAUSES OF COMA AND PREVALENCE

For the physician trying to make sense of it all, there are multifarious causes of coma, but, after an initial evaluation, physicians often have narrowed the range of possibilities. In the initial evaluation of the comatose patient with no apparent cause, the medical history becomes more important and often cues the physician towards a possible explanation. Questions that should be asked to family members or bystanders – when appropriate – are shown in Table 8.1. However, the cause of coma clearly depends on where the patient is seen first. Assessing a patient in a transplant intensive care unit (ICU) is a different environment than consulting in a medical ICU or coronary care unit. Consultation in surgical ICUs for coma is relatively frequent and involves questions about failure to awaken or acute coma in the setting of critical illness. Moreover, the nature of the primary illness for which the patient is admitted may provide sufficient leads. It is likely to be true that intoxications are the predominant cause of coma in patients arriving in the emergency department. Nevertheless, comatose patients may present to the emergency department with no known cause, clinical course and little documentation (Stevens et al., 2015). Many emergency departments in the world are in the midst of a "fentanyl

epidemic" and many survivors have long-term anoxic brain injury. The presentation of a comatose patient in specialized hospital wards and units may also narrow the differential diagnosis of acute coma. It is highly unusual for patients who have been admitted to general medical or surgical wards to suddenly deteriorate and become comatose. Acute coma in the hospital is occasionally a reason for a rapid response team call, and acute metabolic disturbances or an unintentional drug overdose (e.g. post operative opioid treatment) remain most likely. Acute hypo- or hyperglycemia is also often a cause for immediate alarm, but is usually recognized quickly and corrected. In our experience, only a small fraction of comatose patients have no clear explanation on computed tomography (CT) scan or after lumbar puncture (Edlow et al., 2014). In some patients, early magnetic resonance imaging (MRI) has been diagnostic in demonstrating posterior reversible encephalopathy syndrome, fat embolization syndrome (Mijalski et al., 2015), infarcts in the brainstem and thalamus, or acute demyelination disease such as acute disseminated encephalomyelitis (ADEM) or osmotic demyelination. In many others, coma may be a result of an unwitnessed seizure, illicit drug use, or other toxins.

## NEUROPATHOPHYSIOLOGY

Coma is a result of dysfunction or damage of structures that allow normal wakefulness and awareness. Wakefulness is mostly driven by the ascending reticular formation in the brainstem. Becoming aware and thus understanding content requires the thinking parts of the cortex, including the associative parietal areas and frontal lobe. Comatose patients are neither awake nor aware (even if sporadic functional MRI signals may suggest otherwise). Coma may deteriorate to brain death in about 5–10% and simply implies that all brainstem reflexes are permanently lost, including the ability to generate a breath. Hypotension almost always occurs, but the spinal cord may increase sympathetic tone just enough to maintain a pressure which allows circulation. The clinical diagnosis of brain death is conservative and defines a clear point of no return. Once all brainstem reflexes are absent in a demonstrably apneic comatose patient, with no confounding circumstances, recovery does not occur and then fullfills criteria for a neurologic determination of death (Wijdicks 2001, 2011, 2017). In comatose patients with preserved brainstem reflexes, long-term support with a gastrostomy tube for feeding and possibly a tracheostomy and mechanical ventilator is feasible. Patients in a persistent vegetative state (PVS) may be kept alive for decades with no improvement in awareness. Patients in a minimally conscious state may stay in this condition for years or improve marginally. Each of these conditions can be linked to certain degrees of brain injury, but a neuropathologist cannot

*Table 8.1*

Questions to ask in coma of uncertain etiology

Could there have been trauma or assault?
Was the patient breathing when the response team arrived?
Was there noticeable blood loss?
Did the patient use antibiotics for infection?
Was there a rapid onset of fever and headache?
Was a cardiac arrest documented? How long did the efforts last before resumption of circulation?
Has the patient had prior episodes of diabetic ketoacidosis, or severe hypoglycemia, and has there been a recent change in insulin medications?
Is the patient known to have atrial fibrillation or other cardiac disease and be using anticoagulation or has it recently been discontinued?
Was hypertension poorly controlled?
What other pills or over-the-counter drugs does the patient have access to?
Has the patient had prior suicide attempts, a psychiatric consultation, and are there problems at work?
Has anyone complained about the patient's drinking habits?
Has the patient used medications that may increase heat production, such as salicylate drugs with sympathicomimetics such as cocaine, amphetamines, or ecstasy?

*Table 8.2*

**Classification and causes of coma**

| | |
|---|---|
| **Structural brain injury** | Basilar artery occlusion and brainstem infarct |
| *Cerebral hemisphere* | Central pontine myelinolysis |
| UNILATERAL (WITH DISPLACEMENT) | Brainstem contusion |
| Intraparenchymal hematoma | CEREBELLUM (WITH DISPLACEMENT OF BRAINSTEM) |
| Middle cerebral artery ischemic stroke | Cerebellar infarct |
| Intracranial venous thrombosis | Cerebellar hematoma |
| Hemorrhagic contusion | Cerebellar abscess |
| Cerebral abscess | Cerebellar glioma |
| Brain tumor | **Acute metabolic-endocrine disturbance** |
| Subdural or epidural hematoma | Hypoglycemia |
| BILATERAL | Hyperglycemia (nonketotic hyperosmolar) |
| Subarachnoid hemorrhage | Hyponatremia |
| Multiple traumatic brain contusions | Hypernatremia |
| Penetrating traumatic brain injury | Hypocalcemia |
| Anoxic-ischemic encephalopathy | Acute hypothyroidism |
| Multiple cerebral infarcts | Acute panhypopituitarism |
| Bilateral thalamic infarcts | Acute uremia |
| Lymphoma | Hyperammonemia |
| Encephalitis | Hypercapnia |
| Gliomatosis | **Diffuse physiologic brain dysfunction** |
| Acute disseminated encephalomyelitis | Generalized tonic-clonic seizures |
| Cerebral edema | Poisoning, illicit drug use |
| Multiple brain metastases | Hypothermia |
| Acute hydrocephalus | Gas inhalation |
| Acute leukoencephalopathy | Acute catatonia |
| Posterior reversible encephalopathy syndrome | Malignant neuroleptic syndrome |
| Air or fat embolism | **Functional Coma** |
| BRAINSTEM | Pseudostatus epilepticus |
| Pontine hemorrhage | Eyes closed unresponsiveness to stimuli |

predict the clinical state after grading the degree of injury. The neuropathology associated with coma is summarized in Table 8.2.

The neuropathology associated with disorders causing acute or prolonged coma has been well characterized. Several fatal neurologic disorders causing coma have come to autopsy and -mostly in the past-have allowed detailed description of the underlying pathology.

The neuropathology of hypoxic-ischemic injury is a result of damage to the most vulnerable sites, including the first and second frontal gyrus, globus pallidus, cornu ammonis, and the cerebellar cortex affecting predominantly the Purkinje cells. The ischemic alterations in the cornu ammonis involve the CA1 and CA4 sectors. The hippocampus becomes ischemic in CA1 areas after several minutes of global ischemia. The CA4 region requires only minimal ischemic insult for these cells to become damaged. Necrosis of the globus pallidus points to major anoxic-ischemic injury, and is also a common manifestation of carbon monoxide poisoning.

The pathologic changes of anoxic-ischemic injury are typically in the watershed zones and therefore also involve the posterior cerebral regions. With overwhelming ischemia, necrosis of all cortical layers is seen. In most patients, hypoxic-ischemic injury spares the brainstem clinically, but necrosis may occur, especially in the inferior colliculi and tegmental nuclei. Sustained absence of brainstem reflexes after cardiac arrest is relatively uncommon.

Few patients with CT-proven catastrophic stroke come to autopsy. The destruction and mass effect are evident. In patients with large thalamic hemorrhage, blood has tracked deep into the brainstem. In other patients, edema may have caused further deterioration. Edema around an intracerebral hematoma peaks after several days. Edema is a multiphase event and is caused by clot retraction, movement of serum into ambient tissue, followed by activation of coagulation cascade and thrombus, and finally erythrocyte lysis with toxicity from hemoglobin. Edema is perpetuated by disruption of the blood–brain barrier, as well as inflammation and activation of the complement system. Increased production of matrix metalloproteinase iron may also exacerbate cerebral edema.

The neuropathology of traumatic brain injury is diverse but often multiple contusions and subdural hematomas are identified at autopsy, localized on cortical surfaces. Diffuse axonal injury is caused by rotational acceleration following an impact to the head. On gross examination, hemorrhages of the corpus callosum and cerebellar peduncle region are often seen, and there may also be hemorrhages in the deeper structures. So-called "gliding contusions" can sometimes be found in the parasagittal white matter. Small hemorrhagic shear lesions are also commonly found in the hemispheric white matter, perpendicular to the cortical ribbon. Tissue tear hemorrhages are mostly concentrated in the midline structures, such as the corpus callosum, septum pellucidum, fornix, midbrain, pons, and hippocampus. Traumatic brain injury is often in the medial basal cortical areas of the temporal lobes, in the margins of the base of the cerebellar peduncles, due to pressure on the tentorial ridge, and on top of the corpus callosum, due to indentation by the free edge of the falx cerebri.

The neuropathology of bacterial meningitis is fairly characteristic and immediately apparent. At autopsy, purulent meningitis is revealed by pus and yellow and green deposits on the leptomeninges. Generally, the pus follows the distribution of the meningeal blood vessels. Depending on the time elapsed before death, microscopic features include neutrophils, macrophages, and fibrin in the subarachnoid space. Arteritis associated with severe forms of meningitis has now been recognized as one of the most important secondary complications leading to ischemic strokes and much worse outcome, including prolonged coma. Fulminant meningitis may show cerebral edema and relatively little exudate. Acute bacterial meningitis may be a surprising finding in patients who died rapidly, when no real opportunity for the physician existed to obtain cerebrospinal fluid.

Similarly, fulminant viral encephalitis may cause early demise and can be confirmed at autopsy. The findings are generally nonspecific, showing clusters of inflammatory changes. In some regions, there is perivascular chronic inflammation with microglial nodules and neuronophagia. The most common etiology is herpes simplex virus encephalitis, which is characterized by hemorrhagic necrosis, specifically involving the temporal lobes, insula, and posterior orbitofrontal cortex. Cowdry A intranuclear inclusions can be found in herpes simplex virus encephalitis. When ultrastructural findings are examined, viral particles with hexagonal features and a central nucleoid are found. Polymerase chain reaction amplification of viral DNA in cerebrospinal fluid has long replaced brain biopsy in making the diagnosis. Cytomegalovirus encephalitis is more commonly seen in patients who have been infected with the human immunodeficiency virus. Cytomegalovirus has typical microscopic findings of scattered cytomegalic cells with intracytoplasmic viral inclusion. The absence of an inflammatory infiltrate is notable in these infections.

Fungal encephalitis may be difficult to detect microscopically on routine stains, and the fungus may also be challenging to culture. *Aspergillus fumigatus* infection of the CNS is aggressive and destructive. At autopsy, both infarcts and hemorrhages can be found due to angioinvasion.

In acute demyelinated leukoencephalopathies, the acute changes are edema with fibrinoid necrosis of blood vessels, and also infiltration of neutrophils, mononuclear inflammatory cells, sometimes with regions of hemorrhage (particularly in acute hemorrhagic leukoencephalopathy). Another inflammatory demyelinating disease is ADEM, resulting in symmetric subcortical white-matter lesions. Multiple sclerosis may present with an acute mass (tumefactive form of Marburg syndrome). Next to marked demyelinization, the neuropathology findings in this variant are characterized by macrophages, large glial cells with mitosis, and chromatin fragmentation (Creutzfeldt cells).

Coma due to intoxication or poisoning is usually accidental, but can occur intentionally in the setting of suicide or homicide. Many neurotoxins produce no apparent neuropathologic changes in the CNS. In some, such as lithium poisoning, more specific abnormalities are seen, such as spongiform changes in the thalamus, midbrain, and cerebellum, with significant damage to the Purkinje cells (explaining cerebellar ataxia during presentation). Thallium (used in many rat poisons) produces cerebral edema with multiple white matter and cerebellar hemorrhages, but also degenerative changes in the cerebral cortex, hypothalamic nuclei, and olivary complex. An important forensic question is whether death occurred from carbon monoxide poisoning. The morphology is fairly characteristic, with bright redness of brain sections at autopsy that remain after fixation. Often a significant brightness of the dura is seen at exposure of the brain. There is bilateral necrosis of the globus pallidus and pars reticulata of the substantia nigra. Cortical laminar necrosis and involvement of both hippocampi are expected.

Acute fatal alcohol intoxication remains nonspecific, but brain edema and congestion can be found. Equally rare is documented neuropathologic confirmation of Wernicke–Korsakoff syndrome, with its characteristic changes that involve atrophy of the mammillary bodies, periventricular hemorrhages, and also astrogliosis and capillary proliferation in more chronic cases. Far more likely in alcoholics are multiple intracranial hemorrhages, particularly subdural and parenchymal hemorrhages.

## NEUROLOGIC EXAMINATION OF THE COMATOSE PATIENT

The primary goal of the neurologic examination in an unresponsive patient is to localize the lesion and thereby narrow the differential diagnosis. The examination should proceed in a stepwise fashion and is familiar to the neurologist.

Pending a more comprehensive neurologic examination, the depth of coma can be assessed using a coma scale. The Glasgow Coma Scale (GCS) is the most common of such scales and originally developed for victims of traumatic brain injury, and to improve transfer of patients, it consists of three parts: eye opening, best motor response, and best verbal response (Teasdale and Jennett, 1974). Each component is graded on a different scale (maximum 4 for eyes, 5 for verbal, and 6 for motor) and the summation of the scores is used to communicate the depth of coma. The minimum score is 3 and the maximum 15. Although not useful in the diagnosis of coma, the GCS has been shown to have acceptable interobserver reliability through a wide range of trained providers, and has predictive value for outcomes in aneurysmal subarachnoid hemorrhage, traumatic brain injury, and comatose survivors of cardiac arrest. However, the GCS does not account for the presence or absence of brainstem reflexes and does not detect other highly relevant changes in the neurologic examination, findings that could be instrumental in determining a patient's prognosis. GCS is reduced to a raw motor scale if a patient is intubated and has facial injury with swelling.

To address the shortcomings of the GCS, the Full Outline of UnResponsiveness (FOUR) score was developed (Fig. 8.1). To simplify scoring, the FOUR score includes four components – eyes, motor, brainstem, and respiratory – that are each graded on a scale from 0 to 4, producing a maximum combined total score of 16. With an equal to higher interrater reliability than the GCS, as well as validation in multiple patient populations, the FOUR score has proven to be an important initial tool in the evaluation of comatose patients. Perhaps because of its greater emphasis on brainstem reflexes and respiratory patterns, the FOUR score has also been shown to have greater predictive value in terms of eventual progression towards more severe injury, especially in patients with low GCS scores, or the relatively ubiquitous GCS score of 3 T, which is commonly reported by paramedics following intubation in the field after sedatives and paralytics have been given. Brainstem damage and failure to maintain adequate ventilation are reflections of injury severity. The FOUR score does not contain a verbal component, and can be measured with equal accuracy in intubated and nonintubated ICU patients. The FOUR score can be used to evaluate for clinical progression with serial examinations in patients with intracranial mass lesions.

## Cranial nerves

A more formal neurologic evaluation of an unresponsive patient typically begins with the cranial nerves (CNs). Dysfunction of any of these reflexes implies a lesion involving the CNs or the pathways connecting them and thus are indicative of brainstem functioning. Pupil size, shape and reactivity should be examined. Small pupils could be secondary to a pontine lesion that interrupts descending sympathetic outflow. The most common cause of small pupils is prior use of opioids (on the streets, it is most often heroin; in the hospital, it is overuse of opioids and can be related to errors with patient-controlled analgesia pumps or opioid patches). Dilated (>8 mm) pupils are due to disruption of CN III, secondary to either a mesencephalic injury or lesion of the peripheral nerve. Drugs and other toxins such as amphetamines or lidocaine can also result in bilaterally dilated pupils, and must be excluded through the patient's history and laboratory testing. Midsize, fixed pupils are seen in severe midbrain lesions that can be secondary to herniation and are frequently the first sign of impending loss of all brainstem reflexes (Fig. 8.2).

In addition to pupil size and reactivity, any deviation of one or both eyes should also be noted. Spontaneous eye movements, including "ping-pong" eyes or ocular dipping, generally indicate bihemispheric dysfunction. Ocular bobbing, described as a rapid downward deviation of the eyes followed by a slow upward movement, typically implies a pontine lesion. Bihemispheric dysfunction can also lead to the classic "roving eye movements," though metabolic processes and various toxicities can also be responsible. Rather than supporting particular localization or a specific disease process, roving eye movements indicate that the brainstem is relatively intact (Table 8.3). The oculocephalic reflex deserves special mention as several brainstem structures are assessed simultaneously. In a patient with a normally functioning brainstem, eyes will move in a direction opposite the head movement and appear to remain fixated on a point in space (much like a doll's eyes). If a lesion disrupts any of the structures or pathways involved in the reflex, including CNs III, IV, and VI, or the medial longitudinal fasciculus, the eyes will move along with the head, remaining in midposition with respect to the orbits.

Tonic deviation of the eyes, typically in the horizontal plane, may indicate an ipsilateral hemispheric lesion affecting the frontal eye fields or a contralateral pontine lesion. Differentiation between a hemispheric lesion and a pontine lesion can be difficult in comatose patients as hemiparesis is typically not apparent. However, the oculocephalic maneuver will be able to overcome gaze preference from a cortical lesion, since the pontine and midbrain structures responsible for the reflex remain intact.

Horizontal deviation can also be seen with nonconvulsive status epilepticus, and may be one of the few signs to indicate the need for an emergent electroencephalogram (EEG). Skew deviation implies a brainstem injury.

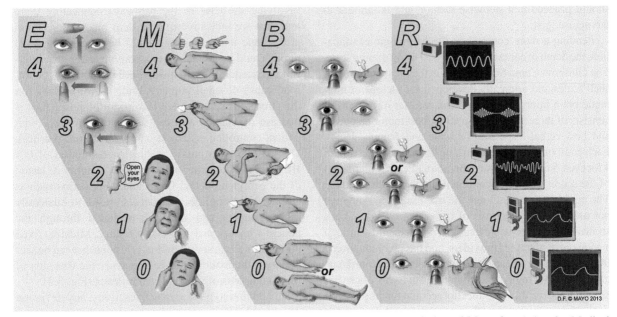

**Fig. 8.1.** The Full Outline of UnResponsiveness (FOUR) score. Used with the permission of Mayo foundation for Medical Education and Research.

Eye response (E)
4 = eyelids open or opened, tracking, or blinking to command
3 = eyelids open but not tracking
2 = eyelids closed but open to loud voice
1 = eyelids closed but open to pain
0 = eyelids remain closed with pain
Motor response (M)
4 = thumbs-up, fist, or peace sign
3 = localizing to pain
2 = flexion response to pain
1 = extension response to pain
0 = no response to pain or generalized myoclonus status

Brainstem reflexes (B)
4 = pupil and corneal reflexes present
3 = one pupil wide and fixed
2 = pupil or corneal reflexes absent
1 = pupil and corneal reflexes absent
0 = absent pupil, corneal, and cough reflex
Respiration (R)
4 = not intubated, regular breathing pattern
3 = not intubated, Cheyne–Stokes breathing pattern
2 = not intubated, irregular breathing pattern
1 = breathes above ventilatory rate
0 = breathes at ventilator rate or apnea

A fundoscopic examination should also be performed once the external examination of the eyes has been completed. Vitreous hemorrhage, often subhyaloid in location, can be indicative of subarachnoid hemorrhage. Fundoscopy may also reveal the presence of papilledema. Though often cited as a manifestation of acutely increased intracranial pressure in subarachnoid hemorrhage or acute meningitis, papilledema is more commonly seen with slowly progressive processes such as an enlarging intracranial mass, and may also be seen with severe hypertensive crisis causing posterior reversible encephalopathy syndrome. The presence of venous pulsations suggests normal intracranial pressure, but their absence is less useful. Measuring the optic nerve sheath with bedside ultrasound using a high-frequency probe is reported to estimate intracranial pressure with some accuracy. This method could be a noninvasive way to detect raised intracranial pressure, allowing earlier and more rational therapeutic interventions, but better validation is needed.

Further testing of the CNs is accomplished through the various reflexes, including the corneal, gag, and cough, but these are the least helpful with localization. Midbrain and pontine lesions can cause central neurogenic hyperventilation. Pontine lesions can cause cluster breathing (brief episodes of tachypnea punctuated by brief spells of apnea). Lower pontine and medullary lesions can produce ataxic breathing or apnea. Sighs or yawns can herald a decrease in level of consciousness resulting from rapidly increasing intracranial pressure.

## Motor responses

Testing of the motor system in an unresponsive patient typically involves applying a noxious stimulus to the supraorbital nerve or the temporomandibular joint, and assessing the patient's reaction. Possible responses include a localizing response, in which the patient reaches towards the stimulus, reflexive responses such as decorticate or decerebrate posturing, or no response at all.

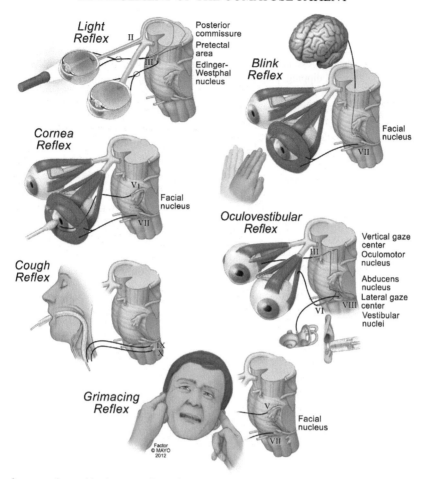

**Fig. 8.2.** Pathways of commonly used brainstem reflexes in assessment of coma. Used with the permission of Mayo foundation for Medical Education and Research. All rights reserved.

*Table 8.3*

**Relevant eye movements in coma examination**

| Type of movement | Lesion location |
| --- | --- |
| Periodic alternating gaze (lateral deviation every few minutes, left and right) | Bihemispheric, midbrain, vermis |
| Ping-pong (lateral deviation every few seconds, left and right) | Bihemispheric, vermis |
| Convergence nystagmus (bilateral abduction, slow with rapid jerk back) | Mesencephalon |
| Retractory nystagmus (retraction orbit) | Mesencephalon |
| Bobbing (rapid down, slow up) | Pons |
| Dipping (slow down, rapid up) | Bihemispheric |

Decorticate posturing involves a slow flexion of the elbow, wrists, and fingers, whereas decerebrate posturing is defined as adduction and internal rotation of the shoulder with arm extension and wrist pronation. Although posturing reflexes have purportedly been useful in lesion localization, these responses can be seen with either focal lesions or global conditions affecting the nervous system. It is also not uncommon for both responses to be present in the same patient at the same time. Given this, the presence of decerebrate or decorticate posturing has relatively little utility in prognostication until the underlying etiology is found.

In addition to movements in response to stimulation, spontaneous movements can also be seen in unresponsive patients, the classic example being generalized myoclonus. Although a predictor of poor outcome following cardiac arrest and resulting anoxic-ischemic injury, generalized myoclonus status can also be seen with various intoxications, including lithium, cephalosporins, and pesticides.

## Classifying coma syndromes

Combinations of physical findings characterize herniation syndromes and their dynamic changes can be used to recognize progression of mass effect (Table 8.4).

*Table 8.4*

**Coma syndromes**

| | |
|---|---|
| Bilateral hemispheric | Spontaneous eye movements (roving, dipping, ping-pong, nystagmoid jerks) |
| | Upward or downward eye deviation |
| | Intact oculovestibular reflexes |
| | Intact pupillary and corneal reflexes |
| | Variable motor responses |
| | Adventitious limb movements (subtle manifestations of seizures, myoclonus, asterixis) |
| Brainstem displacement from a hemispheric mass | Anisocoria or unilateral fixed and dilated pupil (predominant lateral displacement) |
| | Midposition fixed pupils (predominant downward displacement) |
| | Extensor or flexor posturing |
| | Central hyperventilation (diencephalic) |
| Brainstem displacement from a cerebellar mass | Direction-changing or vertical nystagmus from the cerebellar lesion |
| | Ocular bobbing |
| | Absent corneal reflexes with intact pupillary reflexes |
| | Extensor or flexor posturing |
| | Facial or abducens nerve palsy |
| | Skew deviation (vertical misalignment of eyes) |
| | Internuclear ophthalmoplegia |
| Intrinsic brainstem lesion | Vertical nystagmus or bobbing |
| | Miosis (with pontine lesions) |
| | Internuclear ophthalmoplegia |
| | Variable pupillary and corneal reflexes (can both be absent) |
| | Absent oculocephalic and oculovestibular responses |
| | Extensor or flexor posturing |
| | Ataxic breathing (pontomedullary damage) |

Transtentorial herniation classically presents with a dilated pupil ipsilateral to the compressive lesion (ipsilateral CNIII damage) with contralateral hemiplegia (ipsilateral cerebral peduncle compression causing contralateral motor findings). However, either component can be reversed. In up to 10% of cases, the dilated pupil is contralateral (falsely localizing). Because of the Kernohan notch phenomenon (contralateral cerebral peduncle compression), weakness ipsilateral to the lesion can also be falsely localizing. Although increased access to CT has diminished the influence of these false localizing signs, they might still be relevant in hospitals without CT availability, especially if the treating physician is contemplating burrhole trephination. An awake, alert patient with a dilated pupil is unlikely to have uncal herniation as a cause of the anisocoria, but I have seen a partial oculomotor palsy in a relatively awake patient with an acute subdural hematoma. Sixth-nerve palsy from high or low intracranial pressure is also nonlocalizing.

If progressive neurologic disease associated with mass effect goes untreated, brainstem reflexes might fail in a caudal direction. Fixed pupils (midbrain) are followed by disappearance of corneal reflexes and oculocephalic responses (pons), followed by loss of cough response, the development of apnea, and loss of vascular tone (medulla). It defines brain death. Neurologists and neurosurgeons have come to realize that when all brain stem reflexes are absent in a demonstrable apneic patient—and nothing else could explain it—it is irreversible and it is the end of it.

Combinations of physical findings can also characterize toxic syndromes. Pinpoint pupils with hypoventilation suggest opioids. Hypertension, tachycardia, and vertical or rotatory nystagmus suggest a dissociative agent, such as ketamine or phencyclidine. Increased salivation, lacrimation, bronchial secretions, diaphoresis, and incontinence suggest cholinergic agents. Sedative-hypnotic toxicity produces more varied symptoms, including normal vital signs (benzodiazepines), apnea and circulatory collapse (barbiturates), and seizures (gamma hydroxybutyrate).

## LABORATORY TESTS AND NEUROIMAGING

The initial assessment of comatose patients generally includes measurement of serum glucose, complete blood count, coagulation factors, electrolytes, blood urea nitrogen (BUN) and creatinine, liver panel, thyroid function, serum ammonia, and a venous blood gas (Moore and Wijdicks, 2013). Blood should be cultured if infection is suspected. The value of toxicologic testing for ethanol and drugs of abuse is questionable, and poisoning remains a clinical diagnosis. Routine toxicologic testing rarely changes acute management.

In patients with metabolic acidosis, a widened anion gap suggests one of four mechanisms (ketones, uremia, lactate, toxins). Ketosis can occur in diabetes, alcohol misuse, or starvation. Uremia generally produces acidosis only in later stages. Increased serum lactate can occur in sepsis, hypoperfusion, Wernicke's encephalopathy, or with toxins such as cyanide. Toxins can also produce acidosis by other mechanisms (carboxylic acid derivatives in ingestion of methanol or ethylene glycol, pyroglutamic acid in massive ingestion of acetaminophen), or a combination of mechanisms (salicylates).

At most institutions, the CT scan is the fastest and most readily available imaging modality. In the evaluation of an unresponsive patient, CT scans are excellent at detecting hydrocephalus, brain edema or intracranial hemorrhage, with a sensitivity and specificity approaching 100% in conditions such as acute (<12 hours since onset) subarachnoid hemorrhage. Limitations of CT include poor visualization of the posterior fossa secondary to bone artifact, as well as reduced anatomic differentiation in comparison to MRI, which may allow precise determination of etiology.

MRI scans provide greater definition of cortical and subcortical structures and may show cortical injury, laminar necrosis, or white-matter disease that is not apparent on a CT scan. Magnetic resonance angiography allows for excellent visualization of the arterial system and is an appropriate method for visualization of suspected acute basilar artery occlusion; however, this may not be possible at all institutions. In such instances, CT angiogram or conventional angiography can also allow for rapid visualization of the arterial system. The major drawbacks of MRI scans include accessibility, cost, and time necessary to complete the scan but modern neurology cannot and should not do without it. It has resolved many unclear situations in acute neurology.

Hypodensity on CT in comatose patients indicates infarction, edema, and tumor. Very low density indicates air, mostly from penetrating injury. Hyperdensity indicates hemorrhage or calcification. However, in patients with early diffuse cerebral edema (e.g., anoxic-ischemic encephalopathy), the arteries in the basal cisterns are more clearly seen against a hypodense background and may falsely suggest subarachnoid blood (pseudo-subarachnoid hemorrhage). Contrast CT in the acute setting is rarely performed, but could show a ring-enhancing lesion in a poorly defined hypodense area and indicate an abscess or glioma. Epidural or subdural empyema is also much better imaged with contrast, but in all these cases uncertainties in interpretation are best resolved with MRI. A normal CT scan is expected in comatose patients seen immediately after cardiac or respiratory resuscitation, asphyxia, near drowning, most poisonings and intoxications, and acute metabolic disturbance or endocrine crises. CT scans are not sensitive enough to document abnormalities in these conditions, but abnormalities may become apparent later when the patient remains deeply comatose.

MRI is far more revealing in demonstrating anoxic-ischemic injury to the brain. MRI is also superior in documenting acute demyelination, the presence of pus or blood, encephalitis (predominantly herpes simplex virus or limbic encephalitis), and meningitis or ventriculitis. Fat embolism is often clearly seen on early MRI. Sagittal and coronal MRI images are particularly helpful to view brain tissue shifts and brainstem displacement.

Fluid-attenuated inversion recovery (FLAIR) sequences and DWI are the most useful MRI modalities in patients with unexplained coma. MRI usually includes T1- and T2-weighted images and diffusion-weighted imaging (DWI) with mapping of the apparent diffusion coefficient (ADC). DWI measures diffusion of water through tissue; under pathologic circumstances, water accumulates, and in ischemic lesions the decrease in ADC is shown as a hyperintense region on DWI.

Several studies have found that increased signal intensity on FLAIR in the cerebrospinal fluid compartment can indicate subarachnoid hemorrhage or purulent exudate in meningitis. The hyperintensity on FLAIR is explained by the presence of increased protein or pleocytosis and will decrease T1 relaxation time.

## MANAGEMENT OF THE COMATOSE PATIENT

The chance of a favorable outcome in the care of acute brain injury leading to coma can be easily diminished if general principles of high-quality intensive care are not aggressively attended to. An immobile mechanically ventilated patient fed through a percutaneous gastrotomy (PEG) (Fig. 8.3) requires vigilance, specialized nursing care, and stewardship. Every day, infections may present, skin may break down, and fluid shifts may cause rapid imbalance of homeostasis. Drugs (particularly antibiotics) have potential short- and long-term adverse effects. Adequate management of eye, mouth, and skin at compression sites requires frequent change of linens,

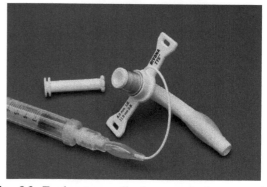

**Fig. 8.3.** Tracheostomy allowing speech for recovering patients.

patches, and protective pads. Splinting of extremities may be needed to avoid contractures. There are few hard data to support any of these interventions. The hard truth is that maintenance of a comatose patient is fraught with difficulties.

Inability to close eyelids completely after trauma and, in particular, nocturnal lagophthalmos are risk factors for conjunctivitis and corneal erosion (Lavrijsen et al., 2005). Polyethylene moisture chambers are required to prevent early epithelial breakdown, but some patients may have to be treated with lateral tarsorrhaphy. Filamentary keratopathy is a common dry-eye syndrome in patients in prolonged coma. Prolonged eyelid contact with the cornea and reduced blinking impair lacrimal fluid turnover and may be contributing factors.

Tracheostomy reduces pulmonary complications and provides easier access for pulmonary toilet. Tracheostomy will reduce length of stay, but it should generally be postponed until approximately 2 weeks in patients who can potentially be liberated from the ventilator if they show early signs of substantial neurologic improvement (Fig. 8.4). Gradually, after the patient is weaned off the ventilator, the tracheostomy can be closed, including in patients with prolonged unconsciousness. Pulmonary care involves frequent culturing of sputum when secretions change in color and texture and immediate antibiotic coverage to treat pneumonia and sepsis. Pleural effusions are frequent as a manifestation of anasarca and large pleural collections may need to be drained. Gastrointestinal problems vary from gastroparesis to paralytic ileus, resulting in distension of the colon and increased risk of perforation. Daily bowel care may include motility agents.

The most common healthcare-related infections are pneumonia, urinary tract infections, or infections of indwelling venous catheters. Potentially difficult to eradicate microorganisms include *Enterococcus*

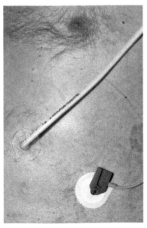

**Fig. 8.4.** Percutaneous gastrostomy.

*faecalis* or *faecium, Staphylococcus aureus, Klebsiella pneumoniae, Acinetobacter baumannii, Pseudomonas aeruginosa,* and *Enterobacter cloacae. Clostridium difficile* infections are also on the rise, particularly in patients with long hospital stays. The dilemma faced by treating physicians is that delayed initiation of antibiotics increases mortality, yet combination therapies to broaden the spectrum may lead to antibiotic resistance. Antibiotic therapy is complex and often changing as a result of infectious disease consultation.

Fever in comatose patients is mostly caused by infections. Lingering infections have to be excluded before attributing fever to the brain injury. However, Paroxysmal sympathetic hyperactivity (PSH) syndrome is a commonly seen in "unexplained" fever of comatose patients. PSH or dysautonomic storming all too frequently remains unrecognized and untreated. These spells are most common in young patients with diffuse axonal traumatic brain injury, but can occur with any major brain injury. Episodes of PSH can begin during the acute phase, often in comatose patients, and continue into the rehabilitation phase. Patients become tachycardic, hypertensive (with widened pulse pressure), tachypneic, febrile, diaphoretic, and often develop markedly increased tone, which may result in dystonic posturing. Pupillary dilatation, piloerection, and skin flushing can also be seen. The manifestations of PSH respond best to bolus doses of morphine sulfate (2–8 mg intravenously). This favorable response is not related to the analgesic effect of opiates, but rather to modulation of central pathways that are responsible for the autonomic dysfunction. The response to morphine is rapid and quite reliable in aborting spells of PSH. Other effective medications for the treatment of PSH include noncardioselective beta-blockers (such as propranolol), clonidine, and dexmedetomidine (central alpha 2-receptor agonists), bromocriptine (a dopamine D2-receptor agonist), baclofen (a $GABA_B$ receptor agonist), benzodiazepines ($GABA_A$ receptor agonist), and gabapentin (which binds GABA receptors and voltage-gated calcium channels in the dorsal horn of the spinal cord). In our experience, beta-blockers and clonidine are useful in controlling the tachycardia and hypertension, but less so for the dystonia. Baclofen and benzodiazepines (especially diazepam) do cause muscle relaxation, but may not improve the other hypersympathetic features.

Continuous volume replacement is needed for long-term care. The adequate intravascular status is determined by satisfactory organ perfusion (urinary output, capillary refill, cold or warm extremities, blood lactate, and mixed venous oxygen saturation). Tissue edema may form over time, possibly as a result of overzealous fluid administration (e.g., failure to adjust intravenous fluid rate while advancing enteral nutrition, failure to concentrate medications). Volume depletion is less common in the longterm but may occur, especially when extravascular compartment is expanded by sepsis. Hypotonic crystalloids, such as lactated Ringer's or half normal saline, should be avoided in traumatic brain injury. Albumin (5%) is a good volume expander, and may have a role in sepsis resuscitation, but the safety in acute brain injury is unclear and may be deleterious in traumatic brain injury. In patients who have developed oliguria and a rise in BUN (BUN/creatinine ratio > 20), dehydration is very likely and should result in discontinuation of all diuretics and administration of normal saline.

Nutrition is eventually provided through a PEG (Fig. 8.3), which is very safe. A study of 674 patients reported only 2% of patient experienced reversible complications (Iizuka and Reding, 2005). Complications include wound infection, leakage, peritonitis, self-extubation or hemorrhage in the first weeks of placement. The risk of gastrointestinal hemorrhage may be increased. Compared with nasogastric tubes, gastroesophageal reflux is lower in patients with a PEG.

A bowel care regimen should be initiated. Bowel incontinence is often present, and the task is to keep the skin clean and dry. Diarrhea may have many causes, but can be attributed to certain nutritional formulas and resolve with reducing fiber content. Antibiotics, as well as *Escherichia coli* or *Clostridium difficile* infections, are other possible causes of diarrhea. Failure to pass stool, or marble-like stools, should be treated with rectal enema or manual removal. Glycerol suppository can be helpful, but senna (10 mL) and lactulose (20 mL) are common maintenance therapies. Comatose patients are at risk of adynamic ileus. Marked abdominal distension and auscultatory silence are early signs. Metoclopramide (10 mg IV) or erythromycin (500 mg orally) can be very effective to resolve the bowel distension.

Nosocomial urinary tract infections will likely occur in comatose patients with long-term indwelling catheters. Bacteriuria involves *Escherichia coli* and *Pseudomonas aeruginosa* in two-thirds of all cases, with less frequent pathogens, including *Enterococcus* spp., *Acinetobacter* spp., *Klebsiella* spp., and *Proteus* spp. Increased risk for bacteriuria in patients admitted to ICU is conveyed by female gender (short urethra and flora contamination), length of ICU stay, antibiotic use, and duration of catheterization; thus, they are to some degree unavoidable. The types of drainage systems, aseptic handling, and other avoidance measures have been successful in reducing infection rates. This includes preventing the catheter tubing from kinking, regular emptying of collection bag, maintaining drainage systems below level of bladder, appropriate meatal care, and use of silver-impregnated urinary catheters or vesical irrigation with

*Table 8.5*

**Daily concerns in care of the comatose patient**

| | |
|---|---|
| Lungs | Mechanical ventilation settings |
| | Weaning option |
| | Tracheostomy care |
| | Chest X-ray for infiltrates |
| Heart | Cardiac arrhythmias |
| | Electrocardiogram changes (i.e., QT prolongation) |
| | Inotropes/vasopressors/beta blockade |
| Gastrointestinal | Oropharyngeal hygiene |
| | Nutrition and choice of formula |
| | Targets glucose/insulin drips |
| | Bowel motility assistance |
| Bladder | Indwelling catheter |
| | Urine analysis |
| Skin | Decubitus |
| | Conjunctiva/eye care |
| Prophylaxis | Unfractionated heparin |
| | Surveillance ultrasound of venous system |
| | Gastrointestinal prophylaxis |
| | Fever control |
| Access | Peripheral catheter |
| | Peripherally inserted central catheter |
| | Subclavian |
| | Peripheral intravenous |
| Medication | Medication reconciliation |
| | Antibiotic stop dates |
| | Drug–drug interaction |
| | Sedation/analgesia needs |

neomycin and polymyxin. The long-term care of the comatose patient is summarized in Table 8.5.

# NEUROREHABILITATION

When a patient awakens from coma, neurorehabilitation can be considered. Criteria to admit patients to rehabilitation centers have been developed. Most generally, patients are not eligible if: (1) there are continuous medical concerns that may lead to an unstable situation; (2) it is unlikely that the patient will be able to improve or make progress in daily therapy sessions; and (3) there is no support system after the patient returns home. Centers for Medicare and Medicaid Services (CMS) criteria are most often applied, as they determine reimbursement. In addition to the patient having brain-related limiting neurologic impairment, the need for multidisciplinary therapies, and the capability to participate and benefit from an intensive intervention (i.e., ≈ 3 hours of daily therapy), CMS requires that: (1) the patient has active medical problems that require physician attendance; (2) the patient has needs specific to specialized rehabilitation nursing; and (3) this care cannot be provided in a less intense medical environment (nursing home). Neurorehabilitation can only function well with a large staff that includes physiatrists, neuropsychologists, speech therapists, occupational and recreational therapists, rehabilitation nurse specialists, social workers, and vocational case counselors. This multidisciplinary team should be carefully orchestrated and often involves a case manager involved in coordinating care. Programs usually involve activities for several hours a day, 5 days a week. Functional independence is best achieved if patients can enter these programs within the first 6 months after acute brain injury. Substantial evidence for remedial interventions involving attention, memory, social communication skills, and executive function remains wanting.

Rating of improvement of patients with disorders of consciousness is needed not only to better measure range of behaviors, but also to assist in research on prognosis in patients with severe brain injury. It has been known that probabilistic models improve accuracy when compared to clinical prediction, but there continues to be an uncertainty about the most meaningful and interpretable score. There is no shortage of scales assessing patients and major competition for practical use. Current scales that are used in practice and research studies are Functional Independence Measure (FIM), Disability Rating Scale (DRS), Glasgow Outcome Scale, Cerebral Performance Scale, Glasgow Outcome Extended Scale, Neurobehavior Rating Scale-Revised and, more recently, Neurologic Outcome Scale for Traumatic Brain Injury. Outcome measures in rehabilitation most commonly are considered in relation to the *International Classification of Functioning, Disability and Health* realms of impairment (how the examination is different from normal), activity limitations (so-called activities of daily living and instrumental activities of daily living), and restrictions to participation (e.g., personal, family, vocational, community roles). The National Institutes of Health toolbox, Patient-Reported Outcomes Measurement Information System (PROMIS) measures, Activity Measure for Post-Acute Care (AM-PAC), and Traumatic Brain Injury Quality of Life (TBI-QOL) are examples of current measures.

Although the FIM is most widely used, the DRS has been used in research studies and requires eight items. The total scores vary from 0 to 30 (a vegetative state has a score of 22 or more, and 30 indicates death). The first three items are the GCS (lowest number is here 0 rather than 1), and the other scores are for self-care activities and level of functioning (physically, mentally, emotionally, and socially). The interrater reliability is good, as is the comparison of ratings by family members and rehabilitation professionals.

Are there therapeutic options in patients with impaired consciousness? Treatment of minimally conscious state has mostly been of interest, and now data suggest that amantadine 100 mg twice daily for 2 weeks followed by 150 mg twice daily at week 3 and 200 mg twice daily at week 4 accelerates recovery in traumatic brain injury. Zolpidem (10 mg) trial may be administered, but the response is variable and mostly absent. Others have tried fluoxetine (selective serotonin reuptake inhibitor) 20 mg daily, with some effect in motor response. Methylphenidate is a dopaminergic agent that improves processing speed, attention, and possibly memory. Another dopaminergic drug (bromocriptine) and a selective norepinephrine reuptake inhibitor (atomoxetine) have been considered in postconcussional cognitive impairment, but not in minimally conscious state.

Interest in deep-brain stimulation has rekindled, and bipolar stimulation of thalamic nuclei has been considered, with variable results. Recent data in 3 patients have not shown clinically evident improvement in consciousness (Magrassi et al., 2016). There is also little evidence that these treatments produce harm in these vulnerable adults (who, I hasten to add, are human beings). On the other hand, one can see that these patients may become perceived as a "neglected" group of patients, while there truly may not be much offered here that will lead to improved functional outcome. It remains unexamined if increased awareness of a major neurologic handicap causes more agony to the patient, who is now becoming more fully aware of the ordeal.

## OUTCOME PREDICTION

Outcome prediction in coma is only possible with disease entities followed for a substantial amount of time, usually 6–12 months. Outcome prediction may not be reliable in young patients who have shown enormous resilience and surprising improvement in functioning. There are some important facts to keep in mind: approximately 50% of poor-grade patients with an aneurysmal subarachnoid hemorrhage improve over time; over 80% of comatose patients with traumatic brain injury awaken; but fewer than 10% of patients who remain comatose 1–2 days after an anoxic-ischemic event improve to better grades of consciousness (Greer et al., 2013).

Prolonged unconsciousness is uncommon, mostly because patients who remain comatose die. This is often because of an intercurrent event (e.g., severe sepsis or decubitus ulcers), but also because family members wish no further life-sustaining interventions as a result of an advance directive (advance directives, used in many countries, are legal documents in which patients have determined what actions should be taken if they are no longer able to make decisions due to illness or incapacity). No neurologist wants to deprive the patient or family of hope or the potential for recovery. Still, families may decide to proceed with withdrawal of life support, even in the setting of some uncertainty. The prospect of a severely disabled person, even if the chance is realistic, might not be commensurate with the patient's wishes. If the patient stays on a ventilator and cannot return home, it may not be the quality of life everyone has hoped for.

The diagnosis of PVS is uncommon because most patients in this condition awaken within 3–6 months. The massive destruction in the cortical layers and thalamus at autopsy, absence of operational modular networks after stimulation using functional MRI, marked reduction in glucose metabolism on positron emission tomography, and markedly depressed EEG in postresuscitation PVS are all test results that confirm a clinical examination showing a nonsapient being. The general rule remains that if the clinical findings of PVS are still present after 3 months in nontraumatic coma (i.e., anoxic-ischemic encephalopathy, hypoglycemia, CNS infections, or status epilepticus), major recovery is not anticipated. In traumatic brain injury, 12 months are needed for certainty; but recovery to a minimally conscious state may occur even beyond this time limit.

## References

Edlow JA, Rabinstein A, Traub SJ et al. (2014). Diagnosis of reversible causes of coma. Lancet 384: 2064–2076.

Greer DM, Yang J, Scripko PD et al. (2013). Clinical examination for prognostication in comatose cardiac arrest patients. Resuscitation 84: 1546–1551.

Iizuka M, Reding M (2005). Use of percutaneous endoscopic gastrostomy feeding tubes and functional recovery in stroke rehabilitation: a case-matched controlled study. Arch Phys Med Rehabil 86: 1049–1052.

Lavrijsen J, vaqn Rens G, van den Bosch H (2005). Filamentary keratopathy as a chronic problem in the long-term care of patients in a vegetative state. Cornea 24: 620–622.

Magrassi L, Maggioni G, Pistarini C et al. (2016 Jan 8). Results of a prospective study (CATS) on the effects of thalamic stimulation in minimally conscious and vegetative state patients. J Neurosurg 1–10.

Mijalski C, Lovett A, Mahajan R et al. (2015). Cerebral fat embolism: a case of rapid-onset coma. Stroke 46: 251–253.

Moore SA, Wijdicks EFM (2013). The acutely comatose patient: clinical approach and diagnosis. Semin Neurol 33: 110–120.

Salottolo K, Carrick M, Levy AS et al. (2016). Aggressive operative neurosurgical management in patients with extra-axial mass lesion and Glasgow Coma Scale of 3 is associated with survival benefit: a propensity matched analysis. Injury 47: 70–76.

Stevens RD, Cadena RS, Pineda J (2015). Emergency neurological life support: approach to the patient with coma. Neurocrit Care 23: 69–75.

Teasdale G, Jennett B (1974). Assessment of coma and impaired consciousness. A practical scale. Lancet 2: 81–84.

Wijdicks EFM (2001). The diagnosis of brain death. N Engl J Med 344: 1215–1221.

Wijdicks EFM (2010). The bare essentials: coma. Pract Neurol 10: 51–60.

Wijdicks EFM, Varelas PN, Gronseth GS et al. (2010). American Academy of N. Evidence-based guideline update: determining brain death in adults: report of the Quality Standards Subcommittee of the American Academy of Neurology. Neurology 74: 1911–1918.

Wijdicks EFM (2014). The Comatose Patient, 2nd edn. Oxford University Press, Oxford.

Wijdicks EFM (2016). Why you may need a neurologist to see a comatose patient in the ICU Critical Care 20: 193.

Wijdicks EFM (2017). Brain Death 3ed Oxford University Press.

*Handbook of Clinical Neurology*, Vol. 140 (3rd series)
*Critical Care Neurology, Part I*
E.F.M. Wijdicks and A.H. Kramer, Editors
http://dx.doi.org/10.1016/B978-0-444-63600-3.00009-X

Chapter 9

# Management of status epilepticus

M. PICHLER[1] AND S. HOCKER[2]*

[1]*Department of Neurology, Mayo Clinic, Rochester, MN, USA*

[2]*Division of Critical Care Neurology, Mayo Clinic, Rochester, MN, USA*

## Abstract

Status epilepticus is a neurologic and medical emergency manifested by prolonged seizure activity or multiple seizures without return to baseline. It is associated with substantial medical cost, morbidity, and mortality. There is a spectrum of severity dependent on the type of seizure, underlying pathology, comorbidities, and appropriate and timely medical management. This chapter discusses the evolving definitions of status epilepticus and multiple patient and clinical factors which influence outcome. The pathophysiology of status epilepticus is reviewed to provide a better understanding of the mechanisms which contribute to status epilepticus, as well as the potential long-term effects. The clinical presentations of different types of status epilepticus in adults are discussed, with emphasis on the hospital course and management of the most dangerous type, generalized convulsive status epilepticus. Strategies for the evaluation and management of status epilepticus are provided based on available evidence from clinical trials and recommendations from the Neurocritical Care Society and the European Federation of Neurological Societies.

Status epilepticus (SE) is a neurologic and medical emergency manifest by prolonged seizure activity or multiple seizures without a return to baseline. It is associated with substantial medical costs, morbidity, and mortality. The mortality of SE ranges from 9% to 22% and increases with age (DeLorenzo et al., 1996; Logroscino et al., 2005; Dham et al., 2014). There is a spectrum of severity dependent on the type of seizure, underlying pathology, comorbidities, and appropriate and timely medical management. SE is broadly categorized as convulsive or nonconvulsive based on the presence or absence of prominent motor activity. Subtypes of SE can be further characterized by seizure semiology, etiology, electroencephalogram (EEG) pattern, duration, or response to medications.

Although the general concept of SE has remained relatively constant, the definition has undergone numerous revisions over the years (Lowenstein et al., 1999). Initial classification by the International League Against Epilepsy (ILAE) in 1964 defined SE as a seizure which "persists for a sufficient length of time or is repeated frequently enough to produce a fixed and enduring epileptic condition" (Arnautova and Nesmeianova, 1964). This ambiguous definition was amended by various organizations and research studies to incorporate specific duration of seizure activity, ranging from 10 to 60 minutes (Lowenstein et al., 1999). A definition of more than 30 minutes of continuous seizure activity or two or more sequential seizures without full recovery of consciousness between was widely adopted, citing neuronal damage in animal models beyond this timeframe (Epilepsy Foundation, 1993). More recently, the duration has been revised to 5 minutes, as clinical or electrographic seizures lasting longer than this are unlikely to stop spontaneously. There is also evidence that pharmacoresistance and neuronal injury may occur when seizures continue beyond this timeframe (Brophy et al., 2012).

Taking these observations into account, the ILAE published an updated classification scheme in 2015, using operational definitions of SE based on specific

*Correspondence to: Sara Hocker, MD, Mayo Clinic, 200 First Street SW, Rochester MN 55905, USA. Tel: +1-507-284-4701, E-mail: Hocker.Sara@mayo.edu

time points of 5 and 30 minutes. To provide a practical guideline for clinicians, generalized tonic-clonic seizures lasting 5 minutes or longer were classified as SE, warranting emergency treatment. Generalized tonic-clonic seizure activity lasting 30 minutes or more was recognized as a risk for irreversible neuronal injury and functional deficits (Trinka et al., 2015). These observations were largely influenced by early studies of convulsive SE in baboons, conducted by Meldrum and colleagues in the 1970s (Meldrum and Horton, 1973; Meldrum et al., 1973a, b). Since then, various animal models and clinical experience in humans have helped to further delineate the sequence of systemic and neuronal complications of convulsive SE. The optimal time points for emergency intervention and risk of irreversible neuronal injury in other seizure subtypes are less defined.

Nonconvulsive SE (NCSE) accounts for approximately 25% of all cases of SE (Cascino, 1993), but the pathophysiology leading to morbidity and mortality in NCSE has not been as well described. Animal models of NCSE indicate that neuronal damage does occur, but the duration and seizure intensity needed to induce damage remain unclear. Additionally, because isolated NCSE is rarely fatal, pathologic studies in humans are lacking (Drislane, 2000).

Refractory SE (RSE) refers to continued clinical or electrographic seizures after adequate dosing of an initial benzodiazepine followed by a second-line antiepileptic drug (AED), and is associated with a worse prognosis than non-RSE (Hocker et al., 2013, 2014). Based on retrospective studies, roughly 20–40% of patients with SE do not respond to initial therapies and become refractory (Mayer et al., 2002; Holtkamp et al., 2005; Rossetti et al., 2005). In a prospective study of RSE, 23% of patients presenting to a tertiary care center with SE were refractory to initial therapies. Refractory cases were associated with higher morbidity and mortality compared to nonrefractory cases (Novy et al., 2010), reproducing the findings of multiple prior retrospective studies. Depending on the underlying etiology and exclusion criteria, mortality rates in RSE can range from 8 to 56% (Mayer et al., 2002; Holtkamp et al., 2005; Rossetti et al., 2005; Drislane et al., 2009; Novy et al., 2010; Hocker et al., 2013; Kantanen et al., 2015). When anoxic-ischemic injury is excluded as an etiology of RSE, the mortality rate is 23–48% (Claassen et al., 2002; Mayer et al., 2002; Holtkamp et al., 2005; Rossetti et al., 2005; Hocker et al., 2013; Sutter et al., 2014; Kantanen et al., 2015).

When RSE occurs in an individual without a history of epilepsy and no immediate underlying etiology is found, it is referred to as new-onset RSE (NORSE). This clinical scenario may be notoriously difficult to treat and by definition does not respond to initial medications (Wilder-Smith et al., 2005; Costello et al., 2009; Gaspard et al., 2015). Recently published data from the global audit of RSE suggest that the largest etiologic category of patients developing superrefractory SE (SRSE) may in fact be cryptogenic; however, this finding must be validated as a selection bias is almost certainly present in registry data (Ferlisi et al., 2015). In a recent retrospective study of NORSE, the majority (52%) of cases remained cryptogenic 2 days after admission. The most commonly identified etiologies were autoimmune (19%) and paraneoplastic (18%) encephalitis (Gaspard et al., 2015). Patient characteristics often seen in NORSE include female gender, young age, extensive negative diagnostic testing, and no prior history of epilepsy (Wilder-Smith et al., 2005).

SRSE has been defined primarily for research purposes as SE that continues or recurs 24 hours or more after the initiation of anesthetic therapy, including cases where SE recurs on the reduction or withdrawal of anesthesia (Shorvon and Ferlisi, 2011). Most studies of SE do not explicitly document the persistence or recurrence of seizures beyond 24 hours of anesthetic treatment, making the exact incidence difficult to assess. Based on limited data, it is estimated that SRSE occurs in 5–15% of all SE episodes (Novy et al., 2010; Shorvon and Ferlisi, 2011; Hocker et al., 2014; Kantanen et al., 2015). SRSE is also associated with a worse prognosis and increased mortality compared with both SE and RSE. While variation in methodology limits direct comparisons, the mortality of SRSE has been reported to range from 25 to 58% (Ferlisi and Shorvon, 2012; Pugin et al., 2014; Ferlisi et al., 2015; Kantanen et al., 2015).

## EPIDEMIOLOGY

SE has an annual incidence of 6–41 per 100 000 people (Oxbury and Whitty, 1971; Aminoff and Simon, 1980; DeLorenzo et al., 1996; Hesdorffer et al., 1998; Coeytaux et al., 2000; Knake et al., 2001; Wu et al., 2002; Vignatelli et al., 2003). There is a bimodal distribution, with increased occurrence during infancy and again after age 60 years (DeLorenzo et al., 1996; Hesdorffer et al., 1998; Wu et al., 2002). Febrile seizures or fever in the setting of infection account for over half of cases of SE in infants and children (Aicardi and Chevrie, 1970; DeLorenzo et al., 1996). Because of the relatively favorable prognosis of these underlying causes, SE in children is associated with low morbidity and mortality (Dunn, 1988; Maytal et al., 1989; DeLorenzo et al., 1996). In contrast, SE in adults is most often due to acute neurologic insults such as cerebrovascular disease, trauma, central nervous system (CNS) infection, or anoxic-ischemic injury (Towne et al., 1994; DeLorenzo et al., 1996; Hesdorffer et al., 1998;

Knake et al., 2001; Legriel et al., 2010). Common causes of SE in adults include low AED levels, stroke, anoxic brain injury, alcohol withdrawal, metabolic dysfunction, brain tumor, infection, drug intoxication, and traumatic brain injury (DeLorenzo et al., 1996). Numerous uncommon causes have also been reported (Tan et al., 2010). Because of the profound differences in patient characteristics and outcomes in children versus adults, this chapter will focus on the management of SE in adults only. Detailed review of SE in children can be found elsewhere (Abend and Loddenkemper, 2014; Freilich et al., 2014).

The incidence in the elderly is approximately three to 10 times higher than in younger adults (Knake et al., 2001; Wu et al., 2002; Vignatelli et al., 2005). In addition, elderly patients have a higher associated mortality (Towne et al., 1994), likely due to a combination of the underlying pathology as well as medical comorbidities. The increasing proportion of elderly individuals in developed countries will likely lead to an even higher overall incidence and mortality of SE in the future.

Several studies in both the USA and Europe have shown a higher incidence (nearly 2:1 in some cases) in males compared with females (Hesdorffer et al., 1998; Coeytaux et al., 2000; Knake et al., 2001; Wu et al., 2002). Hormonal differences may influence seizure threshold via numerous mechanisms, as suggested in animal studies (Moshe et al., 1995; Standley et al., 1995), but this has not been proven in humans.

When stratified by ethnic group, the incidence in American minorities was shown to be substantially higher (57/100 000) than whites (20/100 000) in Richmond, Virginia (DeLorenzo et al., 1996). This racial disparity was supported in a nationwide epidemiologic study in the USA from 1979 to 2010, which found a higher incidence among blacks (13.7/100 000) compared to other minorities (7.4/100 000) and whites (6.9/100 000) (Dham et al., 2014). Despite the higher incidence, SE in blacks and minorities was associated with a lower mortality rate in these studies. The racial variability in mortality has been demonstrated in other studies as well (Towne et al., 1994; Wu et al., 2002), but the cause remains speculative. Differences in socioeconomic, environmental, and cultural factors likely play a role.

Roughly half (43–58%) of patients presenting with SE do not have a prior history of epilepsy (Lowenstein and Alldredge, 1993; DeLorenzo et al., 1996; Hesdorffer et al., 1998; Knake et al., 2001; Novy et al., 2010). SE in these patients is often due to an acute neurologic insult such as trauma, CNS infection, stroke, anoxia, or toxic/metabolic disturbances (Hesdorffer et al., 1998). The other half of cases of SE occurs in patients with epilepsy. It is estimated that more than 15% of patients with epilepsy will experience at least

one episode of SE over their lifetime (Fountain, 2000). Up to 1% of patients with epilepsy will develop SE annually, accounting for approximately 15 000 cases each year in the USA (Hauser, 1990). SE in these patients typically occurs in the setting of low AED levels and is associated with lower mortality than in patients without a history of seizures (Lowenstein and Alldredge, 1993; DeLorenzo et al., 1996; Wu et al., 2002). Identifying the underlying cause of SE is essential and has a large impact on overall mortality. Table 9.1 outlines the most common etiologies associated with SE.

*Table 9.1*

**Common causes of status epilepticus in adults**

**Acute causes**
Stroke: ischemic or hemorrhagic
Metabolic abnormalities: electrolyte disturbances, hypoglycemia, uremia, fulminant hepatic failure
Anoxic ischemic injury
Sepsis
Traumatic brain injury
Brain tumor
Drug effects:
- Acute drug toxicity
- Withdrawal from alcohol, benzodiazepines, baclofen, barbiturates, etc.
- Low antiepileptic drug levels
Central nervous system infection (meningitis, abscess, viral encephalitis)
Hypertensive encephalopathy/posterior reversible encephalopathy syndrome
Antibody-mediated encephalitis: paraneoplastic or nonparaneoplastic

**Chronic causes**
Progressive epilepsy syndromes (e.g., Lennox–Gastaut syndrome)
Congenital malformations (brain or cerebrovascular), or cortical dysplasia
Encephalomalacia due to remote central nervous system structural damage (e.g., stroke, trauma, prior neurosurgery)
Neurodegenerative disorders (e.g., Alzheimer's dementia, amyloid angiopathy)

## NEUROPATHOLOGY

SE occurs when intrinsic brain mechanisms are unable to terminate a seizure or when the neuronal environment becomes conducive to prolonged seizure activity. The specific molecular and cellular mechanisms which contribute to SE are an area of active research. At the time of seizure onset, neurotransmitter release, changes in ion channel configuration, and protein phosphorylation induce a cascade of molecular and cellular changes thought to potentiate seizure activity in some patients. Studies in animals have shown that these changes can quickly lead to internalization of gamma-aminobutyric acid (GABA)$_A$ receptors containing the $\beta_2/\beta_3$ and $\gamma_2$ receptor subunits. This may account for the decreased efficacy of benzodiazepines as the duration of SE lengthens. In animal studies, seizures lasting longer than 30 minutes show a 20-fold decrease in response to diazepam (Wasterlain et al., 2009). Various other receptors have also been implicated in the generation of self-sustaining seizures. Animal models have suggested activity-induced $N$-methyl-D-aspartic acid (NMDA) and $\alpha$-amino-3-hydroxy-5-methyl-4-isoxazolepropionic acid (AMPA) receptor trafficking to synapses. The increase in these excitatory receptors can further perpetuate seizure activity (Chen et al., 2007).

Minutes to hours after seizure onset, changes in neuropeptide expression likely contribute to the hyperexcitable state. Immunocytochemical studies in SE have shown depletion of the inhibitory peptides dynorphin, galanin, somatostatin, and neuropeptide Y, as well as an increase in excitatory substance P and neurokinin B (Chen and Wasterlain, 2006). Days to weeks after seizure onset, genetic and epigenetic changes may become apparent. Excessive neuronal activity may lead to activation of transcription factors, neurotrophic factors, protein synthesis, neurogenesis, and synaptogenesis. There are likely multifaceted interactions which lead to neural reorganization, though the details are poorly understood. Animal models of SE have shown alterations in gene expression, DNA methylation, and regulation of microRNA which may all contribute to ongoing seizure risk (Betjemann and Lowenstein, 2015).

Convulsive SE is a well-described cause of neuronal and systemic injury. Meldrum and Brierley (1973) studied chemically induced SE in baboons, documenting hyperthermia, severe respiratory and metabolic acidosis, hypoxia, and neuronal death. Neuronal damage was seen diffusely in the neocortex and also in the hippocampus and cerebellum. Interestingly, when the animals were paralyzed and mechanically ventilated in an attempt to control the systemic complications associated with convulsive activity, the cerebellum and neocortex seemed to be protected from injury. However, neuronal injury in the hippocampus was observed even in the absence of convulsions, suggesting pathogenesis directly related to excess neuronal firing (Meldrum et al., 1973a, b). Other studies have also supported the theory that prolonged seizure activity can be directly detrimental to neurons. Kainic acid has been used to cause intense electrographic seizures in limbic structures in rats. It is particularly useful because the dose can be adjusted to cause limbic SE without generalized convulsions or significant systemic side-effects. Kainic acid-induced NCSE has been shown to cause hippocampal damage similar to that seen in convulsive SE (Lothman and Collins, 1981). Hippocampal neuronal loss has been demonstrated in animals with frequent limbic seizures or those with limbic SE, but not in those with a shorter duration of seizures (Bertram et al., 1990). An alternative rat model of SE was developed by stimulating an excitatory pathway with electric probes placed in the hippocampus. No generalized convulsions or systemic complications occurred, but the prolonged seizure activity led to hippocampal cell loss and damage to adjacent interneurons (Sloviter, 1987).

Similar pathology has been described in humans following SE. Cell loss in the CA1 region of the hippocampus has been shown in histopathologic examination of patients who died during convulsive SE. These studies have also shown variable neuronal loss in the thalamus, cerebellum, caudate, and middle layers of cortex (Corsellis and Bruton, 1983). Neuron-specific enolase, a marker of neuronal injury, is often elevated following prolonged seizures, a finding which has been documented in all major subtypes of SE (DeGiorgio et al., 1995, 1999; Rabinowicz et al., 1995). Magnetic resonance imaging (MRI) abnormalities may also suggest neuronal injury, sometimes showing edema in the acute setting or atrophy in chronic cases (Nixon et al., 2001; Chen et al., 2007).

Numerous mechanisms are likely involved in neuronal injury, but intracellular calcium concentrations and mitochondrial functioning are felt to be central to the process. Excessive glutamate release and activation of NMDA receptors cause an influx of intracellular calcium and mitochondrial dysfunction. This may subsequently trigger activation of caspases and lead to programmed cell death (Wasterlain et al., 1993; Pollard et al., 1994; Cock et al., 2002; Niquet et al., 2003; Chen et al., 2007). The widespread chemical and structural changes associated with SE are not only important in the acute setting, but also have long-term implications. The risk of a subsequent unprovoked seizure in patients with SE is 3.3 times higher than the risk following a typical self-limited seizure (Hesdorffer et al., 1998). SE in children has been associated with development of epilepsy in over 70% of patients followed for more than 1 year (Aicardi and Chevrie, 1970). Neurologic sequelae and risk of SE recurrence in children are highest in those with nonidiopathic and nonfebrile etiologies (Barnard and Wirrell, 1999). The mechanisms leading to the increased risk is unclear, but may relate to impairment of the blood–brain barrier, glial activation, inflammation, and synaptogenesis (Friedman et al., 2009; Weissberg et al., 2015).

## CLINICAL PRESENTATION

SE is broadly categorized as convulsive or nonconvulsive based on the presence or absence of prominent motor symptoms and the degree of impaired consciousness. The distinction is critical because treatment and outcomes vary depending on seizure semiology. SE with prominent motor symptoms may be further classified as myoclonic (prominent epileptic myoclonic jerks), convulsive (also known as tonic-clonic SE), focal motor, tonic, or hyperkinetic SE (Trinka et al., 2015). These different patterns can overlap or change at times, and can even transition to NCSE. NCSE lacks prominent motor symptoms and can present with varying degrees of impaired consciousness, often making diagnosis difficult. NCSE can be associated with coma, where it is sometimes referred to as "subtle" SE or "nonconvulsive status epilepticus in coma," but can also occur in the absence of coma or present with generalized (absence or myoclonic SE) or focal epileptic activity (with or without impaired consciousness) (Trinka et al., 2015).

## Myoclonic status epilepticus

Myoclonic SE (prominent epileptic myoclonic jerks) can occur with or without coma (Trinka et al., 2015). It is most commonly seen in the setting of anoxic-ischemic injury after a cardiac or respiratory arrest, hanging, or drowning event, and manifests clinically with sudden brief movements of the face, trunk, or extremities. The movements are characteristically arrhythmic, multifocal, and triggered or exacerbated by external stimuli such as repositioning or mechanical ventilation (Hocker, 2015b).

## Convulsive status epilepticus

Patients presenting with convulsive SE are easily recognized because of their prominent motor manifestations. Cortical electric discharges may manifest as sustained muscle contractions (tonic activity), rhythmic jerking of muscles (clonic activity), or a combination of these movements (tonic-clonic activity) (Huff and Fountain, 2011). Catecholamine release during prolonged convulsive seizure activity leads to pupillary dilatation, incontinence, tachycardia, hyperpyrexia, hyperglycemia, and a cascade of other systemic complications (Glaser, 1983; Baumgartner et al., 2001).

Patients often present with metabolic and respiratory acidosis. Metabolic acidosis occurs due to increased lactate production from excessive muscle contraction and conversion to anaerobic glycolysis. Simultaneously, excretion of carbon dioxide is impaired due to altered respiratory function. The development of respiratory acidosis is multifactorial and may include central depression from seizure activity or medication effects, diaphragmatic contraction during seizures, which increases the mechanical load, and impaired gas exchange secondary to aspiration or neurocardiogenic pulmonary edema. Fortunately, the acid–base disturbances are not associated with life-threatening arrhythmias and do not require further intervention (Aminoff and Simon, 1980; Wijdicks and Hubmayr, 1994; Wijdicks, 2013; Hocker, 2015a). Metabolic acidosis is often from barbiturate and lorazepam use and caused by the propylene glycol vehicle (Wijdicks, 2013).

Because of the impaired level of consciousness and medication effects, respiratory complications are frequently encountered in SE and include aspiration pneumonitis, pneumonia, apnea, pulmonary edema, mucous plugging and acute respiratory failure (Hocker, 2015a). Endotracheal intubation is required in around 20% of patients and is more common in the elderly or those with RSE (Vohra et al., 2015).

Cardiac complications may also be apparent at time of presentation. Excess catecholamine release likely plays a role and has been associated with contraction band necrosis in autopsy studies in patients with SE. Contraction bands form when myocardium dies in a hypercontracted state. These pathologic changes occur near insertion of sympathetic end plates, supporting a theory of neurogenic-mediated disease (Manno et al., 2005). Changes on electrocardiogram can include arrhythmias, conduction abnormalities, and ischemic patterns (Boggs et al., 1993). Apical ballooning syndrome (also known as takotsubo cardiomyopathy and stress-induced cardiomyopathy) has also been reported in the setting of SE, in addition to various other acute neurologic insults. This syndrome presents with apical or left ventricular dyskinesis, ST-segment or T-wave abnormalities on electrocardiogram, and a modest troponin elevation, in the absence of obstructive coronary lesions. Treatment is supportive and the prognosis is favorable if the cardiopulmonary systems are appropriately supported (Sakuragi et al., 2007; Legriel et al., 2008; Shimizu et al., 2008).

Musculoskeletal injuries are often detected when the trauma survey is performed and can include fractures of the ribs, vertebrae, or long bones. Posterior shoulder dislocation and tongue lacerations can also occur with convulsive seizure activity. Acute kidney injury may result from prolonged muscle contraction leading to rhabdomyolysis and myoglobinuria. Serial creatinine measurements should be monitored in these cases and, if renal injury is severe, the extremities monitored for compartment syndrome (Hocker, 2015a).

## Nonconvulsive status epilepticus in coma

NCSE in coma is also referred to as "subtle" SE. These terms are most frequently used to describe ongoing electrographic seizures after convulsive SE, but can also be used to describe electrographic SE in a patient who is comatose for other known reasons, such as fulminant bacterial meningitis. During the course of inadequately treated convulsive SE, the initial tonic phase shortens over time and the clonic movements disperse and eventually cease as muscles fatigue and can no longer contract. However, even after the movements have stopped, there may be ongoing subclinical seizure activity, the so-called "subtle" SE (Treiman et al., 1998). In a prospective study by DeLorenzo and colleagues (1998), EEG monitoring showed that, even after controlling convulsive SE, nearly half of patients developed persistent electrographic seizures (48%) or NCSE (14%). These findings highlight the importance of EEG monitoring following treatment of convulsive SE, as the diagnosis of NCSE can be missed by clinical assessment alone. Continuous EEG monitoring should be initiated within 1 hour of SE to rule out NCSE even after convulsive activity has stopped (Brophy et al., 2012).

The diagnosis of NCSE in coma is particularly challenging because the clinical features and EEG patterns are often confounded by the medications used to care for critically ill patients (e.g., analgesics, anesthetics, paralytics). Nonspecific EEG patterns are often of uncertain significance and open to interpretation. Guidelines for diagnosis have been proposed, but not validated or universally applied (Hirsch and Gaspard, 2013). An assessment of the clinical and electrographic response to a rapidly acting antiepileptic medication is often needed to establish the diagnosis. However, clinical improvement may be delayed by several hours following electrographic improvement, and a negative response does not necessarily rule out NCSE. Figure 9.1 illustrates potential EEG findings associated with nonconvulsive status epilepticus in coma and also highlights important differences in outcome depending on the underlying etiology.

## Nonconvulsive status epilepticus without coma

A diagnosis of NCSE should be considered in patients with unexplained or persistent encephalopathy, but it is impractical to perform EEG monitoring in all encephalopathic patients. Patients with risk factors for seizures, such as stroke, intracranial tumor, prior neurosurgery, CNS infection, AED medication noncompliance, and drug intoxication or withdrawal, are most likely to benefit from monitoring (Husain et al., 2003).

### ABSENCE STATUS EPILEPTICUS

Absence SE presents with variable degrees of impaired consciousness, ranging from mild amnesia to stupor. Some patients may still be able to follow simple commands, speak, and even eat and drink, while others are more severely affected and present with hallucinations, behavioral changes, or frank encephalopathy. The duration can vary from minutes to weeks (Andermann and Robb,

1972; Drislane, 2000). EEG typically shows 2–3-Hz spike and wave discharges, though there is more variability in frequency of discharges (0.5–4 Hz) in patients presenting with late-onset absence SE (Granner and Lee, 1994; Baykan et al., 2002; Meierkord and Holtkamp, 2007).

### FOCAL NONCONVULSIVE STATUS EPILEPTICUS WITHOUT IMPAIRED CONSCIOUSNESS

Patients presenting with focal NCSE without impairment of consciousness, also known as simple partial SE, have preserved consciousness by definition. The EEG pattern is variable, with focal spikes and sharp waves localizing to the clinical domain affected. Symptoms can include behavioral changes, sensory symptoms (gustatory, olfactory, visual, tactile), or aphasia (Meierkord and Holtkamp, 2007).

### FOCAL NONCONVULSIVE STATUS EPILEPTICUS WITH IMPAIRED CONSCIOUSNESS

Focal NCSE with impaired consciousness is also known as complex partial SE. Seizure discharges are often more widespread than in patients with simple partial SE, and are usually unilateral. Most cases exhibit gradual evolution of symptoms, beginning with prolonged auras. Symptoms can then progress to include behavioral changes, confusion, and oral or manual automatisms (Meierkord and Holtkamp, 2007).

## Epilepsia partialis continua

Epilepsia partialis continua (EPC) is a distinct disorder characterized by continuous focal clonic motor movements of cortical origin which are confined to one part of the body. EPC is a very specific type of SE which is often refractory to treatment and is not associated with dyscognitive features. This is often considered a separate disorder from SE and managed differently. Classically, EPC is a result of focal lesions involving the motor strip. However, the pathophysiology underlying EPC is not entirely understood and subcortical lesions may be able to cause a similar disease phenotype (Juul-Jensen and Denny-Brown, 1966). A wide range of pathology has been reported to cause EPC, including tumors, focal infections, Rasmussen syndrome, vascular lesions, encephalitis, demyelination, focal cortical dysplasia, mitochondrial disorders, and tuberous sclerosis (Guerrini, 2009).

## NEURODIAGNOSTICS AND IMAGING

Electroencephalography is essential in the diagnosis, localization, and monitoring of patients with SE. Epileptiform discharges should be present and the presence or absence of accompanying motor manifestations will classify patients as convulsive or nonconvulsive, as previously

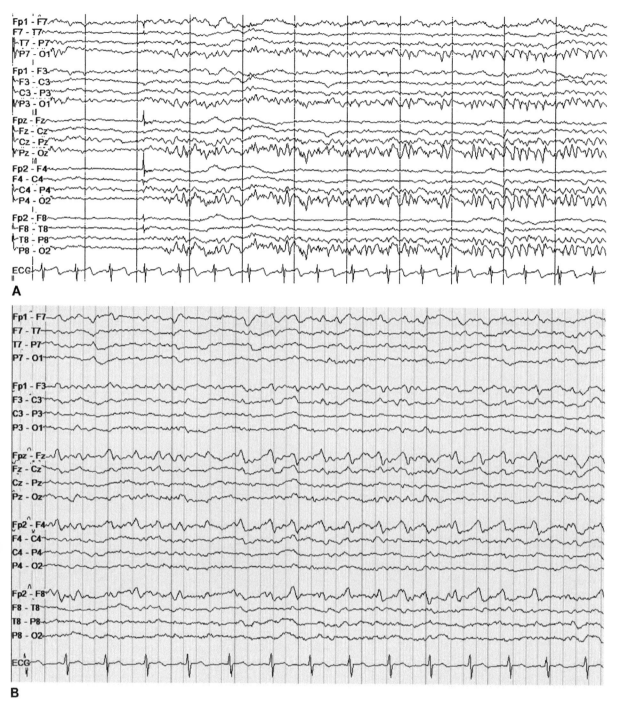

**A**

**B**

**Fig. 9.1.** A 31 year old woman presented following asystolic cardiac arrest. She remained intubated and comatose after arrival. EEG recording shown above is severely suppressed initially, with generalized seizure discharges (maximal in the posterior region) developing at the end of the photograph. The seizure persisted for more than three minutes and EEG continued to fluctuate between periods of suppression and seizure activity. The frequency of discharges clearly becomes greater than 3 Hz and the evolution in frequency, morphology, and location meets criteria for nonconvulsive status epilepticus. She was treated with fosphenytoin followed by a midazolam infusion to achieve a burst suppression pattern. After significant ischemic changes were shown on MRI, family withdrew care and the patient died. High-pass filter: 1 Hz; low-pass filter: 70 Hz; notch filter: 60 Hz.

EEG recording from a 21 year old man initially treated for convulsive status epilepticus in the setting of autoimmune encephalitis. He required intubation and was treated with lorazepam and fosphenytoin. After convulsive seizures stopped, EEG was obtained (B-D) showing nearly continuous right frontal spikes and sharp waves. There was no clear progression in location, but discharges appeared very rhythmic and were treated as nonconvulsive status epilepticus. Twenty minutes after starting midazolam infusion, EEG showed relative seizure cessation (E). He had a prolonged hospitalization and ultimately required numerous antiepileptic medications, plasma exchange, and rituximab before becoming seizure free and discharging to a rehabilitation facility. High-pass filter: 1 Hz; low-pass filter: 70 Hz; notch filter: 60 Hz.

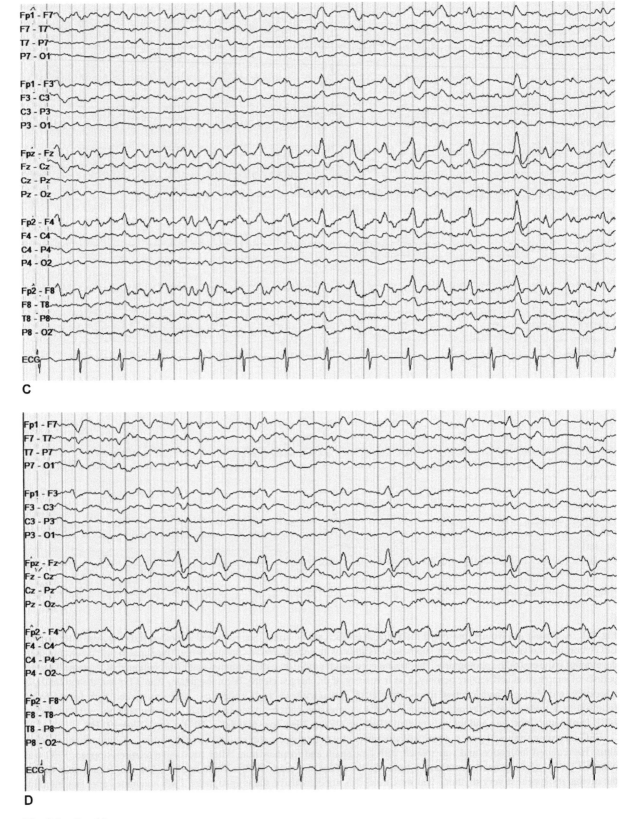

**Fig. 9.1—Cont'd**

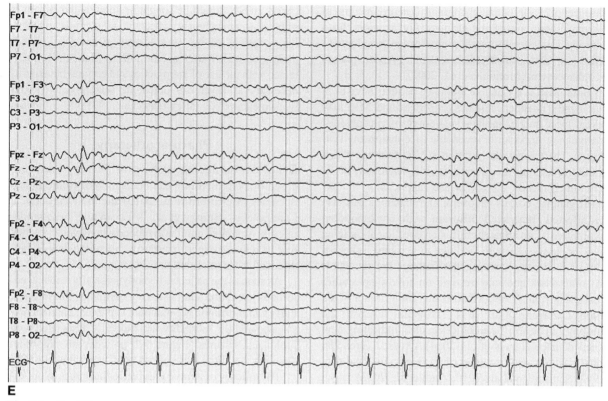

**E**

**Fig. 9.1—Cont'd**

*Table 9.2*

**Criteria for the diagnosis of nonconvulsive status epilepticus (Young et al., 1996; Chong and Hirsch, 2005)**

Altered consciousness with any of the following EEG changes noted for ≥5 minutes:

1. Repetitive focal or generalized epileptiform discharges (spikes, polyspikes, sharp waves, sharp-and-slow-wave complexes) at ≥3Hz
2. Sequential, rhythmic, periodic, or quasiperiodic discharges at ≥1 Hz and unequivocal evolution in frequency, morphology, or location
3. Repetitive focal or generalized epileptiform discharges at ≤3 Hz with significant clinical improvement or appearance of previously absent normal EEG background following administration of a rapidly acting antiepileptic drug

Adapted from Young et al. (1996) and Chong and Hirsch (2005) with permission from Wolters Kluwer Health.
EEG, electroencephalogram.

described. Unfortunately, there are no evidence-based EEG criteria for SE, and the EEG pattern is often nonspecific and difficult to interpret. Criteria for the diagnosis of NCSE are listed in Table 9.2. EEG recordings should be interpreted by someone with specialized training in electroencephalography (Trinka et al., 2015).

Due to the high proportion of electrographic seizures and NCSE following generalized convulsive SE, continuous EEG monitoring should be initiated within 1 hour of onset of SE if ongoing seizures are suspected, even if convulsive seizure activity has been controlled (Brophy et al., 2012). Concomitant video monitoring is often used to assess for clinical correlates, though its utility has not been evaluated prospectively.

Other diagnostic studies include serum laboratory evaluation to check for metabolic abnormalities, urine and serum drug screening, alcohol testing, AED levels (in patients taking AEDs), and lumbar puncture in select patients depending on other presenting symptoms. Serum creatine kinase, lactate, troponin, and arterial blood gas are useful screening markers for systemic injury and should be obtained upon presentation in SE. When the results of initial laboratory testing, neuroimaging, and cerebrospinal fluid (CSF) analysis are not revealing of an etiology, antibody-mediated encephalitides should be considered.

Neuroimaging in SE is primarily obtained to evaluate for an underlying cause of seizures, such as stroke, tumor, abscess, or other structural intracranial abnormalities. In patients without supportive history presenting with SE, noncontrast head computed tomography is typically obtained because it is relatively quick and provides useful information regarding major structural pathologies. In the absence of a structural abnormality, neuroimaging in SE may show nonspecific changes. For example, head computed tomography may be normal or can show hypoattenuation, edema, sulcal effacement, or a gyriform pattern of enhancement (Morimoto et al., 2002).

Brain MRI is a valuable tool once patients have been stabilized if no other cause has been identified. MRI may reveal more subtle findings suggestive of encephalitis, malignancy, or posterior reversible encephalopathy syndrome. There is a wide variation in MRI findings which result from SE and are often reversible. There may be T2 hyperintensities in the cortex and hippocampi, but the basal ganglia, corpus callosum, and thalamus can also be affected. Restricted diffusion with corresponding hypointensity on apparent diffusion coefficient imaging may be seen, similar to findings in cerebral ischemia. Unlike in stroke, however, the findings are reversible in some cases and may resolve on follow-up studies (Lansberg et al., 1999; Szabo et al., 2005; Bauer et al., 2006; Cartagena et al., 2014). Temporal sclerosis and atrophy can be seen as chronic sequelae, indicating neuronal damage (Lewis et al., 2014). Crossed cerebellar diaschisis has also been described (Tien and Ashdown, 1992; Samaniego et al., 2010; Zaidi et al., 2013).

## HOSPITAL COURSE AND MANAGEMENT

SE is a medical emergency and treatment should begin as soon as patients are brought to medical attention. Initial management often starts even before hospital arrival, when paramedics are called. The first priority is to assess and support cardiorespiratory function. Patients may require intubation if there is evidence of impaired gas exchange, ongoing aspiration, or suspected increase in intracranial pressure. Fingerstick glucose is checked with initial vital signs and intravenous thiamine should be given prior to glucose administration to avoid the risk of precipitating an acute Wernicke encephalopathy (Epilepsy Foundation, 1993). Peripheral venous access is needed for administration of medications and fluid resuscitation.

Cerebral autoregulation is severely impaired during SE, and cerebral perfusion is dependent on systemic blood pressure. Patients are often hypertensive initially, but after the first hour may develop relative hypotension, which can create a mismatch between metabolic demand and supply. This mismatch can lead to worsened excitotoxic effects in the form of oxidative stress, ischemia, blood–brain barrier breakdown, and inflammation (Meldrum and Horton, 1973; Lothman, 1990; Gorter et al., 2015). Blood pressure should be maintained in the normal range, with use of pressors if necessary.

Collateral medical history and symptoms prior to onset of SE may offer clues to the underlying etiology. Treatable causes of SE should be sought as soon as the patient is stable. Fever may be associated with infection as an underlying cause of SE, but can also occur as a consequence of prolonged seizure activity. Normothermia should be maintained with the use of antipyretics and cooling blankets as necessary as fever can potentiate seizure activity and worsen excitotoxic injury (Liu et al., 1993).

## Pharmacotherapy

Guidelines on the management of SE have been proposed by both the European Federation of Neurological Societies (Meierkord et al., 2010) and the Neurocritical Care Society (Brophy et al., 2012). While these guidelines incorporated clinical evidence when available, they rely heavily on expert consensus due to the lack of randomized trials in all but the first stage of SE.

As soon as the patient is hemodynamically stable, medications should be administered to terminate the seizures. Early administration is paramount to prevent pharmacoresistance and the morbidity and mortality associated with prolonged seizures. Figure 9.2 provides an algorithm detailing the initial medications used for treatment of SE.

The efficacy of intravenous benzodiazepines in out-of-hospital SE was established in a randomized double-blind trial. Adults with seizures lasting more than 5 minutes or with repetitive generalized convulsive seizures were randomized to treatment with lorazepam (2 mg), diazepam (5 mg), or placebo. The treatment was administered by paramedics and a second identical injection was given after 4 minutes if there was continued seizure activity. Lorazepam and diazepam were both shown to be superior to placebo in terminating SE, and lorazepam was more efficacious than diazepam. Compared to placebo, patients treated with benzodiazepines had lower rates of respiratory or circulatory compromise, likely because of shorter duration of seizures (Alldredge et al., 2001). A subsequent randomized, double-blind trial evaluating prehospital treatment of SE found that intramuscular midazolam was as effective as intravenous lorazepam in termination of SE, with similar rates of intubation and recurrent seizures. Midazolam is thus a viable option and is sometimes used in prehospital administration when intravenous access is not available (Silbergleit et al., 2012). In another randomized, double-blind study of first-line agents for generalized convulsive SE, lorazepam was found to terminate seizures in 65% of cases. Lorazepam was superior to phenytoin alone, and had similar efficacy compared with phenobarbital alone, as well as the combination of diazepam followed by phenytoin (Treiman et al., 1998). Because of the ease of administration and favorable pharmacokinetics, lorazepam is often used as the first-line agent.

If benzodiazepines are not successful with repeat administration, fosphenytoin is typically used as a

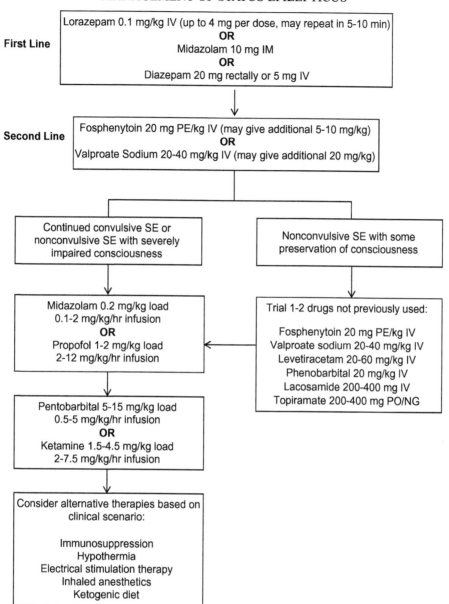

**Fig. 9.2.** Suggested algorithm for the management of generalized convulsive status epilepticus. Adapted from: Hocker SE (2015b). Status Epilepticus. Continuum 21: 1362–1383.

second-line agent. Although fosphenytoin is more expensive, it is typically preferred over phenytoin because it can be administered at a faster rate (up to 150 mg/min vs. 50 mg/min) and carries a lower risk of severe tissue damage in case of extravasation. Both agents have a similar incidence of hypotension and arrhythmia (Betjemann and Lowenstein, 2015). Small randomized studies have suggested that valproic acid is equally effective (Agarwal et al., 2007) or superior (Misra et al., 2006) to phenytoin in benzodiazepine-refractory SE, but with the added benefit of an improved side-effect profile. Valproic acid can be infused rapidly without producing hypotension or cardiac arrhythmias (Naritoku and Mueed, 1999; Venkataraman

and Wheless, 1999; Sinha and Naritoku, 2000; Chen et al., 2011). The Neurocritical Care Society guidelines suggest that valproic acid is an acceptable second-line medication, especially in patients with a history of primary generalized epilepsy (Brophy et al., 2012).

Alternative second-line agents include phenobarbital, midazolam, levetiracetam, and lacosamide. However, the evidence in their favor is less robust. Data supporting the use of one of these medications over another are limited and there is wide variation in clinical practice (Shaner et al., 1988; Treiman et al., 1998; Yoshikawa et al., 2000; Limdi et al., 2005; Peters and Pohlmann-Eden, 2005; Ruegg et al., 2008; Berning et al., 2009;

Eue et al., 2009; Kellinghaus et al., 2011; Hofler and Trinka, 2013). The choice of a particular medication may be influenced by specific clinical circumstances, patient comorbidities, age, and side-effect profiles (Beyenburg et al., 2009; Fattouch et al., 2010; Swisher et al., 2012). Unfortunately, there are no head-to-head large-scale comparisons currently available to guide treatment. To address the lack of evidence regarding second-line treatment agents, the Established Status Epilepticus Treatment Trial (ESETT), which began enrollment in 2015, will compare fosphenytoin, valproic acid, and levetiracetam for the treatment of benzodiazepine-refractory SE. This multicenter, randomized, double-blinded study will include patients over 2 years of age. Primary outcomes will include clinical seizure termination and improving mental status within 1 hour of drug infusion. Serious adverse effects, seizure recurrence, length of hospitalization, and mortality at 30 days will be assessed as secondary endpoints (Bleck et al., 2013).

## Refractory status epilepticus

If one of the second-line AEDs listed above fails, alternative second-line agents may be tried. However, terminating SE early is crucial in preventing seizure propagation and many experts recommend faster transition to an anesthetic agent in the setting of RSE (Brophy et al., 2012; Riviello et al., 2013). The medications most commonly used as a continuous infusion include midazolam, propofol, and barbiturates such as phenobarbital, pentobarbital, or thiopental. Evidence is lacking regarding superiority among these agents and the initial choice often depends on patient comorbidities and physician preference. Retrospective studies have not shown a difference in mortality among these agents, but there are no prospective or large-scale studies available. Having to use an anesthetic agent in order to abort SE has been associated with higher mortality and poorer functional outcomes, even after controlling for other known outcome predictors (Kowalski et al., 2012; Sutter et al., 2014; Marchi et al., 2015). While this is likely in part due to untoward systemic effects of anesthetic agents, the refractoriness of seizures could not be controlled for in these studies and likely remains a driver of the increased mortality.

The anesthetic medications can all cause respiratory depression and typically require mechanical ventilation. Each of these agents has distinct adverse effects which may limit use in certain patients. The barbiturates are associated with lower short-term treatment failure or recurrence, but this comes at the expense of a higher frequency of cardiac depression, hypotension, paralytic ileus, and infection (Claassen et al., 2002; Brophy et al., 2012). Midazolam is renally excreted and should

be used with caution in patients with renal failure. Tachyphylaxis can occur with prolonged use. Propofol can cause a potentially fatal syndrome when given at high doses, known as the propofol infusion syndrome (PRIS). PRIS is characterized by cardiac and renal failure, metabolic acidosis, rhabdomyolysis, and enlarged or fatty liver. Risk factors include carbohydrate depletion, severe illness, mitochondrial dysfunction, and coadministration of catecholamines or steroids. To decrease the chances of developing PRIS, the duration of propofol administration should not exceed 48 hours, and the dose should not be higher than 4 mg/kg/hour (Mirrakhimov et al., 2015). More recently, ketamine has been used as an alternative anesthetic agent. Ketamine has been reported to be relatively safe in a large multicenter series where it was used for the treatment of SRSE, but had to be discontinued in 7% of patients due to suspected treatment-related adverse events, including a syndrome similar to PRIS and cardiac arrhythmias (Gaspard et al., 2013).

## Continuous EEG monitoring

The ideal anesthetic agent is not well established, and the EEG pattern to target also lacks randomized clinical data. Available studies have shown conflicting results regarding the ideal depth of EEG suppression. Relapse of SE after anesthetic treatment has been associated with increased mortality (Krishnamurthy and Drislane, 1996), suggesting that deeper levels of suppression to prevent relapse may be beneficial. However, these deeper levels of suppression require higher doses of anesthetics and associated medication toxicity. Common practice and expert consensus dictate increasing anesthesia to achieve an electrographic burst suppression pattern, characterized by 2–10-second periods of background suppression ($<5\ \mu V$) with interspersed 1–2-second bursts of cerebral activity (Van Ness, 1990; Krishnamurthy and Drislane, 1999; Shorvon, 2011). Continuous EEG monitoring is essential in tracking response to therapy, but the optimal suppression pattern is unclear. In clinical practice and based on available guidelines, suppression is usually continued for 24–48 hours before gradually tapering medications. If seizures occur as anesthetics are weaned, the continuous infusion may be increased to the prior dose and higher doses of maintenance antiepileptics may be needed (Brophy et al., 2012).

Evidence is lacking regarding how long to pursue medically induced EEG suppression when patients do not tolerate weaning of infusions or have recurrent breakthrough seizures. Depending on the underlying etiology, good recovery may still be possible even after weeks to months of treatment (Rossetti et al., 2005; Robakis and

Hirsch, 2006; Cooper et al., 2009; Drislane et al., 2009; Legriel et al., 2010). Aggressive therapy should be continued until there is improvement or until ongoing treatment is considered futile. The underlying cause of SE is the most important factor in predicting morbidity and mortality and prolonged therapy is best suited for otherwise healthy patients with good premorbid function and a treatable or self-limiting cause of SE.

Various adjunctive therapies for RSE have been reported in case reports or small series. These include corticosteroids, inhaled anesthetics, lidocaine, magnesium, ketogenic diet, hypothermia, and electric stimulation therapies such as electroconvulsive therapy, deep-brain stimulation, vagal nerve stimulation, and transcranial magnetic stimulation (Minicucci et al., 2006; Brophy et al., 2012).

## COMPLEX CLINICAL DECISIONS

The management of SE has changed considerably in recent years, influenced by animal models, clinical research, and clinical experience, which has resulted in changes in expert consensus. Even with a greater understanding of the underlying pathophysiology of SE and medical advances, many questions remain unanswered.

## PROGRESS TO ANESTHETICS IN NCSE WITH PRESERVATION OF CONSCIOUSNESS

The decision to pursue anesthetic treatment in SE is influenced by patient age, comorbidities, and prognostic considerations. There are no studies comparing anesthetic therapy with attempting nonanesthetic anticonvulsants as third- or fourth-line therapy. In the absence of these data, and given the relatively favorable outcomes in NCSE with some preservation of consciousness compared to other subtypes of SE, attempting a third- or fourth-line nonanesthetic AED prior to initiation of anesthesia is a reasonable approach. As long as consciousness is at least partially preserved, the risk–benefit analysis favors avoiding anesthesia as long as possible.

## PROGRESS TO ANESTHETICS IN COMATOSE PATIENTS WITH NCSE

The decision to progress to anesthetic treatment for NCSE in coma is determined on a case-by-case basis depending on the degree of certainty regarding the diagnosis (EEG pattern and clinical history). There are no studies available measuring outcomes in patients with varied causes of NCSE in coma, comparing treatment with observation alone, or examining the impact of

aggressiveness of treatment. Thus, it is not possible to predict which, if any, comatose patients with NCSE should be treated aggressively with anesthetic agents. EEG patterns in NCSE are often difficult to interpret, and there is a real risk of excessive sedation and respiratory depression when using anesthetic medications if EEG is not truly reflective of seizure activity. Classification schemes for NCSE in coma have been proposed (Bauer and Trinka, 2010) to guide future studies and outcome evaluation in these situations, but there is still a great deal of uncertainty in clinical practice. Additionally, the type of EEG discharge does not seem to correlate with mortality. The substantial mortality associated with NCSE in coma has been associated with the degree of critical illness and acute systemic illness in particular (Shneker and Fountain, 2003). If there is a clearly established cause for coma, such as anoxic brain injury following cardiac arrest or catastrophic traumatic brain injury, the EEG abnormalities may simply reflect the degree of brain injury rather than be an independent cause of coma. In these cases, treating the EEG pattern would have little impact on the outcome.

In most cases, it is reasonable to treat aggressively to see if there is a clinical and/or electrographic response to antiepileptic medications. Even if there is no improvement, anesthetic treatment is still reasonable if the underlying cause is unknown or if there is a known alternative cause of coma which is thought to be treatable.

## NCSE PATTERNS IN CRITICAL ILLNESS

There are no pathognomonic EEG changes which can definitively diagnose NCSE. This has particular implications in NCSE with impaired consciousness. For example, imagine a patient with sepsis who remains encephalopathic after treatment of the infection. EEG monitoring demonstrates a pattern meeting electrographic criteria for SE. After administration of a short-acting AED the patient becomes more alert and the EEG background improves. The improvement would suggest that the electrographic activity was responsible for the impaired clinical state. However, suppose that after the medication was administered there was instead only a brief improvement in the EEG background before returning to the original pattern, and no clinical improvement. What could one conclude? In this case, the EEG changes may simply indicate an epiphenomenon of the critical illness and further observation may be reasonable before escalating therapy.

## PALLIATIVE CARE IN SUPERREFRACTORY STATUS EPILEPTICUS

Death in the setting of SE may result from systemic complications or directly relate to the etiology (i.e., fulminant bacterial meningitis leading to brain death), but more often stems from withdrawal of life-sustaining treatment after family discussions and a change in the goals of care. The decision to withdraw life-sustaining treatment in the setting of SE should not be taken lightly, and often comes after weeks or months of treatment without improvement. The treatment timeline is influenced by premorbid functional status and whether the underlying etiology is expected to be treatable. In addition to the immediate complications associated with SE, there are systemic and cerebral complications stemming from a prolonged intensive care unit course which may influence ultimate prognosis (Table 9.3).

Goals-of-care discussions with family members are essential to establish realistic expectations based on the perceived wishes of the patient and the quality of life that would be deemed acceptable. In some cases, such as when anoxic-ischemic injury occurs as a result of a cardiac arrest, the underlying cause is known to be associated with a poor prognosis and this can help inform the decision to withdraw life-sustaining treatment. Clear parameters have been developed to assist in prognostication (Wijdicks et al., 2006) and myoclonic SE has been

uniformly associated with a poor prognosis in this setting (Wijdicks et al., 1994; Rossetti et al., 2007).

Prognostication in the setting of other causes of SE is much less clear and additional studies are needed to guide treatment goals for SE based on etiology. In general, in the absence of an acute brain injury or critical illness, which in itself carries a very poor prognosis, treatment should be aggressive and prolonged. Treatment options should be exhausted before considering withdrawing life-sustaining treatment for patients with SE, as excellent outcomes have been reported, even after many months of SRSE.

## IMMUNOSUPPRESSION IN AUTOIMMUNE ENCEPHALITIS AND NORSE

NORSE poses a particular challenge because the underlying etiology is not readily apparent. These patients typically continue to seize for more than 24 hours and respond very poorly to standard treatment algorithms. In cases of NORSE in which an etiology is ultimately found, antibody-mediated disorders are the most common cause (Gaspard et al., 2015). Patients with proven

*Table 9.3*

Systemic and cerebral complications attributable to status epilepticus and to prolonged intensive care unit (ICU) stay

|  | Status epilepticus | Prolonged ICU stay |
|---|---|---|
| **Systemic complications** | **Respiratory** Neurogenic pulmonary edema Aspiration pneumonia/pneumonitis Hypoxemic respiratory failure **Cardiovascular** Hypertension, hypotension, shock Cardiac arrhythmias, cardiac arrest Stress-induced cardiomyopathy **Musculoskeletal** Skeletal fractures, joint dislocations, tongue laceration Rhabdomyolysis **Renal** Acute kidney injury Hyperkalemia **Autonomic system disturbances** Hyperpyrexia Excessive sweating, vomiting, dehydration **Metabolic** Hyperglycemia Acidosis (metabolic and/or respiratory) | **Respiratory** Atelectasis and mucous plugging Ventilator-associated pneumonia Tracheostomy **Immobility** Deep-vein thrombosis/pulmonary embolus Decubitus ulcers **Musculoskeletal** Critical illness myopathy and polyneuropathy **Infection** Catheter-associated urinary tract infection Bacteremia Pneumonia Pseudomembranous colitis |
| **Cerebral complications** | Cerebral edema and dysfunction of blood–brain barrier Temporal sclerosis Cerebral atrophy Epilepsy | Cerebral atrophy |

or suspected autoimmune epilepsy have been shown to respond to intravenous immunoglobulin, intravenous steroids, or both (Toledano et al., 2014). The same may hold true for antibody-mediated SE. However, which patients deserve a trial of immunotherapy is not established and the results of antibody testing may take days to weeks to return. Because the spectrum of autoimmune and paraneoplastic disease is still an area of active research, negative antibody test results do not rule out an immune-mediated process if there is high clinical suspicion. Many autoantibodies have yet to be characterized. Empiric immunosuppression is recommended in cases of suspected autoimmune disease, but only after systemic and CNS infections have been confidently excluded. Patients with an inflammatory CSF profile in which infection has been ruled out are the most likely to benefit from a trial of immunotherapy. Some patients with antibody-mediated encephalitis do not have an inflammatory CSF profile and may also benefit from an empiric trial of immunosuppression while awaiting antibody testing, depending on the degree of clinical suspicion.

Favorable outcomes have been reported when treating NORSE with any immunotherapy compared with those not receiving treatment (Khawaja et al., 2015). Which form of immunotherapy is superior has not been established. There have been reported cases of benefit using intravenous immunoglobulin, plasma exchange, and intravenous steroids. These agents have also been reported in combination, with varying degrees of success (Costello et al., 2009; Gall et al., 2013; Li et al., 2013; Khawaja et al., 2015). No randomized or head-to-head trials are available to guide decisions because of the rarity of this condition. Until randomized or multicenter trial data are available, early initiation of immunotherapy is reasonable in addition to AEDs in patients with no identifiable structural, infectious, metabolic, or toxic (including low AED levels, missed AED doses, or drug/alcohol withdrawal) cause, and after infection has been excluded.

## MANAGEMENT OF STATUS EPILEPTICUS IN PREGNANCY

There is not an increased risk of SE during pregnancy (Harden et al., 2009), but when it occurs it presents a unique set of clinical challenges and can have devastating outcomes for the mother and infant. SE during pregnancy can occur in women with a history of epilepsy prior to conception, new-onset gestational SE, or in the setting of eclampsia. The management of SE during pregnancy depends on the clinical circumstances. In women with SE not related to eclampsia or pre-eclampsia, management is typically the same as for nonpregnant patients and involves aggressive seizure control. Lorazepam or diazepam is typically used as initial emergency therapy

(Karnad and Guntupalli, 2005). Fosphenytoin is typically the next-line agent after benzodiazepines, but phenobarbital may be an acceptable alternative and has been reported to prevent intraventricular hemorrhage in low-birth-weight infants (Morales and Koerten, 1986; Jagoda and Riggio, 1991). Potential birth defects can occur with administration of phenobarbital, phenytoin, or valproate during the first trimester. Data from more recent pregnancy registries suggest decreased risk with some of the newer antiepileptic medications such as levetiracetam, which can be strongly considered in initial management of SE in pregnancy (Molgaard-Nielsen and Hviid, 2011).

Eclampsia is the convulsive stage after pre-eclampsia, which is defined by hypertension and proteinuria after the 20th week of gestation. Eclampsia is associated with increased perinatal mortality and is a medical emergency. Unlike the scenario discussed above, seizures in the setting of eclampsia are best treated with magnesium sulfate rather than antiepileptic medications such as phenytoin or diazepam (Duley et al., 2010a, b). Medications can be used as temporizing measures, but the definitive treatment of SE in the setting of eclamptic seizures is delivery of the fetus. Patients require continuous fetal heart monitoring, obstetric assistance, and pediatric intensive care unit support to care for the mother and child.

## OUTCOME PREDICTION

Because the definition of SE has undergone many changes over the years in terms of duration and qualifying features, patient outcomes described in the literature are often heterogeneous and difficult to interpret. Intuitively, earlier termination of SE should lead to better outcomes. This assertion has been supported in numerous studies but is confounded by varying patient factors, treatment algorithms, and underlying etiologies (Rowan and Scott, 1970; DeLorenzo et al., 1999; Legriel et al., 2010). In a prospective study evaluating outcomes of SE, duration greater than 120 minutes, progression to RSE, and the presence of a cerebral insult were all associated with poor prognosis at 90 days. The presence of all three factors signified an approximately 90% likelihood of moderate disability or death (Legriel et al., 2010).

Even with the wide variation in study methodology, the underlying cause of SE has been consistently validated as a major determinant of morbidity and mortality (Yaffe and Lowenstein, 1993; DeLorenzo et al., 1996; Krishnamurthy and Drislane, 1996; Drislane et al., 2009; Dham et al., 2014). Acute causes of SE are often associated with higher mortality and are likely a reflection of the severity of underlying pathology rather than SE. Patients with anoxic injury, stroke, or systemic infection have higher mortality than causes such as AED noncompliance or alcohol withdrawal (DeLorenzo et al., 1995).

Unfortunately, the underlying etiology is not always readily apparent and some studies have assessed other available clinical parameters to help predict mortality following SE. The Status Epilepticus Severity Score (STESS) was developed based on four variables measured at the time of presentation: history of seizures, age, seizure type, and consciousness impairment. Seizure type was classified as simple partial, complex partial, absence, generalized convulsive, or NCSE in coma. Validation in a small prospective SE series (34 patients) resulted in 100% sensitivity and 64% specificity in predicting survival (Rossetti et al., 2006), and the tool has since been externally validated (Sutter et al., 2013) in 154 patients in a multicenter prospective trial and found an excellent negative predictive value (0.97). A favorable STESS score was highly related to survival. However, there was a poor positive predictive value for death and the tool should therefore not be used to guide decisions on withdrawing life-sustaining treatment (Rossetti et al., 2008).

The Epidemiology-Based Mortality Score in Status Epilepticus (EMSE) was subsequently developed to incorporate EEG findings in addition to patient characteristics of age, comorbidities, and the etiology of SE. Review of mortality risk factors in large systemic reviews of SE (Neligan and Shorvon, 2010, 2011) was used to identify optimal scoring criteria. Ninety-two consecutive patients with various forms of SE were investigated retrospectively using this score. EMSE predicted individual mortality in almost 90% of cases and was superior to the STESS score (Leitinger et al., 2015). Although initial results are promising, prospective validation is still needed.

## CONCLUSIONS

There have been tremendous advances in the understanding and management of SE, yet the disorder remains a neurologic emergency with substantial morbidity and mortality. Animal models have provided a better understanding of the pathophysiology leading to prolonged seizures and pharmacoresistance. These findings have been supported by clinical observations in humans, ultimately leading to adoption of more practical definitions of SE and emphasis on early intervention. Prehospital treatment of SE and earlier transition to anesthetic agents in refractory cases are reflections of the mounting basic and clinical research in this disorder. A better understanding of the cellular and biochemical changes which occur during SE will also pave the way for development of new drug targets.

International guidelines and expert consensus have led to some degree of standardization among treatment protocols, but due to a lack of prospective trials there is still significant variability in clinical practice. The ESETT trial will hopefully clarify the optimal second-line agent in SE not responsive to benzodiazepines, but the management of RSE and SRSE will require additional research and large-scale collaboration. The risks and benefits of various anesthetic agents warrant further investigation, and the role of these agents in various subtypes of SE will need to be better defined.

EEG plays an essential role in SE and improving EEG accessibility and interpretation will be crucial as our understanding of SE evolves. Standardized EEG terminology must be adopted to guide clinical trials and further evaluate the significance of various EEG patterns and their impact on outcomes. SE is a dynamic process with potential for numerous neurologic and systemic complications. Rapid diagnosis and aggressive management based on the most up-to-date evidence provide the best chance for meaningful recovery.

## REFERENCES

Abend NS, Loddenkemper T (2014). Pediatric status epilepticus management. Curr Opin Pediatr 26: 668–674.

Agarwal P, Kumar N, Chandra R et al. (2007). Randomized study of intravenous valproate and phenytoin in status epilepticus. Seizure 16: 527–532.

Aicardi J, Chevrie JJ (1970). Convulsive status epilepticus in infants and children. A study of 239 cases. Epilepsia 11: 187–197.

Alldredge BK, Gelb AM, Isaacs SM et al. (2001). A comparison of lorazepam, diazepam, and placebo for the treatment of out-of-hospital status epilepticus. N Engl J Med 345: 631–637.

Aminoff MJ, Simon RP (1980). Status epilepticus. Causes, clinical features and consequences in 98 patients. Am J Med 69: 657–666.

Andermann F, Robb JP (1972). Absence status. A reappraisal following review of thirty-eight patients. Epilepsia 13: 177–187.

Arnautova EN, Nesmeianova TN (1964). A proposed international classification of epileptic seizures. Epilepsia 5: 297–306.

Barnard C, Wirrell E (1999). Does status epilepticus in children cause developmental deterioration and exacerbation of epilepsy? J Child Neurol 14: 787–794.

Bauer G, Trinka E (2010). Nonconvulsive status epilepticus and coma. Epilepsia 51: 177–190.

Bauer G, Gotwald T, Dobesberger J et al. (2006). Transient and permanent magnetic resonance imaging abnormalities after complex partial status epilepticus. Epilepsy Behav : E&B 8: 666–671.

Baumgartner C, Lurger S, Leutmezer F (2001). Autonomic symptoms during epileptic seizures. Epileptic Disorders : International Epilepsy Journal with Videotape 3: 103–116.

Baykan B, Gokyigit A, Gurses C et al. (2002). Recurrent absence status epilepticus: clinical and EEG characteristics. Seizure 11: 310–319.

Berning S, Boesebeck F, van Baalen A et al. (2009). Intravenous levetiracetam as treatment for status epilepticus. J Neurol 256: 1634–1642.

Bertram EH, Lothman EW, Lenn NJ (1990). The hippocampus in experimental chronic epilepsy: a morphometric analysis. Ann Neurol 27: 43–48.

Betjemann JP, Lowenstein DH (2015). Status epilepticus in adults. The Lancet Neurology 14: 615–624.

Beyenburg S, Reuber M, Maraite N (2009). Intravenous levetiracetam for epileptic seizure emergencies in older people. Gerontology 55: 27–31.

Bleck T, Cock H, Chamberlain J et al. (2013). The established status epilepticus trial 2013. Epilepsia 54 (Suppl 6): 89–92.

Boggs JG, Painter JA, DeLorenzo RJ (1993). Analysis of electrocardiographic changes in status epilepticus. Epilepsy Res 14: 87–94.

Brophy GM, Bell R, Claassen J et al. (2012). Guidelines for the evaluation and management of status epilepticus. Neurocrit Care 17: 3–23.

Cartagena AM, Young GB, Lee DH et al. (2014). Reversible and irreversible cranial MRI findings associated with status epilepticus. Epilepsy Behav : E&B 33: 24–30.

Cascino GD (1993). Nonconvulsive status epilepticus in adults and children. Epilepsia 34 (Suppl 1): S21–S28.

Chen JW, Wasterlain CG (2006). Status epilepticus: pathophysiology and management in adults. The Lancet Neurology 5: 246–256.

Chen JW, Naylor DE, Wasterlain CG (2007). Advances in the pathophysiology of status epilepticus. Acta Neurol Scand Suppl 186: 7–15.

Chen WB, Gao R, Su YY et al. (2011). Valproate versus diazepam for generalized convulsive status epilepticus: a pilot study. Eur J Neurol : The Official Journal of the European Federation of Neurological Societies 18: 1391–1396.

Chong DJ, Hirsch LJ (2005). Which EEG patterns warrant treatment in the critically ill? Reviewing the evidence for treatment of periodic epileptiform discharges and related patterns. Journal of Clinical Neurophysiology : Official Publication of the American Electroencephalographic Society 22: 79–91.

Claassen J, Hirsch LJ, Emerson RG et al. (2002). Treatment of refractory status epilepticus with pentobarbital, propofol, or midazolam: a systematic review. Epilepsia 43: 146–153.

Cock HR, Tong X, Hargreaves IP et al. (2002). Mitochondrial dysfunction associated with neuronal death following status epilepticus in rat. Epilepsy Res 48: 157–168.

Coeytaux A, Jallon P, Galobardes B et al. (2000). Incidence of status epilepticus in French-speaking Switzerland: (EPISTAR). Neurology 55: 693–697.

Cooper AD, Britton JW, Rabinstein AA (2009). Functional and cognitive outcome in prolonged refractory status epilepticus. Arch Neurol 66: 1505–1509.

Corsellis JA, Bruton CJ (1983). Neuropathology of status epilepticus in humans. Adv Neurol 34: 129–139.

Costello DJ, Kilbride RD, Cole AJ (2009). Cryptogenic New Onset Refractory Status Epilepticus (NORSE) in adults – infectious or not? J Neurol Sci 277: 26–31.

DeGiorgio CM, Correale JD, Gott PS et al. (1995). Serum neuron-specific enolase in human status epilepticus. Neurology 45: 1134–1137.

DeGiorgio CM, Heck CN, Rabinowicz AL et al. (1999). Serum neuron-specific enolase in the major subtypes of status epilepticus. Neurology 52: 746–749.

DeLorenzo RJ, Pellock JM, Towne AR et al. (1995). Epidemiology of status epilepticus. Journal of Clinical Neurophysiology : Official Publication of the American Electroencephalographic Society 12: 316–325.

DeLorenzo RJ, Hauser WA, Towne AR et al. (1996). A prospective, population-based epidemiologic study of status epilepticus in Richmond, Virginia. Neurology 46: 1029–1035.

DeLorenzo RJ, Waterhouse EJ, Towne AR et al. (1998). Persistent nonconvulsive status epilepticus after the control of convulsive status epilepticus. Epilepsia 39: 833–840.

DeLorenzo RJ, Garnett LK, Towne AR et al. (1999). Comparison of status epilepticus with prolonged seizure episodes lasting from 10 to 29 minutes. Epilepsia 40: 164–169.

Dham BS, Hunter K, Rincon F (2014). The epidemiology of status epilepticus in the United States. Neurocrit Care 20: 476–483.

Drislane FW (2000). Presentation, evaluation, and treatment of nonconvulsive status epilepticus. Epilepsy Behav : E&B 1: 301–314.

Drislane FW, Blum AS, Lopez MR et al. (2009). Duration of refractory status epilepticus and outcome: loss of prognostic utility after several hours. Epilepsia 50: 1566–1571.

Duley L, Henderson-Smart DJ, Chou D (2010a). Magnesium sulphate versus phenytoin for eclampsia. The Cochrane Database of Systematic Reviews CD000128.

Duley L, Henderson-Smart DJ, Walker GJ et al. (2010b). Magnesium sulphate versus diazepam for eclampsia. The Cochrane Database of Systematic Reviews CD000127.

Dunn DW (1988). Status epilepticus in children: etiology, clinical features, and outcome. J Child Neurol 3: 167–173.

Epilepsy Foundation (1993). Treatment of convulsive status epilepticus. Recommendations of the Epilepsy Foundation of America's Working Group on Status Epilepticus. JAMA 270: 854–859.

Eue S, Grumbt M, Muller M et al. (2009). Two years of experience in the treatment of status epilepticus with intravenous levetiracetam. Epilepsy Behav : E&B 15: 467–469.

Fattouch J, Di Bonaventura C, Casciato S et al. (2010). Intravenous levetiracetam as first-line treatment of status epilepticus in the elderly. Acta Neurol Scand 121: 418–421.

Ferlisi M, Shorvon S (2012). The outcome of therapies in refractory and super-refractory convulsive status epilepticus and recommendations for therapy. Brain : J Neurol 135: 2314–2328.

Ferlisi M, Hocker S, Grade M et al. (2015). Preliminary results of the global audit of treatment of refractory status epilepticus. Epilepsy Behav : E&B 49: 318–324.

Fountain NB (2000). Status epilepticus: risk factors and complications. Epilepsia 41 (Suppl 2): S23–S30.

Freilich ER, Schreiber JM, Zelleke T et al. (2014). Pediatric status epilepticus: identification and evaluation. Curr Opin Pediatr 26: 655–661.

Friedman A, Kaufer D, Heinemann U (2009). Blood–brain barrier breakdown-inducing astrocytic transformation: novel targets for the prevention of epilepsy. Epilepsy Res 85: 142–149.

Gall CR, Jumma O, Mohanraj R (2013). Five cases of new onset refractory status epilepticus (NORSE) syndrome: outcomes with early immunotherapy. Seizure 22: 217–220.

Gaspard N, Foreman B, Judd LM et al. (2013). Intravenous ketamine for the treatment of refractory status epilepticus: a retrospective multicenter study. Epilepsia 54: 1498–1503.

Gaspard N, Foreman BP, Alvarez V et al. (2015). New-onset refractory status epilepticus: etiology, clinical features, and outcome. Neurology 85: 1604–1613.

Glaser GH (1983). Medical complications of status epilepticus. Adv Neurol 34: 395–398.

Gorter JA, van Vliet EA, Aronica E (2015). Status epilepticus, blood–brain barrier disruption, inflammation, and epileptogenesis. Epilepsy Behav : E&B 49: 13–16.

Granner MA, Lee SI (1994). Nonconvulsive status epilepticus: EEG analysis in a large series. Epilepsia 35: 42–47.

Guerrini R (2009). Physiology of epilepsia partialis continua and subcortical mechanisms of status epilepticus. Epilepsia 50 (Suppl 12): 7–9.

Harden CL, Hopp J, Ting TY et al. (2009). Practice parameter update: management issues for women with epilepsy – focus on pregnancy (an evidence-based review): obstetrical complications and change in seizure frequency: report of the Quality Standards Subcommittee and Therapeutics and Technology Assessment Subcommittee of the American Academy of Neurology and American Epilepsy Society. Neurology 73: 126–132.

Hauser WA (1990). Status epilepticus: epidemiologic considerations. Neurology 40: 9–13.

Hesdorffer DC, Logroscino G, Cascino G et al. (1998). Incidence of status epilepticus in Rochester, Minnesota, 1965–1984. Neurology 50: 735–741.

Hirsch LJ, Gaspard N (2013). Status epilepticus. Continuum 19: 767–794.

Hocker S (2015a). Systemic complications of status epilepticus – an update. Epilepsy Behav : E&B 49: 83–87.

Hocker SE (2015b). Status epilepticus. Continuum 21: 1362–1383.

Hocker SE, Britton JW, Mandrekar JN et al. (2013). Predictors of outcome in refractory status epilepticus. JAMA Neurol 70: 72–77.

Hocker S, Tatum WO, LaRoche S et al. (2014). Refractory and super-refractory status epilepticus – an update. Curr Neurol Neurosci Rep 14: 452.

Hofler J, Trinka E (2013). Lacosamide as a new treatment option in status epilepticus. Epilepsia 54: 393–404.

Holtkamp M, Othman J, Buchheim K et al. (2005). Predictors and prognosis of refractory status epilepticus treated in a neurological intensive care unit. J Neurol Neurosurg Psychiatry 76: 534–539.

Huff JS, Fountain NB (2011). Pathophysiology and definitions of seizures and status epilepticus. Emerg Med Clin North Am 29: 1–13.

Husain AM, Horn GJ, Jacobson MP (2003). Non-convulsive status epilepticus: usefulness of clinical features in selecting patients for urgent EEG. J Neurol Neurosurg Psychiatry 74: 189–191.

Jagoda A, Riggio S (1991). Emergency department approach to managing seizures in pregnancy. Ann Emerg Med 20: 80–85.

Juul-Jensen P, Denny-Brown D (1966). Epilepsia partialis continua. Arch Neurol 15: 563–578.

Kantanen AM, Reinikainen M, Parviainen I et al. (2015). Incidence and mortality of super-refractory status epilepticus in adults. Epilepsy Behav : E&B 49: 131–134.

Karnad DR, Guntupalli KK (2005). Neurologic disorders in pregnancy. Crit Care Med 33: S362–S371.

Kellinghaus C, Berning S, Immisch I et al. (2011). Intravenous lacosamide for treatment of status epilepticus. Acta Neurol Scand 123: 137–141.

Khawaja AM, DeWolfe JL, Miller DW et al. (2015). New-onset refractory status epilepticus (NORSE) – the potential role for immunotherapy. Epilepsy Behav : E&B 47: 17–23.

Knake S, Rosenow F, Vescovi M et al. (2001). Incidence of status epilepticus in adults in Germany: a prospective, population-based study. Epilepsia 42: 714–718.

Kowalski RG, Ziai WC, Rees RN et al. (2012). Third-line antiepileptic therapy and outcome in status epilepticus: the impact of vasopressor use and prolonged mechanical ventilation. Crit Care Med 40: 2677–2684.

Krishnamurthy KB, Drislane FW (1996). Relapse and survival after barbiturate anesthetic treatment of refractory status epilepticus. Epilepsia 37: 863–867.

Krishnamurthy KB, Drislane FW (1999). Depth of EEG suppression and outcome in barbiturate anesthetic treatment for refractory status epilepticus. Epilepsia 40: 759–762.

Lansberg MG, O'Brien MW, Norbash AM et al. (1999). MRI abnormalities associated with partial status epilepticus. Neurology 52: 1021–1027.

Legriel S, Bruneel F, Dalle L et al. (2008). Recurrent takotsubo cardiomyopathy triggered by convulsive status epilepticus. Neurocrit Care 9: 118–121.

Legriel S, Azoulay E, Resche-Rigon M et al. (2010). Functional outcome after convulsive status epilepticus. Crit Care Med 38: 2295–2303.

Leitinger M, Holler Y, Kalss G et al. (2015). Epidemiology-based mortality score in status epilepticus (EMSE). Neurocrit Care 22: 273–282.

Lewis DV, Shinnar S, Hesdorffer DC et al. (2014). Hippocampal sclerosis after febrile status epilepticus: the FEBSTAT study. Ann Neurol 75: 178–185.

Li J, Saldivar C, Maganti RK (2013). Plasma exchange in cryptogenic new onset refractory status epilepticus. Seizure 22: 70–73.

Limdi NA, Shimpi AV, Faught E et al. (2005). Efficacy of rapid IV administration of valproic acid for status epilepticus. Neurology 64: 353–355.

Liu Z, Gatt A, Mikati M et al. (1993). Effect of temperature on kainic acid-induced seizures. Brain Res 631: 51–58.

Logroscino G, Hesdorffer DC, Cascino G et al. (2005). Mortality after a first episode of status epilepticus in the United States and Europe. Epilepsia 46 (Suppl 11): 46–48.

Lothman E (1990). The biochemical basis and pathophysiology of status epilepticus. Neurology 40: 13–23.

Lothman EW, Collins RC (1981). Kainic acid induced limbic seizures: metabolic, behavioral, electroencephalographic and neuropathological correlates. Brain Res 218: 299–318.

Lowenstein DH, Alldredge BK (1993). Status epilepticus at an urban public hospital in the 1980s. Neurology 43: 483–488.

Lowenstein DH, Bleck T, Macdonald RL (1999). It's time to revise the definition of status epilepticus. Epilepsia 40: 120–122.

Manno EM, Pfeifer EA, Cascino GD et al. (2005). Cardiac pathology in status epilepticus. Ann Neurol 58: 954–957.

Marchi NA, Novy J, Faouzi M et al. (2015). Status epilepticus: impact of therapeutic coma on outcome. Crit Care Med 43: 1003–1009.

Mayer SA, Claassen J, Lokin J et al. (2002). Refractory status epilepticus: frequency, risk factors, and impact on outcome. Arch Neurol 59: 205–210.

Maytal J, Shinnar S, Moshe SL et al. (1989). Low morbidity and mortality of status epilepticus in children. Pediatrics 83: 323–331.

Meierkord H, Holtkamp M (2007). Non-convulsive status epilepticus in adults: clinical forms and treatment. The Lancet Neurology 6: 329–339.

Meierkord H, Boon P, Engelsen B et al. (2010). EFNS guideline on the management of status epilepticus in adults. European Journal of Neurology : The Official Journal of the European Federation of Neurological Societies 17: 348–355.

Meldrum BS, Brierley JB (1973). Prolonged epileptic seizures in primates. Ischemic cell change and its relation to ictal physiological events. Arch Neurol 28: 10–17.

Meldrum BS, Horton RW (1973). Physiology of status epilepticus in primates. Arch Neurol 28: 1–9.

Meldrum BS, Vigouroux RA, Brierley JB (1973a). Systemic factors and epileptic brain damage. Prolonged seizures in paralyzed, artificially ventilated baboons. Arch Neurol 29: 82–87.

Meldrum BS, Vigouroux RA, Rage P et al. (1973b). Hippocampal lesions produced by prolonged seizures in paralyzed artificially ventilated baboons. Experientia 29: 561–563.

Minicucci F, Muscas G, Perucca E et al. (2006). Treatment of status epilepticus in adults: guidelines of the Italian League against Epilepsy. Epilepsia 47 (Suppl 5): 9–15.

Mirrakhimov AE, Voore P, Halytskyy O et al. (2015). Propofol infusion syndrome in adults: a clinical update. Crit Care Res Prac 2015: 260385.

Misra UK, Kalita J, Patel R (2006). Sodium valproate vs phenytoin in status epilepticus: a pilot study. Neurology 67: 340–342.

Molgaard-Nielsen D, Hviid A (2011). Newer-generation antiepileptic drugs and the risk of major birth defects. JAMA 305: 1996–2002.

Morales WJ, Koerten J (1986). Prevention of intraventricular hemorrhage in very low birth weight infants by maternally administered phenobarbital. Obstet Gynecol 68: 295–299.

Morimoto T, Fukuda M, Suzuki Y et al. (2002). Sequential changes of brain CT and MRI after febrile status epilepticus in a 6-year-old girl. Brain Dev 24: 190–193.

Moshe SL, Garant DS, Sperber EF et al. (1995). Ontogeny and topography of seizure regulation by the substantia nigra. Brain Dev 17 (Suppl): 61–72.

Naritoku DK, Mueed S (1999). Intravenous loading of valproate for epilepsy. Clin Neuropharmacol 22: 102–106.

Neligan A, Shorvon SD (2010). Frequency and prognosis of convulsive status epilepticus of different causes: a systematic review. Arch Neurol 67: 931–940.

Neligan A, Shorvon SD (2011). Prognostic factors, morbidity and mortality in tonic-clonic status epilepticus: a review. Epilepsy Res 93: 1–10.

Niquet J, Baldwin RA, Allen SG et al. (2003). Hypoxic neuronal necrosis: protein synthesis-independent activation of a cell death program. Proc Natl Acad Sci U S A 100: 2825–2830.

Nixon J, Bateman D, Moss T (2001). An MRI and neuropathological study of a case of fatal status epilepticus. Seizure 10: 588–591.

Novy J, Logroscino G, Rossetti AO (2010). Refractory status epilepticus: a prospective observational study. Epilepsia 51: 251–256.

Oxbury JM, Whitty CW (1971). Causes and consequences of status epilepticus in adults. A study of 86 cases. Brain : J Neurol 94: 733–744.

Peters CN, Pohlmann-Eden B (2005). Intravenous valproate as an innovative therapy in seizure emergency situations including status epilepticus – experience in 102 adult patients. Seizure 14: 164–169.

Pollard H, Charriaut-Marlangue C, Cantagrel S et al. (1994). Kainate-induced apoptotic cell death in hippocampal neurons. Neuroscience 63: 7–18.

Pugin D, Foreman B, De Marchis GM et al. (2014). Is pentobarbital safe and efficacious in the treatment of super-refractory status epilepticus: a cohort study. Crit Care 18: R103.

Rabinowicz AL, Correale JD, Bracht KA et al. (1995). Neuron-specific enolase is increased after nonconvulsive status epilepticus. Epilepsia 36: 475–479.

Riviello Jr JJ, Claassen J, LaRoche SM et al. (2013). Treatment of status epilepticus: an international survey of experts. Neurocrit Care 18: 193–200.

Robakis TK, Hirsch LJ (2006). Literature review, case report, and expert discussion of prolonged refractory status epilepticus. Neurocrit Care 4: 35–46.

Rossetti AO, Logroscino G, Bromfield EB (2005). Refractory status epilepticus: effect of treatment aggressiveness on prognosis. Arch Neurol 62: 1698–1702.

Rossetti AO, Logroscino G, Bromfield EB (2006). A clinical score for prognosis of status epilepticus in adults. Neurology 66: 1736–1738.

Rossetti AO, Logroscino G, Liaudet L et al. (2007). Status epilepticus: an independent outcome predictor after cerebral anoxia. Neurology 69: 255–260.

Rossetti AO, Logroscino G, Milligan TA et al. (2008). Status Epilepticus Severity Score (STESS): a tool to orient early treatment strategy. J Neurol 255: 1561–1566.

Rowan AJ, Scott DF (1970). Major status epilepticus. A series of 42 patients. Acta Neurol Scand 46: 573–584.

Ruegg S, Naegelin Y, Hardmeier M et al. (2008). Intravenous levetiracetam: treatment experience with the first 50 critically ill patients. Epilepsy Behav : E&B 12: 477–480.

Sakuragi S, Tokunaga N, Okawa K et al. (2007). A case of takotsubo cardiomyopathy associated with epileptic seizure: reversible left ventricular wall motion abnormality and ST-segment elevation. Heart Vessels 22: 59–63.

Samaniego EA, Stuckert E, Fischbein N et al. (2010). Crossed cerebellar diaschisis in status epilepticus. Neurocrit Care 12: 88–90.

Shaner DM, McCurdy SA, Herring MO et al. (1988). Treatment of status epilepticus: a prospective comparison of diazepam and phenytoin versus phenobarbital and optional phenytoin. Neurology 38: 202–207.

Shimizu M, Kagawa A, Takano T et al. (2008). Neurogenic stunned myocardium associated with status epileptics and postictal catecholamine surge. Intern Med 47: 269–273.

Shneker BF, Fountain NB (2003). Assessment of acute morbidity and mortality in nonconvulsive status epilepticus. Neurology 61: 1066–1073.

Shorvon S (2011). The treatment of status epilepticus. Curr Opin Neurol 24: 165–170.

Shorvon S, Ferlisi M (2011). The treatment of super-refractory status epilepticus: a critical review of available therapies and a clinical treatment protocol. Brain : J Neurology 134: 2802–2818.

Silbergleit R, Durkalski V, Lowenstein D et al. (2012). Intramuscular versus intravenous therapy for prehospital status epilepticus. N Engl J Med 366: 591–600.

Sinha S, Naritoku DK (2000). Intravenous valproate is well tolerated in unstable patients with status epilepticus. Neurology 55: 722–724.

Sloviter RS (1987). Decreased hippocampal inhibition and a selective loss of interneurons in experimental epilepsy. Science 235: 73–76.

Standley CA, Mason BA, Cotton DB (1995). Differential regulation of seizure activity in the hippocampus of male and female rats. Am J Obstet Gynecol 173: 1160–1165.

Sutter R, Kaplan PW, Ruegg S (2013). Independent external validation of the status epilepticus severity score. Crit Care Med 41: e475–e479.

Sutter R, Marsch S, Fuhr P et al. (2014). Anesthetic drugs in status epilepticus: risk or rescue? A 6-year cohort study. Neurology 82: 656–664.

Swisher CB, Doreswamy M, Gingrich KJ et al. (2012). Phenytoin, levetiracetam, and pregabalin in the acute management of refractory status epilepticus in patients with brain tumors. Neurocrit Care 16: 109–113.

Szabo K, Poepel A, Pohlmann-Eden B et al. (2005). Diffusion-weighted and perfusion MRI demonstrates parenchymal changes in complex partial status epilepticus. Brain : J Neurol 128: 1369–1376.

Tan RY, Neligan A, Shorvon SD (2010). The uncommon causes of status epilepticus: a systematic review. Epilepsy Res 91: 111–122.

Tien RD, Ashdown BC (1992). Crossed cerebellar diaschisis and crossed cerebellar atrophy: correlation of MR findings, clinical symptoms, and supratentorial diseases in 26 patients. AJR Am J Roentgenol 158: 1155–1159.

Toledano M, Britton JW, McKeon A et al. (2014). Utility of an immunotherapy trial in evaluating patients with presumed autoimmune epilepsy. Neurology 82: 1578–1586.

Towne AR, Pellock JM, Ko D et al. (1994). Determinants of mortality in status epilepticus. Epilepsia 35: 27–34.

Treiman DM, Meyers PD, Walton NY et al. (1998). A comparison of four treatments for generalized convulsive status epilepticus. Veterans Affairs Status Epilepticus Cooperative Study Group. N Engl J Med 339: 792–798.

Trinka E, Cock H, Hesdorffer D et al. (2015). A definition and classification of status epilepticus – report of the ILAE task force on classification of status epilepticus. Epilepsia 56: 1515–1523.

Van Ness PC (1990). Pentobarbital and EEG burst suppression in treatment of status epilepticus refractory to benzodiazepines and phenytoin. Epilepsia 31: 61–67.

Venkataraman V, Wheless JW (1999). Safety of rapid intravenous infusion of valproate loading doses in epilepsy patients. Epilepsy Res 35: 147–153.

Vignatelli L, Tonon C, D'Alessandro R (2003). Incidence and short-term prognosis of status epilepticus in adults in Bologna, Italy. Epilepsia 44: 964–968.

Vignatelli L, Rinaldi R, Galeotti M et al. (2005). Epidemiology of status epilepticus in a rural area of northern Italy: a 2-year population-based study. European Journal of Neurology : The Official Journal of the European Federation of Neurological Societies 12: 897–902.

Vohra TT, Miller JB, Nicholas KS et al. (2015). Endotracheal intubation in patients treated for prehospital status epilepticus. Neurocrit Care 23: 33–43.

Wasterlain CG, Fujikawa DG, Penix L et al. (1993). Pathophysiological mechanisms of brain-damage from status epilepticus. Epilepsia 34: S37–S53.

Wasterlain CG, Liu HT, Naylor DE et al. (2009). Molecular basis of self-sustaining seizures and pharmacoresistance during status epilepticus: the receptor trafficking hypothesis revisited. Epilepsia 50: 16–18.

Weissberg I, Wood L, Kamintsky L et al. (2015). Albumin induces excitatory synaptogenesis through astrocytic TGF-beta/ALK5 signaling in a model of acquired epilepsy following blood–brain barrier dysfunction. Neurobiol Dis 78: 115–125.

Wijdicks EF (2013). Multifaceted care of status epilepticus. Epilepsia 54 (Suppl 6): 61–63.

Wijdicks EF, Hubmayr RD (1994). Acute acid-base disorders associated with status epilepticus. Mayo Clin Proc 69: 1044–1046.

Wijdicks EF, Parisi JE, Sharbrough FW (1994). Prognostic value of myoclonus status in comatose survivors of cardiac arrest. Ann Neurol 35: 239–243.

Wijdicks EF, Hijdra A, Young GB et al. (2006). Practice parameter: prediction of outcome in comatose survivors after cardiopulmonary resuscitation (an evidence-based review): report of the Quality Standards Subcommittee of the American Academy of Neurology. Neurology 67: 203–210.

Wilder-Smith EP, Lim EC, Teoh HL et al. (2005). The NORSE (new-onset refractory status epilepticus) syndrome: defining a disease entity. Ann Acad Med Singapore 34: 417–420.

Wu YW, Shek DW, Garcia PA et al. (2002). Incidence and mortality of generalized convulsive status epilepticus in California. Neurology 58: 1070–1076.

Yaffe K, Lowenstein DH (1993). Prognostic factors of pentobarbital therapy for refractory generalized status epilepticus. Neurology 43: 895–900.

Yoshikawa H, Yamazaki S, Abe T et al. (2000). Midazolam as a first-line agent for status epilepticus in children. Brain Dev 22: 239–242.

Young GB, Jordan KG, Doig GS (1996). An assessment of nonconvulsive seizures in the intensive care unit using continuous EEG monitoring: an investigation of variables associated with mortality. Neurology 47: 83–89.

Zaidi SA, Haq MA, Bindman D et al. (2013). Crossed cerebellar diaschisis: a radiological finding in status epilepticus not to miss. BMJ Case Reports.

*Handbook of Clinical Neurology, Vol. 140 (3rd series)*
*Critical Care Neurology, Part I*
E.F.M. Wijdicks and A.H. Kramer, Editors
http://dx.doi.org/10.1016/B978-0-444-63600-3.00010-6

Chapter 10

# Critical care in acute ischemic stroke

M. McDERMOTT[1]*, T. JACOBS[2], AND L. MORGENSTERN[1]

[1]*Stroke Program, University of Michigan, Ann Arbor, MI, USA*

[2]*Department of Neurosurgery, University of Michigan, Ann Arbor, MI, USA*

## Abstract

Most ischemic strokes are managed on the ward or on designated stroke units. A significant proportion of patients with ischemic stroke require more specialized care. Several studies have shown improved outcomes for patients with acute ischemic stroke when neurocritical care services are available. Features of acute ischemic stroke patients requiring intensive care unit-level care include airway or respiratory compromise; large cerebral or cerebellar hemisphere infarction with swelling; infarction with symptomatic hemorrhagic transformation; infarction complicated by seizures; and a large proportion of patients require close management of blood pressure after thrombolytics. In this chapter, we discuss aspects of acute ischemic stroke care that are of particular relevance to a neurointensivist, covering neuropathology, neurodiagnostics and imaging, blood pressure management, glycemic control, temperature management, and the selection and timing of antithrombotics. We also focus on the care of patients who have received intravenous thrombolysis or mechanical thrombectomy. Complex clinical decision making in decompressive hemicraniectomy for hemispheric infarction and urgent management of basilar artery thrombosis are specifically addressed.

## INTRODUCTION

Every year in the USA approximately 795 000 people experience a new or recurrent stroke, amounting to about one stroke every 40 seconds (Mozaffarian et al., 2015). Ischemic strokes represent approximately 87% of that total, with the remainder hemorrhagic. In 2011, stroke accounted for approximately one out of every 20 deaths in the USA. In 2013, the US Burden of Disease Collaborators reported that stroke was second only to lung cancer and ischemic heart disease in years of life lost and death (Murray et al., 2013).

Risk factors for acute ischemic stroke include age, sex, hypertension, diabetes mellitus, cardiac dysrhythmias, structural heart disease, smoking, physical inactivity, and family history (Mohr et al., 2004; Meschia et al., 2014). As our population ages and life expectancy increases, the global incidence and prevalence of acute ischemic stroke are expected to increase, perhaps dramatically.

The 2014 Global Burden of Disease Study found that the absolute numbers of people with first stroke, stroke-related deaths, and disability-adjusted life-years had significantly increased from 1990 to 2010, with low- and middle-income countries disproportionately affected (Feigin et al., 2014).

Over the last 20 years, the acute management of stroke patients in many regions has transitioned to designated stroke centers and stroke units. Admission to a dedicated stroke center is associated with increased thrombolysis use (Lattimore et al., 2003; Gropen et al., 2006) and decreased mortality (Xian et al., 2011; Kim et al., 2013). Similarly, admission to a designated stroke unit is associated with improved outcomes, including reduced hospital length of stay and decreased mortality (Candelise et al., 2007; Zhu et al., 2009). However, up to 15–20% of acute stroke patients may benefit from a higher level of care than even a dedicated stroke unit (Coplin, 2012).

*Correspondence to: Mollie McDermott, MD, University of Michigan, Stroke Program, Cardiovascular Center Room 3391, 1500 East Medical Center Drive, Ann Arbor MI 48109-5855, USA. Tel: +1-734-232-4508, E-mail: mcdermom@med.umich.edu

Several studies have shown improved outcomes for acute ischemic stroke patients when neurocritical care services are available. A 2008 prospective study evaluated clinical outcomes in 100 ischemic stroke patients before and after the appointment of a full-time neurointensivist. In the adjusted analysis, patients in the postappointment group had a shorter intensive care unit (ICU) length of stay and hospital length of stay (Varelas et al., 2008). Similarly, a retrospective chart review of 400 patients with acute ischemic stroke managed at a large academic hospital found reductions in ICU and hospital lengths of stay following the institution of a specialized neurocritical care team (Bershad et al., 2008).

In 2005, the Brain Attack Coalition formally recommended that comprehensive stroke centers have an ICU available for acute ischemic stroke patients (Alberts et al., 2005).

In this chapter all aspects of ICU care in the more complicated types of strokes are discussed.

## INDICATIONS FOR ICU STROKE CARE

### Airway management

Patients with acute ischemic stroke complicated by depressed level of consciousness or facial or bulbar weakness may have a reduced ability to protect their airway. Airway compromise can lead to aspiration or respiratory failure. In addition, many ischemic stroke patients have comorbid cardiopulmonary disease that may be exacerbated by the physiologic sequelae of acute stroke (or even by its therapeutics, as in the case of overly aggressive intravenous (IV) fluid hydration). As a result, some acute ischemic stroke patients will require intubation and mechanical ventilation to maintain airway patency and prevent respiratory compromise.

An analysis of 52 acute ischemic stroke patients who required mechanical ventilation found that mechanical ventilation was indicated because of deterioration in consciousness in 47 (90%) and heart insufficiency and/or pneumonia in five (10%) (Berrouschot et al., 2000). The risk of mechanical ventilation was associated with hypertension and an area of hypoattenuation > 66% of the middle cerebral artery (MCA) territory on baseline computed tomography (CT) scan.

The exact proportion of acute ischemic stroke patients who require mechanical ventilation remains unclear, with estimates ranging from < 1% of emergency department (ED) ischemic stroke patients (Petchy et al., 2014) to 24% of stroke patients with hemispheric infarctions (Berrouschot et al., 2000). Furthermore, guidelines regarding which ischemic stroke patients should be intubated are lacking.

## Large cerebral hemisphere or cerebellar hemisphere infarction

Patients with large cerebral hemisphere infarcts tend to experience a significant burden of stroke symptoms, including hemiplegia, sensory/spatial neglect, aphasia, abnormalities of gaze and visual fields, and/or dysphagia. Patients with large cerebral hemisphere infarcts may develop significant cerebral swelling secondary to cytotoxic edema. Such swelling typically begins hours after stroke onset and peaks 2–7 days after stroke onset (Hacke et al., 1996). Swelling and displacement of brain parenchyma can have potentially devastating consequences, such as increased intracranial pressure, hemorrhagic transformation, and uncal herniation.

Because of these risks, patients with large cerebral hemisphere infarcts are often monitored in a neurologic ICU (NICU). In a retrospective analysis of 46 patients treated with IV thrombolysis, infarct volume on magnetic resonance imaging (MRI) obtained within 6 hours of treatment independently predicted requirement for ICU-level care (Faigle et al., 2015). The probability of requiring ICU-level care increased by 3% for every 1 cm$^3$ increase in infarct volume and an infarct volume greater than 3 cm$^3$ predicted ICU-level care with 81.3% sensitivity and 66.7% specificity.

Similarly, patients with large cerebellar hemisphere infarcts are at high risk for brainstem compression, obstructive hydrocephalus, and herniation. These patients are often managed in a NICU with serial neurologic examination as well as neurosurgical consultation. The clinical and radiographic features of patients with cerebellar infarcts who ultimately receive ICU-level care have not been reported.

The 2014 American Heart Association/American Stroke Association (AHA/ASA) scientific statement on management of cerebral and cerebellar infarction with swelling recommends that patients with a large territorial stroke be transferred to an ICU or stroke unit for close monitoring (class I level C recommendation) (Wijdicks et al., 2014). This monitoring includes serial CT scans to recognize swelling early and to anticipate decompressive craniotomy.

## Infarction with hemorrhagic transformation

Development of petechial hemorrhage is a common complication of acute ischemic stroke that is typically clinically silent. A study of 150 consecutive patients with acute anterior circulation infarcts who underwent CT scanning within the first week of stroke found hemorrhagic transformation in 65 patients (43%) (Toni et al., 1996). Of these 65 patients, 58 (89%) had petechial bleeding. Other studies have also found a rate of hemorrhagic transformation of approximately 40% after acute ischemic stroke (Hornig et al., 1986; Okada et al., 1989). Patients with clinically silent or minimally symptomatic hemorrhagic transformation do not typically require ICU-level care.

However, clinically significant hemorrhagic transformation of ischemic stroke is common in ICU patients, particularly after receipt of IV thrombolysis or endovascular revascularization. In a pooled analysis of six randomized placebo-controlled trials of IV tissue plasminogen activator (tPA) involving 2775 patients, hemorrhage was observed in 5.9% of patients treated with IV tPA compared to 1.1% of controls ($p < 0.0001$) (Hacke et al., 2004).

Other risk factors for hemorrhagic transformation include large infarct size, hyperglycemia, and a cardioembolic cause of infarct (Paciaroni et al., 2008; Tan et al., 2014). In a retrospective analysis of the pivotal National Institute of Neurologic Disorders and Stroke (NINDS) tPA trial, baseline serum glucose predicted symptomatic hemorrhage (odds ratio (OR) 2.26; 95% confidence interval (CI) 1.05–4.83) and all hemorrhage (OR 2.26; 95% CI 1.07–4.69) in patients who had received tPA (Demchuk et al., 1999).

Because of the risk of significant clinical worsening, patients with symptomatic hemorrhagic transformation are often monitored in a NICU.

## Seizures

A prospective cohort study of 1632 patients with acute ischemic stroke (excluding patients with previous epilepsy) followed for a median of 9 months found that seizures ultimately occurred in 140 (8.6%) (Bladin et al., 2000). Forty percent of seizures occurred in the first 24 hours, with the risk of first seizure increased by cortical location (hazard ratio (HR) 2.09; 95% CI 1.19–3.68) and severe disability (2.10; 95% CI 1.16–3.82). In a separate study of 609 ischemic stroke patients with first stroke, 24 (4%) had a symptomatic seizure within 7 days of stroke (Beghi et al., 2011).

Patients with seizures are often managed in the ICU given the need for frequent neurologic assessment; the potential necessity of intubation in the setting of ongoing seizures; and side-effects from antiepileptic medications, including sedation, hypotension, and arrhythmia.

## Postendovascular care

Acute ischemic stroke patients who have undergone an endovascular procedure such as intra-arterial (IA) thrombolysis or mechanical thrombectomy are frequently monitored postprocedurally in a NICU. An intensive care setting may allow for increased nursing attention (including frequent neurologic assessment and serial inguinal access site checks) as well as more aggressive blood pressure monitoring and management. Although the 2015 AHA/ASA recommendations regarding endovascular treatment did not specifically recommend postprocedure monitoring in an ICU (Powers et al., 2015), we typically monitor postprocedure patients in the NICU for at least 18–24 hours. Most of the early monitoring relates to control of blood pressure, which may require IV drug infusion.

## Cardiac care

Acute ischemic stroke may lead to cardiac arrhythmias (i.e., atrial fibrillation with rapid ventricular response) or new electrocardiogram (ECG) changes and a rise in serum troponin. Recent carotid stenting (elective or emergent) may be associated with hypotension and bradycardia in the 24–48-hour postprocedure period.

# NEUROPATHOLOGY

Much of the therapy delivered to critically ill acute stroke patients is aimed at limiting the extent of cerebral infarction. A basic appreciation of the pathophysiology of cerebral ischemia and its consequences is helpful in understanding the rationale behind these therapies. This section will briefly address several neuropathologic topics important to neurointensivists: the ischemic penumbra, reperfusion injury and hemorrhagic transformation of infarcted tissue, and cerebral edema.

## Ischemic penumbra

Normal brain cerebral blood flow is approximately 50 mL/100 g of brain tissue per minute (Phillips and Whisnant, 1992; Mohr et al., 2004). Brain tissue becomes infarcted when cerebral blood flow remains lower than 8 mL/100 g/min. Penumbral brain tissue receives cerebral blood flow at a reduced rate between 8 and 20 mL/100 g/min (Baron, 2001). The rate of progression from ischemia to infarction depends largely upon the degree of residual blood flow through the obstructive lesion and on the extent of collateral blood flow (Liebeskind, 2005). Total ischemia results in infarction rapidly, whereas borderline perfusion will maintain tissue viability longer. Most acute stroke therapies aim to preserve this penumbral tissue.

Cerebral ischemia sets off a cascade of detrimental intracellular processes, including the influx of calcium and sodium ions, the promotion of new gene expression, and the generation of nitric oxide and free radicals (Ellison et al., 2004). In animal models of complete MCA occlusion, microscopic changes from ischemia tend to expand from the subcortex outward toward the cortex (Garcia et al., 1993, 1995). Necrosis from ischemia occurs over several hours and affects neurons, glial cells, and endothelial cells (Ogata et al., 2009). In rodent models of MCA occlusion, iatrogenic elevation of blood pressure during the period of induced ischemia is associated with improved cerebral blood flow and oxygenation and reduced infarct volume (Shin et al., 2008) as well as decreased cerebral edema (Cole et al., 1990). Also in animal models of stroke, hyperglycemia is associated with degradation of neurons and expansion of cerebral infarct territory (Gilmore and Stead, 2006). Similarly, hyperthermia is associated with larger infarct volume (Chen et al., 1991; Morikawa et al., 1992) and destruction of microvascular integrity (Meng et al., 2012). Hyperthermia may worsen cerebral ischemia through promotion of neurotransmitter release, production of oxygen free radicals, structural changes in the blood–brain barrier, and degradation of the neuronal cytoskeleton (Ginsberg and Busto, 1998). These findings correlate with the established association between hyperglycemia and hyperthermia and poor outcomes in acute stroke patients.

## Reperfusion injury and hemorrhagic transformation

Restoration of blood flow to ischemic brain tissue incites an inflammatory response involving neutrophil recruitment and upregulation of interleukin-1, tumor necrosis factor-α, and platelet-activating factor (Jean et al., 1998; Emsley et al., 2008). This inflammatory response likely contributes to reperfusion injury, which is characterized by extension of infarct area and degradation of microvasculature. Failure of intracellular calcium regulation and production of reactive oxygen species have also been implicated in reperfusion injury (Pundik et al., 2012).

Reperfusion injury appears to contribute to hemorrhagic transformation after stroke, although the mechanisms underlying hemorrhagic transformation are likely multifactorial (Khatri et al., 2012; Sussman and Connolly, 2013). Ischemia causes damage to or death of endothelial cells, leading to capillary disruption and allowing extravasation of blood into the cerebral parenchyma (Simard et al., 2007). In addition to promoting fibrinolysis, tPA appears to contribute to blood–brain barrier damage (Yepes et al., 2009) via activation of matrix metalloproteinase and degradation of the extracellular membrane, thereby increasing the risk of hemorrhagic transformation (Khatri et al., 2012). These findings correlate with the increased risk of cerebral hemorrhage in ischemic stroke patients who have received IV tPA (NINDS rt-PA Stroke Study Group, 1997).

## Cerebral edema

Cytotoxic edema secondary to cerebral ischemia results from failure of the sodium-potassium adenosine triphosphate pump in neurons and glial cells (Emsley et al., 2008), leading to the intracellular accumulation of osmotically active molecules (such as sodium and chloride) and water (Simard et al., 2007). The degree of cytotoxic edema depends upon the extent and duration of ischemia. Cytotoxic edema is distinct from vasogenic edema, which is a result of fluid leakage through a permeable blood–brain barrier into the extravascular space (Heo et al., 2005). Both cytotoxic and vasogenic edema contribute to cerebral swelling after stroke. However, cytotoxic edema appears to primarily contribute to cerebral edema in the first 12–24 hours after stroke, after which neuronal and glial necrosis occurs. Vasogenic edema predominates later and can lead to mass effect with devastating clinical consequences, such as increased intracranial pressure and herniation.

## CLINICAL PRESENTATION

IV tPA treatment for stroke brought new importance to the fast and accurate diagnosis of acute ischemic stroke (NINDS rt-PA Stroke Study Group, 1995). Much of the initial evaluation of a stroke patient is aimed at quickly determining whether he or she is a candidate for IV tPA or endovascular intervention.

### Emergency department

Because stroke is abrupt in onset, many stroke patients are first evaluated in the ED. Based on several studies suggesting decreased door-to-needle times and increased IV tPA administration rates with "stroke code" teams (Grotta et al., 2001; Tai et al., 2012; Iglesias Mohedano et al., 2015), many large or academic hospitals have moved toward a protocol approach to acute stroke care. This protocol typically includes medical stabilization, rapid point-of-care glucose measurement, peripheral IV catheter placement, ECG assessment, obtainment of routine labs and coagulation factors, noncontrast head CT, and performance of the National Institutes of Health Stroke Scale (NIHSS; Table. 10.1). In addition, blood cultures should be obtained in patients for whom there is concern for endocarditis with cerebral embolism.

### Intensive care unit

For patients who require a higher level of care than a stroke unit, prompt admission to the ICU following medical stabilization and delivery of acute stroke therapy is warranted. One single-center study of 519 ischemic and hemorrhagic stroke patients admitted to the NICU found that an ED length of stay ≥5 hours was associated with an almost fourfold risk of having a modified Rankin scale (mRS) score (Table 10.2) ≥4 at discharge (OR 3.8; 95% CI 1.6–8.8) in the multivariate analysis (Rincon et al., 2010).

*Table 10.1*

**National Institutes of Health Stroke Scale (NIHSS) (From Jauch et al., 2013, with permission from Wolters Kluwer).**

| Tested item | Title | Responses and scores |
|---|---|---|
| 1A | Level of consciousness | 0 Alert<br>1 Drowsy<br>2 Obtunded<br>3 Coma/unresponsive |
| 1B | Orientation questions (2) | 0 Answers both correctly<br>1 Answers one correctly<br>2 Answers neither correctly |
| 1C | Response to commands (2) | 0 Performs both tasks correctly<br>1 Performs one task correctly<br>2 Performs neither |
| 2 | Gaze | 0 Normal horizontal movements<br>1 Partial gaze palsy<br>2 Complete gaze palsy |
| 3 | Visual fields | 0 No visual field deficit<br>1 Partial hemianopia<br>2 Complete hemianopia<br>3 Bilateral hemianopia |
| 4 | Facial movement | 0 Normal<br>1 Minor facial weakness<br>2 Partial facial weakness<br>3 Complete unilateral palsy |
| 5 | Motor function (arm)<br>a. Left<br>b. Right | 0 No drift<br>1 Drift before 5 seconds<br>2 Falls before 10 seconds<br>3 No effort against gravity<br>4 No movement |
| 6 | Motor function (leg)<br>a. Left<br>b. Right | 0 No drift<br>1 Drift before 5 seconds<br>2 Falls before 5 seconds<br>3 No effort against gravity<br>4 No movement |
| 7 | Limb ataxia | 0 No ataxia<br>1 Ataxia in one limb<br>2 Ataxia in two limbs |
| 8 | Sensory | 0 No sensory loss<br>1 Mild sensory loss<br>2 Severe sensory loss |
| 9 | Language | 0 Normal<br>1 Mild aphasia<br>2 Severe aphasia<br>3 Mute or global aphasia |
| 10 | Articulation | 0 Normal<br>1 Mild dysarthria<br>2 Severe dysarthria |
| 11 | Extinction of inattention | 0 Absent<br>1 Mild (one sensory modality lost)<br>2 Severe (two sensory modalities lost) |

*Table 10.2*

*Table 10.2*

**The modified Rankin scale (mRS) score is a six-point scale frequently used to quantify disability in stroke clinical trials (From van Swieten et al., 1988, with permission from Wolters Kluwer)**

| mRS | Description of disability |
|---|---|
| 0 | Asymptomatic |
| 1 | Able to carry out all usual duties and activities despite symptoms |
| 2 | Unable to carry out all previous activities but independent in looking after own affairs |
| 3 | Requiring help, but able to walk without assistance |
| 4 | Unable to walk without assistance; unable to take care of own bodily needs without assistance |
| 5 | Bedridden, incontinent, and fully dependent on nursing care and attention |

In addition to patients with acute ischemic stroke presenting from the ED, patients from outside institutions may present in transfer to the NICU. A retrospective cohort analysis comparing 448 patients with acute ischemic stroke or intracerebral hemorrhage (ICH) who presented to an ICU from an outside ED versus the study center's own ED found that outside ED transfer was associated with a twofold increased rate of a poor outcome, defined as death or fully dependent status (65% vs. 34%, $p = 0.05$). In the multivariate analysis, outside ED presentation predicted a poor outcome (OR 1.36; 95% CI 1.02–1.83) (Rincon et al., 2011). While these findings likely reflect selected transfer of sicker patients, other factors such as discontinuity of care or complications of transfer may be involved.

## Postthrombolysis transfers

Of particular note are so called "drip and ship" transfers – patients who receive IV tPA at their local ED or hospital and are transferred to a larger center for continued care. One study evaluated the safety of the "drip and ship" practice using registry data from 44 667 acute ischemic stroke patients treated with IV tPA in 1440 hospitals (Sheth et al., 2015). After risk adjustment, "drip and ship" patients had a higher in-hospital mortality (OR 1.46; 95% CI 1.22–1.46) and a higher rate of symptomatic ICH (OR 1.41; 95% CI 1.25–1.58). These results may be influenced by selection bias, with sicker or more medically complex patients being transferred to larger centers. Thrombolytic administration through the "drip and ship" method occurs in approximately 20% of patients treated with IV tPA in the USA (Tekle et al., 2012; Sheth et al., 2015).

## NEURODIAGNOSTICS AND NEUROIMAGING

This section will primarily focus on diagnostic and imaging modalities that are of use in the evaluation of acute and critically ill ischemic stroke patients. For example, we will not discuss long-term ambulatory cardiac ECG (event) monitoring, which is typically employed after a patient has left the ICU setting. We will not separately discuss carotid Doppler ultrasound, which is used to screen for carotid artery stenosis and occlusion but not typically relevant to acute stroke ICU decision making.

### Noncontrast head CT

The initial imaging modality in most acute stroke patients is a noncontrasted head CT, typically obtained in the ED. Head CT scans can be obtained quickly and are relatively easy to interpret in the acute setting. Noncontrasted head CTs help to immediately exclude the presence of hemorrhage in patients who would otherwise be candidates for IV thrombolysis or endovascular therapy. The initial CT scan may demonstrate early changes that can help to predict the age, distribution, and size of an infarct, thereby informing expectations regarding the clinical course of the patient.

In the NINDS tPA study group trial, 194 of 616 patients (31%) had early ischemic changes on CT scan obtained within 3 hours of symptom onset (Patel et al., 2001). Early ischemic change does not preclude treatment with IV thrombolysis; however, frank hypodensity composing more than one-third of the MCA distribution represents a contraindication to treatment (Jauch et al., 2013). In addition to screening for hemorrhage and frank infarct, a CT scan may help identify alternative causes of neurologic change, such as hydrocephalus or tumor.

Current ASA/AHA guidelines recommend obtaining a head CT within 25 minutes of a stroke patient's arrival in the ED (Jauch et al., 2013). Some hospitals have moved toward diffusion-weighted MRI as the initial imaging modality of choice for acute ischemic stroke patients, but this technology is not widely available in the acute setting and may delay treatment.

Early ischemia typically remains occult on head CT, particularly if the area of ischemia is small. In addition, CT scans are relatively insensitive at detecting posterior fossa ischemic changes due to the degree of artifact in that region. One common radiographic change in early MCA territory ischemia includes loss of gray–white differentiation, particularly in the basal ganglia, insular region, and cortical convexities. In about one-third of patients with an acute large artery occlusion, an early vessel sign (such as the "hyperdense MCA") can be seen on noncontrast CT (Tomsick et al., 1996) (Fig. 10.1), representing thrombus in that vessel. The hyperdense MCA sign predicts poor outcome after stroke (Manno et al., 2003; Smith et al., 2006).

The Alberta Stroke Program Early CT Score (ASPECTS) provides a 1–10-point scale for grading the degree of early ischemic change (Barber et al., 2000), where a score of 10 indicates no early changes in the relevant ischemic hemisphere (Fig. 10.2). One point is subtracted for evidence of early ischemic change in each of 10 places (seven cortical and three subcortical): anterior MCA cortex, middle MCA cortex, and posterior MCA cortex at the level of the basal ganglia; anterior, middle, and posterior MCA cortex directly superior to those at the basal ganglia level; insular ribbon; internal capsule; caudate; and lentiform nucleus. The ASPECTS score was used to help determine patient candidacy in several of the recent trials of mechanical thrombectomy (Goyal et al., 2015; Jovin et al., 2015; Saver et al., 2015). In our experience, the usefulness of ASPECTS is limited by interrater variability and questions surrounding the importance of when, in relation to stroke onset, imaging is acquired. Early infarction as defined by ASPECT <7 indicates a considerable area of infarction and reduces the chance of improvement after clot retrieval and thus may be used to select patients for IV thrombolysis or endovascular treatment.

In addition to their value in the acute setting, noncontrast head CT scans are useful for evaluating ICU patients with clinical deterioration and for performing radiographic surveillance in patients at risk for cerebral swelling or hemorrhagic transformation after ischemic stroke. A portable CT scanner is available in some NICUs, obviating the potentially unsafe transfer of critically ill stroke patients to a fixed scanner. Use of a portable CT scanner as opposed to transporting a patient to a fixed scanner may also result in reduced NICU staff workload (Gunnarsson et al., 2000). However, due to radiation exposure and expense, repeated CT imaging should only be performed if clinically indicated.

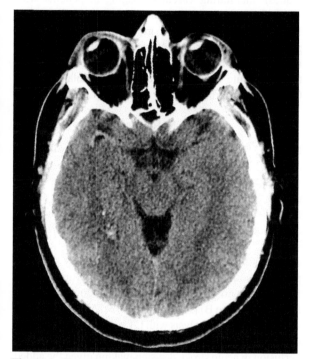

**Fig. 10.1.** Hyperdense right middle cerebral artery indicating active thrombus within that vessel.

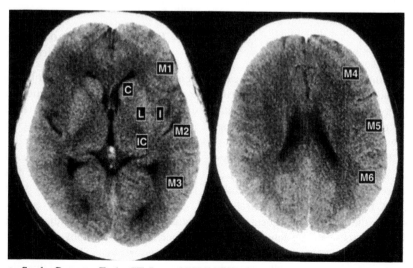

**Fig. 10.2.** The Alberta Stroke Program Early CT Score (ASPECTS). One point is subtracted for evidence of early ischemic changes in the anterior middle cerebral artery (MCA) cortex (M1), middle MCA cortex (M2), and posterior MCA cortex (M3) at the level of the basal ganglia; anterior (M4), middle (M5), and posterior MCA cortex (M6) directly superior to M1–M3; insular ribbon (I), internal capsule (IC); caudate (C), and lentiform nucleus (L) (Barber et al., 2000; Hill et al., 2003), with permission from Wolters Kluwer.

# MRI of the brain

Unlike CT scans and T1 and T2 MRI sequences, the diffusion-weighted MRI sequence is sensitive and specific for acute ischemia, with sensitivity estimates ranging from 88 to 100% (Lovblad et al., 1998; Gonzalez et al., 1999; Fiebach et al., 2002). Given its sensitivity, the MRI is useful in ruling out stroke when there is diagnostic ambiguity. In addition, MRI with susceptibility imaging is equivalent to CT in evaluating for acute cerebral hemorrhage (Fiebach et al., 2002; Kidwell et al., 2004) and can thus be used to rule out ICH prior to IV tPA or endovascular therapies (Jauch et al., 2013).

MRI is typically more useful than CT in clarifying the size of an infarct and stroke mechanism, the latter given that MRI is superior in demonstrating multifocal infarcts that may point to a proximal source of embolism. MRI is also superior to CT in visualizing areas of ischemia or infarct in the posterior fossa. The extent of MRI diffusion restriction can diminish with thrombolysis, suggesting that the area of diffusion restriction represents both infarcted and penumbral tissue (Kidwell et al., 2000).

# CT and MR angiography

CT angiography (CTA) uses a standard CT scanner to obtain contrasted images of the extracranial and intracranial vasculature. In acute ischemic stroke care, CTA is used primarily for the rapid identification of large-artery occlusion. The importance of this imaging modality is underscored by its use in the five recent trials of mechanical thrombectomy (Berkhemer et al., 2015; Campbell et al., 2015; Goyal et al., 2015; Jovin et al., 2015; Saver et al., 2015). Critically, the acquisition of vascular imaging should not delay the administration of IV tPA for appropriate thrombolysis candidates.

Compared to conventional angiography, CTA can identify large intracranial occlusions with nearly 100% sensitivity and specificity (Skutta et al., 1999; Lev et al., 2001; Nguyen-Huynh et al., 2008) and ≥50% stenosis with 97.1% sensitivity and 99.5% specificity (Nguyen-Huynh et al., 2008). CTA is superior to MR angiography (MRA) in detecting intracranial vessel irregularities, including stenosis, occlusion, and dissection (Bash et al., 2005). Although CTA requires the administration of iodinated contrast dye, the risk of consequent renal injury and renal failure appears relatively low. In 1075 patients who underwent routine CTA and CT perfusion at a single institution, creatinine rise ≥0.5 mg/dL occurred in only 5% and renal failure in only 0.37% (Josephson et al., 2005). Regardless, in patients with kidney disease who are likely to be candidates for mechanical thrombectomy based on their clinical presentation, it may be advisable to skip CTA in favor of empiric conventional angiography to reduce the overall dye load the patient receives.

Compared to CTA, MRA is less frequently used in the acute setting given the significantly longer time for image acquisition. However, unlike CTA, MRA can be performed without contrast (using time-of-flight techniques), facilitating vascular imaging in patients with a significant iodine allergy or renal disease. As above, MRA is inferior to CTA in identifying intracranial pathology; however, MRA is adequate for evaluating large-artery stenosis and occlusion and can thus be used to make acute decisions regarding revascularization if CTA is contraindicated.

# CT and MR perfusion

CT and MR perfusion scans are increasingly utilized in early ischemic stroke management in an attempt to provide revascularization therapy to those who may still benefit but are outside of the treatment time window. Perfusion scans allow for the measurement of blood flow and blood volume, which can be used to differentiate the ischemic penumbra from infarcted tissue (Wintermark et al., 2006). The 2013 AHA/ASA guidelines state that perfusion studies may be considered for selecting patients for IV tPA who are outside the time window (class IIB; level of evidence B) (Jauch et al., 2013). Although patient selection for thrombolysis with CT perfusion appears safe (Burton et al., 2015), we do not typically use CT or MR perfusion in acute stroke decision making given the added time for acquisition and interpretation and because of concerns regarding interoperator variability (Wintermark et al., 2008).

# Transthoracic and transesophageal echocardiograms

Echocardiography in acute stroke patients is useful for evaluating overall pump function and chamber sizes; detecting left-to-right shunting (such as from a patent foramen ovale); and identifying atrial or ventricular thrombus. In addition to potentially assisting with the diagnosis of stroke etiology, echocardiography provides a measure of diastolic and systolic function, which can be important in managing a NICU patient's volume status.

Surface echocardiography is typically sufficient for patients at low risk for cardioembolic stroke. However, surface echocardiography is inferior to transesophageal echocardiography (TEE) in viewing the left atrial appendage, a common site of thrombus, and in assessing for valvular vegetations or perivalvular abscesses in patients for whom endocarditis is a concern. One study evaluated the utility of TEE in 212 acute ischemic stroke patients with cryptogenic stroke despite standard workup (including surface echocardiogram) who would be candidates for oral anticoagulation; TEE identified a high-risk source for stroke implicating anticoagulation in 17 (8%) (Harloff et al., 2006).

## HOSPITAL COURSE AND MANAGEMENT

This section focuses on many of the largest issues facing neurointensivists in the management of acute ischemic stroke patients. The first part addresses acute management, including IV thrombolysis and endovascular therapies. The second part covers management of acute ischemic stroke patients in the ICU setting, including blood pressure, glycemic, and temperature management.

### Intravenous thrombolysis trials

The US Food and Drug Administration (FDA) approved IV tPA for use in acute ischemic stroke patients in 1996. This approval was based on results from the NINDS tPA Stroke Study Group trial published the previous year (NINDS rt-PA Stroke Study Group, 1995). The NINDS trial consisted of two parts. Inclusion criteria included acute ischemic stroke patients with clear time of symptom onset and NIHSS $\geq 1$. Exclusion criteria included (but were not limited to) initial CT scan showing hemorrhage; history of stroke or serious head trauma within the prior 3 months; major surgery within the prior 14 days; history of ICH; systolic blood pressure (SBP) $> 185$ mmHg or diastolic blood pressure (DBP) $>110$ mmHg; arterial puncture at a noncompressible site within the previous 21 days; platelet count $< 100\ 000/cm^3$, elevated partial thromboplastin time or international normalized ratio; and glucose $< 50$ mg/dL or $> 400$ mg/dL.

In the first part of the trial, 291 ischemic stroke patients were randomized to receive IV tPA versus placebo within 3 hours of stroke onset. IV tPA was dosed at 0.9 mg/kg (maximum dose of 90 mg) administered as a 10% bolus followed by a 60-minute infusion of the remaining 90%. The primary endpoint, intended to represent immediate benefit of therapy, was complete resolution of neurologic deficits or improvement of $\geq 4$ points on the NIHSS at 24 hours. No statistically significant difference was found between the tPA and placebo groups.

In the second part, 333 ischemic stroke patients were randomized to IV tPA versus placebo, with a primary endpoint designed to evaluate delayed benefit of thrombolysis. This primary outcome was a global test statistic created from a combination of outcome measures, including NIHSS $\leq 1$ and mRS $\leq 1$ at 90 days. In this second part, patients were treated with IV tPA did better than patients who received placebo (OR 1.7; 95% CI 1.2–2.6). More patients in the thrombolysis group had a very good outcome (90-day mRS $\leq 1$) than in the placebo group

(39 vs. 26%, $p = 0.019$). The authors calculated a number needed to treat of 8–11 to achieve minimal to no disability.

When NINDS trial parts one and two were combined, a greater number of patients in the IV tPA group developed symptomatic intracranial hemorrhage during the first 36 hours after treatment (6 vs. 1%, $p < 0.001$). However, no difference in mortality was found between the two groups.

Subsequent randomized controlled trials studied the safety and efficacy of IV tPA administered beyond the 3-hour time window. The European Cooperative Acute Stroke Study (ECASS) II trial evaluated IV tPA compared to placebo when treatment was provided within a 6-hour window (Hacke et al., 1998). No difference between groups was found in the primary outcome of 90-day mRS dichotomized to favorable (0–1) or unfavorable (2–6). Significantly more intracerebral bleeding was found in the thrombolysis group. The Alteplase Thrombolysis for Acute Noninterventional Therapy in Ischemic Stroke (ATLANTIS) trial evaluated tPA administered between 3 and 5 hours after stroke onset (Clark et al., 1999). Similar to ECASS II, no significant difference was found between groups in the primary outcome of NIHSS $\leq 1$ at 90 days, and there was more symptomatic ICH in the thrombolysis group.

A subsequent pooled analysis of ECASS I (a neutral trial evaluating treatment with tPA 1.1 mg/kg within 6 hours of ischemic stroke onset) (Hacke et al., 1995), the NINDS tPA trial, ECASS II, and ATLANTIS suggested that a benefit of tPA may persist up to 4½ hours after symptom onset (Hacke et al., 2004). Subsequently, ECASS III enrolled 821 patients randomized to IV tPA 0.9 mg/kg versus placebo provided within 3–4½ hours of symptom onset (Hacke et al., 2008). The primary outcome was mRS 0–1 at 90 days. Unlike the NINDS trial, ECASS III excluded patients $> 80$ years, with NIHSS $> 25$, with a history of both previous stroke and diabetes mellitus, and patients on oral anticoagulation treatment, regardless of coagulation parameters. The thrombolysis group showed a "modest but significant" increase in the favorable outcome compared to the placebo group (OR 1.42; 95% CI 1.02–1.98) with a number needed to treat calculated at 14. Symptomatic ICH within 36 hours occurred more often in the thrombolysis group (2.4 vs. 0.2%, $p = 0.008$), but there was no significant difference in mortality.

In 2009, the AHA/ASA guidelines changed to reflect the results of ECASS III, stating that IV tPA should be administered to eligible patients in the time period of 3–4½ hours if they did not meet one of the four additional ECASS III exclusion criteria (Del Zoppo et al., 2009). However, the authors were sure to note that thrombolysis should be delivered as rapidly as possible to appropriate

*Table 10.3*

American Heart Association/American Stroke Asociation-recommended exclusion criteria for tissue plasminogen activator administration (From Jauch et al., 2013, with permission from Wolters Kluwer)

| | |
|---|---|
| **Absolute exclusion criteria** | |
| Active internal bleeding | Current use of direct thrombin inhibitors or direct factor Xa inhibitors |
| CT scan with hemorrhage | Heparin received within 48 hours with PTT > upper limit of normal |
| CT scan shows hypodensity > one-third of cerebral hemisphere | Aggressive measures require to bring blood pressure < 185/110 mmHg |
| History of stroke or serious head trauma within the previous 3 months | INR > 1.7 or PT > 15 seconds |
| History of previous intracranial hemorrhage | Platelet count < 100 000/cm$^3$ |
| SBP > 185 mmHg or DBP > 110 mmHg | Glucose level < 50 mg/dL |
| Symptoms suggestive of subarachnoid hemorrhage | Recent intracranial or intraspinal surgery |
| Intracranial neoplasm, arteriovenous malformation, or aneurysm | Arterial puncture at a noncompressible site within the previous 7 days |
| **Relative exclusion criteria** | |
| Minor or rapidly improving stroke symptoms | Seizure at onset with postictal residual neurologic impairment |
| Major surgery or serious trauma within the previous 14 days | Recent gastrointestinal or urinary tract hemorrhage (within previous 21 days) |
| Acute myocardial infarction within previous 3 months | |
| **Additional exclusion criteria for patients in the 3–4.5-hour window** | |
| Age > 80 | NIHSS > 25 |
| Taking an oral anticoagulant regardless of INR | History of both diabetes and prior ishcemic stroke |

CT, computed tomography; PTT, partial thromboplastin time; INR, international normalized ratio; PT, prothrombin time; SBP, systolic blood pressure; DBP, diastolic blood pressure; NIHSS, National Institutes of Health Stroke Scale.

patients, despite the extended time window. Of note, the FDA declined to amend the alteplase (tPA) package insert to reflect the longer treatment window. NINDS and ECASS III inclusion and exclusion criteria are used in clinical practice to inform decision making regarding a patient's candidacy for IV tPA (Table 10.3). Timely administration of IV tPA to eligible acute ischemic stroke patients is now considered standard of care.

## Patient management prior to IV tPA

Urgent IV access is indicated for all acute ischemic stroke patients. IV access is required for the administration of tPA, administration of contrast dye if CTA is indicated, and to provide IV fluids when required to maintain euvolemia and normotension. The placement of two peripheral IV catheters is recommended.

SBP > 185 mmHg and/or DBP > 110 mmHg are contraindications to treatment with IV tPA. However, if blood pressure decreases independently or without aggressive pharmacologic treatment, tPA can be administered. To treat elevated blood pressure prior to tPA, AHA/ASA guidelines recommend labetalol 10–20 mg IV administered over 1–2 minutes, repeated once if needed, or a nicardipine infusion, started at 5 mg/h and titrated up by 2.5 mg/h every 5–15 minutes to a maximum dose of 15 mg/h (Jauch et al., 2013). Other agents such as hydralazine and enalaprilat can also be considered.

Prior to IV tPA administration, the stroke patient should be evaluated for the necessity of an indwelling bladder catheter. If required, the catheter should be placed prior to tPA administration given the potential for urinary tract bleeding with placement following tPA (Jauch et al., 2013).

## Patient management after IV tPA

The most feared complication of tPA administration is symptomatic hemorrhagic transformation of ischemic or infarcted brain tissue, most frequently occurring in the first 24 hours after treatment (NINDS rt-PA Stroke Study Group, 1997). Hemorrhagic transformation is associated with early major worsening after ischemic stroke (Ntaios et al., 2013), particularly in the setting of large hematoma (Fiorelli et al., 1999).

Posttreatment blood pressure can predict hemorrhagic transformation after tPA (Butcher et al., 2010). In the Safe Implementation of Thrombolysis in Stroke International Stroke Thrombolysis Register (SITS-ISTR) of 11 080 patients treated with IV thrombolysis for acute ischemic stroke, the association between SBP and symptomatic ICH was almost linear (Ahmed et al., 2009). Given this association, frequent blood pressure checks are recommended in patients who have received IV tPA. Blood pressure should be checked every 15 minutes for 2 hours from the start of tPA treatment, followed by every 30 minutes for 6 hours, and then every hour until 24 hours have elapsed since the tPA bolus. Blood pressure during and after treatment with IV tPA should be maintained at 180/105 mmHg or below. Elevated blood pressure should be treated as recommended above (for elevated pressures prior to IV tPA), with the additional recommendation that IV sodium nitroprusside can be considered for refractory hypertension or DBP > 140 mmHg.

Hemorrhagic transformation should be managed by discontinuing tPA if still infusing, performing serial CT imaging to assess for extension or mass effect, and potentially by involving neurosurgery for consideration of decompressive surgery or hematoma evacuation if consistent with patient goals of care (Kirkman et al., 2014). Hematology consultation may be advisable to assist with correction of coagulopathy. The identification of hemorrhagic transformation should prompt lowering of blood pressure goals. Maintenance of SBP < 160 mmHg in patients with sizable or symptomatic hemorrhagic transformation following ischemic stroke is reasonable.

Placement of a nasogastric tube, indwelling bladder catheter, or arterial line should be delayed after administration of tPA to reduce the risk of bleeding (Jauch et al., 2013). We typically avoid such instrumentation until 24 hours have elapsed from administration of the tPA bolus. However, in patients with acute urinary retention who require an indwelling catheter, placement delayed at least 30 minutes following the end of the infusion is reasonable (Quality Standards Subcommittee of the AAN, 1996). Antiplatelet therapy should also be deferred for 24 hours after tPA administration, and anticoagulation for at least that long (see section on complex clinical decisions, below). We typically obtain a surveillance CT or MRI prior to restarting anticoagulation; we do not always obtain surveillance imaging before restarting antiplatelet therapy as long as the patient is clinically stable.

Neurointensivists should also be aware of the risk of angioedema following tPA administration. Angioedema, or swelling of the lips and tongue, occurs in approximately 1% of tPA-treated patients (Hill and Buchan, 2005), with the risk likely increased by concurrent angiotensin-converting enzyme inhibitor use (Hill et al., 2003). Treatment of angioedema may include antihistamines and glucocorticoids. Although the course is typically self-limited, patients with severe or progressive angioedema may require intubation (Fugate et al., 2012).

## Intra-arterial thrombolysis

After the FDA approval of IV tPA in 1996, investigators sought to evaluate the safety and efficacy of IA thrombolysis, the delivery of a high dose of a thrombolytic at the site of thrombus while potentially minimizing systemic complications. The largest trial to address this question was Prolyse in Acute Cerebral Thromboembolism (PROACT) II, which randomized 180 patients with a proximal MCA occlusion to receive IA pro-urokinase plus IV heparin versus IV heparin alone (Furlan et al., 1999). Clinical outcomes were better in the IA arm, with 40% of IA patients demonstrating an mRS of 0–2 at 90 days compared to 25% of control (OR 2.13; 95% CI 1.02–4.42). However, a trend toward a higher rate of symptomatic hemorrhage was found in the treatment arm (10 vs. 2%, $p = 0.06$). As a result, the FDA did not approve IA pro-urokinase, recommending a confirmatory study. Such a study has not been performed, largely due to a shift in the stroke community's collective attention to a new generation of mechanical endovascular devices. IA thrombolytics are currently not FDA-approved for acute ischemic stroke.

Specific evidence regarding the ICU care of patients who have received IA thrombolysis is lacking (Tarlov et al., 2012). However, adherence to blood pressure recommendations as defined for IV tPA-treated patients is reasonable.

## Intra-arterial thrombectomy

Early trials of the first generation of FDA-approved clot retrieval devices (Merci and Penumbra) did not show a clinical benefit of intervention (Broderick et al., 2013; Ciccone et al., 2013; Kidwell et al., 2013). However, these trials did not require that all subjects undergo pretreatment vascular imaging to establish a large artery occlusion and permitted a relatively long interval between symptom onset and treatment (Berkhemer et al., 2015). Furthermore, these trials did not involve frequent use of the newer generation of mechanical thrombectomy devices, including the stent retrievers, the Solitaire Flow Restoration (FR) device and Trevo. Solitaire FR and Trevo gained FDA approval in 2012 based on trials showing superior revascularization by angiography when compared to the earlier-generation Merci device (Nogueira et al., 2012; Saver et al., 2012).

In 2015, five trials of endovascular stroke therapy were published, all showing benefit of mechanical thrombectomy over standard care (Berkhemer et al., 2015; Campbell et al., 2015; Goyal et al., 2015; Jovin et al., 2015; Saver et al., 2015). MR CLEAN, the first published and perhaps most pragmatic of the trials, enrolled 500 patients with occlusion of the distal internal carotid artery (ICA), proximal MCA (M1 or M2 branches), or proximal ACA (A1 or A2 branches) established by CTA, MRA, or conventional angiography who could have endovascular treatment initiated within 6 hours of stroke onset. IV tPA was received by 89% of all patients. Stent retrievers were used in 81.5% of patients in the thrombectomy arm. The primary outcome, a favorable shift in the mRS at 90 days, was achieved significantly more frequently in the intervention group (OR 1.67; 95% CI 1.21–2.30) (Berkhemer et al., 2015). The

*Table 10.4*

**A comparison of five trials of mechanical thrombectomy for acute ischemic stroke published in 2015**

| | n | Selected exclusion criteria | IV tPA | Goal timing re: symptom onset | Median onset to GP | Safety outcomes | Efficacy outcomes |
|---|---|---|---|---|---|---|---|
| MR CLEAN | 500 | plt <40, INR >3 | 89% of all patients prior to randomization | Initiate treatment within 6 hours | 4 hours 20 minutes | No difference in mortality or sICH | Adj OR that intervention leads to lower mRS = 1.7 |
| ESCAPE | 316 | ASPECTS ≤5, poor collateral circulation by CTA | 73% of intervention arm | Randomize within 12 hours | 3 hours | No difference in sICH; lower mortality in intervention group | Adj OR that intervention leads to lower mRS = 3.1 |
| EXTEND-IA | 70 | CTP mismatch; tPA exclusions | 100% | GP within 6 hours | 3 hours 30 minutes | No difference in mortality or sICH | ≥8-point reduction on NIHSS or a score of 0–1 at day 3 = 37% in control vs. 80% in intervention |
| SWIFT-PRIME | 196 | ASPECTS ≤5, tPA exclusions | 100% | Initiate endovascular treatment within 6 hours | 3 hours 40 minutes | No difference in mortality or sICH | Median 90-day mRS 2 in intervention compared to 3 in control |
| REVASCAT | 206 | ASPECTS ≤6 | 68% of intervention arm | Initiate endovascular treatment within 8 hours | 4 hours 30 minutes | No difference in mortality or sICH | Adj OR that intervention leads to 1-point improvement on mRS = 1.7 |

n, number of patients; IV tPA, intravenous tissue plasminogen activator; GP, groin puncture; plt, platelets; INR, international normalized ratio; sICH, symptomatic intracerebral hemorrhage; Adj, adjusted; OR, odds ratio; mRS, modified Rankin scale; CTA, computed tomography angiography; CTP, computed tomography perfusion scan; NIHSS, National Institutes of Health Stroke Scale.

incidence of symptomatic intracranial hemorrhage did not differ between the two groups.

Relevant details of MR CLEAN and the other 2015 endovascular stroke trials are shown in Table 10.4. Based on these positive trials, the AHA/ASA now recommend endovascular thrombectomy for appropriate patients with a causative occlusion of the ICA or proximal MCA who can undergo groin puncture within 6 hours of stroke onset (class I; level of evidence A) (Powers et al., 2015).

### Patient management after endovascular therapy

In light of the recent positive endovascular studies, neurointensivists may more frequently manage patients who have undergone mechanical thrombectomy. The ideal blood pressure range following mechanical thrombectomy has not been established, but maintaining blood pressure < 180/105 mmHg is reasonable. Any deterioration in the patient's clinical status should be evaluated

with a noncontrast head CT to evaluate for hemorrhagic transformation or cerebral swelling. The access site sheath should be removed as soon as possible to reduce the risk of thrombosis and infection (Tarlov et al., 2012), and frequent monitoring of the site for hematoma or pseudoaneurysm development is recommended.

## INTENSIVE CARE OF THE ACUTE ISCHEMIC STROKE PATIENT

### Blood pressure management

In acute ischemic stroke patients, blood pressure can be considered a surrogate for cerebral perfusion pressure, given that intracranial pressure changes are usually insignificant (Sheth and Sims, 2012). Hypotension is rarely associated with acute ischemic stroke and, when present, is usually the result of a medication effect or a comorbid medical issue such as sepsis, aortic dissection, or unstable arrhythmia (Jauch et al., 2013). As such, the identification of hypotension should spur a search for other causative factors. Hypertension, on the other hand, is a frequent feature of acute ischemic stroke presentation and subsequent hospital course. An analysis of 17 398 patients from the first International Stroke Trial (IST) (International Stroke Trial Collaborative Group, 1997) found that 81.6% of patients had a pre-randomization SBP > 140 mmHg with a mean SBP at enrollment of 160 mmHg (Leonardi-Bee et al., 2002).

Unfortunately, a specific goal blood pressure range for acute ischemic stroke patients has not been established; such a range may vary substantially by individual (Jauch et al., 2013). Patients who suffer from ischemic stroke may have baseline hypertension that shifts their autoregulation curve to the right compared to nonhypertensive individuals. In the first IST, the lowest frequency of poor outcome occurred in patients with a baseline SBP of 140–179 mmHg, with the nadir around 150 mmHg (Leonardi-Bee et al., 2002).

Several large studies have found no clinical benefit of early blood pressure lowering in acute ischemic stroke patients. Three older trials of nimodipine found no benefit of early administration of nimodipine in acute ischemic stroke (Kaste et al., 1994; Ahmed et al., 2000; Horn et al., 2001). The Scandinavian Candesartan Acute Stroke Trial (SCAST) randomized 2029 acute ischemic and hemorrhagic stroke patients with SBP ≥140 mmHg to candesartan versus placebo for 7 days (Sandset et al., 2011). Although blood pressures were significantly lower in the candesartan group, no significant difference was found between groups in mRS at 6 months or in the composite endpoint of vascular death, myocardial infarct, or stroke during the first 6 months.

The Continue or Stop PostStroke Antihypertensives Collaborative Study (COSSACS) trial in the UK randomized 763 of an intended 2900 patients with acute ischemic or hemorrhagic stroke to either continue or stop their pre-existing antihypertensive regimen (Robinson et al., 2010). A significant difference in blood pressure was found between the two groups at 3 weeks. However, no significant difference in the primary outcome of death or dependency (mRS > 3) was found between groups at 2 weeks, although the trial was underpowered.

Similarly, the China Antihypertensive Trial in Acute Ischemic Stroke (CATIS) enrolled 4071 ischemic stroke patients with nonthrombolysed acute ischemic stroke and SBP between 140 and 220 mmHg (He et al., 2014). The patients were randomized to either an antihypertensive arm, wherein blood pressure was lowered by 10–25% within the first 24 hours after randomization, achieving a blood pressure less than 140/90 mmHg within 7 days, or discontinuation of all antihypertensives during hospitalization. No difference was found between groups in the primary outcome of death or mRS ≥3 at

2 weeks or hospital discharge. Most recently, the ENOS trial randomized 4011 ischemic or hemorrhagic stroke patients with an SBP 140–220 mmHg to 7 days of transdermal nitrate therapy at 5 mg/day versus placebo (Bath et al., 2015). No difference was found between groups in the primary outcome of 90-day mRS.

At present, AHA/ASA guidelines recommend tolerating blood pressures up to 220/120 mmHg in acute ischemic stroke patients who have not received thrombolysis and who have no indication for blood pressure lowering, such as myocardial ischemia or heart failure (class I; level of evidence C) (Jauch et al., 2013). A short period of discontinuation or reduction of outpatient antihypertensive medications is recommended given the risk of an unpredictable response to medications in the acute poststroke period. The optimal time for restarting home antihypertensives after acute stroke remains unknown, although AHA/ASA guidelines state that restarting antihypertensives after the first 24 hours is reasonable in patients who have pre-existing hypertension and are neurologically stable (class IIa; level of evidence B). As mentioned above, patients who have been treated with IV tPA, IA tPA, or endovascular thrombectomy should have their blood pressure maintained below 180/105 mmHg for at least 24 hours after receipt of tPA.

An important feature of neurocritical care is the management of blood pressure in acute ischemic stroke patients at the time of procedures, such as mechanical thrombectomy, TEE, or tracheostomy. Few data exist to guide periprocedural blood pressure management (Sheth and Sims, 2012). Deferring elective procedures to reduce the risk of iatrogenic hypotension (from medications or anesthesia) after ischemic stroke is advisable. Treating symptomatic periprocedural hypotension with fluids and even vasopressors may be indicated.

## Glycemic management

Hypoglycemia (blood glucose < 60 mg/dL) can cause neurologic symptoms, including altered mental status, stroke mimics, and seizure. As a result, blood glucose <50 mg/dL (2.7 mmol/L) is an absolute contraindication to IV thrombolysis. Primary hypoglycemia is uncommon among acute ischemic stroke patients and, when present, is typically due to antiglycemic medications (Jauch et al., 2013).

Unlike hypoglycemia, hyperglycemia is frequently encountered in the setting of acute ischemic stroke, with approximately one-third of patients demonstrating a blood glucose level > 140 mg/dL (Williams et al., 2002; Gentile et al., 2006). Hyperglycemia in stroke patients in the NICU may be a result of underlying insulin resistance, a stress response, or receipt of dextrose-containing fluids or total parenteral nutrition (Godoy et al., 2010).

Hyperglycemia is associated with worse clinical outcomes after stroke. One observational study of 476 patients with acute ischemic stroke found that a blood glucose of ≥155 mg/dL at any time during the first 48 hours after admission was associated with an almost threefold increase in having an mRS > 2 at 3 months after adjustment (OR 2.73; 95% CI 1.43–5.24) and greater than threefold increase in mortality at 3 months (HR 3.80; 95% CI 1.79–8.10) (Fuentes et al., 2009).

In a systematic review of 26 studies, an admission glucose of 110–126 mg/dL was associated with an increased risk of in-hospital or 30-day mortality in nondiabetic patients but not diabetic patients (relative risk for nondiabetic patients 3.28; 95% CI, 2.32–4.64) (Capes et al., 2001). In the NINDS tPA trial, the risk of symptomatic ICH increased with increasing admission glucose (OR 1.75 per 100 mg/dL increase in admission glucose; 95% CI 1.11–2.78) in both tPA-treated patients and untreated patients in the multivariate analysis (Bruno et al., 2002).

In the UK Glucose Insulin in Stroke Trial (GIST-UK), 933 of an intended 2355 patients with acute ischemic stroke with admission glucose between 108 and 306 mg/dL were randomized to an insulin infusion (with variable dosing to achieve glucose 72–126 mg/dL) versus placebo for 24 hours (Gray et al., 2007). No significant difference between groups was found in the primary outcome of 90-day mortality; however, the study was underpowered. The multicenter Stroke Hyperglycemia Insulin Network Effort (SHINE) study, intended to randomize 1400 hyperglycemic patients to sliding-scale insulin to maintain glucose < 180 mg/dL or continuous insulin infusion to maintain glucose 80–130 mg/dL, is currently ongoing; the primary outcome is a 90-day mRS adjusted for baseline stroke severity (Bruno et al., 2014).

Current AHA/ASA guidelines recommend treating blood glucose < 60 mg/dL in acute ischemic stroke patients with a goal of achieving normoglycemia (class I; level of evidence C) as well as treating hyperglycemia in the first 24 hours after stroke to achieve blood glucose levels in the range of 140–180 mg/dL (class IIa; level of evidence C) (Jauch et al., 2013).

## Temperature management

Approximately 25–40% of patients develop fever (temperature ≥37.9°C) in the first several days to 1 week following acute ischemic stroke (Azzimondi et al., 1995; Grau et al., 1999; Indredavik et al., 2008). Fever is most often due to lung infection or inflammation, but urinary tract and viral infections are also common (Grau et al., 1999).

Hyperthermia is associated with increased morbidity and mortality in stroke patients (Reith et al., 1996; Hajat et al., 2000; Phipps et al., 2011). One meta-analysis of six cohort studies including 2986 patients found that acute ischemic stroke patients with a temperature ≥37.4°C within the first 24 hours of hospitalization had twice the mortality of afebrile patients (Prasad and Krishnan, 2010).

To evaluate the empiric administration of acetaminophen to acute stroke patients, the Paracetamol (Acetaminophen) in Stroke (PAIS) trial enrolled 1500 (of an intended 2500) patients with baseline temperature 36–39°C (den Hertog et al., 2009). The patients were randomized to acetaminophen 6 g/day versus placebo administered within 12 hours of stroke onset. The groups did not differ in the primary outcome of improvement beyond expectation on the mRS at 3 months. However, in a *post hoc* analysis, patients in the treatment group who had a baseline temperature of 37–39°C did better than the placebo group (OR 1.43; 95% CI 1.02–1.97). PAIS II, which will evaluate empiric acetaminophen in patients with baseline temperature > 36.5°C, is ongoing (de Ridder et al., 2015).

At this time, AHA/ASA guidelines make no recommendations regarding empiric antipyretic treatment in afebrile stroke patients (Jauch et al., 2013). However, the guidelines recommend that sources of fever should be identified and fever should be treated with antipyretics (class I; level of evidence C).

In many medical ICUs, induced hypothermia is used to treat comatose cardiac arrest survivors for 12–24 hours after ventricular fibrillation arrest. Induced hypothermia is an attractive prospect for the treatment of acute ischemic stroke given the association of hyperthermia with worse outcomes after stroke. At present, induced hypothermia for treatment of ischemic stroke is considered experimental (Jauch et al., 2013).

## Antiplatelet management

Two very large randomized controlled trials, the IST and the Chinese Acute Stroke Trial (CAST), examined the effectiveness of early aspirin use in acute ischemic stroke (Chinese Acute Stroke Trial Collaborative Group, 1997; International Stroke Trial Collaborative Group, 1997). In each trial aspirin was started within 48 hours of stroke onset. In CAST, which used an aspirin dose of 162 mg, aspirin-allocated patients had lower mortality and fewer recurrent ischemic strokes. In IST, which used an aspirin dose of 300 mg, aspirin-allocated patients had fewer recurrent ischemic strokes but no significant difference was found in mortality. When the results of the two trials were combined (with a total of about 40 000 patients), aspirin appeared to reduce the overall risk of recurrent stroke or death in the hospital by 9 per 1000 patients (Chen et al., 2000).

Although aspirin is the most widely used antiplatelet agent, other agents such as dipyridamole and clopidogrel have been evaluated in trials of acute ischemic stroke patients, both as monotherapy and in combination with aspirin. In the Fast Assessment of Stroke and Transient Ischemic Attack to Prevent Early Recurrence (FASTER) trial, 392 patients with recent stroke or transient ischemic attack (TIA) with NIHSS < 4 were randomized to clopido-grel (300 mg loading dose followed by 75 mg daily) ver-sus placebo; no significant difference in ischemic or hemorrhagic stroke within 90 days was found between the two groups (Kennedy et al., 2007). In the EARLY trial, 543 acute ischemic stroke patients were randomized to receive either aspirin 100 mg or aspirin 25 mg plus extended-release dipyridamole 200 mg, either within 24 hours of stroke or TIA or after 7 days of aspirin mono-therapy (Dengler et al., 2010). No significant difference in mRS at 90 days was found between the combination and the aspirin monotherapy groups.

More recently, the CHANCE trial found that patients with TIA or minor stroke (NIHSS ≤ 3) benefit when trea-ted with clopidogrel (initial dose 300 mg followed by 75 mg daily) plus aspirin (75 mg daily) compared to aspirin monotherapy if the treatment is started within 24 hours of symptom onset and continued for 90 days after onset (Wang et al., 2013). In 90-day follow-up, ischemic or hemorrhagic stroke occurred in 8.2% of the combination group compared to 11.7% in the aspirin group (HR 0.68; 95% CI 0.57–0.81). The ongoing Platelet-Oriented Inhibition in New TIA and Minor Ischemic Stroke (POINT) trial will address the benefit of clopidogrel (initial dose 600 mg followed by 75 mg daily) plus aspirin taken within 12 hours of symptom onset versus aspirin alone (Johnston et al., 2013).

Based on the results of CAST and IST, the AHA/ASA recommend oral administration of aspirin (with an initial dose of 325 mg) within 24–48 hours after stroke onset, cit-ing a small but statistically significant decline in mortality and unfavorable outcomes (class I; level of evidence A) (Jauch et al., 2013). The current guidelines state that the usefulness of clopidogrel is not well established.

Several IV antiplatelet agents, including abciximab, tirofiban, and eptifibatide, have been studied for acute ischemic stroke in clinical trials. At this time the AHA/ASA state that "considerably more research" is required before these agents can be considered part of the routine management of acute ischemic stroke.

## Deep vein thrombosis prophylaxis

Deep vein thrombosis (DVT) is a common and often pre-ventable complication of acute ischemic stroke. In a prospective study of 489 patients with acute ischemic or hemorrhagic stroke managed in a comprehensive stroke unit, DVT occurred in 0.6% within 1 week and 2.5% within 3 months of stroke (Indredavik et al., 2008). DVT prophylaxis can include early mobilization, systemic anticoagulation, and mechanical compression. DVT prophylaxis is associated with a decreased risk of a combined outcome of in-hospital mortality, discharge to hospice, or discharge to a skilled nursing facility (OR 0.60; 95% CI 0.37–0.96) (Bravata et al., 2010).

In the PREVAIL study, 1762 patients with acute ischemic stroke who were unable to walk without assis-tance were randomized within 48 hours of stroke onset to enoxaparin 40 mg delivered subcutaneously daily versus unfractionated heparin 1500 units delivered subcutane-ously twice daily (Sherman et al., 2007). The enoxaparin group was less likely to develop DVT or pulmonary embolism compared to the heparin group (relative risk 0.57; 95% CI 0.44–0.76) with no significant difference in bleeding. The authors concluded that enoxaparin is preferable to twice-daily heparin for venous thromboem-bolism prophylaxis in acute ischemic patients. However, it should be noted that the observed benefit of enoxa-parin in preventing symptomatic venous thromboem-bolism was offset by more episodes of major bleeding (O'Donnell and Kearon, 2007). In addition, three-times-daily dosing of subcutaneous heparin, a common regi-men for hospitalized stroke patients, was not studied.

In the CLOTS III trial, acute ischemic stroke patients who were immobile on the day of admission were ran-domized to usual care versus usual care plus intermittent pneumatic compression devices (Dennis et al., 2015). The primary outcome, DVT in popliteal or femoral veins within 30 days, was less common in the pneumatic com-pression group (OR 0.65; 95% CI 0.51–0.84).

Currently, AHA/ASA guidelines call for subcutane-ous anticoagulation for immobilized patients to prevent DVT (class I; level of evidence A) as well as aspirin (class IIa; level of evidence A) and possibly intermittent pneumatic compression devices (class IIa; level of evi-dence B) for patients who cannot receive anticoagulation (Jauch et al., 2013). It is our practice to use unfractio-nated heparin at a dose of 5000 IU three times daily and pneumatic compression devices for DVT prophy-laxis in routine acute stroke patients.

## Anemia management

Anemia is a frequent complication in ICU patients (Corwin et al., 2004). Anemia may be particularly detri-mental to acute ischemic stroke patients in whom cere-bral hypoxia may cause secondary ischemic injury (Kramer and Zygun, 2009). In patients with acute ische-mic stroke managed in an ICU, low hemoglobin level is

associated with prolonged ICU length of stay and duration of mechanical ventilation (Kellert et al., 2014). At
present no hemoglobin goal or transfusion parameter
has been defined in acute ischemic stroke patients
(Leal-Noval et al., 2008), and AHA/ASA guidelines
do not specifically comment on the management of anemia in acute ischemic stroke patients. We typically maintain a hemoglobin level greater than 7 g/dL unless a
higher level is indicated (such as in patients with acute
coronary syndromes).

## CLINICAL TRIALS AND GUIDELINES

A number of important clinical trials involving acute
ischemic stroke patients are discussed in the above
and proceeding text. The AHA/ASA guidelines for
the early management of patients with acute ischemic
stroke, which is frequently cited above, provide a
comprehensive summary of early acute ischemic stroke
care building on clinical trial results and expert
opinion (Jauch et al., 2013). This publication is a
critical resource for neurointensivists managing acute
ischemic stroke patients. Class I level of evidence
A recommendations relevant to the intensive care of
acute ischemic stroke patients included in the guidelines are as follows:

- Emergency imaging of the brain (CT or MRI) is
  recommended before treatment with IV thrombolysis or endovascular therapies.
- Vascular imaging (such as CTA) is recommended if
  endovascular therapy is being considered, but this
  imaging should not delay administration of IV
  thrombolysis.
- Rapid treatment with IV thrombolysis is recommended for patients without exclusion criteria who
  can be treated within 3 hours of symptom onset.
  (Treatment in the 3–4½-hour window in those without exclusion criteria is a class I; level of evidence
  B recommendation.)
- Aspirin at a dose of 325 mg should be administered
  orally to most acute ischemic stroke patients within
  24–48 hours of stroke onset.
- DVT prophylaxis with subcutaneous anticoagulation
  is recommended for immobilized patients.
- In patients with large infarction, close monitoring
  and efforts to reduce brain edema are recommended.

After the publication of the five recent mechanical
thrombectomy trials, the AHA/ASA released a focused
update to the 2013 guidelines (Powers et al., 2015).
An additional relevant class I level A recommendation
was presented.

Patients with acute ischemic stroke should receive
endovascular thrombectomy with a stent retriever device

if they meet the following criteria: (1) premorbid mRS
0–1; (2) receive IV tPA within 4½ hours of stroke onset;
(3) have a causative occlusion identified in the ICA or
proximal MCA; (4) are ≥18 years old; (5) have an
NIHSS ≥6; (6) have an ASPECTS (on noncontrast head
CT) of ≥6; and (7) groin puncture can be achieved within
6 hours of stroke onset.

## COMPLEX CLINICAL DECISIONS

A common decision encountered by neurointensivists is
when to initiate or resume anticoagulation in patients
with a clinical indication (such as atrial fibrillation) after
acute ischemic stroke. The risk of recurrent stroke must
be weighed against the risk of hemorrhagic transformation, particularly in patients with large infarcts.

A 2008 Cochrane review addressed this question,
analyzing 24 trials enrolling 23 748 patients who were randomized to early anticoagulation (started within 2 weeks
of stroke onset) versus control (Sandercock et al., 2008).
Early anticoagulation was associated with fewer recurrent
ischemic strokes, but it was also associated with a comparable increase in symptomatic intracranial hemorrhage.
The authors concluded that there was no evidence that
early anticoagulation improved outcomes after ischemic
stroke. Similarly, a 2007 meta-analysis of seven trials
enrolling 4624 patients found no benefit of early anticoagulation started within 48 hours of stroke as compared to
aspirin or placebo (Paciaroni et al., 2007).

On the other hand, a cohort analysis of data from
10 304 ischemic stroke patients with atrial fibrillation
included in the Virtual International Stroke Trials Archive
(VISTA) found that initiation of anticoagulation (with or
without an antiplatelet) at a median of 2 days after acute
ischemic stroke was associated with a lower risk of recurrent stroke (OR 0.60; 95% CI 0.40–0.91) and death (OR
0.58; 95% CI 0.43–0.78) after adjustment (Abdul-Rahim
et al., 2015). In an attempt to clarify the best time for starting anticoagulation, the Early Recurrence and Cerebral
Bleeding in Patients with Acute Ischemic Stroke and
Atrial Fibrillation (RAF) study enrolled 1029 patients with
atrial fibrillation and acute ischemic stroke (Paciaroni
et al., 2015). In an adjusted analysis, patients who started
anticoagulation between 4 and 14 days after stroke had a
significant reduction in a composite primary outcome of
stroke, TIA, symptomatic systemic embolism, symptomatic cerebral bleeding, and major extracranial bleeding
within 90 days of stroke when compared to patients treated
before 4 days or after 14 days.

It should be noted that the results of both VISTA and
RAF are limited by their lack of randomization and the
possibility of selection bias. No randomized trials have
addressed the best timing for anticoagulation after acute
cardioembolic stroke. The timing of anticoagulation is a

decision that should be individualized for each patient. Factors that should influence this decision include the patient's medical status, infarct size, and daily risk of recurrent ischemic stroke (which can be estimated with the CHADS2VASC tool: Lip et al., 2010).

Another complex decision is timing of decompressive hemicraniectomy in patients with a swollen hemispheric infarct. The term "malignant MCA stroke" refers to a space-occupying infarct involving the entirety of the MCA territory (Hacke et al., 1996). Malignant MCA strokes occur in approximately 10% of stroke patients and have a mortality rate of nearly 80%. Almost all deaths are related to brain herniation, which tends to occur between the second and fifth day after stroke onset. Standard antiedema agents such as hypertonic saline and mannitol are ineffective in preventing neurologic decline in malignant MCA strokes.

Several case series and small studies in the 1990s and early 2000s suggested that hemicraniectomy reduced mortality in patients with malignant MCA stroke (Carter et al., 1997; Schwab et al., 1998). Hemicraniectomy involves the removal of a bone flap of at least 12 cm with dural opening to allow extracranial herniation of edematous brain tissue.

The first randomized trials (DESTINY, DECIMAL, and HAMLET) to address the utility of hemicraniectomy for stroke were published in 2007 (Juttler et al., 2007; Vahedi et al., 2007b; Hofmeijer et al., 2009). The three trials enrolled patients less than 60 years old. Each trial individually found a significant mortality benefit for patients who underwent hemicraniectomy. The primary endpoint for each of the trials was a 6-month mRS of 0–3 versus 4–6, a dichotomization that drew some criticism given that an mRS of 3 is generally not considered a favorable outcome in stroke research. The primary endpoint was not found to be different between the two groups in any of the trials. Notably, in none of the studies did a patient have an mRS of 0 or 1 at 90 days.

A subsequent pooled analysis of the 93 patients enrolled in the three trials found that mortality rate differed significantly between the surgery and medical care groups (22 compared to 71%; $p < 0.0001$) (Vahedi et al., 2007a). The surgical group was less likely to have an mRS $> 4$ at 12 months (OR 0.10; 95% CI 0.04–0.27) and an mRS $> 3$ at 12 months (OR 0.33; 95% CI 0.13–0.86). The authors calculated a number needed to treat of 4 for survival with an mRS $\leq 3$. The best mRS score achieved was 2, by one patient of 42 in the medical care group (2%) and by seven of 51 in the surgical treatment group (14%). The risk of surviving with an mRS of 4 increased from 2% in the control group to 31% in the surgery group.

A subsequent study (DESTINY II) investigated outcomes of hemicraniectomy in 112 patients with large MCA territory stroke $> 60$ years of age (Juttler et al., 2014). The primary outcome of 6-month mRS 0–4 in the surgical group was almost threefold that of the control group (OR 2.91; 95% CI 1.06–7.49). The best mRS achieved at 12 months was three, by seven of 49 (13%) in the surgical group and three of 63 (5%) in the control group.

The ideal timing for hemicraniectomy remains unknown (Neugebauer and Juttler, 2014). In the pooled analysis of DESTINY, DECIMAL, and HAMLET, outcome was not affected by treatment on the first versus second day after stroke (Vahedi et al., 2007a). However, HAMLET, which assessed the effect of decompressive surgery within 4 days of stroke, found no benefit of surgical treatment over medical treatment for those randomized after 48 hours from symptom onset (Hofmeijer et al., 2009).

Discussions regarding the pursuit of hemicraniectomy for malignant MCA strokes involve an individualized decision based on the patient's preferences and values. In discussions with families, the responsible medical provider must clearly communicate that hemicraniectomy is considered a life-saving procedure and that, based on the best evidence we have, the family's loved one will never return to his or her baseline level of function. If the patient survives hemicraniectomy, he or she has about the same chance of being able to walk independently (mRS of 3) as of being unable to independently manage his or her own bodily needs (mRS of 4).

The degree of acceptable disability after hemicraniectomy remains a point of debate. A meta-analysis of 382 patients who had undergone hemicraniectomy for stroke found that, of the 209 for whom satisfaction data was available, 77% of the patients and/or caregivers reported that they would give consent for the procedure again (Rahme et al., 2012).

Current AHA/ASA guidelines state that, for patients $<60$ years with unilateral MCA infarctions and neurologic deterioration within 48 hours, decompressive hemicraniectomy is effective; craniectomy after 48 hours should be strongly considered (class I; level of evidence B) (Wijdicks et al., 2014). The guidelines further state that clinicians may wish to relay to family members that half of patients with malignant MCA stroke who survive decompressive hemicraniectomy are severely disabled and one-third are fully dependent on others for care (class IIb; level of evidence C).

Finally, a commonly misinterpreted and mishandled stroke is an acute basilar artery embolus. Acute basilar artery embolus is a neurologic emergency that is associated with a mortality rate of up to 90% (Baird et al., 2004). Because the symptoms of basilar artery thrombosis can be nonspecific, including dizziness, nausea, altered respiration, and impaired consciousness, rapid diagnosis can be difficult (Demel and Broderick, 2015).

Providers must maintain a high index of suspicion for this potentially catastrophic clinical entity. The clinical consequences of basilar thrombosis reflect the site of thrombosis and infarction. With mid-basilar occlusion, bilateral pontine infarcts can lead to a "locked-in" state, characterized by whole-body paralysis with retained awareness and eye movements.

A systematic analysis comparing IV tPA with IA thrombolysis in 420 patients with basilar artery occlusion found no difference in death or dependency, although recanalization occurred more frequently in the IA group (65 vs. 53%, $p = 0.04$) (Lindsberg and Mattle, 2006). A prospective registry study of 619 patients at 48 centers found similar outcomes between patients treated with IV versus IA thrombolysis (Schonewille et al., 2009). Notably, 402 patients (68%) had an mRS of 4, 5, or death at 1 month.

Randomized controlled trials of thrombolysis and thrombectomy in basilar artery thrombosis have not been performed given low patient numbers and concerns regarding high mortality in untreated patients. Patients with basilar artery thrombosis have been excluded from many acute ischemic stroke trials. However, general consensus holds that patients with acute basilar thrombosis who are candidates for IV thrombolysis should receive it (Demel and Broderick, 2015).

The ENDOSTROKE multicenter registry evaluated outcomes in 148 consecutive patients with acute basilar occlusion treated with endovascular therapy, 59% of whom had received IV tPA previously (Singer et al., 2015). Mortality was 35%; an mRS of 0–2 was achieved by 34% and an mRS of 0–3 was achieved by 42%. Given the potentially devastating consequences of this condition, the time window for thrombectomy is often extended beyond what would be considered for an anterior circulation stroke, even up to 48 hours in some cases (Strbian et al., 2013). We typically consider basilar artery thrombectomy up to 24 hours from stroke onset.

## NEUROREHABILITATION

In this section we will briefly address three topics that may be useful to NICU teams managing acute ischemic stroke patients.

## Early mobilization

Mobility programs in the NICU have been associated with decreased ICU length of stay, decreased hospital length of stay, and decreased ventilator-associated pneumonia (Titsworth et al., 2012). Early mobilization after stroke has been advocated given its potential to promote recovery of motor function and prevent DVT and skin breakdown. However, limited clinical evidence exists to support its safety and efficacy.

A Very Early Rehabilitation Trial (AVERT), the largest clinical trial to address the efficacy of early mobilization, randomized 2104 patients to either early mobilization (typically within 24 hours) or usual care (Bernhardt et al., 2015). Somewhat surprisingly, fewer patients in the early mobilization group had a favorable outcome (defined as having no symptoms, minimal symptoms, or slight disability) at 3 months compared to the usual care group (OR 0.73; 95% CI 0.59–0.90). However, it should be noted that the difference between the intervention and control group was not substantial, with the intervention group receiving on average 201.5 minutes of rehab per patient starting within 18.5 hours and the control group receiving on average 70 minutes of rehabilitation starting within 22.4 hours.

Current AHA/ASA guidelines recommend the use of comprehensive specialized stroke care that incorporates rehabilitation (class I; level of evidence A) and early mobilization of less severely affected patients (class I; level of evidence C).

## Treatment of dysphagia

Dysphagia after acute ischemic stroke is common, resulting from a number of causes such as altered mentation, oropharyngeal weakness, disturbed gag reflex, and/or neglect. A 2005 systematic review of stroke patients treated in acute or longer-term settings found that 64–78% of ischemic and hemorrhagic stroke patients demonstrated poststroke dysphagia on videofluoroscopic assessment (Martino et al., 2005). Current AHA/ASA guidelines recommend assessment of swallowing before a stroke patient begins eating, drinking, or receiving oral medications (class I; level of evidence B) (Jauch et al., 2013). It is our practice to perform a bedside swallow screening evaluation for every acute ischemic stroke patient.

In the acute setting, many ischemic stroke patients are unable to safely take in food orally. These patients are typically provided nutrition through nasogastric or orogastric routes pending improvement in mental status or dysphagia. For those whose swallow function does not improve sufficiently (or sufficiently quickly), placement of a percutaneous endoscopic gastrostomy (PEG) tube may be indicated, ideally depending on the patient's previously stated wishes. One study of 49 patients who received a PEG tube for poststroke dysphagia found that 8 (16.3%) patients had had the tube removed at a mean of 4.8 months after insertion (Yi et al., 2012). Eventual PEG independence may be associated with left hemispheric strokes (Crisan et al., 2014). For dysphagic patients, the AHA/ASA guidelines recommend nasogastric feeding over PEG tube placement for 2–3 weeks after stroke onset (class IIA; level of evidence B) to allow time for swallow recovery.

## Tracheostomy

Institutions and providers differ in their philosophies regarding the timing of tracheostomy in acute ischemic stroke complicated by airway compromise. The benefits of early tracheostomy over prolonged endotracheal intubation include lower risk of ventilator-associated pneumonia (Villwock et al., 2014), patient comfort, an improved ability to communicate, and decreased ICU length of stay (Rumbak et al., 2004; Griffiths et al., 2005). However, too early tracheostomy may expose the patient to a potentially unnecessary procedure.

In one single-center pilot trial, 60 patients with ischemic or hemorrhagic stroke and a foreseen requirement for ≥2 weeks of mechanical ventilation were randomized to either early tracheostomy (performed 1–3 days after intubation) versus standard tracheostomy (performed 7–14 days from intubation) (Bosel et al., 2013). The primary outcome of ICU length of stay did not differ between the groups, but the early tracheostomy group had lower ICU mortality (10 vs. 47%) and 6-month mortality (27 vs. 60%). Current AHA/ASA guidelines do not make recommendations regarding tracheostomy in acute ischemic stroke patients.

## REFERENCES

Abdul-Rahim AH, Fulton RL, Frank B et al. (2015). Association of improved outcome in acute ischaemic stroke patients with atrial fibrillation who receive early antithrombotic therapy: analysis from VISTA. Eur J Neurol 22: 1048–1055.

Ahmed N, Nasman P, Wahlgren NG (2000). Effect of intravenous nimodipine on blood pressure and outcome after acute stroke. Stroke 31: 1250–1255.

Ahmed N, Wahlgren N, Brainin M et al. (2009). Relationship of blood pressure, antihypertensive therapy, and outcome in ischemic stroke treated with intravenous thrombolysis: retrospective analysis from Safe Implementation of Thrombolysis in Stroke-International Stroke Thrombolysis Register (SITS-ISTR). Stroke 40: 2442–2449.

Alberts MJ, Latchaw RE, Selman WR et al. (2005). Recommendations for comprehensive stroke centers: a consensus statement from the Brain Attack Coalition. Stroke 36: 1597–1616.

Azzimondi G, Bassein L, Nonino F et al. (1995). Fever in acute stroke worsens prognosis: a prospective study. Stroke 26: 2040–2043.

Baird TA, Muir KW, Bone I (2004). Basilar artery occlusion. Neurocrit Care 1: 319–329.

Barber PA, Demchuk AM, Zhang J et al. (2000). Validity and reliability of a quantitative computed tomography score in predicting outcome of hyperacute stroke before thrombolytic therapy. Lancet 355: 1670–1674.

Baron JC (2001). Perfusion thresholds in human cerebral ischemia: historical perspective and therapeutic implications. Cerebrovasc Dis 11: 2–8.

Bash S, Villablanca JP, Jahan R et al. (2005). Intracranial vascular stenosis and occlusive disease: evaluation with CT angiography, MR angiography, and digital subtraction angiography. Am J Neuroradiol 26: 1012–1021.

Bath PM, Woodhouse L, Scutt P et al. (2015). Efficacy of nitric oxide, with or without continuing antihypertensive treatment, for management of high blood pressure in acute stroke (ENOS): a partial-factorial randomised controlled trial. Lancet 385: 617–628.

Beghi E, D'Alessandro R, Beretta S et al. (2011). Incidence and predictors of acute symptomatic seizures after stroke. Neurology 77: 1785–1793.

Berkhemer OA, Fransen PS, Beumer D et al. (2015). A randomized trial of intraarterial treatment for acute ischemic stroke. N Engl J Med 372: 11–20.

Bernhardt J, Langhorne P, Lindley RI et al. (2015). Efficacy and safety of very early mobilisation within 24 h of stroke onset (AVERT): a randomised controlled trial. Lancet 386: 46–55.

Berrouschot J, Rossler A, Koster J et al. (2000). Mechanical ventilation in patients with hemispheric ischemic stroke. Crit Care Med 28: 2956–2961.

Bershad EM, Feen ES, Hernandez OH et al. (2008). Impact of a specialized neurointensive care team on outcomes of critically ill acute ischemic stroke patients. Neurocrit Care 9: 287–292.

Bladin CF, Alexandrov AV, Bellavance A et al. (2000). Seizures after stroke: a prospective multicenter study. Arch Neurol 57: 1617–1622.

Bosel J, Schiller P, Hook Y et al. (2013). Stroke-related Early Tracheostomy versus Prolonged Orotracheal Intubation in Neurocritical Care Trial (SETPOINT): a randomized pilot trial. Stroke 44: 21–28.

Bravata DM, Wells CK, Lo AC et al. (2010). Processes of care associated with acute stroke outcomes. Arch Intern Med 170: 804–810.

Broderick JP, Palesch YY, Demchuk AM et al. (2013). Endovascular therapy after intravenous t-PA versus t-PA alone for stroke. N Engl J Med 368: 893–903.

Bruno A, Levine SR, Frankel MR et al. (2002). Admission glucose level and clinical outcomes in the NINDS rt-PA Stroke Trial. Neurology 59: 669–674.

Bruno A, Durkalski VL, Hall CE et al. (2014). The Stroke Hyperglycemia Insulin Network Effort (SHINE) trial protocol: a randomized, blinded, efficacy trial of standard vs. intensive hyperglycemia management in acute stroke. Int J Stroke 9: 246–251.

Burton KR, Dhanoa D, Aviv RI et al. (2015). Perfusion CT for selecting patients with acute ischemic stroke for intravenous thrombolytic therapy. Radiology 274: 103–114.

Butcher K, Christensen S, Parsons M et al. (2010). Postthrombolysis blood pressure elevation is associated with hemorrhagic transformation. Stroke 41: 72–77.

Campbell BC, Mitchell PJ, Kleinig TJ et al. (2015). Endovascular therapy for ischemic stroke with perfusion-imaging selection. N Engl J Med 372: 1009–1018.

Candelise L, Gattinoni M, Bersano A et al. (2007). Stroke-unit care for acute stroke patients: an observational follow-up study. Lancet 369: 299–305.

Capes SE, Hunt D, Malmberg K et al. (2001). Stress hyperglycemia and prognosis of stroke in nondiabetic and diabetic patients: a systematic overview. Stroke 32: 2426–2432.

Carter BS, Ogilvy CS, Candia GJ et al. (1997). One-year outcome after decompressive surgery for massive nondominant hemispheric infarction. Neurosurgery 40: 1168–1176.

Chen H, Chopp M, Welch KM (1991). Effect of mild hyperthermia on the ischemic infarct volume after middle cerebral artery occlusion in the rat. Neurology 41: 1133–1135.

Chen ZM, Sandercock P, Pan HC et al. (2000). Indications for early aspirin use in acute ischemic stroke: a combined analysis of 40 000 randomized patients from the Chinese acute stroke trial and the international stroke trial. Stroke 31: 1240–1249.

Chinese Acute Stroke Trial Collaborative Group (1997). CAST: randomised placebo-controlled trial of early aspirin use in 20,000 patients with acute ischaemic stroke. Lancet 349: 1641–1649.

Ciccone A, Valvassori L, Nichelatti M et al. (2013). Endovascular treatment for acute ischemic stroke. N Engl J Med 368: 904–913.

Clark WM, Wissman S, Albers GW et al. (1999). Recombinant tissue-type plasminogen activator (Alteplase) for ischemic stroke 3 to 5 hours after symptom onset: a randomized controlled trial. JAMA 282: 2019–2026.

Cole DJ, Drummond JC, Osborne TN et al. (1990). Hypertension and hemodilution during cerebral ischemia reduce brain injury and edema. Am J Physiol 259: 211–217.

Coplin WM (2012). Critical care management of acute ischemic stroke. Continuum 18: 547–559.

Corwin HL, Gettinger A, Pearl RG et al. (2004). The CRIT study: anemia and blood transfusion in the critically ill – current clinical practice in the United States. Crit Care Med 32: 39–52.

Crisan D, Shaban A, Boehme A et al. (2014). Predictors of recovery of functional swallow after gastrostomy tube placement for dysphagia in stroke patients after inpatient rehabilitation: a pilot study. Ann Rehabil Med 38: 467–475.

de Ridder IR, de Jong FJ, den Hertog HM et al. (2015). Paracetamol (Acetaminophen) In Stroke 2 (PAIS 2): protocol for a randomized, placebo-controlled, double-blind clinical trial to assess the effect of high-dose paracetamol on functional outcome in patients with acute stroke and a body temperature of 36.5 degrees C or above. Int J Stroke 10: 457–462.

Del Zoppo GJ, Saver JL, Jauch EC et al. (2009). Expansion of the time window for treatment of acute ischemic stroke with intravenous tissue plasminogen activator: a science advisory from the American Heart Association/American Stroke Association. Stroke 40: 2945–2948.

Demchuk AM, Morgenstern LB, Krieger DW et al. (1999). Serum glucose level and diabetes predict tissue plasminogen activator-related intracerebral hemorrhage in acute ischemic stroke. Stroke 30: 34–39.

Demel SL, Broderick JP (2015). Basilar occlusion syndromes: an update. Neurohospitalist 5: 142–150.

den Hertog HM, van der Worp HB, van Gemert HM et al. (2009). The Paracetamol (Acetaminophen) In Stroke (PAIS) trial: a multicentre, randomised, placebo-controlled, phase III trial. Lancet Neurol 8: 434–440.

Dengler R, Diener HC, Schwartz A et al. (2010). Early treatment with aspirin plus extended-release dipyridamole for transient ischaemic attack or ischaemic stroke within 24 h of symptom onset (EARLY trial): a randomised, open-label, blinded-endpoint trial. Lancet Neurol 9: 159–166.

Dennis M, Sandercock P, Graham C et al. (2015). The Clots in Legs Or sTockings after Stroke (CLOTS) 3 trial: a randomised controlled trial to determine whether or not intermittent pneumatic compression reduces the risk of post-stroke deep vein thrombosis and to estimate its cost-effectiveness. Health Technol Assess 19: 1–90.

Ellison D, Love S, Chimelli L et al. (2004). Neuropathology: a reference text of CNS pathology. Elsevier, Amsterdam, pp. 173–206.

Emsley HC, Smith CJ, Tyrrell PJ et al. (2008). Inflammation in acute ischemic stroke and its relevance to stroke critical care. Neurocrit Care 9: 125–138.

Faigle R, Wozniak AW, Marsh EB et al. (2015). Infarct volume predicts critical care needs in stroke patients treated with intravenous thrombolysis. Neuroradiology 57: 171–178.

Feigin VL, Forouzanfar MH, Krishnamurthi R et al. (2014). Global and regional burden of stroke during 1990-2010: findings from the Global Burden of Disease Study 2010. Lancet 383: 245–254.

Fiebach JB, Schellinger PD, Jansen O et al. (2002). CT and diffusion-weighted MR imaging in randomized order: diffusion-weighted imaging results in higher accuracy and lower interrater variability in the diagnosis of hyperacute ischemic stroke. Stroke 33: 2206–2210.

Fiorelli M, Bastianello S, von Kummer R et al. (1999). Hemorrhagic transformation within 36 hours of a cerebral infarct: relationships with early clinical deterioration and 3-month outcome in the European Cooperative Acute Stroke Study I (ECASS I) cohort. Stroke 30: 2280–2284.

Fuentes B, Castillo J, San Jose B et al. (2009). The prognostic value of capillary glucose levels in acute stroke: the GLycemia in Acute Stroke (GLIAS) study. Stroke 40: 562–568.

Fugate JE, Kalimullah EA, Wijdicks EF (2012). Angioedema after tPA: what neurointensivists should know. Neurocrit Care 16: 440–443.

Furlan A, Higashida R, Wechsler L et al. (1999). Intra-arterial prourokinase for acute ischemic stroke. The PROACT II study: a randomized controlled trial Prolyse in Acute Cerebral Thromboembolism. JAMA 282: 2003–2011.

Garcia JH, Yoshida Y, Chen H et al. (1993). Progression from ischemic injury to infarct following middle cerebral artery occlusion in the rat. Am J Pathol 142: 623–635.

Garcia JH, Liu KF, Ho KL (1995). Neuronal necrosis after middle cerebral artery occlusion in Wistar rats progresses at different time intervals in the caudoputamen and the cortex. Stroke 26: 636–643.

Gentile NT, Seftchick MW, Huynh T et al. (2006). Decreased mortality by normalizing blood glucose after acute ischemic stroke. Acad Emerg Med 13: 174–180.

Gilmore RM, Stead LG (2006). The role of hyperglycemia in acute ischemic stroke. Neurocrit Care 5: 153–158.

Ginsberg MD, Busto R (1998). Combating hyperthermia in acute stroke: a significant clinical concern. Stroke 29: 529–534.

Godoy DA, Di Napoli M, Rabinstein AA (2010). Treating hyperglycemia in neurocritical patients: benefits and perils. Neurocrit Care 13: 425–438.

Gonzalez RG, Schaefer PW, Buonanno FS et al. (1999). Diffusion-weighted MR imaging: diagnostic accuracy in patients imaged within 6 hours of stroke symptom onset. Radiology 210: 155–162.

Goyal M, Demchuk AM, Menon BK et al. (2015). Randomized assessment of rapid endovascular treatment of ischemic stroke. N Engl J Med 372: 1019–1030.

Grau AJ, Buggle F, Schnitzler P et al. (1999). Fever and infection early after ischemic stroke. J Neurol Sci 171: 115–120.

Gray CS, Hildreth AJ, Sandercock PA et al. (2007). Glucose-potassium-insulin infusions in the management of post-stroke hyperglycaemia: the UK Glucose Insulin in Stroke Trial (GIST-UK). Lancet Neurol 6: 397–406.

Griffiths J, Barber VS, Morgan L et al. (2005). Systematic review and meta-analysis of studies of the timing of tracheostomy in adult patients undergoing artificial ventilation. BMJ 330: 1243.

Gropen TI, Gagliano PJ, Blake CA et al. (2006). Quality improvement in acute stroke: the New York State Stroke Center Designation Project. Neurology 67: 88–93.

Grotta JC, Burgin WS, El-Mitwalli A et al. (2001). Intravenous tissue-type plasminogen activator therapy for ischemic stroke: Houston experience 1996 to 2000. Arch Neurol 58: 2009–2013.

Gunnarsson T, Theodorsson A, Karlsson P et al. (2000). Mobile computerized tomography scanning in the neurosurgery intensive care unit: increase in patient safety and reduction of staff workload. J Neurosurg 93: 432–436.

Hacke W, Kaste M, Fieschi C et al. (1995). Intravenous thrombolysis with recombinant tissue plasminogen activator for acute hemispheric stroke (ECASS). JAMA 274: 1017–1025.

Hacke W, Schwab S, Horn M et al. (1996). 'Malignant' middle cerebral artery territory infarction: clinical course and prognostic signs. Arch Neurol 53: 309–315.

Hacke W, Kaste M, Fieschi C et al. (1998). Randomised double-blind placebo-controlled trial of thrombolytic therapy with intravenous alteplase in acute ischaemic stroke (ECASS II). Lancet 352: 1245–1251.

Hacke W, Donnan G, Fieschi C et al. (2004). Association of outcome with early stroke treatment: pooled analysis of ATLANTIS, ECASS, and NINDS rt-PA stroke trials. Lancet 363: 768–774.

Hacke W, Kaste M, Bluhmki E et al. (2008). Thrombolysis with alteplase 3 to 4.5 hours after acute ischemic stroke. N Engl J Med 359: 1317–1329.

Hajat C, Hajat S, Sharma P (2000). Effects of poststroke pyrexia on stroke outcome : a meta-analysis of studies in patients. Stroke 31: 410–414.

Harloff A, Handke M, Reinhard M et al. (2006). Therapeutic strategies after examination by transesophageal echocardiography in 503 patients with ischemic stroke. Stroke 37: 859–864.

He J, Zhang Y, Xu T et al. (2014). Effects of immediate blood pressure reduction on death and major disability in patients with acute ischemic stroke: the CATIS randomized clinical trial. JAMA 311: 479–489.

Heo JH, Han SW, Lee SK (2005). Free radicals as triggers of brain edema formation after stroke. Free Radic Biol Med 39: 51–70.

Hill MD, Buchan AM (2005). Thrombolysis for acute ischemic stroke: results of the Canadian Alteplase for Stroke Effectiveness Study. CMAJ 172: 1307–1312.

Hill MD, Lye T, Moss H et al. (2003). Hemi-orolingual angioedema and ACE inhibition after alteplase treatment of stroke. Neurology 60: 1525–1527.

Hill MD, Rowley HA, Adler F et al. (2003). Selection of acute ischemic stroke patients for intra-arterial thrombolysis with pro-urokinase by using ASPECTS. Stroke 34: 1925–1931.

Hofmeijer J, Kappelle LJ, Algra A et al. (2009). Surgical decompression for space-occupying cerebral infarction (the Hemicraniectomy After Middle Cerebral Artery infarction with Life-threatening Edema Trial [HAMLET]): a multicentre, open, randomised trial. Lancet Neurol 8: 326–333.

Horn J, de Haan RJ, Vermeulen M et al. (2001). Very Early Nimodipine Use in Stroke (VENUS): a randomized, double-blind, placebo-controlled trial. Stroke 32: 461–465.

Hornig CR, Dorndorf W, Agnoli AL (1986). Hemorrhagic cerebral infarction: a prospective study. Stroke 17: 179–185.

Iglesias Mohedano AM, Garcia Pastor A, Garcia Arratibel A et al. (2015). Factors associated with in-hospital delays in treating acute stroke with intravenous thrombolysis in a tertiary centre. Neurologia (14). http://dx.doi.org/10.1016/j.nrl.2014.12.004. pii: S0213-4853(14)00266-7. (Epub ahead of print).

Indredavik B, Rohweder G, Naalsund E et al. (2008). Medical complications in a comprehensive stroke unit and an early supported discharge service. Stroke 39: 414–420.

International Stroke Trial Collaborative Group (1997). The International Stroke Trial (IST): a randomised trial of aspirin, subcutaneous heparin, both, or neither among 19435 patients with acute ischaemic stroke. Lancet 349: 1569–1581.

Jauch EC, Saver JL, Adams Jr HP et al. (2013). Guidelines for the early management of patients with acute ischemic stroke: a guideline for healthcare professionals from the American Heart Association/American Stroke Association. Stroke 44: 870–947.

Jean WC, Spellman SR, Nussbaum ES et al. (1998). Reperfusion injury after focal cerebral ischemia: the role of inflammation and the therapeutic horizon. Neurosurgery 43: 1382–1396.

Johnston SC, Easton JD, Farrant M et al. (2013). Platelet-oriented inhibition in new TIA and minor ischemic stroke (POINT) trial: rationale and design. Int J Stroke 8: 479–483.

Josephson SA, Dillon WP, Smith WS (2005). Incidence of contrast nephropathy from cerebral CT angiography and CT perfusion imaging. Neurology 64: 1805–1806.

Jovin TG, Chamorro A, Cobo E et al. (2015). Thrombectomy within 8 hours after symptom onset in ischemic stroke. N Engl J Med 372: 2296–2306.

Juttler E, Schwab S, Schmiedek P et al. (2007). Decompressive Surgery for the Treatment of Malignant Infarction of the Middle Cerebral Artery (DESTINY): a randomized, controlled trial. Stroke 38: 2518–2525.

Juttler E, Unterberg A, Woitzik J et al. (2014). Hemicraniectomy in older patients with extensive middle-cerebral-artery stroke. N Engl J Med 370: 1091–1100.

Kaste M, Fogelholm R, Erila T et al. (1994). A randomized, double-blind, placebo-controlled trial of nimodipine in acute ischemic hemispheric stroke. Stroke 25: 1348–1353.

Kellert L, Schrader F, Ringleb P et al. (2014). The impact of low hemoglobin levels and transfusion on critical care patients with severe ischemic stroke (STRAIGHT): an observational study. J Crit Care 29: 236–240.

Kennedy J, Hill MD, Ryckborst KJ et al. (2007). Fast assessment of stroke and transient ischaemic attack to prevent early recurrence (FASTER): a randomised controlled pilot trial. Lancet Neurol 6: 961–969.

Khatri R, McKinney AM, Swenson B et al. (2012). Blood–brain barrier, reperfusion injury, and hemorrhagic transformation in acute ischemic stroke. Neurology 79: 52–57.

Kidwell CS, Saver JL, Mattiello J et al. (2000). Thrombolytic reversal of acute human cerebral ischemic injury shown by diffusion/perfusion magnetic resonance imaging. Ann Neurol 47: 462–469.

Kidwell CS, Chalela JA, Saver JL et al. (2004). Comparison of MRI and CT for detection of acute intracerebral hemorrhage. JAMA 292: 1823–1830.

Kidwell CS, Jahan R, Gornbein J et al. (2013). A trial of imaging selection and endovascular treatment for ischemic stroke. N Engl J Med 368: 914–923.

Kim DH, Cha JK, Bae HJ et al. (2013). Organized comprehensive stroke center is associated with reduced mortality: analysis of consecutive patients in a single hospital. J Stroke 15: 57–63.

Kirkman MA, Citerio G, Smith M (2014). The intensive care management of acute ischemic stroke: an overview. Intensive Care Med 40: 640–653.

Kramer AH, Zygun DA (2009). Anemia and red blood cell transfusion in neurocritical care. Crit Care 13: R89.

Lattimore SU, Chalela J, Davis L et al. (2003). Impact of establishing a primary stroke center at a community hospital on the use of thrombolytic therapy: the NINDS Suburban Hospital Stroke Center experience. Stroke 34: 55–57.

Leal-Noval SR, Munoz-Gomez M, Murillo-Cabezas F (2008). Optimal hemoglobin concentration in patients with subarachnoid hemorrhage, acute ischemic stroke and traumatic brain injury. Curr Opin Crit Care 14: 156–162.

Leonardi-Bee J, Bath PM, Phillips SJ et al. (2002). Blood pressure and clinical outcomes in the International Stroke Trial. Stroke 33: 1315–1320.

Lev MH, Farkas J, Rodriguez VR et al. (2001). CT angiography in the rapid triage of patients with hyperacute stroke to intraarterial thrombolysis: accuracy in the detection of large vessel thrombus. J Comput Assist Tomogr 25: 520–528.

Liebeskind DS (2005). Collaterals in acute stroke: beyond the clot. Neuroimaging Clin N Am 15: 553–573.

Lindsberg PJ, Mattle HP (2006). Therapy of basilar artery occlusion: a systematic analysis comparing intra-arterial and intravenous thrombolysis. Stroke 37: 922–928.

Lip GY, Nieuwlaat R, Pisters R et al. (2010). Refining clinical risk stratification for predicting stroke and thromboembolism in atrial fibrillation using a novel risk factor-based approach: the Euro heart survey on atrial fibrillation. Chest 137: 263–272.

Lovblad KO, Laubach HJ, Baird AE et al. (1998). Clinical experience with diffusion-weighted MR in patients with acute stroke. Am J Neuroradiol 19: 1061–1066.

Manno EM, Nichols DA, Fulgham JR et al. (2003). Computed tomographic determinants of neurologic deterioration in patients with large middle cerebral artery infarctions. Mayo Clin Proc 78: 156–160.

Martino R, Foley N, Bhogal S et al. (2005). Dysphagia after stroke: incidence, diagnosis, and pulmonary complications. Stroke 36: 2756–2763.

Meng Q, He C, Shuaib A et al. (2012). Hyperthermia worsens ischaemic brain injury through destruction of microvessels in an embolic model in rats. Int J Hyperthermia 28: 24–32.

Meschia JF, Bushnell C, Boden-Albala B et al. (2014). Guidelines for the primary prevention of stroke: a statement for healthcare professionals from the American Heart Association/American Stroke Association. Stroke 45: 3754–3832.

Mohr JP, Choi DW, Grotta JC et al. (2004). Stroke: pathophysiology, diagnosis, and management. Elsevier, Philadelphia, PA.

Morikawa E, Ginsberg MD, Dietrich WD et al. (1992). The significance of brain temperature in focal cerebral ischemia: histopathological consequences of middle cerebral artery occlusion in the rat. J Cereb Blood Flow Metab 12: 380–389.

Mozaffarian D, Benjamin EJ, Go AS et al. (2015). Heart disease and stroke statistics 2015 update: a report from the American Heart Association. Circulation 131: 29–322.

Murray CJ, Atkinson C, Bhalla K et al. (2013). The state of US health, 1990–2010: burden of diseases, injuries, and risk factors. JAMA 310: 591–608.

National Institute of Neurological Disorders and Stroke rt-PA Stroke Study Group (1995). Tissue plasminogen activator for acute ischemic stroke. N Engl J Med 333: 1581–1587.

National Institute of Neurological Disorders and Stroke rt-PA Stroke Study Group (1997). Intracerebral hemorrhage after intravenous t-PA therapy for ischemic stroke. Stroke 28: 2109–2118.

Neugebauer H, Juttler E (2014). Hemicraniectomy for malignant middle cerebral artery infarction: current status and future directions. Int J Stroke 9: 460–467.

Nguyen-Huynh MN, Wintermark M, English J et al. (2008). How accurate is CT angiography in evaluating intracranial atherosclerotic disease? Stroke 39: 1184–1188.

Nogueira RG, Lutsep HL, Gupta R et al. (2012). Trevo versus Merci retrievers for thrombectomy revascularisation of large vessel occlusions in acute ischaemic stroke (TREVO 2): a randomised trial. Lancet 380: 1231–1240.

Ntaios G, Lambrou D, Cuendet D et al. (2013). Early major worsening in ischemic stroke: predictors and outcome. Neurocrit Care 19: 287–292.

O'Donnell M, Kearon C (2007). Thromboembolism prevention in ischaemic stroke. Lancet 369: 1413–1415.

Ogata J, Yamanishi H, Pantoni L (2009). Neuropathology of ischemic brain injury. Handb Clin Neurol 92: 93–116.

Okada Y, Yamaguchi T, Minematsu K et al. (1989). Hemorrhagic transformation in cerebral embolism. Stroke 20: 598–603.

Paciaroni M, Agnelli G, Micheli S et al. (2007). Efficacy and safety of anticoagulant treatment in acute cardioembolic stroke: a meta-analysis of randomized controlled trials. Stroke 38: 423–430.

Paciaroni M, Agnelli G, Corea F et al. (2008). Early hemorrhagic transformation of brain infarction: rate, predictive factors, and influence on clinical outcome: results of a prospective multicenter study. Stroke 39: 2249–2256.

Paciaroni M, Agnelli G, Falocci N et al. (2015). Early recurrence and cerebral bleeding in patients with acute ischemic stroke and atrial fibrillation: effect of anticoagulation and its timing: The RAF Study. Stroke 46: 2175–2182.

Patel SC, Levine SR, Tilley BC et al. (2001). Lack of clinical significance of early ischemic changes on computed tomography in acute stroke. JAMA 286: 2830–2838.

Petchy MF, Bounes V, Dehours E et al. (2014). Characteristics of patients with acute ischemic stroke intubated before imaging. Eur J Emerg Med 21: 145–147.

Phillips SJ, Whisnant JP (1992). Hypertension and the brain. Arch Intern Med 152: 938–945.

Phipps MS, Desai RA, Wira C et al. (2011). Epidemiology and outcomes of fever burden among patients with acute ischemic stroke. Stroke 42: 3357–3362.

Powers WJ, Derdeyn CP, Biller J et al. (2015). 2015 American Heart Association/American Stroke Association focused update of the 2013 guidelines for the early management of patients with acute ischemic stroke regarding endovascular treatment: a guideline for healthcare professionals from the American Heart Association/American Stroke Association. Stroke 46: 3020–3035.

Prasad K, Krishnan PR (2010). Fever is associated with doubling of odds of short-term mortality in ischemic stroke: an updated meta-analysis. Acta Neurol Scand 122: 404–408.

Pundik S, Xu K, Sundararajan S (2012). Reperfusion brain injury: focus on cellular bioenergetics. Neurology 79: 44–51.

Quality Standards Subcommittee of the American Academy of Neurology (1996). Practice advisory: thrombolytic therapy for acute ischemic stroke – summary statement. Neurology 47: 835–839.

Rahme R, Zuccarello M, Kleindorfer D et al. (2012). Decompressive hemicraniectomy for malignant middle cerebral artery territory infarction: is life worth living? J Neurosurg 117: 749–754.

Reith J, Jorgensen HS, Pedersen PM et al. (1996). Body temperature in acute stroke: relation to stroke severity, infarct size, mortality, and outcome. Lancet 347: 422–425.

Rincon F, Mayer SA, Rivolta J et al. (2010). Impact of delayed transfer of critically ill stroke patients from the emergency department to the neuro-ICU. Neurocrit Care 13: 75–81.

Rincon F, Morino T, Behrens D et al. (2011). Association between out-of-hospital emergency department transfer and poor hospital outcome in critically ill stroke patients. J Crit Care 26: 620–625.

Robinson TG, Potter JF, Ford GA et al. (2010). Effects of antihypertensive treatment after acute stroke in the Continue or Stop Post-Stroke Antihypertensives Collaborative Study (COSSACS): a prospective, randomised, open, blinded-endpoint trial. Lancet Neurol 9: 767–775.

Rumbak MJ, Newton M, Truncale T et al. (2004). A prospective, randomized, study comparing early percutaneous dilational tracheotomy to prolonged translaryngeal intubation (delayed tracheotomy) in critically ill medical patients. Crit Care Med 32: 1689–1694.

Sandercock PA, Counsell C, Kamal AK (2008). Anticoagulants for acute ischaemic stroke. Cochrane Database Syst Rev. CD 000024.

Sandset EC, Bath PM, Boysen G et al. (2011). The angiotensin-receptor blocker candesartan for treatment of acute stroke (SCAST): a randomised, placebo-controlled, double-blind trial. Lancet 377: 741–750.

Saver JL, Jahan R, Levy EI et al. (2012). Solitaire flow restoration device versus the Merci Retriever in patients with acute ischaemic stroke (SWIFT): a randomised, parallel-group, non-inferiority trial. Lancet 380: 1241–1249.

Saver JL, Goyal M, Bonafe A et al. (2015). Stent-retriever thrombectomy after intravenous t-PA vs. t-PA alone in stroke. N Engl J Med 372: 2285–2295.

Schonewille WJ, Wijman CA, Michel P et al. (2009). Treatment and outcomes of acute basilar artery occlusion in the Basilar Artery International Cooperation Study (BASICS): a prospective registry study. Lancet Neurol 8: 724–730.

Schwab S, Steiner T, Aschoff A et al. (1998). Early hemicraniectomy in patients with complete middle cerebral artery infarction. Stroke 29: 1888–1893.

Sherman DG, Albers GW, Bladin C et al. (2007). The efficacy and safety of enoxaparin versus unfractionated heparin for the prevention of venous thromboembolism after acute ischaemic stroke (PREVAIL study): an open-label randomised comparison. Lancet 369: 1347–1355.

Sheth KN, Sims JR (2012). Neurocritical care and periprocedural blood pressure management in acute stroke. Neurology 79: 199–204.

Sheth KN, Smith EE, Grau-Sepulveda MV et al. (2015). Drip and ship thrombolytic therapy for acute ischemic stroke: use, temporal trends, and outcomes. Stroke 46: 732–739.

Shin HK, Nishimura M, Jones PB et al. (2008). Mild induced hypertension improves blood flow and oxygen metabolism in transient focal cerebral ischemia. Stroke 39: 1548–1555.

Simard JM, Kent TA, Chen M et al. (2007). Brain oedema in focal ischaemia: molecular pathophysiology and theoretical implications. Lancet Neurol 6: 258–268.

Singer OC, Berkefeld J, Nolte CH et al. (2015). Mechanical recanalization in basilar artery occlusion: the ENDOSTROKE study. Ann Neurol 77: 415–424.

Skutta B, Furst G, Eilers J et al. (1999). Intracranial stenoocclusive disease: double-detector helical CT angiography versus digital subtraction angiography. Am J Neuroradiol 20: 791–799.

Smith WS, Tsao JW, Billings ME et al. (2006). Prognostic significance of angiographically confirmed large vessel intracranial occlusion in patients presenting with acute brain ischemia. Neurocrit Care 4: 14–17.

Strbian D, Sairanen T, Silvennoinen H et al. (2013). Thrombolysis of basilar artery occlusion: impact of baseline ischemia and time. Ann Neurol 73: 688–694.

Sussman ES, Connolly Jr ES (2013). Hemorrhagic transformation: a review of the rate of hemorrhage in the major clinical trials of acute ischemic stroke. Front Neurol 4: 69.

Tai YJ, Weir L, Hand P et al. (2012). Does a 'code stroke' rapid access protocol decrease door-to-needle time for thrombolysis? Intern Med J 42: 1316–1324.

Tan S, Wang D, Liu M et al. (2014). Frequency and predictors of spontaneous hemorrhagic transformation in ischemic stroke and its association with prognosis. J Neurol 261: 905–912.

Tarlov N, Nien YL, Zaidat OO et al. (2012). Periprocedural management of acute ischemic stroke intervention. Neurology 79: 182–191.

Tekle WG, Chaudhry SA, Hassan AE et al. (2012). Drip-and-ship thrombolytic treatment paradigm among acute ischemic stroke patients in the United States. Stroke 43: 1971–1974.

Titsworth WL, Hester J, Correia T et al. (2012). The effect of increased mobility on morbidity in the neurointensive care unit. J Neurosurg 116: 1379–1388.

Tomsick T, Brott T, Barsan W et al. (1996). Prognostic value of the hyperdense middle cerebral artery sign and stroke scale score before ultraearly thrombolytic therapy. Am J Neuroradiol 17: 79–85.

Toni D, Fiorelli M, Bastianello S et al. (1996). Hemorrhagic transformation of brain infarct: predictability in the first 5 hours from stroke onset and influence on clinical outcome. Neurology 46: 341–345.

Vahedi K, Hofmeijer J, Juettler E et al. (2007a). Early decompressive surgery in malignant infarction of the middle cerebral artery: a pooled analysis of three randomised controlled trials. Lancet Neurol 6: 215–222.

Vahedi K, Vicaut E, Mateo J et al. (2007b). Sequential-design, multicenter, randomized, controlled trial of early decompressive craniectomy in malignant middle cerebral artery infarction (DECIMAL trial). Stroke 38: 2506–2517.

van Swieten JC, Koudstaal PJ, Visser MC et al. (1988). Interobserver agreement for the assessment of handicap in stroke patients. Stroke 19: 604–607.

Varelas PN, Schultz L, Conti M et al. (2008). The impact of a neuro-intensivist on patients with stroke admitted to a neurosciences intensive care unit. Neurocrit Care 9: 293–299.

Villwock JA, Villwock MR, Deshaies EM (2014). Tracheostomy timing affects stroke recovery. J Stroke Cerebrovasc Dis 23: 1069–1072.

Wang Y, Wang Y, Zhao X et al. (2013). Clopidogrel with aspirin in acute minor stroke or transient ischemic attack. N Engl J Med 369: 11–19.

Wijdicks EF, Sheth KN, Carter BS et al. (2014). Recommendations for the management of cerebral and cerebellar infarction with swelling: a statement for healthcare professionals from the American Heart Association/American Stroke Association. Stroke 45: 1222–1238.

Williams LS, Rotich J, Qi R et al. (2002). Effects of admission hyperglycemia on mortality and costs in acute ischemic stroke. Neurology 59: 67–71.

Wintermark M, Flanders AE, Velthuis B et al. (2006). Perfusion-CT assessment of infarct core and penumbra: receiver operating characteristic curve analysis in 130 patients suspected of acute hemispheric stroke. Stroke 37: 979–985.

Wintermark M, Albers GW, Alexandrov AV et al. (2008). Acute stroke imaging research roadmap. Stroke 39: 1621–1628.

Xian Y, Holloway RG, Chan PS et al. (2011). Association between stroke center hospitalization for acute ischemic stroke and mortality. JAMA 305: 373–380.

Yepes M, Roussel BD, Ali C et al. (2009). Tissue-type plasminogen activator in the ischemic brain: more than a thrombolytic. Trends Neurosci 32: 48–55.

Yi Y, Yang EJ, Kim J et al. (2012). Predictive factors for removal of percutaneous endoscopic gastrostomy tube in post-stroke dysphagia. J Rehabil Med 44: 922–925.

Zhu HF, Newcommon NN, Cooper ME et al. (2009). Impact of a stroke unit on length of hospital stay and in-hospital case fatality. Stroke 40: 18–23.

*Handbook of Clinical Neurology*, Vol. 140 (3rd series)
*Critical Care Neurology, Part I*
E.F.M. Wijdicks and A.H. Kramer, Editors
http://dx.doi.org/10.1016/B978-0-444-63600-3.00011-8

Chapter 11

# Management of intracerebral hemorrhage

A.M. THABET[1], M. KOTTAPALLY[2], AND J. CLAUDE HEMPHILL III[1]*

[1]*Department of Neurology, University of California, San Francisco, CA, USA*

[2]*Department of Neurology, University of Miami, Miami, FL, USA*

## Abstract

Intracerebral hemorrhage (ICH) is a potentially devastating neurologic injury representing 10–15% of stroke cases in the USA each year. Numerous risk factors, including age, hypertension, male gender, coagulopathy, genetic susceptibility, and ethnic descent, have been identified. Timely identification, workup, and management of this condition remain a challenge for clinicians as numerous factors can present obstacles to achieving good functional outcomes. Several large clinical trials have been conducted over the prior decade regarding medical and surgical interventions. However, no specific treatment has shown a major impact on clinical outcome. Current management guidelines do exist based on medical evidence and consensus and these provide a framework for care. While management of hypertension and coagulopathy are generally considered basic tenets of ICH management, a variety of measures for surgical hematoma evacuation, intracranial pressure control, and intraventricular hemorrhage can be further pursued in the emergent setting for selected patients. The complexity of management in parenchymal cerebral hemorrhage remains challenging and offers many areas for further investigation. A systematic approach to the background, pathology, and early management of spontaneous parenchymal hemorrhage is provided.

## INTRODUCTION

Intracerebral hemorrhage (ICH) is a potentially devastating neurologic injury representing 10–15% of stroke cases in the USA each year. Timely identification, workup, and management of this condition remain a challenge for clinicians as numerous factors can present obstacles to achieving good functional outcomes. Current management guidelines do exist based on medical evidence and consensus and these provide a framework for care. While management of hypertension and coagulopathy are generally considered basic tenets of ICH management, a variety of measures for surgical hematoma evacuation, intracranial pressure (ICP) control, and intraventricular hemorrhage (IVH) can be further pursued in the emergent setting for selected patients. A systematic approach to the background, pathology, and early management of spontaneous parenchymal hemorrhage is provided.

## EPIDEMIOLOGY

ICH represents 10–15% of all 700 000 strokes in the USA every year (Qureshi et al., 2001). The incidence of ICH is estimated to be 24.6 cases per 100 000 person-years (van Asch et al., 2010); incidence increases with age (relative risk increase of 1.97 per decade) (Ariesen et al., 2003) and is expected to rise with the increase in the overall population age (Qureshi et al., 2001). African American and Asian people have a higher incidence of ICH (relative risk 1.89 for African Americans) (Sturgeon et al., 2007), possibly due to the higher incidence of hypertension and cerebrovascular anomalies respectively in these ethnicities (Gunel et al., 1996). Male gender is associated with a higher incidence of ICH and with deep more than lobar ICH, possibly due to the higher incidence of hypertension (Labovitz et al., 2005). The risk of recurrence of ICH is higher in cases associated with cerebral amyloid angiopathy (CAA) (10–20% per year and tripled in cases of

*Correspondence to: J. Claude Hemphill III, M.D., M.A.S., Department of Neurology, Building 1, Room 101, San Francisco General Hospital, 1001 Potrero Avenue, San Francisco CA 94939, USA. Tel: +1-415-206-3213, Fax: +1-415-206-4055, E-mail: claude.hemphill@ucsf.edu

apolipoprotein 4 gene E2 and E4 alleles) (O'Donnell et al., 2000) as compared to cases associated with hypertension (less than 2% per year, if hypertension is well controlled) (Hypertension Detection and Follow-up Program Cooperative Group, 1982). ICH is one of the most devastating medical emergencies, with long-term functional independence achieved in only 12–39% of cases and mortality rates of 40% at 1 month and 54% at 1 year (van Asch et al., 2010). Large retrospective cohort studies in the USA and UK have shown a significant improvement in mortality rates since 2000 (Liotta and Prabhakaran, 2013), although a meta-analysis of studies between 1980 and 2008 did not show a significant difference in those rates (Gonzalez-Perez et al., 2013). The aggregate lifetime cost of first ICH in the USA in 1990 was estimated to be $6.0 billion and the lifetime cost per person of first ICH in the same year was estimated to be $123 565 (Taylor et al., 1996).

## NEUROPATHOLOGY

Hypertension is the most common risk factor for primary ICH, accounting for 60–70% of all cases (McCormick and Rosenfield, 1973) (relative risk 3.68 and an increase with the worsening in the degree of hypertension) (Ariesen et al., 2003). Chronic hypertension leads to lipohyalinosis, a process of fibroblast proliferation, macrophage deposition, and smooth-muscle cell replacement with collagen in the wall of deep small arterioles, leading to reduced elasticity and increased spontaneous rupture susceptibility (Fisher, 1971). Common locations for hypertension-related ICH are the putamen (46% of all ICH patients), thalamus (18%), caudate (4%), pons (13%), and cerebellum (4%) (Fig. 11.1) (Ziai, 2013).

CAA is the second most common risk factor for primary ICH (Fig. 11.2). It is a process involving β-amyloid peptide deposition in the wall of cortical

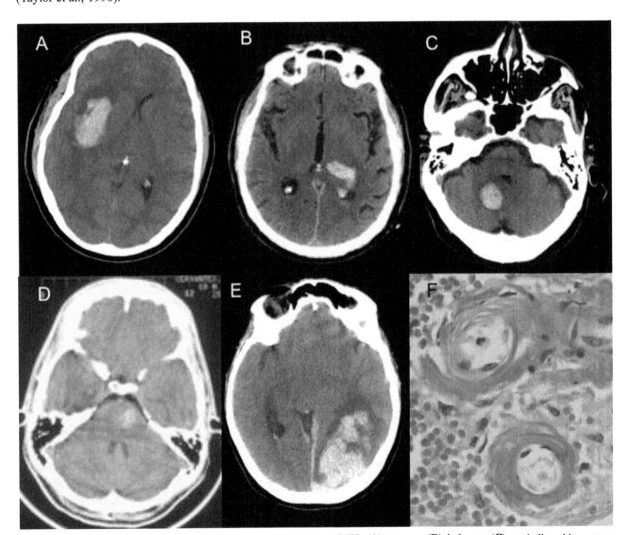

**Fig. 11.1.** Typical locations for hypertensive intracerebral hemorrhage (ICH). (**A**) putamen; (**B**) thalamus; (**C**) cerebellar white matter; (**D**) pontine tegmentum; (**E**) lobar white matter. (**F**) Hematoxylin and eosin photomicrograph demonstrating lipohyalinosis of small penetrating arteries that weaken the arterial wall and are the source of typical hypertensive ICH. (**F**, courtesy of Han Lee, M.D., Ph.D. and Andrew W. Bollen, M.D., D.V.M., UCSF Neuropathology.) (Reproduced from Elijovich et al., 2008, with permission.)

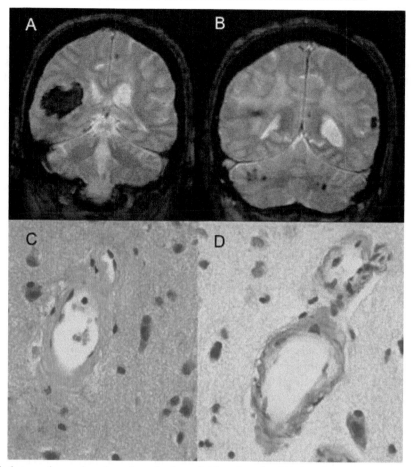

**Fig. 11.2.** Histopathology and neuroimaging of cerebral amyloid angiopathy (CAA). (**A, B**) Magnetic resonance imaging T2 susceptibility-weighted images demonstrating a parieto-occipital lobar hemorrhage with several asymptomatic microhemorrhages scattered throughout the cerebral and cerebellar hemispheres. (**C**) Hematoxylin and eosin photomicrograph of a cerebral arteriole demonstrating medial thickening secondary to amyloid deposition. (**D**) Congo red staining of β-amyloid deposition in the media diagnostic of CAA. (**C, D** courtesy of Han Lee, M.D., Ph.D. and Andrew W. Bollen, M.D., D.V.M., UCSF Neuropathology). (Reproduced from Elijovich et al., 2008, with permission.)

small arterioles (Greenberg and Vonsattel, 1997), leading to lobar ICH most commonly (9% of all ICH patients) (Ziai, 2013) and microhemorrhages. Common locations for CAA-related ICH are the occipital lobes, followed by the frontal, temporal, and parietal lobes. CAA is a disease of the elderly and is the most common risk factor for lobar ICH in patients >70 years (Charidimou et al., 2012).

Coagulopathy is a common risk factor for primary ICH. A total of 6.6% of ICH patients in the USA from 2005 to 2008 were using warfarin (Liotta and Prabhakaran, 2013). New oral anticoagulants have a lower risk of ICH than warfarin; apixaban is the most favorable, with a bleeding risk approaching that of aspirin. The combination of aspirin plus clopidogrel has a lower risk of ICH than warfarin and aspirin alone has a lower risk of major hemorrhage than aspirin plus clopidogrel (Culebras et al., 2014). Although low levels of

both low-density lipoproteins and triglycerides as well as high-dose statin therapy have been thought to be risk factors for the occurrence of primary ICH (Amarenco et al., 2006; Sturgeon et al., 2007), a recent retrospective cohort study of 3481 patients with ICH found that cessation of statin use was associated with worse outcomes in acute ICH patients (Flint et al., 2014). Heavy alcohol intake and sympathomimetic drug abuse are also risk factors for primary ICH (Thrift et al., 1999; Elijovich et al., 2008). Further differential diagnoses for secondary ICH include vascular malformations (arteriovenous malformation, dural arteriovenous fistula, cavernous malformation, and aneurysm), hemorrhagic conversion of ischemic stroke, dural sinus thrombosis, moyamoya disease, vasculitis, and tumors (Elijovich et al., 2008).

The primary injury from ICH is mostly due to direct brain tissue damage from the initial hematoma following blood vessel rupture, with larger hematoma volume being associated with worse outcomes (Broderick et al., 1993). Secondary injury can follow the primary one and lead to further neurologic deterioration. The secondary injury can be due to hematoma expansion (defined in many studies as growth >33% of the initial volume). This is a common occurrence and has been reported in 38% of patients within 3 hours after the time of symptom onset and 26% of patients within 1 hour after initial computed tomography (CT) scan (Brott et al., 1997) as well as 50% of patients on anticoagulation (Flibotte et al., 2004). The higher volume of hematoma expansion is associated with worse outcomes (Davis et al., 2006). Although the precise mechanism of hematoma expansion is unclear, it may be attributable to persistent bleeding or rebleeding from the initial blood vessel rupture or new foci of bleeding at the periphery of the lesion, often attributed to ischemia, poor venous flow, and local coagulopathy (due to release of plasmin and fibrin degradation products) (Mayer et al., 1998; Mayer, 2003).

Additional mechanisms of secondary injury that are being increasingly appreciated are perihematomal edema and inflammation. These may develop as early as 1 hour after ICH, show peak growth by 7 days, may last for weeks postinjury, and have been associated with worse outcomes (Gebel et al., 2002; Staykov et al., 2011). The causes for these are likely multifactorial and include blood–brain barrier damage, lysis of red blood cells, and white blood cell recruitment, in addition to release of plasma proteins, thrombin, hemoglobin, iron, matrix metalloproteinases, interleukins, and other inflammatory mediators (Power et al., 2003; Butcher et al., 2004; Xi et al., 2006; Levine et al., 2007; Tejima et al., 2007; Wagner, 2007; Ziai, 2013).

## CLINICAL PRESENTATION

ICH patients usually present with a sudden onset of focal neurologic deficits, often associated with symptoms and signs of elevated ICP, including headache, nausea, vomiting, hypertension, tachycardia or bradycardia, and decreased level of consciousness which may progress into coma from cerebral herniation (Elijovich et al., 2008). More than 20% of ICH patients will deteriorate by 2 or more points in their Glasgow Coma Scale (GCS) score between initial assessment by emergency medical services (EMS) and arrival to an emergency department (ED) (Moon et al., 2008). Another 15–23% of patients will continue to deteriorate within the first few hours of their hospitalization (Fan et al., 2012). It is therefore critical that rapid assessment, diagnosis, and management of ICH

patients occur without delay. A focused medical history should include time of symptom onset, symptom progression, screening for risk factors, as mentioned above, as well as recent trauma or surgery (Hemphill et al., 2015). General localization of clinical findings may be important for early triage and assessment; however, the most important distinction in this regard is to identify cerebellar ICH, since these patients may require particularly early surgical hematoma evacuation. In addition to a focused neurologic examination, standardized disease severity scores such as the GCS, National Institutes of Health Stroke Scale, and the ICH Score should be utilized to help facilitate clear communication between medical providers (Hemphill et al., 2015).

## NEURODIAGNOSTICS AND IMAGING

Initial laboratory workup includes a complete blood count, coagulation profile, basic metabolic panel, cardiac troponin, and a toxicology screen. Blood cultures are appropriate if endocarditis is considered. An electrocardiogram should also be done to rule out associated cardiac injury (Hemphill et al., 2015). In addition, a pregnancy test should be performed for all female patients of childbearing age.

While sudden onset of symptoms is usually suggestive of a vascular etiology, it is almost impossible to reliably differentiate between ICH and ischemic infarct based on clinical presentation only (Andrews et al., 2012). Though symptoms of elevated ICP are usually suggestive of ICH, they are not specific enough to definitely diagnose ICH without imaging (e.g., headache can be present in 30% of acute ischemic stroke patients) (Tentschert et al., 2005). Neuroimaging studies have made the diagnosis of ICH straightforward and should not be delayed as time from symptom onset to initial neuroimaging study correlates with mortality rates (Falcone et al., 2013; Hemphill et al., 2015). CT without contrast is the most commonly used initial study to diagnose ICH due to its wide availability and high sensitivity and specificity (Fiebach et al., 2004). Magnetic resonance imaging (MRI) without contrast (gradient echo and T2* susceptibility-weighted sequences) is another reasonable alternative due to its high sensitivity and specificity for ICH, but its use is limited by availability, duration, and often poor tolerance by critically ill hyperacute patients (Fiebach et al., 2004; Singer et al., 2004; Chalela et al., 2007).

MRI is more sensitive than CT for old cortical or subcortical microhemorrhages consistent with CAA. The burden of these cerebral microbleeds has been associated with increased risk of hematoma expansion and ICH recurrence (Marti-Fabregas et al., 2013). According to the Boston Criteria for CAA-related ICH, a definitive diagnosis of CAA can only be made after a postmortem examination showing severe CAA with vasculopathy. A diagnosis of probable CAA can be made in patients with multiple cortical or subcortical hemorrhages, who are 55 years or older, and with no other cause of ICH. A diagnosis of possible CAA can be made in patients with a single lobar, cortical, or cortical/subcortical hemorrhage without another cause, who are 55 years or older, and with no other cause of ICH (Knudsen et al., 2001).

CT and MRI can also evaluate hematoma location, volume, mass effect, perihematomal edema, IVH, and hydrocephalus. Because hematoma volume is a strong predictor of outcome and hematoma expansion is a common occurrence, the ability to quickly assess hematoma volume is strongly desired. While planimetric computerized methods can be used, hematoma volume can be "hand calculated" quite accurately using the ABC/2 method to estimate the volume of a spheroid (Kothari et al., 1996; Hussein et al., 2013). In the ABC/2 method, three dimensions of the hematoma are estimated and used in a calculation. A is the maximum diameter of the hematoma on a reference axial slice that appears to have the largest hematoma area. B is the maximum hematoma diameter perpendicular to A on this slice, and C is the number of slices of hematoma in the vertical plane multiplied by slice thickness. In order to appropriately consider the hematoma as a spheroid rather than a cube, slices for the C dimension which are < 25% in hematoma area of the reference slice are ignored, those 25–75% of the reference slice are considered as a half-slice, and those > 75% are considered a full slice (Chan and Hemphill, 2014) (Fig. 11.3).

Contrast extravasation within the hematoma ("spot sign") is a radiographic finding that can help identify high-risk patients, having been shown to have a 60% association with hematoma expansion (Rizos et al., 2013; Hemphill et al., 2015) (Fig. 11.4).

Large hematoma volume and a heterogeneous pattern can also be predictive of potential expansion (Barras et al., 2013; Takeda et al., 2013). Repeat imaging can show delayed findings up to 72 hours from time of symptom onset (Maas et al., 2013) and should be performed routinely as well as in the setting of clinical neurologic deterioration. The timing and number of scans are usually individualized, based on the clinical presentation and findings on initial imaging. ICH cases without a clear primary inciting factor (hypertension, coagulopathy) should be further investigated for secondary causes including vascular malformations, neoplasm, and infectious etiologies. This is often pursued through contrast-based imaging, including CT, MRI, or formal cerebral angiography (Hemphill et al., 2015). CT angiography

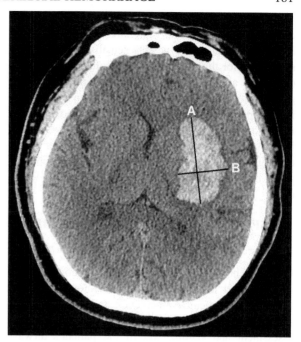

**Fig. 11.3.** Acute left basal ganglia hematoma measured by the ABC/2 method. A is 6 cm, B is 4 cm, and C is 3 cm (hematoma is seen on 12 slices (10 full and four half) with a slice thickness of 0.25 cm). Hematoma volume is 36 cc ($(6 \times 4 \times 3)/2$).

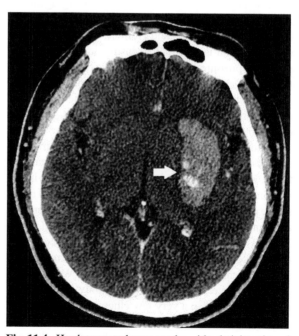

**Fig. 11.4.** Head computed tomography with administration of intravenous contrast demonstrating two spot signs (at tip of white arrow) due to contrast extravasation into an acute left basal ganglia hematoma.

and venography are the most commonly used vascular neuroimaging studies as they are widely available, noninvasive, and have a 97% sensitivity and 98.9% specificity for the diagnosis of vascular abnormalities (Wong et al., 2012). However, conventional angiography should always be considered when a high clinical suspicion remains despite negative noninvasive radiographic workup (Hemphill et al., 2015). Delayed MRI (often with contrast) can show utility in determining etiologies for ICH that may not be apparent given initial hematoma volume on presentation (Wong et al., 2012).

## HOSPITAL COURSE AND MANAGEMENT

### Prehospital management

In the prehospital setting the differentiation between ischemic and hemorrhagic stroke cannot be reliably made. ICH is a medical emergency, and first responders should follow well-established guidelines for immediate assessment and stabilization of the patient's airway, breathing, and circulatory function before management options are considered.

Rapid-sequence intubation is often pursued due to the risk of early neurologic decline and is appropriate when consciousness is threatened. Propofol and etomidate are preferred induction agents in this setting due to their relatively short half-lives (Diringer, 1993; Lummel et al., 2012). Nondepolarizing neuromuscular paralytics (e.g., rocuronium) are preferred over depolarizing agents in order to minimize risk of ICP elevation and hyperkalemia (Booij, 2001; Reynolds and Heffner, 2005). Avoidance of hypotension is essential to ensure adequate cerebral perfusion pressure (CPP), with the use of isotonic solutions and vasopressors as needed. Dextrose-containing solutions should be avoided, considering the association of hyperglycemia with worse outcomes (Passero et al., 2003).

Following initial stabilization, emergency medical services providers should obtain a focused medical history as mentioned above, including family contact information, and notify the receiving ED of the potential acute stroke patient in order to allow them to start the appropriate acute stroke management pathway (Hemphill et al., 2015). Getting a prehospital CT scan in a CT-equipped ambulance has the potential to help triage potential acute stroke patients faster (Walter et al., 2010; Weber et al., 2013). However, this technology is only beginning to become available in a very few cities worldwide. Acute stroke patients should be transferred to an ED with the resources to treat them or to transfer them to a stroke center, but management of urgent issues such as hypertension or coagulopathy should be undertaken in the presenting ED and not be delayed pending patient transfer. Telemedicine may help provide expert consultation for the initial management of these patients until they are transferred to a stroke center (Schwamm et al., 2009; Angileri et al., 2012).

### Management of hypertension

Hypertension is a common finding during the initial presentation of ICH (Qureshi et al., 2007) and in some studies has been associated with hematoma expansion and worse outcomes (Rodriguez-Luna et al., 2013; Sakamoto et al., 2013). While it was initially thought that there may be a perihematomal ischemic penumbra that could be worsened by lowering the blood pressure, numerous studies have found that ischemia is not the major mechanism of perihematomal injury (Mayer et al., 1998; Siddique et al., 2000; Kidwell et al., 2001). Acute blood pressure lowering therefore appears to be generally safe in most patients (Anderson et al., 2008; Qureshi et al., 2010; Sakamoto et al., 2013). The Intensive Blood Pressure Reduction in Acute Cerebral Hemorrhage 2 (INTERACT2) trial was a phase III randomized clinical trial of acute blood pressure lowering in ICH. It enrolled 2794 ICH patients with a systolic blood pressure (SBP) 150–220 mmHg, within 6 hours from time of symptom onset, and evaluated the efficacy of targeting an SBP goal of less than 140 mmHg with an SBP goal less than 180 mmHg. Treatment was for 7 days and used an antihypertensive agent of the treatment physician's choosing. The primary outcome was severe disability, defined as a score of 3–6 on the modified Rankin Scale (mRS). An additional prespecified analysis looked at the entire ordinal analysis of the mRS. Overall there were slightly better functional outcomes in the group of patients with an SBP goal of less than 140 mmHg and this was statistically significant in the ordinal analysis of the entire mRS. There was no difference in adverse events or hematoma expansion between groups (Anderson et al., 2013). Antihypertensive Treatment of Acute Cerebral Hemorrhage II (ATACH II) is a similar multicenter blood pressure-lowering trial funded by the National Institutes of Health. Differences from INTERACT2 include that ATACH II uses intravenous (IV) nicardipine as the sole blood pressure-lowering agent and that the treatment phase is for only 24 hours. Enrollment has been completed but results are not available at the time of this writing (Qureshi and Palesch, 2011).

The current 2015 American Heart Association/ American Stroke Association (AHA/ASA) guidelines for the management of spontaneous ICH recommend targeting an SBP goal of less than 140 mmHg for ICH patients with a presenting SBP between 150 and 220 mmHg and no contraindication for treatment. This is considered safe and can improve functional outcome.

(Hemphill et al., 2015). Short-acting IV beta-blockers (e.g., labetalol) and calcium channel blockers (e.g., nicardipine) are preferred in the initial stages of management. Antihypertensives that cause significant venodilation, impaired autoregulation, and ICP elevation such as hydralazine and nitrates should be avoided (Elijovich et al., 2008). Early arterial line placement for close blood pressure monitoring is frequently required for careful titration of antihypertensive therapy (Honner et al., 2011).

## Management of coagulopathy

Coagulopathy is a common risk factor for primary ICH and is associated with worse outcomes, commonly in the setting of the use of vitamin K antagonists (VKAs) such as warfarin ((Flibotte et al., 2004; Rosand et al., 2004; Liotta and Prabhakaran, 2013). Other causes of coagulopathy include new oral anticoagulants (NOACs) such as dabigatran (direct thrombin inhibitor), rivaroxaban, apixaban, and edoxaban (anti-Xa), heparin, congenital or acquired coagulation factor deficiencies, and liver disease. Antiplatelet agents as well as platelet deficiency and dysfunction may also create a coagulopathic state (Hemphill et al., 2015). The risk for ICH occurrence and expansion is higher with warfarin and the NOAC than with antiplatelet agents (Culebras et al., 2014).

Table 11.1 summarizes the 2015 AHA/ASA guidelines for reversal of coagulopathy in ICH patients. For VKA-related ICH in which the international normalized ratio (INR) is elevated, several agents such as IV vitamin K, fresh frozen plasma (FFP), and recombinant activated factor VIIa (rFVIIa) have previously been used for reversal of coagulopathy, but all have significant disadvantages. The efficacy of IV vitamin K peaks at 24 hours, thus it is poor for urgent coagulopathy reversal. In rare cases it may also cause an allergic reaction (Dentali et al., 2006). FFP takes time to cross-match and thaw and large volumes may be needed to fully correct an elevated INR; FFP also carries a risk of blood-borne infection (Goldstein et al., 2006). rFVIIa does not replenish all of the vitamin K-dependent factors and this may lead to a normalized INR on laboratory testing, even if coagulopathy is not actually corrected and bleeding continues (Tanaka et al., 2008). Prothrombin complex concentrates (PCCs) are now the generally preferred approach to VKA coagulopathy reversal. There are various preparations of PCC, some of which include primarily three factors (II, IX, and X) and more recent preparations that include four factors (II, VII, IX, and X). PCCs can be reconstituted quickly, given in small volume intravenously, and correct the INR rapidly (Riess et al., 2007; Leissinger et al., 2008; Pabinger et al., 2008). Four-factor PCC is preferred. Even so, there have not been

*Table 11.1*

**Summary of the 2015 American Heart Association/American Stroke Association intracerebral hemorrhage guidelines for reversal of coagulopathy (Hemphill et al., 2015)**

| Etiology of coagulopathy | Management |
| --- | --- |
| VKA and elevated INR | Vitamin K-dependent factor replacement for INR correction and IV vitamin K. PCCs are favored over FFP. rFVIIa is not recommended |
| Dabigatran, rivaroxaban, or apixaban | PCCs, FEIBA, or rFVIIa might be used on an individual basis. Activated charcoal might be used if the last dose was taken within 2 hours. Hemodialysis might be used for dabigatran |
| Heparin | Protamine sulfate might be used |
| Antiplatelets | Platelet transfusion use is uncertain |
| Severe coagulation factor deficiency or thrombocytopenia | Appropriate coagulation factor or platelet replacement respectively |

VKA, vitamin K antagonist; INR, international normalized ratio; IV, intravenous; PCC, prothrombin complex concentrate; FFP, fresh frozen plasma; rFVIIa, recombinant factor VIIa; FEIBA, factor VIII inhibitor bypassing activity.

prospective randomized clinical trials that have assessed whether PCC (over FFP) or even coagulopathy correction at all clearly improves clinical outcomes (Fredriksson et al., 1992; Cartmill et al., 2000; Sjoblom et al., 2001). However, given the morbidity of coagulopathy-related ICH, correction is recommended. Guidelines thus recommend that, for VKA-related ICH, either PCC or FFP should be given (generally favoring PCC) and that IV vitamin K should also be given concurrently in order to avoid rebound coagulopathy. The ideal goal INR is not clear, but commonly used goals are to correct the INR to less than 1.3, and certainly less than 1.5 (Hemphill et al., 2015). Recombinant factor VIIa is not recommended.

A recent large cohort study found that the combination of SBP below 160 mmHg and reversal of an elevated INR to below 1.3 within 4 hours of admission were associated with reduced rates of hematoma enlargement in VKA-related ICH (Kuramatsu et al., 2015). This suggests that aggressive intervention for both elevated blood pressure and coagulopathy correction may interact to limit hematoma expansion more than either intervention individually. This also sets a time benchmark for coagulopathy reversal that is reasonable to target.

There are limited data regarding reversal of coagulopathy related to NOACs (Majeed and Schulman, 2013). Of note, half-lives of the various NOACs range between 5 and 15 hours (Hemphill et al., 2015). PCCs, factor VIII inhibitor bypassing activity, and rFVIIa may be considered on an individual basis in these cases. Activated charcoal may be considered if the last dose of the NOAC was taken within 2 hours and hemodialysis may be considered in cases of dabigatran (Kaatz et al., 2012; Hemphill et al., 2015).

Antidotes for NOACs are currently being developed. The efficacy and safety of idarucizumab, a monoclonal antibody directed against dabigatran, were recently evaluated in a prospective cohort study of 90 patients with serious bleeding or requiring an urgent procedure. Idarucizumab normalized dilute thrombin time and/or ecarin clotting time in 88–98% of patients within minutes. It restored hemostasis in patients with serious bleeding at a median of 11.4 hours and maintained it in 33 out of 36 patients who had an urgent procedure. Only one thrombotic event within 72 hours was reported (Pollack et al., 2015).

In cases of heparin-related ICH, protamine sulfate should be considered for reversal of coagulopathy (Hemphill et al., 2015), especially if heparin was administered within the previous 4 hours or low-molecular-weight heparin (LMWH) within 8 hours. Reversal may be incomplete in cases of LMWH (Andrews et al., 2012). Regarding antiplatelet agents, studies have found differing results regarding their impact on hematoma expansion and clinical outcome (Broderick, 2009; Naidech et al., 2009a, c; Sansing et al., 2009; Campbell et al., 2011). Overall, antiplatelet agents such as aspirin and clopidogrel probably worsen hematoma expansion in patients with acute ICH, but to a lesser degree than warfarin or NOACs. It remains unclear whether strategies to improve platelet function in acute ICH patients, such as platelet transfusion or administration of desmopressin, lessen hematoma expansion or improve clinical outcome in ICH patients who have been receiving antiplatelet medications. The efficacy of platelet transfusion in cases of antiplatelet-associated ICH is being considered for evaluation in randomized clinical trials (de Gans et al., 2010). In cases of severe coagulation factor deficiency or thrombocytopenia-related ICH, the appropriate coagulation factor or platelets should be replaced respectively (Hemphill et al., 2015).

The use of hemostatic agents has also been studied in noncoagulopathic ICH patients in order to target a decrease in hematoma expansion. Recombinant factor VIIa was studied in the Factor Seven for Acute Hemorrhagic Stroke (FAST) phase III randomized trial. FAST enrolled 841 nonanticoagulation-related ICH patients within 4 hours from time of symptom onset. It compared the efficacy of rFVIIa versus placebo on improving severe disability and mortality rates (mRS 5–6) at 90 days. There were no differences in severe disability or mortality rates between the two groups even though rFVIIa did reduce hematoma expansion (Mayer et al., 2008). Therefore, rFVIIa is not recommended in these cases (Hemphill et al., 2015) (Table 11.2).

## Management of seizures

There are variable data regarding the incidence and impact of seizures associated with ICH. Several studies have shown that clinical and especially electrographic seizures are common in ICH (Bladin et al., 2000; Passero et al., 2002; Vespa et al., 2003; Claassen et al., 2007; Szaflarski et al., 2008; Beghi et al., 2011; De Herdt et al., 2011). Seizures are more common early after ICH and with cortical hematomas (Bladin et al., 2000; Passero et al., 2002). Therefore, guidelines recommend that ICH patients with an unexpected decreased level of consciousness should be screened for electrographic seizures with continuous electroencephalographic monitoring (Hemphill et al., 2015). Some studies have found that seizures in the setting of acute ICH do not negatively affect outcomes (Passero et al., 2002; Vespa et al., 2003; Mullen et al., 2013), while others have found that they were associated with worse outcomes (De Herdt et al., 2011; Mullen et al., 2013). Likewise, studies of the impact of anticonvulsant medications in ICH have had conflicting results. Findings have included that antiepileptic drugs (AEDs) did not influence outcome (Battey et al., 2012), that they reduced seizures in lobar ICH only (Vespa et al., 2003), and that they were associated with worse outcomes (Messe et al., 2009; Naidech et al., 2009b). The 2015 AHA/ASA ICH guidelines recommend against prophylactic AEDs, but do recommend that clinical and electrographic seizures in patients with a decreased level of consciousness should be treated with AEDs (Hemphill et al., 2015).

## Management of fever

Fever is commonly encountered in ICH patients and has been associated with both hematoma expansion and worse outcomes (Schwarz et al., 2000; Rincon et al., 2013). Although current studies have failed to show improved outcomes with controlled normothermia in this setting (Broessner et al., 2009; Middleton et al., 2011), guidelines recommend that fever be treated and this is generally accepted as appropriate clinical practice (Hemphill et al., 2015). Of note, a small study involving 12 patients with large supratentorial ICH found that the use of mild hypothermia to 35°C for 10 days reduced

*Table 11.2*

**Selected ongoing clinical trials or large studies of intracerebral hemorrhage**

| Treatment target | Mechanism being investigated | Study title | ClinicalTrials.gov identifier |
|---|---|---|---|
| Hematoma expansion | | | |
| | Aggressive blood pressure control | Antihypertensive Treatment in Acute Cerbral Hemorrhage II (ATACH-II) | NCT01176565 |
| | | The Second Intensive Blood Pressure Reduction in Acute Cerebral Hemorrhage Trial (INTERACT 2) | NCT00716079 |
| | Hemostatic therapy | The Spot Sign for Predicting and Treating ICH Growth Study (STOP-IT) | NCT00810888 |
| | | "Spot Sign" Selection of Intracerebral Hemorrhage to Guide Hemostatic Therapy (SPOTLIGHT) | NCT01359202 |
| | | Tranexamic Acid for Acute ICH Growth prEdicted by Spot Sign (TRAIGE) | NCT02625948 |
| Secondary injury | | | |
| | Surgical treatment | Comparison between stereotactic aspiration and intra-endoscopic surgery to treat intracerebral hemorrhage | NCT02515903 |
| | | Decompressive hemicraniectomy in intracerebral hemorrhage (SWITCH) | NCT02258919 |
| | | Surgical trial in lobar intracerebral hemorrhage | NCT01320423 |
| | Minimally invasive surgery | Minimally Invasive Surgery plus rt-PA for ICH Evacuation (MISTIE) | NCT01827046 |
| | Hematoma clearance | Safety of piolglitazone for Hematoma Resolution in Intracerebral Hemorrhage (SHRINC) | NCT00827892 |
| | Iron chelation | Intracerebral hemorrhage Deferoxamine trial (iDEF) | NCT02175225 |
| | Platelet dysfunction | Platelet transfusion in acute intracerebral hemorrhage | NCT00699621 |
| | | Improving Platelet Activity for Cerebral hemorrhage Treatment – DDAVP proof of concept (IMPACT) | NCT00961532 |
| | Epilepsy | Prevention of Epileptic seizures in Acute intracerebral Hemorrhage (PEACH) | NCT02631759 |
| | Temperature modulation | Systemic Normothermia in Intracerebral Hemorrhage (SNICH) | NCT02078037 |
| | | Targeted temperature management after intracerebral hemorrhage | NCT01866384 |
| Other | | | |
| | Atrial fibrillation | Apixaban versus antiplatelet drugs or no antithrombotic drugs after Anticoagulation-associated intracerebral Hemorrhage in patients with Atrial Fibrillation (APACHE-AF) | NCT02565693 |
| | Intraventricular hemorrhage | Clot Lysis: Evaluating Accelerated Resolution of intraventricular hemorrhage phase III (CLEAR III) | NCT00784134 |
| | | Intraventricular hemorrhage and post hemorrhagic ventricular dilation: natural course, treatment, and outcome | NCT00957840 |

perihematomal edema (Kollmar et al., 2010) and a phase II clinical trial is currently ongoing (Kollmar et al., 2012).

## Management of hyperglycemia

Hyperglycemia in ICH patients has been associated with worse outcomes in several studies (Passero et al., 2003; Fogelholm et al., 2005; Kimura et al., 2007). However, the concern has been raised that aggressive treatment of elevated blood glucose may lead to systemic or cerebral hypoglycemia and potentially worsen outcomes (Vespa et al., 2006; Oddo et al., 2008; Vespa, 2008). Current guidelines recommend close monitoring of the glucose level and avoiding either hyperglycemia or hypoglycemia (Hemphill et al., 2015). However, the specific optimal target glucose and whether continuous insulin infusions should be used remain unclarified.

## Management of venous thromboembolism

ICH patients are at high risk for thromboembolic complications (Gregory and Kuhlemeier, 2003). Several studies have shown the efficacy of intermittent pneumatic compression and the inefficacy of graduated compression stockings in reducing deep venous thrombosis (DVT) in ICH patients (Lacut et al., 2005; Dennis et al., 2009, 2013). Although historically there has been reluctance to use heparin early after ICH for fear of worsening intracranial bleeding, low-dose unfractionated heparin and LMWH have both shown safety in reducing the incidence of pulmonary embolism (PE) without affecting ICH hematoma volume (Paciaroni et al., 2011). LMWH or unfractionated heparin for DVT or PE prophylaxis may be considered in immobile ICH patients after demonstration of hematoma stabilization 1–4 days after onset according to the 2015 AHA/ASA ICH guidelines (Hemphill et al., 2015). There are very few data regarding the management of DVT and PE in ICH patients, but treatment with anticoagulation or inferior vena cava filter placement is probably indicated (Kelly et al., 2003a). Factors that should be taken into consideration before treating are the time of onset of ICH, its location (lobar ICH has a higher rate of recurrence), hematoma stability, and the patient's general condition (Hemphill et al., 2015).

## COMPLEX CLINICAL DECISIONS

### Surgical management

The role of surgery for ICH remains controversial, although much less so in cases of cerebellar ICH. Observational studies have found that patients with cerebellar ICH may do well after hematoma evacuation and that specific characteristics of these patients may include those with cerebellar ICH 3 cm or greater in diameter, presence of obstructive hydrocephalus, or with brainstem compression (Da Pian et al., 1984; Firsching et al., 1991; van Loon et al., 1993). Though there are no randomized clinical trials confirming these findings, there is generally not considered to be equipoise as to whether cerebellar surgery in these patients is beneficial. The 2015 AHA/ASA guidelines recommend evacuation of cerebellar hematomas in cases of neurologic deterioration, hydrocephalus, and/or brainstem compression. Treatment solely by placing an external ventricular drain (EVD) to treat obstructive hydrocephalus caused by compression from a cerebellar hematoma is not recommended, although this may be reasonable after surgical hematoma evacuation (Hemphill et al., 2015).

On the contrary, though, there are two large randomized clinical trials, Surgical Trial in Intracerebral Hemorrhage I and II (STICH and STICH II), which evaluated the efficacy of evacuation of supratentorial ICH. However, because of specific aspects related to the design of these clinical trials, their ability to answer the fundamental question of whether surgery is beneficial for supratentorial ICH is limited. Theoretically, hematoma evacuation may improve mass effect and surrounding inflammation, reduce ICP, and prevent herniation (Andrews et al., 2012). The STICH trial enrolled 1033 patients with supratentorial ICH and in which the local treating neurosurgeon had clinical equipoise regarding whether surgery should be performed in the specific patient at hand. STICH compared the efficacy of a policy of early hematoma evacuation versus a policy of medical treatment only on improving functional outcome at 6 months as measured by the extended Glasgow Outcome Scale. STICH showed no difference in functional outcomes or mortality rates between the two groups, but subgroup analyses suggested that patients with superficial (less than 1 cm from the cortical surface) lobar hematomas might benefit from surgery and that comatose patients (GCS 8 or less) at presentation might not (Mendelow et al., 2005). Importantly, about one in four of the patients who were randomized to the medical treatment arm were treated with surgery in a delayed fashion and this high crossover rate limits the ability of STICH to address whether the outcome was due to lack of benefit of surgery itself, the timing of surgery, or other aspects related to patient selection.

STICH II trial was designed based on these analyses, enrolling 601 patients with supratentorial ICH (superficial, lobar, hematoma size 10–100 mL, no IVH, and conscious at presentation) within 48 hours of time of symptom onset. STICH II also compared early hematoma evacuation and medical treatment versus medical treatment alone. STICH II also showed no difference in functional outcomes between the two groups, but a *post hoc* analysis suggested that patients with a poor prognosis, as determined by a specific equation based on several patient characteristics, might benefit from surgery (Mendelow et al., 2013). About one in five patients in the medical group in STICH II crossed over to surgery. While both trials have been criticized for their narrow inclusion criteria, use of early surgery only, and a high rate of crossover from the medical to delayed surgery, STICH and STICH II should be considered landmark studies that demonstrated that large surgical trials can be performed in ICH. The 2015 AHA/ASA guidelines acknowledge both the accomplishments and the limitations of STICH and STICH II. Thus, while a policy of early surgery for patients meeting the inclusion criteria for STICH or STICH II seems to be neither harmful nor beneficial, hematoma evacuation might still be considered as a life-saving measure in deteriorating patients (Hemphill et al., 2015).

Building on the legacy of STICH and STICH II, which largely involved open craniotomy and hematoma evacuation, several other surgical interventions are now being considered and studied in clinical trials. Minimally invasive techniques to evacuate ICH include simple aspiration, endoscopic removal, and mechanical aspiration with or without instillation of thrombolytic agents (Backlund and von Holst, 1978; Tanikawa et al., 1985; Auer et al., 1989; Niizuma et al., 1989; Vespa et al., 2005). Several small studies have compared the efficacy of different techniques of minimally invasive hematoma evacuation to craniotomy, suggesting better outcomes with minimally invasive techniques (Cho et al., 2006; Wang et al., 2009; Mould et al., 2013). The Minimally Invasive Surgery and rt-PA for Intracerebral Hemorrhage Evacuation II trial (MISTIE II) enrolled 118 ICH patients and showed an improvement in perihematomal edema in the group that underwent minimally invasive evacuation and thrombolysis compared to the group that had medical treatment only (Mould et al., 2013). MISTIE III is an ongoing phase III clinical trial funded by the National Institutes of Health to assess whether minimally invasive aspiration with adjunctive thrombolysis improves patient outcome.

Although decompressive craniectomy has been shown of benefit in patients with large hemispheric ischemic infarction, its role in supratentorial ICH remains unclarified and controversial. Studies have suggested that it may have a role in the management of comatose patients, those with large hematomas, those with significant midline shift, or ICH patients with refractory elevated ICP (Fung et al., 2012; Hayes et al., 2013; Heuts et al., 2013; Takeuchi et al., 2013).

## Management of intracranial pressure and cerebral perfusion pressure

Elevated ICP can be seen in ICH due to a variety of factors, including mass effect, cerebral edema, and hydrocephalus from IVH (Hemphill et al., 2015). ICP monitoring through an EVD or an intraparenchymal monitor can help guide management, although there is some risk of infection and catheter-associated hemorrhage (Hemphill et al., 2015). Younger age, supratentorial ICH, and IVH have been found to be risk factors for elevated ICP (Mendelow et al., 2005; Kamel and Hemphill, 2012). Several retrospective studies have associated elevated ICP and low CPP with worse outcomes (Ko et al., 2011; Nikaina et al., 2012; Ziai et al., 2012).

There are limited data on management of ICP and CPP in ICH patients. Therefore, the current approach to ICP management in ICH is mostly borrowed from the approach recommended for traumatic brain injury

(TBI) patients. ICP monitoring could be considered for patients with a GCS of 8 or less with treatment recommended to maintain ICP below 20 mmHg and CPP between 50 and 70 mmHg depending on the cerebral autoregualtion status of the patient (Bratton et al., 2007a, b, c). The 2015 AHA/ASA ICH guidelines recommend considering ICP monitoring for ICH patients with GCS 8 or less, transtentorial herniation, or significant IVH or hydrocephalus. Placement of an EVD in patients with hydrocephalus should be undertaken, especially if they have a decreased level of consciousness (Hemphill et al., 2015).

Elevated ICP can be treated using a variety of measures including elevation of the head of bed to 30°, administration of sedative agents, the use of hypertonic saline or mannitol as osmotherapy, and drainage of cerebrospinal fluid via an EVD. Refractory elevated ICP can be treated with neuromuscular paralytics, hypothermia, deep sedation with propofol or barbiturate coma, or surgery (e.g., hematoma evacuation or decompressive craniectomy). However, the safety and efficacy of these interventions have not been formally studied in ICH.

## Management of intraventricular hemorrhage

IVH is common in ICH patients and is secondary to parenchymal ICH extending to the ventricles. It is present in about 45% of ICH patients and is consistently associated with worse outcomes across studies (Bhattathiri et al., 2006; Hallevi et al., 2008; Gaberel et al., 2012).

IVH can lead to obstructive hydrocephalus and elevated ICP, which can present clinically with decreased range of vertical eye movements and a decreased level of consciousness from the mass effect on the midbrain. This can progress to brainstem herniation and death. Therefore, the emergent placement of an EVD to measure and treat elevated ICP and drain cerebrospinal fluid and intraventricular blood in ICH patients with decreased level of consciousness, IVH, or hydrocephalus can be life saving (Gates et al., 1986; Hemphill et al., 2015).

The possibility of facilitating the clearance of IVH by instilling thombolytic agents into the ventricles via an EVD has been assessed preliminarily in several studies (Dunatov et al., 2011; Gaberel et al., 2011; King et al., 2012; Castano Avila et al., 2013). The largest published experience to date come from the phase II trial, CLEAR IVH, which enrolled 100 ICH patients with significant IVH and parenchymal hematoma volumes less than 30 cc. This study tested the safety of the instillation of recombinant tissue plasminogen activator (rt-PA) through an EVD. The use of rt-PA was associated with a higher rate of IVH resolution, lower ICP, and fewer EVD obstructions requiring replacement. However, there was also a higher rate of secondary intraparenchymal hemorrhage, although this was not statistically significant. There was no difference in functional outcome, mortality, or the rate of infection (Naff et al., 2011). CLEAR III is a phase III pivotal trial testing the efficacy of intrathecal rt-PA for IVH. As of this writing, it has completed enrollment but results have not been reported. Endoscopic evacuation of IVH is another procedure that has been reported on a smaller scale and shown variable results (Yadav et al., 2007; Zhang et al., 2007; Chen et al., 2011; Basaldella et al., 2012). Current guidelines considered the safety and efficacy of using rt-PA through an EVD or endoscopic evacuation of IVH as uncertain (Hemphill et al., 2015). However, the results of CLEAR III may provide increased clarity regarding the value of this treatment.

## OUTCOME PREDICTION

Only about 12–39% of ICH patients regain long-term functional independence and the mortality rate of ICH is consistently around 40% at 1 month and 54% at 1 year across numerous studies (van Asch et al., 2010). Given this profound morbidity and mortality associated with ICH and the fact that many patients present with a significantly depressed level of consciousness, it is common for families to desire prognostication regarding possible outcomes for acute ICH patients. Additionally, physicians often desire to use initial prognostic models as a way of considering triage for ongoing care decisions. Many different clinical grading scales have been developed with the goal of providing a prediction of likely outcome based on characteristics of ICH patients at the time of initial presentation (Hemphill et al., 2001; Rost et al., 2008). The most widely used scale is the ICH Score, which was developed as a way of standardizing and improving communication among providers about ICH but not to specifically predict outcome precisely. Components of the ICH Score include aspects related to patient characteristics, including patient age and GCS score, as well as factors identified from initial neuroimaging from CT, including hematoma volume and location and the presence of IVH. The total ICH Score is the sum of points provided for each component (Table 11.3). Each increase in the ICH Score is associated with an increase in risk of 30-day mortality and a decrease in the likelihood of long-term functional independence (Hemphill et al., 2001, 2009).

The lack of a panoply of highly effective therapies for acute ICH has allowed heterogeneity regarding overall care to exist. This heterogeneity has included wide variation in the utilization of aggressive measures such as surgery as well as nonaggressive measures such as early "do not resuscitate" (DNR) orders (Gregson et al., 2003; Hemphill et al., 2004). Perception of a poor prognosis without possibility of good recovery may lead to a decision to limit care or withdraw medical support. Palliative

*Table 11.3*

Determination of the intracerebral hemorrhage (ICH) score (Hemphill et al., 2001)

| Component | | ICH score points |
|---|---|---|
| Glasgow Coma Scale (GCS) | 3–4 | 2 |
| | 5–12 | 1 |
| | 13–15 | 0 |
| ICH volume (cc) | ≥30 | 1 |
| | <30 | 0 |
| Intraventricular hemorrhage | Yes | 1 |
| | No | 0 |
| Infratentorial origin of ICH | Yes | 1 |
| | No | 0 |
| Age (years) | ≥80 | 1 |
| | <80 | 0 |
| Total ICH score | | 0-6 |

GCS score on initial presentation (or after resuscitation); ICH volume, volume on initial computed tomography (CT) calculated using ABC/2 method; and IVH, presence of any IVH on initial CT.

care is an important aspect of end-of-life care and is appropriate to provide in stroke patients, including those with ICH, in this context (Holloway et al., 2014). However, there is also the possibility that early care limitations may allow patients to die who would otherwise have the potential for an acceptable outcome. This leads to the possibility that withdrawal of care could lead to a self-fulfilling prophecy of poor outcome (Becker et al., 2001). It has also been demonstrated that care limitations in the form of early DNR orders are associated with a lower likelihood of favorable outcome, even adjusting for other patient and treating hospital characteristics (Hemphill et al., 2004). Balancing the need for realistic decision making with the potential for the self-fulfilling prophecy of poor outcome is one of the major challenges in the care of patients with ICH.

No ICH outcome prediction model to date has effectively taken into account the impact of care limitations such as early DNR orders or withdrawal of medical support (Zahuranec et al., 2010; Creutzfeldt et al., 2011). A recent multicenter study found that patients cared for without DNR orders for at least the first 5 days had a significantly higher rate of survival than predicted using the point estimates often quoted from the original ICH Score publication (Morgenstern et al., 2015). However, each point increase in the ICH Score was still associated with an increased risk of mortality. This suggests that clinical grading scales such as the ICH Score remain useful with regard to overall patient severity stratification but should not be used to provide an assumed precise numeric prediction of outcome. Given these concerns, current guidelines recommend a trial of aggressive treatment in all ICH patients without pre-existing advance directives stating otherwise, and to postpone new DNR orders until at least the second full day of hospitalization (Hemphill et al., 2015).

## NEUROREHABILITATION

Though only less than one-third of ICH patients achieve long-term functional independence (van Asch et al., 2010), several studies have shown that ICH patients may recover greater and faster than ischemic stroke patients and that this may continue for months after initial presentation (Chae et al., 1996; Kelly et al., 2003b; Schepers et al., 2008; Katrak et al., 2009; Wei et al., 2010). It is thus considered imperative that rehabilitation begin as soon as possible for functional recovery. Multidisciplinary care of stroke patients has been proven to improve outcomes and to be cost-effective. This includes comprehensive stroke units, which can provide inpatient rehabilitation services before discharge, and home-based rehabilitation services, which can help accelerate hospital discharge and patient recovery (Outpatient Service Trialists, 2003; Chan et al., 2013; Stroke Group, 2013). Early inpatient and outpatient multidisciplinary rehabilitation is recommended by the 2015 AHA/ASA ICH guidelines (Hemphill et al., 2015).

## REFERENCES

Amarenco P, Bogousslavsky J, Callahan 3rd A et al. (2006). High-dose atorvastatin after stroke or transient ischemic attack. N Engl J Med 355: 549–559.

Anderson CS, Huang Y, Wang JG et al. (2008). Intensive blood pressure reduction in acute cerebral haemorrhage trial (INTERACT): a randomized pilot trial. Lancet Neurol 7: 391–399.

Anderson CS, Heeley E, Huang Y et al. (2013). Rapid blood-pressure lowering in patients with acute intracerebral hemorrhage. N Engl J Med 368: 2355–2365.

Andrews CM, Jauch EC, Hemphill 3rd JC et al. (2012). Emergency neurological life support: intracerebral hemorrhage. Neurocrit Care 17 (Suppl 1): S37–S46.

Angileri FF, Cardali S, Conti A et al. (2012). Telemedicine-assisted treatment of patients with intracerebral hemorrhage. Neurosurg Focus 32. E6.

Ariesen MJ, Claus SP, Rinkel GJ et al. (2003). Risk factors for intracerebral hemorrhage in the general population: a systematic review. Stroke 34: 2060–2065.

Auer LM, Deinsberger W, Niederkorn K et al. (1989). Endoscopic surgery versus medical treatment for spontaneous intracerebral hematoma: a randomized study. J Neurosurg 70: 530–535.

Backlund EO, von Holst H (1978). Controlled subtotal evacuation of intracerebral haematomas by stereotactic technique. Surg Neurol 9: 99–101.

Barras CD, Tress BM, Christensen S et al. (2013). Quantitative CT densitometry for predicting intracerebral hemorrhage growth. AJNR Am J Neuroradiol 34: 1139–1144.

Basaldella L, Marton E, Fiorindi A et al. (2012). External ventricular drainage alone versus endoscopic surgery for severe intraventricular hemorrhage: a comparative retrospective analysis on outcome and shunt dependency. Neurosurg Focus 32:E4.

Battey TW, Falcone GJ, Ayres AM et al. (2012). Confounding by indication in retrospective studies of intracerebral hemorrhage: antiepileptic treatment and mortality. Neurocrit Care 17: 361–366.

Becker KJ, Baxter AB, Cohen WA et al. (2001). Withdrawal of support in intracerebral hemorrhage may lead to self-fulfilling prophecies. Neurology 56: 766–772.

Beghi E, D'Alessandro R, Beretta S et al. (2011). Incidence and predictors of acute symptomatic seizures after stroke. Neurology 77: 1785–1793.

Bhattathiri PS, Gregson B, Prasad KS et al. (2006). Intraventricular hemorrhage and hydrocephalus after spontaneous intracerebral hemorrhage: results from the STICH trial. Acta Neurochir Suppl 96: 65–68.

Bladin CF, Alexandrov AV, Bellavance A et al. (2000). Seizures after stroke: a prospective multicenter study. Arch Neurol 57: 1617–1622.

Booij LH (2001). Is succinylcholine appropriate or obsolete in the intensive care unit? Crit Care 5: 245–246.

Bratton SL, Chestnut RM, Ghajar J et al. (2007a). Guidelines for the management of severe traumatic brain injury. IX. Cerebral perfusion thresholds. J Neurotrauma 24 (Suppl 1): S59–S64.

Bratton SL, Chestnut RM, Ghajar J et al. (2007b). Guidelines for the management of severe traumatic brain injury. VI. Indications for intracranial pressure monitoring. J Neurotrauma 24 (Suppl 1): S37–S44.

Bratton SL, Chestnut RM, Ghajar J et al. (2007c). Guidelines for the management of severe traumatic brain injury. VIII. Intracranial pressure thresholds. J Neurotrauma 24 (Suppl 1): S55–S58.

Broderick JP (2009). Evidence against rapid reversal of antiplatelet medications in acute intracerebral hemorrhage. Neurology 72: 1376–1377.

Broderick JP, Brott TG, Duldner JE et al. (1993). Volume of intracerebral hemorrhage. A powerful and easy-to-use predictor of 30-day mortality. Stroke 24: 987–993.

Broessner G, Beer R, Lackner P et al. (2009). Prophylactic, endovascularly based, long-term normothermia in ICU patients with severe cerebrovascular disease: bicenter prospective, randomized trial. Stroke 40: e657–e665.

Brott T, Broderick J, Kothari R et al. (1997). Early hemorrhage growth in patients with intracerebral hemorrhage. Stroke 28: 1–5.

Butcher KS, Baird T, MacGregor L et al. (2004). Perihematomal edema in primary intracerebral hemorrhage is plasma derived. Stroke 35: 1879–1885.

Campbell PG, Yadla S, Sen AN et al. (2011). Emergency reversal of clopidogrel in the setting of spontaneous intracerebral hemorrhage. World Neurosurg 76: 100–104. discussion 159–160.

Cartmill M, Dolan G, Byrne JL et al. (2000). Prothrombin complex concentrate for oral anticoagulant reversal in neurosurgical emergencies. Br J Neurosurg 14: 458–461.

Castano Avila S, Corral Lozano E, Vallejo De La Cueva A et al. (2013). Intraventricular hemorrhage treated with intraventricular fibrinolysis. A 10-year experience. Med Intensiva 37: 61–66.

Chae J, Zorowitz RD, Johnston MV (1996). Functional outcome of hemorrhagic and nonhemorrhagic stroke patients after in-patient rehabilitation. Am J Phys Med Rehabil 75: 177–182.

Chalela JA, Kidwell CS, Nentwich LM et al. (2007). Magnetic resonance imaging and computed tomography in emergency assessment of patients with suspected acute stroke: a prospective comparison. Lancet 369: 293–298.

Chan S, Hemphill 3rd JC (2014). Critical care management of intracerebral hemorrhage. Crit Care Clin 30: 699–717.

Chan DK, Cordato D, O'Rourke F et al. (2013). Comprehensive stroke units: a review of comparative evidence and experience. Int J Stroke 8: 260–264.

Charidimou A, Gang Q, Werring DJ (2012). Sporadic cerebral amyloid angiopathy revisited: recent insights into pathophysiology and clinical spectrum. J Neurol Neurosurg Psychiatry 83: 124–137.

Chen CC, Liu CL, Tung YN et al. (2011). Endoscopic surgery for intraventricular hemorrhage (IVH) caused by thalamic hemorrhage: comparisons of endoscopic surgery and external ventricular drainage (EVD) surgery. World Neurosurg 75: 264–268.

Cho DY, Chen CC, Chang CS et al. (2006). Endoscopic surgery for spontaneous basal ganglia hemorrhage: comparing endoscopic surgery, stereotactic aspiration, and craniotomy in noncomatose patients. Surg Neurol 65: 547–555. discussion 555–546.

Claassen J, Jette N, Chum F et al. (2007). Electrographic seizures and periodic discharges after intracerebral hemorrhage. Neurology 69: 1356–1365.

Creutzfeldt CJ, Becker KJ, Weinstein JR et al. (2011). Do-not-attempt-resuscitation orders and prognostic models for intraparenchymal hemorrhage. Crit Care Med 39: 158–162.

Culebras A, Messe SR, Chaturvedi S et al. (2014). Summary of evidence-based guideline update: prevention of stroke in nonvalvular atrial fibrillation: report of the Guideline Development Subcommittee of the American Academy of Neurology. Neurology 82: 716–724.

Da Pian R, Bazzan A, Pasqualin A (1984). Surgical versus medical treatment of spontaneous posterior fossa haematomas: a cooperative study on 205 cases. Neurol Res 6: 145–151.

Davis SM, Broderick J, Hennerici M et al. (2006). Hematoma growth is a determinant of mortality and poor outcome after intracerebral hemorrhage. Neurology 66: 1175–1181.

de Gans K, de Haan RJ, Majoie CB et al. (2010). PATCH: platelet transfusion in cerebral haemorrhage: study protocol for a multicentre, randomised, controlled trial. BMC Neurol 10: 19.

De Herdt V, Dumont F, Henon H et al. (2011). Early seizures in intracerebral hemorrhage: incidence, associated factors, and outcome. Neurology 77: 1794–1800.

Dennis M, Sandercock PA, Reid J et al. (2009). Effectiveness of thigh-length graduated compression stockings to reduce the risk of deep vein thrombosis after stroke (CLOTS trial 1): a multicentre, randomised controlled trial. Lancet 373: 1958–1965.

Dennis M, Sandercock P, Reid J et al. (2013). Effectiveness of intermittent pneumatic compression in reduction of risk of deep vein thrombosis in patients who have had a stroke (CLOTS 3): a multicentre randomised controlled trial. Lancet 382: 516–524.

Dentali F, Ageno W, Crowther M (2006). Treatment of coumarin-associated coagulopathy: a systematic review and proposed treatment algorithms. J Thromb Haemost 4: 1853–1863.

Diringer MN (1993). Intracerebral hemorrhage: pathophysiology and management. Crit Care Med 21: 1591–1603.

Dunatov S, Antoncic I, Bralic M et al. (2011). Intraventricular thrombolysis with rt-PA in patients with intraventricular hemorrhage. Acta Neurol Scand 124: 343–348.

Elijovich L, Patel PV, Hemphill 3rd JC (2008). Intracerebral hemorrhage. Semin Neurol 28: 657–667.

Falcone GJ, Biffi A, Brouwers HB et al. (2013). Predictors of hematoma volume in deep and lobar supratentorial intracerebral hemorrhage. JAMA Neurol 70: 988–994.

Fan JS, Huang HH, Chen YC et al. (2012). Emergency department neurologic deterioration in patients with spontaneous intracerebral hemorrhage: incidence, predictors, and prognostic significance. Acad Emerg Med 19: 133–138.

Fiebach JB, Schellinger PD, Gass A et al. (2004). Stroke magnetic resonance imaging is accurate in hyperacute intracerebral hemorrhage: a multicenter study on the validity of stroke imaging. Stroke 35: 502–506.

Firsching R, Huber M, Frowein RA (1991). Cerebellar haemorrhage: management and prognosis. Neurosurg Rev 14: 191–194.

Fisher CM (1971). Pathological observations in hypertensive cerebral hemorrhage. J Neuropathol Exp Neurol 30: 536–550.

Flibotte JJ, Hagan N, O'Donnell J et al. (2004). Warfarin, hematoma expansion, and outcome of intracerebral hemorrhage. Neurology 63: 1059–1064.

Flint AC, Conell C, Rao VA et al. (2014). Effect of statin use during hospitalization for intracerebral hemorrhage on mortality and discharge disposition. JAMA Neurol 71: 1364–1371.

Fogelholm R, Murros K, Rissanen A et al. (2005). Admission blood glucose and short term survival in primary intracerebral hemorrhage: a population based study. J Neurol Neurosurg Psychiatry 76: 349–353.

Fredriksson K, Norrving B, Stromblad LG (1992). Emergency reversal of anticoagulation after intracerebral hemorrhage. Stroke 23: 972–977.

Fung C, Murek M, Z'Graggen WJ et al. (2012). Decompressive hemicraniectomy in patients with supratentorial intracerebral hemorrhage. Stroke 43: 3207–3211.

Gaberel T, Magheru C, Parienti JJ et al. (2011). Intraventricular fibrinolysis versus external ventricular drainage alone in intraventricular hemorrhage: a meta-analysis. Stroke 42: 2776–2781.

Gaberel T, Magheru C, Emery E (2012). Management of non-traumatic intraventricular hemorrhage. Neurosurg Rev 35: 485–494. discussion 494–485.

Gates PC, Barnett HJ, Vinters HV et al. (1986). Primary intra-ventricular hemorrhage in adults. Stroke 17: 872–877.

Gebel Jr JM, Jauch EC, Brott TG et al. (2002). Relative edema volume is a predictor of outcome in patients with hypera-cute spontaneous intracerebral hemorrhage. Stroke 33: 2636–2641.

Goldstein JN, Thomas SH, Frontiero V et al. (2006). Timing of fresh frozen plasma administration and rapid correction of coagulopathy in warfarin-related intracerebral hemor-rhage. Stroke 37: 151–155.

Gonzalez-Perez A, Gaist D, Wallander MA et al. (2013). Mortality after hemorrhagic stroke: data from general prac-tice (The Health Improvement Network). Neurology 81: 559–565.

Greenberg SM, Vonsattel JP (1997). Diagnosis of cerebral amyloid angiopathy. Sensitivity and specificity of cortical biopsy. Stroke 28: 1418–1422.

Gregory PC, Kuhlemeier KV (2003). Prevalence of venous thromboembolism in acute hemorrhagic and thromboem-bolic stroke. Am J Phys Med Rehabil 82: 364–369.

Gregson BA, Mendelow AD, Investigators (2003). International variations in surgical practice for spontaneous intracerebral hemorrhage. Stroke 34: 2593–2597.

Gunel M, Awad IA, Finberg K et al. (1996). A founder muta-tion as a cause of cerebral cavernous malformation in Hispanic Americans. N Engl J Med 334: 946–951.

Hallevi H, Albright KC, Aronowski J et al. (2008). Intraventricular hemorrhage: anatomic relationships and clinical implications. Neurology 70: 848–852.

Hayes SB, Benveniste RJ, Morcos JJ et al. (2013). Retrospective comparison of craniotomy and decompres-sive craniectomy for surgical evacuation of nontraumatic, supratentorial intracerebral hemorrhage. Neurosurg Focus 34. E3.

Hemphill 3rd JC, Bonovich DC, Besmertis L et al. (2001). The ICH score: a simple, reliable grading scale for intracerebral hemorrhage. Stroke 32: 891–897.

Hemphill 3rd JC, Newman J, Zhao S et al. (2004). Hospital usage of early do-not-resuscitate orders and outcome after intracerebral hemorrhage. Stroke 35: 1130–1134.

Hemphill 3rd JC, Farrant M, Neill Jr TA (2009). Prospective validation of the ICH Score for 12-month functional out-come. Neurology 73: 1088–1094.

Hemphill 3rd JC, Greenberg SM, Anderson CS et al. (2015). Guidelines for the management of spontaneous intracere-bral hemorrhage: a guideline for healthcare professionals from the American Heart Association/American Stroke Association. Stroke 46: 2032–2060.

Heuts SG, Bruce SS, Zacharia BE et al. (2013). Decompressive hemicraniectomy without clot evacuation in dominant-sided intracerebral hemorrhage with ICP crisis. Neurosurg Focus 34. E4.

Holloway RG, Arnold RM, Creutzfeldt CJ et al. (2014). Palliative and end-of-life care in stroke: a statement for healthcare professionals from the American Heart Association/American Stroke Association. Stroke 45: 1887–1916.

Honner SK, Singh A, Cheung PT et al. (2011). Emergency department control of blood pressure in intracerebral hem-orrhage. J Emerg Med 41: 355–361.

Hussein HM, Tariq NA, Palesch YY et al. (2013). Reliability of hematoma volume measurement at local sites in a mul-ticenter acute intracerebral hemorrhage clinical trial. Stroke 44: 237–239.

Hypertension Detection and Follow-up Program Cooperative Group (1982). Five-year findings of the hypertension detection and follow-up program. III. Reduction in stroke incidence among persons with high blood pressure. Jama 247: 633–638.

Kaatz S, Kouides PA, Garcia DA et al. (2012). Guidance on the emergent reversal of oral thrombin and factor Xa inhibitors. Am J Hematol 87 (Suppl 1): S141–S145.

Kamel H, Hemphill 3rd JC (2012). Characteristics and sequelae of intracranial hypertension after intracerebral hemorrhage. Neurocrit Care 17: 172–176.

Katrak PH, Black D, Peeva V (2009). Do stroke patients with intracerebral hemorrhage have a better functional outcome than patients with cerebral infarction? PM R 1: 427–433.

Kelly J, Hunt BJ, Lewis RR et al. (2003a). Anticoagulation or inferior vena cava filter placement for patients with pri-mary intracerebral hemorrhage developing venous throm-boembolism? Stroke 34: 2999–3005.

Kelly PJ, Furie KL, Shafqat S et al. (2003b). Functional recov-ery following rehabilitation after hemorrhagic and ische-mic stroke. Arch Phys Med Rehabil 84: 968–972.

Kidwell CS, Saver JL, Mattiello J et al. (2001). Diffusion-perfusion MR evaluation of perihematomal injury in hyperacute intracerebral hemorrhage. Neurology 57: 1611–1617.

Kimura K, Iguchi Y, Inoue T et al. (2007). Hyperglycemia independently increases the risk of early death in acute spontaneous intracerebral hemorrhage. J Neurol Sci 255: 90–94.

King NK, Lai JL, Tan LB et al. (2012). A randomized, placebo-controlled pilot study of patients with spontaneous intraventricular haemorrhage treated with intraventricular thrombolysis. J Clin Neurosci 19: 961–964.

Knudsen KA, Rosand J, Karluk D et al. (2001). Clinical diag-nosis of cerebral amyloid angiopathy: validation of the Boston criteria. Neurology 56: 537–539.

Ko SB, Choi HA, Parikh G et al. (2011). Multimodality mon-itoring for cerebral perfusion pressure optimization in comatose patients with intracerebral hemorrhage. Stroke 42: 3087–3092.

Kollmar R, Staykov D, Dorfler A et al. (2010). Hypothermia reduces perihemorrhagic edema after intracerebral hemor-rhage. Stroke 41: 1684–1689.

Kollmar R, Juettler E, Huttner HB et al. (2012). Cooling in intracerebral hemorrhage (CINCH) trial: protocol of a ran-domized German-Austrian clinical trial. Int J Stroke 7: 168–172.

Kothari RU, Brott T, Broderick JP et al. (1996). The ABCs of measuring intracerebral hemorrhage volumes. Stroke 27: 1304–1305.

Kuramatsu JB, Gerner ST, Schellinger PD et al. (2015). Anticoagulant reversal, blood pressure levels, and anticoagulant resumption in patients with anticoagulation-related intracerebral hemorrhage. JAMA 313: 824–836.

Labovitz DL, Halim A, Boden-Albala B et al. (2005). The incidence of deep and lobar intracerebral hemorrhage in whites, blacks, and Hispanics. Neurology 65: 518–522.

Lacut K, Bressollette L, Le Gal G et al. (2005). Prevention of venous thrombosis in patients with acute intracerebral hemorrhage. Neurology 65: 865–869.

Leissinger CA, Blatt PM, Hoots WK et al. (2008). Role of prothrombin complex concentrates in reversing warfarin anticoagulation: a review of the literature. Am J Hematol 83: 137–143.

Levine JM, Snider R, Finkelstein D et al. (2007). Early edema in warfarin-related intracerebral hemorrhage. Neurocrit Care 7: 58–63.

Liotta EM, Prabhakaran S (2013). Warfarin-associated intracerebral hemorrhage is increasing in prevalence in the United States. J Stroke Cerebrovasc Dis 22: 1151–1155.

Lummel N, Lutz J, Bruckmann H et al. (2012). The value of magnetic resonance imaging for the detection of the bleeding source in non-traumatic intracerebral haemorrhages: a comparison with conventional digital subtraction angiography. Neuroradiology 54: 673–680.

Maas MB, Nemeth AJ, Rosenberg NF et al. (2013). Delayed intraventricular hemorrhage is common and worsens outcomes in intracerebral hemorrhage. Neurology 80: 1295–1299.

Majeed A, Schulman S (2013). Bleeding and antidotes in new oral anticoagulants. Best Pract Res Clin Haematol 26: 191–202.

Marti-Fabregas J, Delgado-Mederos R, Granell E et al. (2013). Microbleed burden and hematoma expansion in acute intracerebral hemorrhage. Eur Neurol 70: 175–178.

Mayer SA (2003). Ultra-early hemostatic therapy for intracerebral hemorrhage. Stroke 34: 224–229.

Mayer SA, Lignelli A, Fink ME et al. (1998). Perilesional blood flow and edema formation in acute intracerebral hemorrhage: a SPECT study. Stroke 29: 1791–1798.

Mayer SA, Brun NC, Begtrup K et al. (2008). Efficacy and safety of recombinant activated factor VII for acute intracerebral hemorrhage. N Engl J Med 358: 2127–2137.

McCormick WF, Rosenfield DB (1973). Massive brain hemorrhage: a review of 144 cases and an examination of their causes. Stroke 4: 946–954.

Mendelow AD, Gregson BA, Fernandes HM et al. (2005). Early surgery versus initial conservative treatment in patients with spontaneous supratentorial intracerebral hematomas in the International Surgical Trial in Intracerebral Hemorrhage (STICH): a randomized trial. Lancet 365: 387–397.

Mendelow AD, Gregson BA, Rowan EN et al. (2013). Early surgery versus initial conservative treatment in patients with spontaneous supratentorial lobar intracerebral

haematomas (STICH II): a randomized trial. Lancet 382: 397–408.

Messe SR, Sansing LH, Cucchiara BL et al. (2009). Prophylactic antiepileptic drug use is associated with poor outcome following ICH. Neurocrit Care 11: 38–44.

Middleton S, McElduff P, Ward J et al. (2011). Implementation of evidence-based treatment protocols to manage fever, hyperglycaemia, and swallowing dysfunction in acute stroke (QASC): a cluster randomised controlled trial. Lancet 378: 1699–1706.

Moon JS, Janjua N, Ahmed S et al. (2008). Prehospital neurologic deterioration in patients with intracerebral hemorrhage. Crit Care Med 36: 172–175.

Morgenstern LB, Zahuranec DB, Sanchez BN et al. (2015). Full medical support for intracerebral hemorrhage. Neurology 84: 1739–1744.

Mould WA, Carhuapoma JR, Muschelli J et al. (2013). Minimally invasive surgery plus recombinant tissue-type plasminogen activator for intracerebral hemorrhage evacuation decreases perihematomal edema. Stroke 44: 627–634.

Mullen MT, Kasner SE, Messe SR (2013). Seizures do not increase in-hospital mortality after intracerebral hemorrhage in the nationwide inpatient sample. Neurocrit Care 19: 19–24.

Naff N, Williams MA, Keyl PM et al. (2011). Low-dose recombinant tissue-type plasminogen activator enhances clot resolution in brain hemorrhage: the intraventricular hemorrhage thrombolysis trial. Stroke 42: 3009–3016.

Naidech AM, Bernstein RA, Levasseur K et al. (2009a). Platelet activity and outcome after intracerebral hemorrhage. Ann Neurol 65: 352–356.

Naidech AM, Garg RK, Liebling S et al. (2009b). Anticonvulsant use and outcomes after intracerebral hemorrhage. Stroke 40: 3810–3815.

Naidech AM, Jovanovic B, Liebling S et al. (2009c). Reduced platelet activity is associated with early clot growth and worse 3-month outcome after intracerebral hemorrhage. Stroke 40: 2398–2401.

Niizuma H, Shimizu Y, Yonemitsu T et al. (1989). Results of stereotactic aspiration in 175 cases of putaminal hemorrhage. Neurosurgery 24: 814–819.

Nikaina I, Paterakis K, Paraforos G et al. (2012). Cerebral perfusion pressure, microdialysis biochemistry, and clinical outcome in patients with spontaneous intracerebral hematomas. J Crit Care 27: 83–88.

Oddo M, Schmidt JM, Carrera E et al. (2008). Impact of tight glycemic control on cerebral glucose metabolism after severe brain injury: a microdialysis study. Crit Care Med 36: 3233–3238.

O'Donnell HC, Rosand J, Knudsen KA et al. (2000). Apolipoprotein E genotype and the risk of recurrent lobar intracerebral hemorrhage. N Engl J Med 342: 240–245.

Outpatient Service Trialists (2003). Therapy-based rehabilitation services for stroke patients at home. Cochrane Database Syst Rev: Cd002925.

Pabinger I, Brenner B, Kalina U et al. (2008). Prothrombin complex concentrate (Beriplex P/N) for emergency anticoagulation reversal: a prospective multinational clinical trial. J Thromb Haemost 6: 622–631.

Paciaroni M, Agnelli G, Venti M et al. (2011). Efficacy and safety of anticoagulants in the prevention of venous thromboembolism in patients with acute cerebral hemorrhage: a meta-analysis of controlled studies. J Thromb Haemost 9: 893–898.

Passero S, Rocchi R, Rossi S et al. (2002). Seizures after spontaneous supratentorial intracerebral hemorrhage. Epilepsia 43: 1175–1180.

Passero S, Ciacci G, Ulivelli M (2003). The influence of diabetes and hyperglycemia on clinical course after intracerebral hemorrhage. Neurology 61: 1351–1356.

Pollack Jr CV, Reilly PA, Eikelboom J et al. (2015). Idarucizumab for dabigatran reversal. N Engl J Med 373: 511–520.

Power C, Henry S, Del Bigio MR et al. (2003). Intracerebral hemorrhage induces macrophage activation and matrix metalloproteinases. Ann Neurol 53: 731–742.

Qureshi AI, Palesch YY (2011). Antihypertensive Treatment of Acute Cerebral Hemorrhage (ATACH) II: design, methods, and rationale. Neurocrit Care 15: 559–576.

Qureshi AI, Tuhrim S, Broderick JP et al. (2001). Spontaneous intracerebral hemorrhage. N Engl J Med 344: 1450–1460.

Qureshi AI, Ezzeddine MA, Nasar A et al. (2007). Prevalence of elevated blood pressure in 563,704 adult patients with stroke presenting to the ED in the United States. Am J Emerg Med 25: 32–38.

Qureshi AI, Palesch YY, Martin R et al. (2010). Effect of systolic blood pressure reduction on hematoma expansion, perihematomal edema, and 3-month outcome among patients with intracerebral hemorrhage: results from the antihypertensive treatment of acute cerebral hemorrhage study. Arch Neurol 67: 570–576.

Reynolds SF, Heffner J (2005). Airway management of the critically ill patient: rapid-sequence intubation. Chest 127: 1397–1412.

Riess HB, Meier-Hellmann A, Motsch J et al. (2007). Prothrombin complex concentrate (Octaplex) in patients requiring immediate reversal of oral anticoagulation. Thromb Res 121: 9–16.

Rincon F, Lyden P, Mayer SA (2013). Relationship between temperature, hematoma growth, and functional outcome after intracerebral hemorrhage. Neurocrit Care 18: 45–53.

Rizos T, Dorner N, Jenetzky E et al. (2013). Spot signs in intracerebral hemorrhage: useful for identifying patients at risk for hematoma enlargement? Cerebrovasc Dis 35: 582–589.

Rodriguez-Luna D, Pineiro S, Rubiera M et al. (2013). Impact of blood pressure changes and course on hematoma growth in acute intracerebral hemorrhage. Eur J Neurol 20: 1277–1283.

Rosand J, Eckman MH, Knudsen KA et al. (2004). The effect of warfarin and intensity of anticoagulation on outcome of intracerebral hemorrhage. Arch Intern Med 164: 880–884.

Rost NS, Smith EE, Chang Y et al. (2008). Prediction of functional outcome in patients with primary intracerebral hemorrhage: the FUNC score. Stroke 39: 2304–2309.

Sakamoto Y, Koga M, Yamagami H et al. (2013). Systolic blood pressure after intravenous antihypertensive treatment and clinical outcomes in hyperacute intracerebral hemorrhage: the stroke acute management with urgent risk-factor assessment and improvement-intracerebral hemorrhage study. Stroke 44: 1846–1851.

Sansing LH, Messe SR, Cucchiara BL et al. (2009). Prior antiplatelet use does not affect hemorrhage growth or outcome after ICH. Neurology 72: 1397–1402.

Schepers VP, Ketelaar M, Visser-Meily AJ et al. (2008). Functional recovery differs between ischaemic and hemorrhagic stroke patients. J Rehabil Med 40: 487–489.

Schwamm LH, Audebert HJ, Amarenco P et al. (2009). Recommendations for the implementation of telemedicine within stroke systems of care: a policy statement from the American Heart Association. Stroke 40: 2635–2660.

Schwarz S, Hafner K, Aschoff A et al. (2000). Incidence and prognostic significance of fever following intracerebral hemorrhage. Neurology 54: 354–361.

Siddique MS, Fernandes HM, Arene NU et al. (2000). Changes in cerebral blood flow as measured by HMPAO SPECT in patients following spontaneous intracerebral haemorrhage. Acta Neurochir Suppl 76: 517–520.

Singer OC, Sitzer M, du Mesnil de Rochemont R et al. (2004). Practical limitations of acute stroke MRI due to patient-related problems. Neurology 62: 1848–1849.

Sjoblom L, Hardemark HG, Lindgren A et al. (2001). Management and prognostic features of intracerebral hemorrhage during anticoagulant therapy: a Swedish multicenter study. Stroke 32: 2567–2574.

Staykov D, Wagner I, Volbers B et al. (2011). Natural course of perihemorrhagic edema after intracerebral hemorrhage. Stroke 42: 2625–2629.

Stroke Group (2013). Organised inpatient (stroke unit) care for stroke. Cochrane Database Syst Rev 9: Cd000197.

Sturgeon JD, Folsom AR, Longstreth Jr WT et al. (2007). Risk factors for intracerebral hemorrhage in a pooled prospective study. Stroke 38: 2718–2725.

Szaflarski JP, Rackley AY, Kleindorfer DO et al. (2008). Incidence of seizures in the acute phase of stroke: a population-based study. Epilepsia 49: 974–981.

Takeda R, Ogura T, Ooigawa H et al. (2013). A practical prediction model for early hematoma expansion in spontaneous deep ganglionic intracerebral hemorrhage. Clin Neurol Neurosurg 115: 1028–1031.

Takeuchi S, Wada K, Nagatani K et al. (2013). Decompressive hemicraniectomy for spontaneous intracerebral hemorrhage. Neurosurg Focus 34. E5.

Tanaka KA, Szlam F, Dickneite G et al. (2008). Effects of prothrombin complex concentrate and recombinant activated factor VII on vitamin K antagonist induced anticoagulation. Thromb Res 122: 117–123.

Tanikawa T, Amano K, Kawamura H et al. (1985). CT-guided stereotactic surgery for evacuation of hypertensive intracerebral hematoma. Appl Neurophysiol 48: 431–439.

Taylor TN, Davis PH, Torner JC et al. (1996). Lifetime cost of stroke in the United States. Stroke 27: 1459–1466.

Tejima E, Zhao BQ, Tsuji K et al. (2007). Astrocytic induction of matrix metalloproteinase-9 and edema in brain hemorrhage. J Cereb Blood Flow Metab 27: 460–468.

Tentschert S, Wimmer R, Greisenegger S et al. (2005). Headache at stroke onset in 2196 patients with ischemic stroke or transient ischemic attack. Stroke 36: e1–e3.

Thrift AG, Donnan GA, McNeil JJ (1999). Heavy drinking, but not moderate or intermediate drinking, increases the risk of intracerebral hemorrhage. Epidemiology 10: 307–312.

van Asch CJ, Luitse MJ, Rinkel GJ et al. (2010). Incidence, case fatality, and functional outcome of intracerebral haemorrhage over time, according to age, sex, and ethnic origin: a systematic review and meta-analysis. Lancet Neurol 9: 167–176.

van Loon J, Van Calenbergh F, Goffin J et al. (1993). Controversies in the management of spontaneous cerebellar haemorrhage. A consecutive series of 49 cases and review of the literature. Acta Neurochir (Wien) 122: 187–193.

Vespa PM (2008). Intensive glycemic control in traumatic brain injury: what is the ideal glucose range? Crit Care 12: 175.

Vespa PM, O'Phelan K, Shah M et al. (2003). Acute seizures after intracerebral hemorrhage: a factor in progressive midline shift and outcome. Neurology 60: 1441–1446.

Vespa P, McArthur D, Miller C et al. (2005). Frameless stereotactic aspiration and thrombolysis of deep intracerebral hemorrhage is associated with reduction of hemorrhage volume and neurological improvement. Neurocrit Care 2: 274–281.

Vespa P, Boonyaputthikul R, McArthur DL et al. (2006). Intensive insulin therapy reduces microdialysis glucose values without altering glucose utilization or improving the lactate/pyruvate ratio after traumatic brain injury. Crit Care Med 34: 850–856.

Wagner KR (2007). Modeling intracerebral hemorrhage: glutamate, nuclear factor-kappa B signaling and cytokines. Stroke 38: 753–758.

Walter S, Kostpopoulos P, Haass A et al. (2010). Bringing the hospital to the patient: first treatment of stroke patients at the emergency site. PLoS One 5. e13758.

Wang WZ, Jiang B, Liu HM et al. (2009). Minimally invasive craniopuncture therapy vs. conservative treatment for spontaneous intracerebral hemorrhage: results from a randomized clinical trial in China. Int J Stroke 4: 11–16.

Weber JE, Ebinger M, Rozanski M et al. (2013). Prehospital thrombolysis in acute stroke: results of the PHANTOM-S pilot study. Neurology 80: 163–168.

Wei JW, Heeley EL, Wang JG et al. (2010). Comparison of recovery patterns and prognostic indicators for ischemic and hemorrhagic stroke in China: the ChinaQUEST (QUality Evaluation of Stroke Care and Treatment) Registry study. Stroke 41: 1877–1883.

Wong GK, Siu DY, Abrigo JM et al. (2012). Computed tomographic angiography for patients with acute spontaneous intracerebral hemorrhage. J Clin Neurosci 19: 498–500.

Xi G, Keep RF, Hoff JT (2006). Mechanisms of brain injury after intracerebral haemorrhage. Lancet Neurol 5: 53–63.

Yadav YR, Mukerji G, Shenoy R et al. (2007). Endoscopic management of hypertensive intraventricular hemorrhage with obstructive hydrocephalus. BMC Neurol 7: 1.

Zahuranec DB, Morgenstern LB, Sanchez BN et al. (2010). Do-not-resuscitate orders and predictive models after intracerebral hemorrhage. Neurology 75: 626–633.

Zhang Z, Li X, Liu Y et al. (2007). Application of neuroendoscopy in the treatment of intraventricular hemorrhage. Cerebrovasc Dis 24: 91–96.

Ziai WC (2013). Hematology and inflammatory signaling of intracerebral hemorrhage. Stroke 44: S74–S78.

Ziai WC, Melnychuk E, Thompson CB et al. (2012). Occurrence and impact of intracranial pressure elevation during treatment of severe intraventricular hemorrhage. Crit Care Med 40: 1601–1608.

*Handbook of Clinical Neurology*, Vol. 140 (3rd series)
*Critical Care Neurology, Part I*
E.F.M. Wijdicks and A.H. Kramer, Editors
http://dx.doi.org/10.1016/B978-0-444-63600-3.00012-X

Chapter 12

# Management of aneurysmal subarachnoid hemorrhage

N. ETMINAN[1] AND R.L. MACDONALD[2]*

[1]*Department of Neurosurgery, University Hospital Mannheim, University of Heidelberg, Mannheim, Germany*

[2]*Division of Neurosurgery, St. Michael's Hospital, Toronto, Ontario, Canada*

## Abstract

Spontaneous subarachnoid hemorrhage (SAH) affects people with a mean age of 55 years. Although there are about 9/100 000 cases per year worldwide, the young age and high morbidity and mortality lead to loss of many years of productive life. Intracranial aneurysms account for 85% of cases. Despite this, the majority of survivors of aneurysmal SAH have cognitive deficits, mood disorders, fatigue, inability to return to work, and executive dysfunction and are often unable to return to their premorbid level of functioning. The main proven interventions to improve outcome are aneurysm repair in a timely fashion by endovascular coiling rather than neurosurgical clipping when feasible and administration of nimodipine. Management also probably is optimized by neurologic intensive care units and multidisciplinary teams. Improved diagnosis, early aneurysm repair, administration of nimodipine, and advanced neurointensive care support may be responsible for improvement in survival from SAH in the last few decades.

## EPIDEMIOLOGY

Aneurysmal subarachnoid hemorrhage (aSAH) accounts for 2–5% of all strokes. Population-based studies reported a global incidence of SAH of 9 per 100 000 person-years (95% confidence interval (CI) 8.8–9.5), with distinct differences in Central and South America (4.3 per 100 000 person-years), Europe or Northern America (7.8 per 100 000 person-years), Finland (19.7 per 100 000 person-years), and Japan (23 per 100 000 person-years) (de Rooij et al., 2007). The incidence of SAH increases with increasing age, peaking at 50–60 years, with only 20% of cases occurring in patients younger than 45 years old (Ingall et al., 2000). The incidence of SAH may be declining, likely due to the lower incidence of modifiable risk factors for SAH as opposed to preventive treatment of unruptured intracranial aneurysms (UIAs), but robust data to support this are lacking (de Rooij et al., 2007). There is a female preponderance in the incidence of SAH (male-to-female ratio: 1:1.5), but only after the fifth life decade. In 2007 in the USA, there were 2 423 712 deaths (Centers for Disease Control and Prevention, 2016). A total of 135 952 were due to cerebrovascular disease (5.6%) and 5708 were attributed to SAH (0.2% or 1 in 500 of all deaths, 4% of cerebrovascular deaths). The increased incidence in mainly postmenopausal females has been hypothesized to be due to lack of estrogen and progesterone as protective factors, although a meta-analysis found the data were conflicting and no firm conclusions could be drawn (Algra et al., 2012).

### Natural history of aneurysmal SAH

Patients began to have their ruptured aneurysms repaired in the 1960s, at least in a delayed fashion, so there are few data on the natural history of aSAH. Pakarinen (1967) collected 589 cases of spontaneous SAH from Helsinki between 1954 and 1961. Most of these cases were probably aneurysmal SAH. Seventy-six of 554 patients with their first SAH (14%, a third of all deaths) died before hospital admission. Death occurred in another 115 (21%) on day 1 (half of all deaths) for a total of 25–30% mortality in the first day, 40–45% in the first

*Correspondence to: R. Loch Macdonald, M.D., Ph.D., Division of Neurosurgery, Department of Surgery, University of Toronto, 30 Bond Street, Toronto, Ontario, Canada M5B 1 W8. Tel: +1-416-864-5452, Fax: +1-416-864-5634, E-mail: macdonaldlo@smh.ca

week, and 50–60% in the first month. There was a cumulative mortality from the initial hemorrhage within a month of 43% and 30–35% were alive after 5 years.

## ETIOLOGY

### Subtypes of SAH

About 85% of cases of spontaneous SAH are aneurysmal and 10% are nonaneurysmal perimesencephalic SAH. The remaining 5% have diverse etiologies (Table 12.1 and Fig. 12.1) (van Gijn et al., 2007). Among 352 patients with SAH admitted to hospitals in Greater Cincinnati between 1998 and 2004, 285 (81%) had ruptured aneurysms, 43 (12%) had nonaneurysmal, non-perimesencephalic SAH (often in the subarachnoid space over the cerebral convexities), and 24 (7%) had nonaneurysmal perimesencephalic SAH (Flaherty et al., 2005; Refai et al., 2008). Nonaneurysmal perimesencephalic SAH has a specific pattern on initial computed tomography (CT: Fig. 12.1). Patients with nonaneurysmal perimesencephalic SAH tend to more often be male, younger, and hypertensive than aneurysmal cases.

### Weather and climate

There are at least 48 studies including 72 694 patients that examined the risk of SAH in relation to season, temperature, atmospheric pressure, and relative humidity (de Steenhuijsen Piters et al., 2013). Meta-analysis found SAH was less common in summer than in winter (relative risk (RR) 0.89, 95% CI 0.83–0.96), but the magnitude of this effect was small. There is no consistent relation to barometric pressure, temperature, or humidity. The usual explanation for the increase in SAH in winter is that cold weather is associated with increased blood pressure, blood viscosity, serum lipids, and sympathetic nervous system activity. Blood clotting time is altered, fibrinogen concentration decreases, and there is increased fibrinolytic activity. Furthermore, behaviors may be different in the winter, with more smoking, drinking alcohol, and work people are unaccustomed to due to snow and ice.

## NEUROPATHOLOGY

The neuropathology of SAH can be categorized based on the mechanisms of aneurysm formation and rupture and then the consequences of aneurysm rupture. Aneurysm rupture causes brain damage in two phases (Fig. 12.2). There is early brain injury that is reflected in the neurologic grade of the patient, and that is secondary to transient global ischemia, toxicity of subarachnoid blood, herniations, and intracerebral hemorrhage (ICH) (Matz et al., 2001; Fujii et al., 2013). There is a delayed phase of brain injury 3–14 days after the SAH when delayed neurologic

*Table 12.1*

**Causes of subarachnoid hemorrhage (SAH)**

| Category | Causes |
|---|---|
| Idiopathic | Nonaneurysmal perimesencephalic SAH |
| Infections | Bacterial, tuberculous, and fungal meningitis, syphilis, herpes simplex or other viral encephalitis, leptospirosis, listeriosis, brucellosis, yellow fever, typhoid fever, dengue, malaria, anthrax |
| Trauma | Closed head injury, electric injury, gunshot wounds and other penetrating cranial trauma, heat injury, strangulation, high altitude, caisson disease, radiation, germinal matrix hemorrhage in neonates |
| Toxins | Amphetamines, cocaine, monoamine oxidase inhibitors, epinephrine, alcohol, ether, carbon monoxide, morphine, nicotine, lead, quinine, phosphorus, pentylenetetrazol, hydrocyanic acid, insulin, snake venom |
| Vascular | Intracranial saccular, fusiform, or dissecting aneurysm, reversible cerebral vasoconstriction syndrome, rupture of hypertensive, amyloid, or other type of intracerebral hemorrhage into the cerebrospinal fluid, hemorrhagic transformation of ischemic infarction, ruptured arteriovenous or other vascular malformation, vasculitis from systemic lupus erythematosus, polyarteritis nodosa or other cause, eclampsia, intracranial venous thrombosis, oral contraceptives, volume depletion, hypercoagulable states, trauma, infection |
| Blood diseases | Leukemia, hemophilia, sickle-cell anemia, pernicious anemia, aplastic anemia, agranulocytosis, thrombocytopenic purpura, polycythemia vera, Waldenström's macroglobulinemia, lymphoma, myeloma, hereditary spherocytosis, afibrinogenemia, liver diseases associated with coagulopathy, disseminated intravascular coagulation, acquired coagulopathies due to anticoagulant drugs, other congenital or acquired platelet vessel or coagulation disorders |
| Neoplasms | Glioma, meningioma, hemangioblastoma, choroid plexus papilloma, chordoma, hemangioma, pituitary adenoma, sarcoma, osteochondroma, ependymoma, neurofibroma, schwannoma, bronchogenic carcinoma, choriocarcinoma, melanoma, numerous other cranial and spinal tumors |

Modified from Weir (1987).

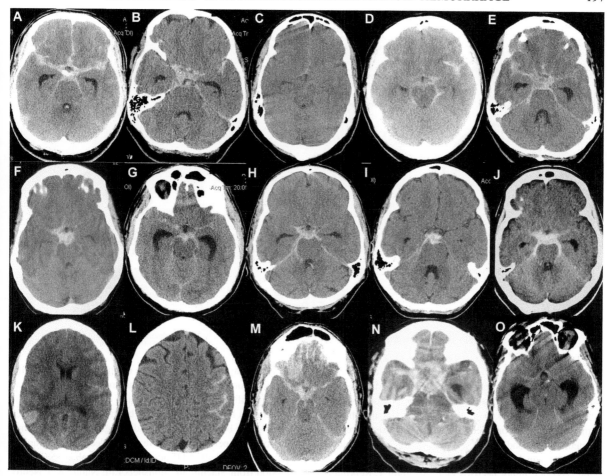

**Fig. 12.1.** Computed tomography (CT) of different types of subarachnoid hemorrhage (SAH). The CT scans of patients with aneurysmal SAH from aneurysms of the right middle cerebral artery (**A**), right internal carotid artery (**B**), anterior communicating artery (**C**), left middle cerebral artery (**D**), and right superior cerebellar artery (**E**) are shown. CT of patients with nonaneurysmal perimesencephalic SAH (**F–H, J**) resemble aneurysmal SAH from a basilar bifurcation aneurysm (**I**), showing that CT and/or catheter angiography are necessary in all patients with nonaneurysmal perimesencephalic SAH. Nonaneurysmal SAH due to cerebral venous thrombosis (**K, L**), trauma (**M**), pituitary apoplexy (**N**), and pseudo-SAH due to increased intracranial pressure, brain swelling, and compression of the basal cisterns (**O**) are shown. Reprinted from The Lancet, Macdonald RL, Schweizer TA, Spontaneous subarachnoid haemorrhage, advance online publication, 2016, with permission from Elsevier.

deterioration can occur due to delayed cerebral ischemia (DCI) in up to a third of patients (Macdonald, 2014).

Almost all aneurysm ruptures cause some SAH (Fig. 12.1). There also commonly is bleeding into the ventricles (intraventricular hemorrhage (IVH)) and brain tissue (ICH). Bleeding into the subdural space is uncommon.

A systemic response to SAH is typical and can affect the lungs (pulmonary edema, acute respiratory distress syndrome), heart (arrhythmias, contractility abnormalities) and fluid and electrolyte balance (Chen et al., 2014). A systemic inflammatory response develops in up to a third of patients and is associated with poor outcome. Mechanisms of the systemic response to SAH are hypothesized to include increased sympathetic nervous system activity with increased catecholamines, natriuretic peptides, renin–angiotensin system activation, and inflammatory cytokines.

## Aneurysm formation and rupture

Intracranial, saccular aneurysms are acquired and develop at major branching cerebral arteries in response to hemodynamic stress-induced degeneration of the internal elastic lamina with secondary thinning and loss of the tunica media (Fig. 12.3) (Etminan et al., 2014b). The pathophysiologic mechanisms involved in aneurysm formation are theoretic since there are few molecular manipulations or alterations in humans that are known to affect aneurysm formation and few studies of risk factors and hemodynamics before and after aneurysm formation. The average size of a ruptured aneurysm

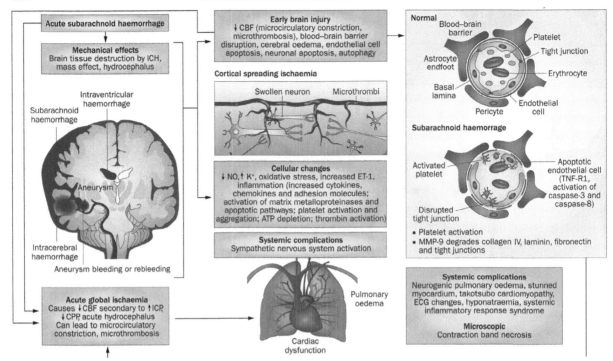

**Fig. 12.2.** Early pathophysiology of subarachnoid hemorrhage. Acute hemorrhage from an aneurysm can physically damage the brain and lead to acute transient global ischemia. Transient global ischemia secondary to increased intracranial pressure (ICP) can also trigger sympathetic nervous system activation, leading to systemic complications. The contribution of each process to the pathophysiology is unknown, but transient global ischemia and subarachnoid blood result in early brain injury, characterized by microcirculation constriction, microthrombosis, disruption of the blood–brain barrier, cytotoxic and vasogenic cerebral edema, and neuronal and endothelial cell death. CBF, cerebral blood flow; CPP, cerebral perfusion pressure; ECG, electrocardiographic; ET-1, endothelin-1; ICH, intracranial hemorrhage; MMP-9, matrix metalloproteinase-9; ATP, adenosine triphosphate; NO, nitric oxide; TNF-R1, tumor necrosis factor receptor 1. Reprinted by permission from Macmillan Publishers Ltd: Nature Rev Neurol (Macdonald, 2014), copyright 2014.

is 6–7 mm, which is smaller than in older studies (8–10 mm), where probably the size was less accurately determined (Weir et al., 2002; Beck et al., 2006).

The prevalence of UIA in the adult population is 3.2% (Vlak et al., 2011a). Risk factors for aneurysm formation (and growth/progression) and risk factors associated with aneurysm rupture are similar, but there are conflicting data due in part to differences in study design, as well as because the factors that lead to aneurysm formation may differ from those leading to aneurysm rupture (Table 12.2). For example, smoking is strongly linked to SAH and to aneurysm growth, but it was not a risk factor for rupture of UIA, suggesting it is more important in aneurysm formation than rupture (Wiebers et al., 2003; Feigin et al., 2005; Morita et al., 2012; Backes et al., 2016). The mechanisms of aneurysm formation due to smoking are postulated to include increased circulating carbon monoxide and cigarette toxins, increased blood proteases, fibrinogen and inflammation, inhibition of $\alpha_1$-antitrypsin, antiestrogen effects, and acute elevations of blood pressure.

Risk factors for SAH are most easily documented (Table 12.2). In addition to smoking, modifiable risk

factors include hypertension and excess alcohol intake, each of which doubles the risk (Weir, 2002; Feigin et al., 2005; Andreasen et al., 2013). Hypertension may contribute to aneurysm formation and rupture by damage to endothelium and vasa vasorum and altered collagen and elastin formation by smooth-muscle cells. Alcohol can damage endothelial cells, induce oxidative stress, elevate blood pressure, induce tumor necrosis factor-$\alpha$, and increase hematocrit, plasma osmolarity, and fibrinogen. Regular exercise may be protective against SAH; it reduces blood pressure, decreases vascular oxidative stress, and increases endothelial nitric oxide (NO). The above modifiable risk factors for SAH account for 70% of cases of SAH. Serum lipids may influence the risk of SAH but data are conflicting (Lindbohm et al., in press). Nonmodifiable risk factors for SAH include increasing age, female sex, family history, possibly Japanese or Finnish ethnicity, and history of SAH (de Rooij et al., 2007).

Risk factors for rupture of UIA have been derived from studies of the natural history of selected subgroups of these patients, which results in various limitations in

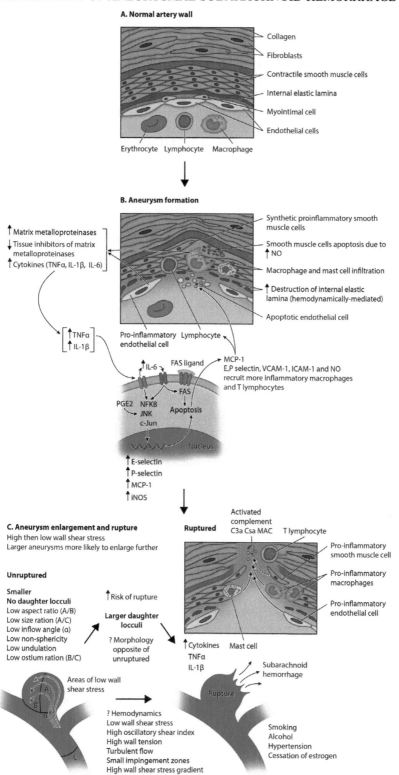

**Fig. 12.3.** See legend on next page.

the data (Table 12.2) (Korja and Kaprio, 2016). Pooled analysis of six prospective cohort studies, including data on 8382 persons and 10 272 aneurysms, established six risk factors for aneurysm rupture: previous SAH from another aneurysm, Finnish or Japanese ethnicity, older age, hypertension, and aneurysm size and location (Wiebers et al., 2003; Morita et al., 2012; Greving et al., 2014). Irregular aneurysm shape was a risk factor for UIA rupture in one study (Morita et al., 2012). Compared to risk factors for SAH, smoking, alcohol intake, exercise, higher serum cholesterol, and female sex seem less important in predicting UIA rupture. Data from case-control studies also identified family history (two or more first-degree relatives with a previous SAH or UIA), stimulants such as cocaine or amphetamines, and aneurysm wall inflammation or aneurysm growth and *de novo* formation on serial imaging as additional risk factors (Juvela, 2002; Feigin et al., 2005; Morita et al., 2012; Hasan et al., 2013; Etminan et al., 2014a; Korja et al., 2014; Backes et al., 2015).

The few population-based studies of risk factors for aneurysm formation suggest that aneurysms are more likely in females, with increasing age, autosomal-dominant polycystic kidney disease, family history, and in patients with a history of SAH (Table 12.2) (Taylor et al., 1995; Horikoshi et al., 2002; Weir, 2002; Li et al., 2013b; Vlak et al., 2013a).

A genetic risk score for presence of UIA could not be identified in the population-based Rotterdam study (Peymani et al., 2015). Genomewide association studies identified six definite and one probable loci with common variants associated with UIA and/or SAH. These are 4q31.23 (*EDNRA*, odds ratio (OR) 1.22), 8q11.23-q12.1 (*SOX17,* OR 1.28), 9p21.3 (*CDKN2A/CDKN2B*, OR 1.31), 10q24.32 (*CNNM2*, OR 1.29), 12q22 (*NDUFA12/NR2C1/FGD6/VEZT*, OR 1.16), 13q13.1 (*KL/STARD13*, OR 1.20), and 18q11.2 (*RBBP8*, OR 1.22) (Yasuno et al., 2011; Kurki et al., 2014). These loci explain 5% of genetic risk. This seems lower than the well-documented increased risk of identifying a UIA and of SAH when screening family members of patients with UIA or prior SAH (Kojima et al., 1998; Horikoshi et al., 2002; Teasdale et al., 2005). The prevalence of UIA in families with at least two members who have been diagnosed with UIA is 20% (compared to 2–3% in the general population) (Brown and Broderick, 2014). A familial intracranial aneurysm study screened 548 high-risk relatives (smokers and/or hypertensive) of patients with two affected siblings or $\geq 3$ affected first- or second-degree relatives and found 21% had aneurysms (Broderick et al., 2009). The risk of rupture of these UIA was 1.2% per year (95% CI 0.14–4.3%). This was compared to a historic matched nonfamilial cohort and the rupture risk was 17 times higher in familial cases (Wiebers et al., 2003). This was based on only two ruptures, however, so, while family history is associated with UIA and SAH, whether a familial UIA has a higher risk of rupture is less certain. These data do suggest that familial clustering may be related to common environmental factors at least as much as to genetic ones (Korja et al., 2010).

One other genetic association is that patients with the *APOE4* allele have increased risk of DCI (OR 2.0, 95% CI 1.3–3.3) and poor outcome (OR 2.6, 95% CI 1.6–4.1) after SAH (Lanterna et al., 2007).

**Fig. 12.3—cont'd** Pathogenesis of cerebral saccular aneurysm formation, enlargement, and rupture. Clinical factors such as smoking, hypertension, and cessation of estrogen interact with high wall shear stress and increased wall shear stress gradient near major cerebral artery bifurcations (**A**) to form aneurysms (**B**) (Kulcsar et al., 2011). These factors are hypothesized to lead to activation of endothelial cell molecules, including cyclooxygenase-mediated production of prostaglandin $E_2$ ($PGE_2$) and others. These activate proinflammatory signaling pathways such as NF-kappaB and C-Jun amino-terminal kinase. These in turn lead to increased monocyte chemoattractant protein 1 (MCP-1), cell adhesion molecules (intercellular adhesion molecule 1, vascular cell adhesion molecule 1, E-selectin, P-selectin), and proinflammatory cytokines (tumor necrosis factor-$\alpha$, interleukin-6 (IL-6), IL-1$\beta$). Cytokines and cell adhesion molecules can lead to endothelial cell apoptosis by activation of Fas-associated death domain pathway. They also attract macrophages and mast cells that infiltrate the artery wall, incite further inflammation by producing similar mediators, and increase matrix metalloproteinases and reduce activity of tissue inhibitors of metalloproteinase. Smooth-muscle cells are induced to undergo similar changes, becoming proinflammatory and less contractile. Endothelial cells produce more inducible nitric oxide synthase that produces high noxious levels of nitric oxide which can cause smooth-muscle cell apoptosis. Aneurysm growth and rupture are also associated clinically with smoking, hypertension, alcohol, and cessation of estrogen. Aneurysm enlargement was associated with low wall shear stress and with larger initial aneurysm size (Shojima et al., 2004; Lall et al., 2009). Rupture is associated with increased size and daughter loculi (**C**) (Morita et al., 2012). Other studies only compare ruptured with unruptured aneurysms and report ruptured ones tend to have areas of lower wall shear stress, high oscillatory shear index, higher wall tension, more turbulent flow, small flow impingement zones, and high wall shear stress gradient. Morphologic features associated with ruptured compared to unruptured aneurysms include increased size, daughter loculi, higher aspect ratio, size ratio, inflow angle, nonsphericity index, ellipticity index, undulation index, and ostium ratio (Dhar et al., 2008; Francis et al., 2013). Molecular pathways that may be associated with rupture status include more T cells, more proinflammatory macrophages and mast cells, C3a and C5a and complement activation, and inflammatory cytokines and activation of cyclooxygenase 2 and microsomal prostaglandin $E_2$ synthase-1, enzymes involved in inflammation and defects in polycystin (Hudson et al., 2013). From Macdonald and Schweizer (2016).

*Table 12.2*

**Risk factors for cerebral aneurysms and subarachnoid hemorrhage (SAH)**

| Risk factor | Formation of an unruptured aneurysm | Rupture of known unruptured aneurysm | Subarachnoid hemorrhage |
|---|---|---|---|
| **Modifiable** | | | |
| Smoking | Case-control study suggests smoking associated with unruptured aneurysms (OR 3.0, 95% CI 2.0–4.5) (Vlak et al., 2013b). Screening of a population in China did not find an association (Li et al., 2013b) | Not significant in meta-analysis, ISUIA, UCAS or PHASES (Wiebers et al., 2003; Rinkel 2008; Morita et al., 2012; Greving et al., 2014). Smoking increased risk of rupture in case-control study (OR 1.9, 95% CI 1.2–3.0) (Vlak et al., 2013b) | Significantly associated with smoking in multiple studies, RR for current smokers 2.2 (95% CI 1.3–3.6), OR 3.1 (95% CI 2.7–3.5) (Weir; Feigin et al., 2005). Population attributable risk 20–40% (Andreasen et al., 2013) |
| Hypertension | Not significant in one screened population in China but significant in Japan in a selected population (Horikoshi et al., 2002; Li et al., 2013b). Associated with aneurysms in another study and in a case-control study (Taylor et al., 1995; Vlak et al., 2013b) | History of hypertension did not independently influence the risk in case-control study (Vlak et al., 2013b). Also was not independently predictive in ISUIA or UCAS but was in PHASES (Wiebers et al., 2003; Morita et al., 2012; Greving et al., 2014) | More common in patients with SAH in multiple studies and a meta-analysis of epidemiologic studies (RR 2.5, 95% CI 2.0–3.1, OR 2.6, 95% CI 2.0–3.1) (Feigin et al., 2005). Population attributable risk 17–28% (Andreasen et al., 2013) |
| Alcohol intake | Not significant in a screened population or a case-control study (Li et al., 2013b; Vlak et al., 2013b) | Was not a predictor of rupture in ISUIA or PHASES and was not assessed in UCAS (Wiebers et al., 2003; Morita et al., 2012; Greving et al., 2014) | Increased risk of SAH (RR 2.1, 95% CI 1.5–2.8, OR 1.5, 95% CI 1.3–1.8) (Feigin et al., 2005). Population attributable risk 11–21% (Andreasen et al., 2013) |
| Regular physical exercise | Reduced the risk in one study (OR 0.6, 95% CI 0.3–0.9) (Vlak et al., 2013b). | Was not assessed in most studies; chronic exercise unlikely a risk for rupture (Wiebers et al., 2003; Morita et al., 2012; Greving et al., 2014) | Rigorous exercise associated with reduced risk of SAH (RR 0.5, 95% CI 0.3–1.0, OR 1.2, 95% CI 1.0–1.6) (Feigin et al., 2005). Increased risk of SAH during high-intensity exercise (Vlak et al., 2013b) |
| Cholesterol | Hyperlipidemia associated with aneurysms in a population-based study (Li et al., 2013b). Hypercholesterolemia reduced the risk in a case-control study (OR 0.5, 95% CI 0.3–0.9) (Vlak et al., 2013b) | Hypercholesterolemia decreased the risk in case-control studies (OR 0.4, 95% CI 0.2–1.0) (Vlak et al., 2013b). Not significant in ISUIA or UCAS, not assessed in PHASES (Wiebers et al., 2003; Morita et al., 2012; Greving et al., 2014) | Hypercholesterolemia reduced the risk of SAH, (RR 0.8, 95% CI 0.6–1.2, OR 0.6, 95% CI 0.4–0.9) (Feigin et al., 2005) |
| **Not modifiable** | | | |
| Age | Autopsy studies show increased prevalence with increasing age, that may or may not level off in later decades (Weir). Increased prevalence with age in screening of populations and in meta-analysis (Horikoshi et al., 2002; Li et al., 2013b; Harada et al., 2013; Vlak et al., 2013b) | Not significant in ISUIA or UCAS; increased age increased risk of rupture in PHASES (Wiebers et al., 2003; Morita et al., 2012; Greving et al., 2014). Age > 60 associated with increased risk in meta-analysis (RR 2.0, 95% CI 1.1–3.7) (Wermer et al., 2007) | Incidence of SAH rises with age (de Rooij et al., 2007) |

*Continued*

**Table 12.2**

Continued

| Risk factor | Formation of an unruptured aneurysm | Rupture of known unruptured aneurysm | Subarachnoid hemorrhage |
|---|---|---|---|
| Sex | Autopsy studies show more aneurysms in females (Weir). Increased prevalence in females in populations and meta-analysis (Horikoshi et al., 2002; Li et al., 2013b; Harada et al., 2013; Vlak et al., 2013b) | Female sex increased risk in one study (RR 1.6, 95% CI 1.1–2.4) (Wermer et al., 2007), not significant in ISUIA, UCAS, or PHASES (Wiebers et al., 2003; Morita et al., 2012; Greving et al., 2014) | More common in females overall, about equal until age 50–55, after which females increasingly predominate (de Rooij et al., 2007) |
| Family history | Screening of first-degree relatives in families with one or two first-degree relatives shows increased prevalence of aneurysms (Kojima et al., 1998; Horikoshi et al., 2002). Meta-analysis also suggests increased prevalence in families (Vlak et al., 2013b) | A familial intracranial aneurysm study suggested patients with familial aneurysms had a 17-times higher risk of rupture than nonfamilial incidental aneurysms based on two cases (Broderick et al., 2009) | Increased risk in families with two or more first-degree relatives (Teasdale et al., 2005) |
| Ethnicity | There was no difference in prevalence of aneurysms in various regions (Vlak et al., 2013b) | 3.6 times increased risk in Finnish and 2.8 times increased risk in Japanese in PHASES (Greving et al., 2014). Japanese or Finnish descent had increased risk of rupture (RR 3.4, 95% CI 2.6–4.4) (Wermer et al., 2007) | Risk of nonwhite ethnicity was marginal in one meta-analysis (RR 1.8, 95% CI 0.8–4.2, OR 3.4, 95% CI 1.0–11.9) (Feigin et al., 2005). Increased risk in Japan and Finland in another meta-analysis (de Rooij et al., 2007) |
| Genetics | Population-based Rotterdam study developed genetic risk score based on genetic variants associated with aneurysms. This score was not associated with aneurysms but with size of aneurysms (Peymani et al., 2015). Other studies identify various loci that explain 2% of heritability in Finland (Kurki et al., 2014) | Studies generally have not separated risks for unruptured aneurysms or SAH. Six definite and one probable loci identified associated with unruptured aneurysms or aneurysmal SAH were 4q31.23 (*EDNRA*, OR 1.22), 8q11.23-q12.1 (*SOX17*, OR 1.28), 9p21.3 (*CDKN2A/CDKN2B*, OR 1.31), 10q24.32 (*CNNM2*, OR 1.29), 12q22 (*NDUFA12/NR2C1/FGD6/VEZT*, OR 1.16), 13q13.1 (*KL/STARD13*, OR 1.20), and 18q11.2 (*RBBP8*, OR 1.22) (Yasuno et al., 2011; Kurki et al., 2014) | |
| Autosomal-dominant polycystic kidney disease | Increased prevalence of aneurysms in these patients when they are screened (Weir). Also increased prevalence in meta-analysis (Vlak et al., 2013b) | Not well studied; retrospective reviews suggest there is no increased risk of SAH (Kemp et al., 2013) | Limited data suggest increased incidence of SAH due to increased prevalence of aneurysms rather than increased risk of rupture of known unruptured aneurysm (Schievink et al., 1992; Perrone et al., 2015) |
| Aneurysm size | Most were <3 mm (41%) in one population, with a mean of 3.5 and 3.4 mm (Harada et al., 2013; Li et al., 2013b) and <6 mm (74%) in another (Horikoshi et al., 2002). 66% were <5 mm in a meta-analysis (Vlak et al., 2013b) | Increasing aneurysm size is consistently a significant factor associated with rupture risk, including in ISUIA, UCAS, and PHASES (Wiebers et al., 2003; Morita et al., 2012; Greving et al., 2014) | Ruptured aneurysms are slightly larger than unruptured ones, but there are many small ruptured aneurysms (Weir) |

| | | | |
|---|---|---|---|
| Aneurysm location | Middle cerebral > internal carotid = anterior communicating artery in autopsy studies and one large screening study (Weir; Horikoshi et al., 2002; Harada et al., 2013). Internal carotid > anterior cerebral > middle cerebral artery in a population (Li et al., 2013b). Internal carotid > middle cerebral > anterior cerebral in a meta-analysis (Vlak et al., 2013b) | Anterior or posterior communicating or posterior circulation aneurysms at higher risk of rupture in PHASES, fairly consistent with ISUIA and UCAS (Wiebers et al., 2003; Morita et al., 2012; Greving et al., 2014) | In series of SAH patients, most common locations are anterior communicating = internal carotid artery > middle cerebral artery (Weir) |
| Aneurysm shape | Not applicable | Aneurysms with daughter loculus were more likely to rupture in UCAS (hazard ratio 1.6, 95% CI 1.1–2.5) (Morita et al., 2012) | Comparative studies of unruptured and ruptured aneurysms only, suggest irregularity correlated with rupture status (Francis et al., 2013) |
| Aneurysm growth | Not applicable | Increased risk of rupture if aneurysm growing (Juvela et al., 2001). Growth not included in ISUIA, UCAS, or PHASES (Wiebers et al., 2003; Morita et al., 2012; Greving et al., 2014) | Not applicable |
| Symptomatic aneurysm | Not applicable | Symptomatic aneurysm more likely to rupture in one meta-analysis (RR 4.4, 95% CI 2.8–6.8) (Werner et al., 2007). Symptoms were not predictive in ISUIA or UCAS, and not included in PHASES (Wiebers et al., 2003; Morita et al., 2012; Greving et al., 2014) | Not applicable |
| History of SAH | New aneurysm formation more common in patients with history of SAH (Horikoshi et al., 2002) | Significant in ISUIA and PHASES but not in UCAS (Morita et al., 2012; Wiebers et al., 2003; Greving et al., 2014) | Recurrent SAH and death from SAH are probably more common in patients with history of SAH based on long-term follow-up in several studies, but this is not well documented (Molyneux et al., 2009; Huttunen et al., 2011) |

OR, odds ratio; CI, confidence interval; ISUIA, International Study of Unruptured Intracranial Aneurysms; UCAS; Unruptured Cerebral Aneurysm Study; PHASES, Population Hypertension Age Size Earlier Subarachnoid hemorrhage site; RR, relative risk.

## Early brain injury

At the time of aneurysm rupture, blood pulses under arterial pressure into the subarachnoid or subdural space, ventricles, and/or brain itself. These different patterns of hemorrhage can result in a transient or prolonged increase of intracranial pressure (ICP) and transient global ischemia. The brain can be damaged by ICH and herniation. Subarachnoid blood itself also damages the brain, since application of blood or hemolyzed erythrocytes to the pial surface of the brain induces blood–brain barrier breakdown, edema, and brain injury (Matz et al., 2001). The pathophysiology of this initial phase of SAH has been called early brain injury and comprises microcirculatory constriction, endothelial cell apoptosis, blood–brain barrier disruption, edema formation, and excitotoxicity (Fujii et al., 2013; Suzuki, 2015). Excitotoxicity involves biomechanical processes such as sodium, potassium, or calcium channel dysfunction and increase of inflammation or matrix metalloproteinases resulting in neuronal and other brain cell damage or loss. The extent of early brain injury is reflected in the initial neurologic presentation (Glasgow Coma Scale (GCS) or World Federation of Neurologic Surgeons (WFNS) grading scale), the ICP, and the extent of hemorrhage into the different brain compartments (modified Fisher scale) (Drake et al., 1988; Frontera et al., 2006).

## Delayed cerebral ischemia

DCI occurs 3–14 days after a single SAH. The pathophysiology is hypothesized to be due to combined effects of angiographic vasospasm, microcirculatory dysfunction, microthromboembolism, cortical spreading ischemia (CSI), capillary transit time heterogeneity, and other processes (Fig. 12.4) (Vergouwen et al., 2007; Dreier, 2011; Ostergaard et al., 2013; Budohoski et al., 2014; Macdonald, 2014).

### ANGIOGRAPHIC VASOSPASM

The onset of angiographic vasospasm is 3–4 days, with a peak 6–8 days and resolution 12–14 days after SAH (Weir et al., 1978). About 70% of patients with aneurysmal SAH have some degree of angiographic vasospasm, although it is severe in only 30% (Dorsch and King, 1994; Macdonald, 2014). The vasoconstriction of the large subarachnoid arteries encased in the SAH is due to subarachnoid blood and depends on the location, volume, density, and duration of presence of the SAH (Reilly et al., 2004). It originates from hemolysis,

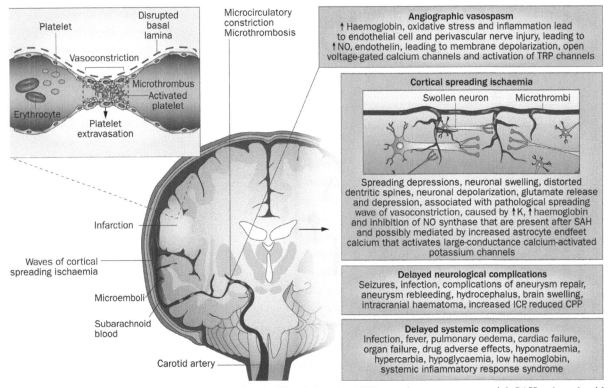

**Fig. 12.4.** Pathophysiology of delayed cerebral ischemia. NO, nitric oxide; TRP, transient receptor potential; SAH, subarachnoid hemorrhage; ICP, intracranial pressure; CPP, cerebral perfusion pressure. Reprinted by permission from Macmillan Publishers Ltd: Nature Rev Neurol (Macdonald, 2014), copyright 2014.

resulting in release of oxyhemoglobin, which incites a complex cascade of increased smooth-muscle intracellular calcium, endothelin-1 (ET-1) modulation, and impairment of physiologic NO regulation (Macdonald and Weir, 1991). An increase of intracellular calcium ultimately leads to contraction of vascular smooth-muscle cells (Jahromi et al., 2008). Further, ET-1 is one of three known endothelin peptides that are produced in vascular smooth muscle and endothelial cells. They bind to two receptor subtypes. Activation of the $ET_A$ receptor leads to vasoconstriction, typically via ET-1 and ET-2. The $ET_B$ receptor can induce vasodilation via NO and other dilatory factors, such as ET, endothelium-derived relaxing factor, or various eicosanoids (Roman et al., 2006; Pluta and Oldfield, 2007; Xie et al., 2007; Vatter et al., 2011; Rasmussen et al., 2015). The current hypothesis regarding the pathogenesis of vasospasm is that it is a subarachnoid blood/hemoglobin-induced inflammatory- and free-radical-mediated generation of an imbalance between vasoconstrictors (ET acting on $ET_A$ and $ET_B$, resulting in $ET_A$-derived vasoconstriction) and vasodilation (reduced NO vasodilation) (Macdonald, 2014).

### MICROCIRCULATORY DYSFUNCTION

Up to 5–10% of SAH patients develop DCI without angiographic macrovascular spasm (Crowley et al., 2011). In some cases this may be due to lack of angiographic imaging performed when DCI develops. In other patients, microvascular spasm or microcirculatory dysfunction has been hypothesized to cause DCI (Uhl et al., 2003; Friedrich et al., 2012). One possible mechanism for microcirculatory dysfunction is ET-1-mediated vasoconstriction or endothelial dysfunction of small cerebral arteries, which is correlated with the amount of subarachnoid blood (Park et al., 2001).

### MICROTHROMBOEMBOLISM

In addition to microvascular spasm/dysfunction, microthromboemboli have been reported as an additional mechanism for DCI in the absence of angiographic vasospasm (Giller et al., 1998; Stein et al., 2006; Weidauer et al., 2008). The role of microemboli in the pathogenesis of DCI is supported by transcranial Doppler studies that have detected microemboli in patients with SAH and pathology studies showing microthrombi in arterioles and small infarcts in brains of humans dying after SAH (Stoltenburg-Didinger and Schwarz, 1987; Giller et al., 1998). Platelets aggregate in small brain blood vessels after experimental SAH, leading to breakdown of the basal lamina mediated by matrix metalloproteinases (Friedrich et al., 2010). Additionally, there is some evidence suggesting that nimodipine exerts fibrinolytic activity, which could reduce DCI by reducing microthrombi, independent of angiographic vasospasm (Roos et al., 2001). This could explain the beneficial effect of nimodipine when an effect on angiographic vasospasm in randomized clinical trials (RCT) has been difficult to document (Dorhout Mees et al., 2007).

### CORTICAL SPREADING DEPOLARIZATION/ISCHEMIA

Cortical spreading depolarization describes an electrophysiologic phenomenon in the gray matter, characterized by slow electric depolarizing potentials. The physiologic response to this neuronal activation is vasodilation to increase cerebral blood flow. Under conditions such as SAH, there may be a vasoconstrictive response, leading to near-complete breakdown of ion gradients, sustained depolarization in neurons, and cerebral ischemia. These waves of depolarization and ischemia spreading over the cortex are documented in humans with SAH (Dreier, 2011; Sakowitz et al., 2013). Cortical spreading depolarization and CSI have been described in association with DCI in SAH patients (Dreier, 2011; Woitzik et al., 2012; Sakowitz et al., 2013). Nimodipine reversed CSI into normal cortical spreading hyperemia in experimental models in vivo, which could also explain the beneficial effect of nimodipine on DCI and outcome (Dreier, 2011).

## CLINICAL PRESENTATION

The most common clinical symptom of SAH is sudden onset of very severe headache, often referred to as thunderclap headache, defined as reaching maximum severity within a flash of a second (Hop et al., 1999). The headache may resolve spontaneously or following consumption of analgesic drugs, which may explain why patients sometimes fail to consult a physician following aneurysm rupture. Less than 10% of patients presenting with only a severe headache actually have SAH (Table 12.1) (Perry et al., 2013). Other symptoms of SAH include nausea, vomiting, photophobia, nuchal rigidity, or meningismus and loss of consciousness or coma (Edlow and Caplan, 2000). However, these symptoms are nonspecific, headache may be the only symptom, and focal neurologic deficits after SAH are uncommon – all of which increase the difficulty in diagnosing SAH (Edlow and Caplan, 2000; Kowalski et al., 2004). The Ottawa SAH rule (age > 40 years, neck pain or stiffness, witnessed loss of consciousness, onset of headache during exertion, instantaneous onset of headache, or limited neck flexion on examination) detected SAH with 100% sensitivity (95% CI 97–100%) and 15% specificity (95% CI 14–17%) (Perry et al., 2013). Such decision rules need to be individualized and a low threshold for investigation of patients suspected to have SAH should be maintained because of the potentially severe consequences of missing the diagnosis.

A commonly used clinical classification of SAH is the WFNS grading scale. This scale is based on the level of consciousness, as measured by the GCS and the presence of focal neurologic deficits (Table 12.3) (Drake et al., 1988). The Prognosis on Admission of Aneurysmal SAH (PAASH) scale is similar to the WFNS (van Heuven et al., 2008). Another scale that is used mainly in the USA is the Hunt and Hess scale, but this scale has higher interobserver variability than the WFNS and PAASH scales (Hunt and Hess, 1968; Degen et al., 2011). Clinical grading is important because it

*Table 12.3*

Clinical grading scales include the Hunt and Hess, World Federation of Neurologic Surgeons (WFNS), and Prognosis on Admission of Aneurysmal Subarachnoid Hemorrhage (PAASH) scales (Hunt and Hess, 1968; Drake et al., 1988; van Heuven et al., 2008; Degen et al., 2011). The WFNS and PAASH scores rely on the Glasgow Coma Scale (GCS) and have similar interobserver agreement that is higher than the Hunt and Hess scale (Degen et al., 2011)

| | Hunt and Hess (Hunt and Hess, 1968) | WFNS (Drake et al., 1988) | PAASH (Degen et al., 2011) |
|---|---|---|---|
| 1 | Asymptomatic or mild headache and slight nuchal rigidity | GCS 15 | GCS 15 |
| 2 | Moderate to severe headache, nuchal rigidity, no focal neurologic deficit other than cranial nerve palsy | GCS 14–13 without major focal deficit (aphasia or hemiparesis/ hemiplegia) | GCS 11–14 |
| 3 | Confusion, lethargy, or mild focal neurologic deficit other than cranial-nerve palsy | GCS 14–13 with major focal deficit | GCS 8–10 |
| 4 | Stupor or moderate to severe hemiparesis | GCS 12–7 with or without major focal deficit | GCS 4–7 |
| 5 | Coma, extensor posturing, moribund appearance | GCS 6–3 with or without major focal deficit | GCS 3 |

influences recommendations for the acute management of SAH and is the most powerful prognostic factor for outcome (Jaja et al., 2013).

Although half of SAH cases in one series occurred during sleep or rest, 19% occurred during or within 2 hours of moderate or heavy exercise (OR 2.7, 95% CI 1.6–4.6) (Anderson et al., 2003). Various other activities and dietary intakes may trigger SAH, the theory being this is because they cause blood pressure fluctuations (Vlak et al., 2011b).

# NEURODIAGNOSTICS AND IMAGING

## Computed tomography

Any patient with suspected SAH should be referred to a hospital for further diagnostic testing and preferably to a neurovascular center. The test of choice for detection of SAH is nonenhanced CT. It is fast, safe, and widely available. Acute blood in the basal cisterns appears hyperdense and the hemorrhage pattern may indicate the location of the ruptured aneurysm, show other acute complications of SAH such as hydrocephalus and ICH, or suggest other etiologies for SAH (Perry et al., 2011). The sensitivity depends on the quality of the CT scanner and the time between headache onset and image acquisition. In a prospective, multicenter study, 3132 asymptomatic patients with nontraumatic headache reaching maximum intensity within 1 hour underwent CT for suspected SAH. For 953 patients scanned within 6 hours after headache onset, sensitivity of CT was 100%, declining with increasing time from ictus. In the first 3 days after ictus, the sensitivity of CT for detection of SAH is still greater than 97% but only 50% after 5 days.

A widely used radiologic (CT) classification of SAH is the Fisher or modified Fisher score, although there are several others (Table 12.4) (Fisher et al., 1980; Hijdra et al., 1990; Claassen et al., 2001; Frontera et al., 2006). The clinical importance of the modified Fisher score is its ability to predict DCI due to the association of increasing blood clot volumes and IVH with increasing risk of DCI.

## Magnetic resonance imaging

Magnetic resonance imaging (MRI) plays a secondary role in the acute diagnosis of SAH because of its more limited availability, longer acquisition time, and difficulty of use in critically ill patients (Pierot et al., 2013). The sensitivity of MRI increases by 48–72 hours after SAH (Ogawa et al., 1995). Gradient-echo T2*- weighted and susceptibility-weighted images are very sensitive to detecting hemosiderin and may be useful to diagnose SAH in patients who present weeks after onset (Lummel et al., 2015). MRI and MR angiography

*Table 12.4*

The amount of subarachnoid (SAH) and intraventricular hemorrhage (IVH) on the initial computed tomography scan is the most important factor predicting delayed cerebral ischemia and cerebral infarction is a prognostic factor for outcome (Frontera et al., 2006). Qualitative, semiquantitative, and quantitative scales have been proposed to measure this (Fisher et al., 1980; Hijdra et al., 1990; Claassen et al., 2001)

| Grade for entire brain except for Hijdra scale | Fisher scale (Fisher et al., 1980) | Claassen scale (Claassen et al., 2001) | Modified Fisher scale (Frontera et al., 2006) | Hijdra scale, grade each of 10 cisterns and each of the four ventricles (Hijdra et al., 1990) |
|---|---|---|---|---|
| 0 | | No SAH or IVH | No SAH or IVH | No blood in cistern, no blood in ventricle |
| 1 | No SAH or IVH | Minimum or thin SAH, no IVH in either lateral ventricle | Localized or diffuse thin SAH with no IVH | Small amount of blood in cistern, sedimentation of blood in posterior part of ventricle |
| 2 | Diffuse deposition of thin layer with all vertical layers of blood (interhemispheric fissure, insular cistern, ambient cistern) < 1 mm thick | Minimal or thin SAH, with IVH in both lateral ventricles | No or localized or diffuse thin SAH but with IVH | Moderate amount of blood in cistern, ventricle partly filled with blood |
| 3 | Vertical layers of blood ≥1 mm thick or localized clots (clots defined as > 3 × 5 mm) | Thick SAH completely filling two or more cisterns or fissures, no IVH in both lateral ventricles | Localized or diffuse thick SAH with no IVH | Cistern completely filled with blood, ventricle completely filled with blood |
| 4 | Diffuse or no subarachnoid blood, but with intracerebral or intraventricular clots | Thick SAH completely filling two or more cisterns or fissures, with IVH in both lateral ventricles | Localized or diffuse thick SAH with IVH | |

also are used for investigation of SAH of unknown cause, follow-up of coiled aneurysms to assess for recanalization, for vessel wall imaging and as a research tool to examine brain structure and function after SAH (Schweizer et al., 2012).

## Lumbar puncture

If CT or MRI does not demonstrate SAH or a cause for the patient's symptoms and signs, then a lumbar puncture is recommended. It is one of the most sensitive tests to confirm SAH by detecting xanthochromia in cerebrospinal fluid (CSF). Xanthochromia is yellow discoloration of CSF more than 12 hours after SAH due to formation *in vivo* of bilirubin (Backes et al., 2012). The CSF sample should be centrifuged immediately, stored in the dark, and analyzed as soon as possible. Visual inspection of the CSF can be done but it is less reliable than spectrophotometry (Arora et al., 2010). A traumatic lumbar puncture can be difficult to differentiate from SAH; there

are exceptions to and caveats for every criteria (Table 12.5). If SAH cannot be excluded, a CT angiogram (CTA) may be done to exclude an aneurysm.

## Determining the cause of SAH

If SAH is diagnosed, angiography is recommended to identify the source of hemorrhage (Fig. 12.5). The most sensitive diagnostic tool is catheter angiography. However, catheter angiography is invasive, time consuming, expensive, and carries a risk of transient or permanent complications of up to 2.6% (Kaufmann et al., 2007). CTA is thus increasingly used to detect aneurysms and meta-analyses report a pooled sensitivity of CTA of 97–98% (95% CI 95–98%) compared to catheter angiography or three-dimensional catheter angiography (Westerlaan et al., 2011; Liu et al., 2013). Neurosurgical clipping can be performed based on CTA in many cases but catheter angiography is required for endovascular coiling, complex aneurysms, and in case of negative

*Table 12.5*

**Differentiating subarachnoid hemorrhage (SAH) from traumatic lumbar puncture (Shah and Edlow, 2002)**

| Criteria | SAH | Traumatic puncture |
|---|---|---|
| Erythrocyte count | No change from first to subsequent tubes; some suggest $> 5 \times 10^6$ erythrocytes/L, although any erythrocytes are technically abnormal | Decreasing number of erythrocytes, although no specific decline has been shown to rule out SAH |
| Clotting | Does not clot | May clot |
| Xanthochromia, free hemoglobin, bilirubin (Brunell et al., 2013) | Present $> 12$ hours after ictus in supernatant fluid of a centrifuged tube that has been kept refrigerated in the dark, processed expeditiously and subjected to spectrophotometry, free hemoglobin $> 0.04$ AU, bilirubin $> 350$ nmol/L | No xanthochromia, free hemoglobin $< 0.04$ AU, bilirubin $< 350$ nmol/L |
| Crenated erythrocytes | Present | Absent |
| Erythrocyte/leukocyte ratio | May be decreased due to inflammation | Same as peripheral blood |
| D-dimer | Present | Absent |
| Protein | May be increased | Normal in relation to number of erythrocytes |
| Hemosiderin-laden macrophages | Present weeks after an SAH | Not present |
| Cerebrospinal fluid pressure | Normal or increased in 60% of cases | Normal |
| Repeat lumbar puncture | SAH | Usually clear |

AU, absorption units.

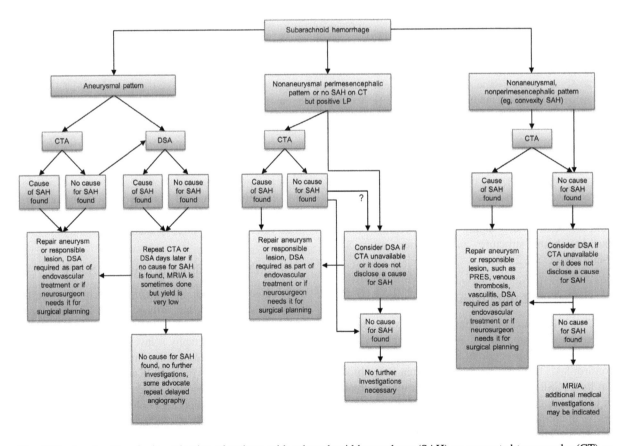

**Fig. 12.5.** An algorithm for investigation of patients with subarachnoid hemorrhage (SAH) on computed tomography (CT) or lumbar puncture (LP). CTA, computed tomography angiography; DSA, digital subtraction angiography; MRI, magnetic resonance imaging; MRA, magnetic resonance angiography; PRES, posterior reversible encephalopathy syndrome. Reprinted with modification from The Lancet, Macdonald RL, Schweizer TA, Spontaneous subarachnoid haemorrhage, advance online publication, 2016, with permission from Elsevier.

CTA and an aneurysmal or convexity pattern of SAH or SAH only detected by lumbar puncture. In case of an initial negative catheter angiogram, this is often repeated within 2 weeks, with a yield of 10% (95% CI 7.4–13.6%) (Agid et al., 2010; Bakker et al., 2014).

Imaging for perimesencephalic SAH is controversial because only 10% of such hemorrhages are caused by posterior circulation aneurysms and about 10% of posterior circulation aneurysms bleed with a perimesencephalic pattern (Alen et al., 2003). Since CTA is nearly as sensitive as catheter angiography for detection of the source of hemorrhage, it has been argued that patients with perimesencephalic SAH and a negative CTA do not need to undergo catheter angiography (Ruigrok et al., 2000).

## HOSPITAL COURSE AND MANAGEMENT

### Initial management and prevention of rebleeding

Following detection of SAH and the ruptured aneurysm, patients should be monitored in an intermediate or intensive care unit until endovascular or surgical repair of the aneurysm. Patients with impaired consciousness usually receive an external ventricular drain for CSF drainage and ICP monitoring (Diringer et al., 2011; Connolly et al., 2012; Steiner et al., 2013). Patients with acute hydrocephalus also may require a ventricular catheter as a life-saving acute treatment. Patients with space-occupying acute subdural (commonly due to internal carotid artery aneurysms) and/or ICH (commonly due to middle cerebral artery aneurysms) are usually treated immediately by surgical clot removal and clipping of the ruptured aneurysm. Not treating the aneurysm at the time of clot removal is associated with worse outcomes due to more frequent rebleeding (Fig. 12.6) (Wheelock et al., 1983).

Rebleeding from the ruptured aneurysm occurs in 8–23% of patients (Larsen and Astrup, 2013). Up to 90% of rehemorrhages occur within the first 6 hours. The most commonly reported risk factors for rebleeding are poor neurologic grade, amount of subarachnoid blood (Fisher grade), admission hypertension, larger aneurysm, CSF drainage, and possibly antiplatelet drugs (Larsen and Astrup, 2013; van Donkelaar et al., 2015). Catheter angiography performed within 6 hours of SAH is also associated with rebleeding, but whether this is related to the natural history or to angiography is uncertain (Fujii et al., 1996). Preventing acute hypertension and reducing the blood pressure on admission are recommended to reduce the risk of rebleeding. Since rebleeding has a detrimental effect on neurologic outcome, it is likely that early aneurysm repair improves outcome and current data, including those from an RCT on early

versus delayed aneurysm repair in SAH patients, highlight that aneurysm repair should be performed as soon as possible or within 72 hours (Ohman and Heiskanen, 1989; Connolly et al., 2012; van Donkelaar et al., 2015). On the other hand, the adjusted risk ratio for poor outcome for aneurysm repair within 24 hours compared to 24–72 hours was 1.37 (95% CI 1.11–1.68) in two case series (Oudshoorn et al., 2014). While early aneurysm repair makes sense, its beneficial effect on outcome thus has been difficult to confirm.

Another strategy to reduce rebleeding is to administer antifibrinolytic drugs. The rationale is data suggesting that aneurysm rupture is associated with activation of fibrinolysis in clot surrounding the aneurysm. A meta-analysis of 10 RCTs including 1904 patients treated with or without tranexamic acid or ε-aminocaproic acid reported a significant reduction in rebleeding but an increase of cerebral infarctions such that there was no overall effect on outcome (Baharoglu et al., 2013). Since these data are derived from long-term antifibrinolytic treatment (usually at least 14 days) and the era before early aneurysm repair, there is a rationale to investigate short courses of antifibrinolytic drugs until aneurysm repair (Germans et al., 2013).

### Aneurysm repair

Patients with SAH and intractable increases in ICP (usually WFNS grade 5) without space-occupying hematomas are usually managed supportively until they improve neurologically or the ICP can be controlled (de Oliveira Manoel et al., in press). This is based on the poor prognosis in such cases. On the other hand, aggressive supportive care and early aneurysm repair in WFNS grade 4 and selected grade 5 patients resulted in favorable outcome in up to 28% of cases (de Oliveira Manoel et al., in press).

The method of aneurysm repair is usually decided by an interdisciplinary neurovascular team and depends on factors such as patient age, clinical condition, pre-existing medical illnesses, aneurysm location, size, and morphology. Further, the presence of multiple aneurysms, the estimated risk of treatment associated with each modality, and the need for additional devices such as stents or flow diverters requiring dual antiplatelet therapy influence the choice of treatment (Molyneux et al., 2009; Spetzler et al., 2013). When either treatment is possible, endovascular repair is recommended. A meta-analysis of four RCTs of clipping versus coiling of ruptured aneurysms found that coiling reduced the risk of poor outcome to 23% compared to 34% after clipping (OR 1.48, 95% CI 1.24–1.76), with no difference in mortality (Li et al., 2013a). Endovascular coiling was associated with a lower risk of seizures, DCI, a reduced degree of complete aneurysm occlusion, and a higher risk of rebleeding.

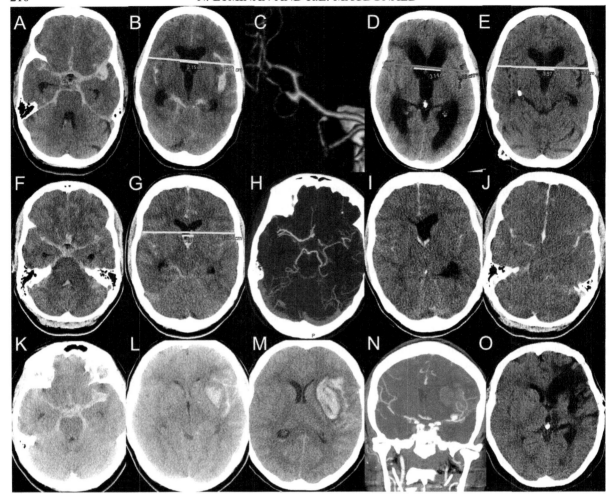

**Fig. 12.6.** Management of acute and chronic hydrocephalus and intracerebral hemorrhage in three cases. A 56-year-old female collapsed and was brought to hospital. Initial modified Glasgow Coma Scale was 6 T or 9 (imputed). She was intubated and computed tomography (CT) scan showed subarachnoid hemorrhage (SAH: **A**) and acute hydrocephalus (**B**), measured as above the 95th percentile for age by the ventriculocranial ratio (VCR 2.15/10.11 = 0.21) or bicaudate ratio (width of the frontal horns at the level of the foramen of Monro where the lateral walls of the frontal horns are parallel, divided by the internal diameter of the skull at the same level) (van Gijn et al., 1985). The upper 95th percentile is 0.16 for < 30 years old, 0.18 for 50 years old, 0.19 at 60 years old, 0.21 for 80 years old, and 0.25 for 100 years old. A ventricular catheter was inserted 11 hours after the ictus and the left middle cerebral aneurysm clipped through a pterional craniotomy 17 hours after the ictus. Preoperative CT angiography (CTA: **C**) demonstrated the aneurysm that was repaired, as confirmed by intraoperative indocyanine green angiography. The patient remained in poor condition and was transferred to chronic care. The patient remained bedridden and minimally responsive to her family 3 months later, when a CT scan showed chronic hydrocephalus (**D**, VCR 3.14/9.86 = 0.32). A ventriculoperitoneal shunt was inserted. Eight months later, a year after SAH, the patient almost fully recovered and was at home, independent, and functioning, according to her and her family, essentially normally apart from fatigue and anxiety about having another SAH (**E**, VCR 1.97/9.99 = 0.20). A 28-year-old female had sudden-onset severe headache. She had a modified Glasgow Coma Scale of 15 and a CT scan showed diffuse SAH with mild ventricular enlargement (**F**, **G**, VCR 1.42/11.34 = 0.13). A CTA showed an anterior communicating artery aneurysm (**H**). Her level of consciousness deteriorated 11 hours later. A CT scan showed dilation of the left lateral ventricle and obliteration of the subarachnoid sulci (**I**). Mannitol did not result in improvement. Both pupils became dilated 14 hours later and a ventricular catheter was inserted. The intracranial pressure progressively increased, was intractable to medical management, and the patient was brain-dead 2 days later (**J**). A 49-year-old female developed sudden headache and right hemiparesis. Modified Glasgow Coma Scale was 12 and CT scan showed SAH and intracerebral hemorrhage (**K**, **L**) consistent with left middle cerebral artery aneurysm. During transport to the neurosurgical center, she deteriorated and had a modified Glasgow Coma Scale of 4. She was intubated and on arrival 4 hours after ictus underwent CT and CTA that showed increase in the left intracerebral hemorrhage and a left middle cerebral artery aneurysm (**M**, **N**). She underwent immediate craniotomy, clipping of the aneurysm, evacuation of the hemorrhage, insertion of a ventricular catheter, and decompressive craniectomy. The bone flap was replaced 3 months later (**O**). She was ambulatory with a cane but had residual dysphasia and hemiparesis and was unable to resume work 30 months later. From Macdonald and Schweizer (2016).

# Complications and secondary treatment

The most common neurologic complications of SAH are rebleeding, DCI, early or delayed hydrocephalus, and seizures. Rebleeding and DCI decreased as causes of death between the cooperative study on timing of aneurysm surgery that accrued patients between 1980 and 1984 (7% each) to 1% and 3%, respectively, in a prospective database of patients collected between 1996 and 2006 (Komotar et al., 2009). Up to 80% of patients develop a serious medical complication, which may increase the risk of secondary brain injury and DCI (Wartenberg et al., 2006). This makes medical complications an increasingly important factor in outcome. Common medical complications are cardiopulmonary dysfunction or failure due to acute heart or renal failure and acute lung injury (acute respiratory distress syndrome) (Komotar et al., 2009; Beseoglu et al., 2013). The incidence of cardiopulmonary complications is increased in patients with cardiovascular (smoking, hypertension) risk factors. Electrocardiographic alterations and cardiac enzyme elevations are present in up to 20% of SAH patients and are significant surrogates for clinical outcome (Manavalan et al., 1997; Naidech et al., 2005). Patients with SAH frequently have left ventricular and cardiac output failure, hypotension, and pulmonary edema, which may then result in cerebral infarction due to reduced cerebral perfusion pressure (Bruder and Rabinstein, 2011; Ranieri et al., 2012). Aneurysmal SAH causes salt wasting (natriuresis) and elevated natriuretic peptides, renin activity, aldosterone, catecholamines, and arginine vasopressin that cause hypovolemia (Fig. 12.2) (Gress, 2011). Hypovolemia is believed to be detrimental so it is recommended to maintain euvolemia and normal serum sodium, but how to monitor for and accomplish this requires further study.

# Delayed cerebral ischemia

SAH is unique in that there is a secondary phase, commonly 3–14 days after ictus, during which DCI can result in cerebral infarction (Fig. 12.4). While angiographic vasospasm is correlated with delayed cerebral infarction after SAH, the relationship is complex. Seventy percent of patients with SAH develop angiographic vasospasm, whereas only 30% of those patients develop clinical symptoms for DCI and/or cerebral infarction (Vergouwen et al., 2011b; Etminan et al., 2013c). This is hypothesized to be because angiographic vasospasm has to be severe enough to reduce cerebral blood flow, other factors occur with angiographic vasospasm to cause DCI, and other factors influence cerebral blood flow after SAH. Review of RCTs showed effective pharmacologic reduction of angiographic vasospasm but less or no effect on delayed cerebral infarction or clinical outcome (Macdonald et al., 2008; Etminan et al., 2011). Other causes of deterioration, such as early brain injury, loss of consciousness at ictus, hyponatremia, and seizures, may contribute to and exacerbate DCI (Macdonald, 2014). Cerebral infarction from DCI remains the most important cause of mortality and morbidity in patients surviving the initial SAH (Vergouwen et al., 2011a). The main predictors of DCI are the amount of SAH on admission CT scan (i.e., Fisher grade) and poor neurologic grade, but multiple factors contribute and prediction remains inaccurate (Macdonald, 2014).

## DIAGNOSIS

The diagnosis of DCI relies on exclusion of other causes for neurologic deterioration (Table 12.6). It is even more difficult in sedated or already neurologically impaired patients. DCI is diagnosed when other causes of neurologic deterioration are ruled out. The most sensitive surrogate for DCI is the clinical condition. A multidisciplinary expert group defined clinical deterioration due to DCI as:

*occurrence of focal neurologic impairment (such as hemiparesis, aphasia, apraxia, hemianopia, or neglect), or a decrease of at least 2 points on the GCS (either on the total score or on one of its individual components [eye, motor on either side, verbal]). This should last for at least 1 hour, is not apparent immediately after aneurysm occlusion, and cannot be attributed to other causes by means of clinical assessment, CT or MRI scanning of the brain, and appropriate laboratory studies (Vergouwen et al., 2010).*

A study using Markov modeling and patient data from previous RCTs highlighted that additional radiologic exams in patients with clinical features of DCI may not be helpful in selecting patients requiring treatment for DCI (Rawal et al., 2015). Although there are no proven treatments for DCD, radiologic exams for detection or monitoring of DCI are still widely used. Screening protocols vary among institutions from clinical examination alone to invasive monitoring and frequent CTA and CT perfusion (CTP) and even routine catheter angiography (Hanggi, 2011; Macdonald, 2014). DCI is hypothesized to involve interaction of angiographic vasospasm, microcirculatory constriction, impaired autoregulation, microthrombosis, capillary transit time heterogeneity, and CSI. Radiologic detection of DCI is focused on imaging of the cerebral vasculature and/or quantification of cerebral blood flow, since these are the only two of the above processes that are clinically easily detectable (Macdonald, 2014).

*Table 12.6*

**Causes of deterioration after subarachnoid hemorrhage (SAH)**

| Neurological | | Systemic | |
|---|---|---|---|
| Secondary to SAH | Delayed cerebral ischemia | Systemic infection | |
| | Hydrocephalus | Hepatic, renal failure | |
| | Rebleeding | Drugs | Corticosteroids |
| | Seizures | | Sedation |
| | Intracranial hematoma (subdural, intracerebral) | | Alcohol withdrawal |
| | Cerebral edema/increased intracranial pressure | Other drug reactions | Anticonvulsants |
| | Enlargement/thrombosis of aneurysm | Metabolic | Hyponatremia, syndrome of inappropriate antidiuretic hormone, cerebral salt wasting |
| Postoperative complications | Major arterial occlusion | | Hypernatremia, diabetes insipidus |
| | Venous infarction | | Metabolic acidosis or alkalosis |
| | Perforator injury | | Hypocalcemia |
| | Intracranial hematoma | | Hypomagnesemia |
| | Cerebral edema/increased intracranial pressure | Pulmonary | Hypoxemia |
| | Retraction injury | | Respiratory acidosis or alkalosis |
| | Hypotension, hypoxic brain injury | | Venous thromboembolism |
| | Aseptic or infectious meningitis | Cardiovascular | Hypotension |
| | Seizures | | Hypertension |
| Complications of angiography | Thromboembolism | | Arrhythmias |
| | | | Takotsubo cardiomyopathy/low cardiac output |

Data from Peerless (1979).

Since angiographic vasospasm is one contributor to DCI, catheter or CTA are the most common diagnostic tools. The latter is increasingly used because it is less invasive, has low risk, and can be combined with CTP (Wintermark et al., 2006; Turowski et al., 2007; Wittsack et al., 2008; Washington and Zipfel, 2011). CTP measures the time of passage of a contrast agent bolus from the arterial to the venous side of the brain, which gives an indication of cerebral blood flow (Wintermark et al., 2006; Wittsack et al., 2008). In contrast to MR perfusion, CTP is more practical in critically ill patients and permits serial imaging and establishment of perfusion thresholds in DCI screening in patients with SAH (Fig. 12.1) (Etminan et al., 2013b).

Transcranial Doppler sonography also is used to measure blood flow velocities that are a surrogate for arterial diameters. The assessment is generally limited to the middle cerebral artery and is characterized by high interoperator variability and relatively low sensitivity and specificity for DCI (Carrera et al., 2009).

### PROPHYLAXIS AND TREATMENT

The principles for prevention of DCI are to optimize cerebral blood flow (and thus delivery of oxygen and glucose to the brain) and to avoid reduction of cerebral blood flow. Management includes maintaining normal body oxygenation, temperature, body fluid volumes, hemoglobin, glucose, electrolytes, particularly sodium and magnesium, adequate cerebral perfusion pressure and adequate nutrition, and mobilizing the patient as tolerated (Darby et al., 1994; Dankbaar et al., 2010; Diringer et al., 2011).

The only pharmacologic agent recommended with a high level of evidence in most countries is enteral nimodipine, a dihydropyridine L-type calcium channel antagonist (Dorhout Mees et al., 2007; Connolly et al., 2012; Steiner et al., 2013). The main side-effect of nimodipine is systemic hypotension, which is deleterious to patients with SAH because it may lower cerebral perfusion pressure and worsen DCI (Darby et al., 1994; Dankbaar et al., 2010). According to a multinational, multidisciplinary neurocritical care consensus conference, oral nimodipine should be administered to patients with SAH but it is strongly recommended that if nimodipine results in hypotension, then dosing intervals should be changed to more frequent lower doses and, if hypotension continues, nimodipine may be discontinued (Diringer et al., 2011). Even though nimodipine had minimal effect on angiographic vasospasm in RCTs, oral nimodipine improved outcome after SAH, presumably due to additional beneficial effects, such as inhibition of CSI and of microthromboembolism (Vergouwen et al., 2007; Dreier et al., 2009). In Japan, nimodipine is not available, whereas fasudil is commonly administered to patients with SAH (Liu et al., 2012).

Prophylactic induction of hypervolemia, hypertension, hemodilution, hypermagnesemia, and hypothermia has not been beneficial for improving outcome after SAH and is currently not recommended.

If, despite the management outlined above, a patient deteriorates due to DCI, the most commonly instituted so-called rescue therapies are induced hypertension, balloon angioplasty, or selective intra-arterial administration of vasodilators such as calcium channel antagonists (verapamil, nimodipine, nicardipine) or milrinone (Hanggi et al., 2009; Abruzzo et al., 2012; Lannes et al., 2012).

Studies using focal brain tissue monitors suggest that induced hypertension increases cerebral blood flow and brain oxygen delivery in areas with impaired autoregulation and that it is more effective and has fewer complications than hypervolemia (Raabe et al., 2005). On the other hand, induced hypertension with dopamine reduced regional cerebral blood flow in other studies (Darby et al., 1994). Effects of fluid bolus, induced hypertension, or transfusion on global and focal cerebral blood flow and brain oxygen delivery have been studied using positron emission tomography (Dhar et al., 2012). Transfusion was most effective at increasing oxygen delivery to regions with initially low oxygen delivery, followed by induced hypertension and, lastly, fluid bolus. How these effects translate to clinical benefit has not been adequately assessed. Overall, induced hypertension is reported to reverse symptoms and signs of DCI in up to two-thirds of treated patients (Treggiari, 2011). There is no vasopressor of choice, blood pressure should be raised gradually, and the target level based on clinical improvement. The limitations of hemodynamic therapies for DCI are that all evidence is based on small, unblinded, nonrandomized retrospective or prospective case series. An RCT of induced hypertension for DCI showed no benefit of treatment on CTP, which calls into question the use of induced hypertension in the absence of additional RCTs (Gathier et al., 2015).

Endovascular treatment may be used when patients do not improve with medical treatment of DCI, or when there is concern or inability to use hemodynamic rescue therapy due to cardiac disease. Another suggested indication is in poor-grade patients with severe angiographic vasospasm or CTP deficits in the absence of neurologic deterioration (Abruzzo et al., 2012). There are no RCTs to guide its use and all evidence is anecdotal. Balloon angioplasty results in angiographic improvement in >80% of arteries treated and clinical improvement in 31–77% (Abruzzo et al., 2012). Risks include arterial rupture in 1% and thromboembolic complications in 5%. The effect tends to be durable. Pharmacologic angioplasty resulted in angiographic improvement in 29–44% and clinical improvement in a similar percent and has lower risks (hypotension, seizures, and ICP) than balloon angioplasty (Abruzzo et al., 2012). Nicardipine, verapamil, nimodipine, and milrinone are used most widely. These therapies should be subjected to study in an RCT because of lack of rigorous evidence of efficacy as well as their substantial risk of side-effects, expense, and labor intensity (Chou et al., 2010; Connolly et al., 2012).

The site of drug administration (local versus systemic) may play a role in the benefit:risk ratio for prophylaxis or treatment of DCI. Delivery of sustained-release formulations of dihydropyridines, such as nicardipine, into the subarachnoid space next to cerebral arteries reduced DCI and improved outcome (Kasuya et al., 2002; Barth et al., 2007). An RCT entered 32 patients with SAH to undergo aneurysm clipping with or without intracisternal administration of up to 40 mg nicardipine pellets (Barth et al., 2007). Angiographic vasospasm was significantly reduced in patients treated with nicardipine pellets (7% vs. 73% in the control group). Patients treated with pellets had less delayed cerebral infarction (14% vs. 47% in the control group) and death (6% vs. 38% in the control group). Since treatment with nicardipine pellets is restricted to patients undergoing surgical aneurysm repair, more recent pharmacologic strategies delivered nimodipine microparticles, either intracisternally or intraventricularly (Hanggi et al., 2015).

## Acute hydrocephalus

Twenty percent of patients with aneurysmal SAH develop acute hydrocephalus (Fig. 12.6) (Germanwala et al., 2010). In patients who are WFNS 2 or worse, insertion of a ventricular catheter can be life-saving (Gigante et al., 2010). Neurologic deterioration can be due to hydrocephalus and can be rapidly fatal unless treated (Lu et al., 2012). Factors associated with acute hydrocephalus include increased SAH on admission CT scan, IVH, and poor neurologic grade on admission (Germanwala et al.,

2010). Acute hydrocephalus is often, but not uniformly, reported as an adverse prognostic factor for neurologic outcome after SAH (Rosengart et al., 2007). Methods to quantify hydrocephalus are commonly based on CT imaging and include the measurement of the bicaudate or ventriculocranial ratio (Fig. 12.6) (van Gijn et al., 1985; Dupont and Rabinstein, 2013).

Reluctance to insert a ventricular drain is based on the risks of this procedure, that include infection and intracranial hemorrhage. The pooled infection and hemorrhage incidence rates were 7.9% (95% CI 6.3–8.4%) and 8.4% (95% CI 5.7–11.1), respectively, in 9667 patients from 33 studies (Dey et al., 2015). Most infections do not cause permanent morbidity and symptomatic ventricular drain-associated hemorrhage is rare (incidence rate 0.7%, 95% CI 0.4–1.1) (Dey et al., 2015). Rebleeding from the aneurysm is associated with ventricular drainage in 0–43% of cases, but this is thought to be due to the natural history of rebleeding and not to the ventricular drainage itself (Gigante et al., 2010).

Up to 7% of patients with SAH cannot tolerate removal of the ventricular drain or develop delayed hydrocephalus and thus require permanent CSF diversion. The rate varies between centers due to the underlying factors (e.g., actual amount of CSF drainage versus imaging-derived diagnosis of hydrocephalus) used to determine the indication for shunting (Lai and Morgan, 2013). Poor admission grade, acute hydrocephalus, IVH, ruptured vertebral artery aneurysm, meningitis, and prolonged ventricular drainage are independent predictors of shunt dependency (Lai and Morgan, 2013). Intrathecal thrombolysis has not been efficacious to reduce the incidence of permanent hydrocephalus and understanding of the pathophysiology of chronic hydrocephalus is limited (Etminan et al., 2013a).

## Seizures

Focal or generalized seizures occur in 4–26% of patients at the time of hemorrhage and in 1–28% of patients later in the acute hospital course (Lanzino et al., 2011). In an RCT, 65% of seizures which occurred after admission but before aneurysm repair were associated with aneurysm rerupture. Long-term epilepsy develops in about 2% of patients but varies with functional outcome, with a >25% risk in patients with poor outcome. Risk factors for seizures in hospital and for long-term epilepsy include younger age, loss of consciousness at ictus, history of hypertension, middle cerebral artery aneurysm, more SAH on CT, ICH, subdural hematoma, aneurysm repair by clipping compared to coiling, and DCI (Lanzino et al., 2011; Ibrahim et al., 2013).

There is limited evidence upon which to guide pharmacologic treatment of seizures after SAH. One

argument for prophylactic treatment is that seizure activity increases cerebral metabolic demand and sometimes ICP and may precipitate irreversible neurologic injury. However, anticonvulsants, particularly phenytoin, have been associated with poor outcome after SAH (Rosengart et al., 2007). Phenytoin increases activity of CYP450, which can increase nimodipine metabolism, resulting in reduced plasma concentrations and drug effect of the latter, which could account in part for the association of phenytoin and worse clinical outcome. In general, the authors administer drugs such as levetiracetam to patients with SAH only if they have documented clinical or electroencephalographic seizures.

## Increased intracranial pressure

Increased ICP (>20 mmHg) occurs in 50% of Hunt–Hess grade 1–3 patients and was increasingly likely with worsening grade and if there was more SAH, ICH, or IVH (Voldby and Enevoldsen, 1982; Heuer et al., 2004). Acute hydrocephalus, cerebral infarction, and cerebral edema also contribute to increased ICP. Ventricular drainage for acute hydrocephalus and craniotomy to evacuate/decompress large ICH can be life saving and associated with good outcome and probably are beneficial, in part due to their ability to reduce ICP and improve cerebral perfusion pressure (Kolias et al., 2013).

Guidelines for management of SAH have generally not addressed treatment of increased ICP since there are few studies specific to this population. Some authors have made recommendations based on studies in traumatic brain injury and thus, these may not be appropriate for SAH. One suggestion was to maintain some combination of ICP < 20 mmHg and cerebral perfusion pressure between 50 and 70 mmHg (Mak et al., 2013).

In SAH, decompressive craniectomy has been used at the time of aneurysm clipping in patients with brain swelling or ICH or days after SAH when patients deteriorate from brain swelling or cerebral infarction (Guresir et al., 2009). Also it has been suggested that more sophisticated measures of ICP and compliance, such as the cardiac-induced ICP waves (mean ICP wave amplitude) that reflect intracranial compliance are better measures to monitor. Eide et al. (2011) randomized 97 patients with SAH to management by ICP or by mean ICP wave amplitude and found better outcome on the modified Rankin scale at 1 year with the latter method.

## CLINICAL TRIALS AND GUIDELINES

About 150 RCTs on pharmacologic treatment or other maneuvers for SAH included 29 181 patients (Macdonald, 2014). Only nimodipine reduced the risk of DCI and guidelines suggest oral nimodipine be started within 96 hours of SAH (Diringer et al., 2011; Connolly et al., 2012; Steiner et al., 2013). The only other highly recommended management of SAH is to repair the aneurysm in a timely fashion. Meta-analyses of fasudil, intrathecal fibrinolytics, and cilostazol suggest these may be beneficial, but these findings are based on limited RCTs and require further study (Amin-Hanjani et al., 2004; Liu et al., 2011; Niu et al., 2014). To understand why many treatments have not demonstrated efficacy, individual patient data from multiple RCTs and databases were pooled. Recommendations from this exercise include a need to develop common data elements for SAH and to conduct multicenter RCTs (Button et al., 2013; Jaja et al., 2014). Current SAH management guidelines are derived from many national and international organizations, including the American Heart Association, the Neurocritical Care Society, and the European Stroke Organization (Table 12.7) (Diringer et al., 2011; Connolly et al., 2012; Steiner et al., 2013).

## COMPLEX CLINICAL DECISIONS

Complex clinical decisions include the method of repair for complex ruptured aneurysms. This may require surgical clip reconstruction, endovascular stenting plus coiling, or the use of flow-diverting stents. Studies, predominantly from the USA, and one meta-analysis suggest that outcome from SAH is better in centers that manage more patients (Connolly et al., 2012; Boogaarts et al., 2014). Although it is unclear whether patients at different sites are matched for prognostic factors for outcome, referral to high-volume centers is recommended since they are more likely to have experience with complex aneurysms. Also, stenting requires dual antiplatelet treatment, which is associated with an increased risk of hemorrhagic cerebral complications (Mahaney et al., 2013). Therefore, stent-assisted coiling for ruptured aneurysms should only be considered when there are no or only high-risk surgical or endovascular options (Connolly et al., 2012).

The risk–benefit ratio of rescue therapy (i.e., hemodynamic therapy and/or intra-arterial pharmaceutical or mechanical vasodilation) for patients with DCI and/or severe angiographic vasospasm remains highly controversial. An RCT comparing induced hypertension to normotension in patients with DCI was stopped due to insufficient recruitment (Gathier et al., 2015). Randomization of 36 patients found a trend towards improvement of cerebral blood flow in areas with impaired perfusion based on CTP but no overall increase of CBF (Gathier et al., 2015). Current guidelines recommend induced hypertension for patients with DCI unless patients already have elevated blood pressure during admission or present with cardiac status which precludes induced

hypertension or simply that there is no evidence for the use of induced hypertension (Connolly et al., 2012; Steiner et al., 2013).

No strong evidence for efficacy of pharmacologic or mechanical vasodilation exists. Guidelines do not mention endovascular therapy for DCI or simply state that until better evidence comes available either pharmaceutical or mechanical vasodilation is reasonable in patients with DCI refractory to induced hypertension (Connolly et al., 2012; Steiner et al., 2013).

## OUTCOME PREDICTION

Meta-analysis of 33 population-based studies reported a reduction of 30-day mortality after SAH of 0.9% (95% CI 0.3–1.5%) per year between 1980 and 2005, cumulating in a 50% decrease (Lovelock et al., 2010). Case fatality remains 15% prior to hospitalization and 20% in hospital for a total of 35% (Nieuwkamp et al., 2009; Korja et al., 2013). About 30% of SAH patients develop DCI, and 15% of SAH patients die or sustain permanent disability from DCI. Morbidity is less well defined. One meta-analysis reported that, in those who survive, 75% have permanent neurologic or neurocognitive impairment (Al-Khindi et al., 2010). Thus, only about 20% of all aneurysmal SAH patients survive and resume their previous lifestyle after 3–6 months. The most common deficits in survivors of SAH are cognitive deficits (verbal memory, language, and executive function), decreased decision-making capacity (cognitive inflexibility and enhanced risk-taking behavior), and decreased quality of life (Al-Khindi et al., 2010). Mood disorders, fatigue, and sleep disturbances also are common (Al-Khindi et al., 2010).

Many outcome scales have been developed to assess neurologic and cognitive outcome and quality of life after brain injury, including the Glasgow and extended Glasgow Outcome Scales, modified Rankin scale, Short Form-36, and Montreal cognitive assessment (Rankin, 1957; Deane et al., 1996; Wilson et al., 1998; Nasreddine et al., 2005). None were developed specifically for SAH, although they are commonly used for this disease.

Prognostic factors for unfavorable outcome include worse admission neurologic condition, older age, aneurysm repair by clipping rather than coiling, more SAH on CT scan, history of hypertension, larger aneurysm, and posterior circulation aneurysm (Jaja et al., 2013). Only 25% of the variation in outcome is explained by these variables, demonstrating that other factors (genetic, epigenetic, disease-related) have substantial effects on outcome and/or that outcome scales are imprecise.

Long-term outcome in patients who survive SAH shows many have persistent deficits in cognition and

*Table 12.7*

**Summary of guidelines from different countries and committees**

| Management | Neurocritical Care Society (Diringer et al., 2011) | American Heart Association (Connolly et al., 2012) | European Guidelines (Steiner et al., 2013) |
|---|---|---|---|
| Diagnosis | CTA recommended over DSA if endovascular therapy not planned initially (very-low-quality evidence, weak recommendation) | Maintain high level of suspicion for SAH in patients with acute headache (class 1, level of evidence B). Perform CT scan and, if negative, lumbar puncture (class 1, level of evidence B). CTA can be done initially after diagnosis of SAH, but if it does not show a cause for SAH, DSA is recommended except possibly in perimesencephalic SAH (class 2b, level of evidence C). 3D DSA recommended unless CTA shows an aneurysm and it is not needed to guide aneurysm repair (class 1, level of evidence B) | CT/CTA and MRI/A equally suitable for diagnosis and to find underlying SAH etiology (class 2, level B). Lumbar puncture indicated if SAH suspected and CT/MRI does not show SAH (class 2, level B). DSA indicated if CTA/MRA does not show a cause for SAH and a typical basal SAH pattern is seen (class 2, level B). If no aneurysm is found, repeat CTA or DSA (class 3, level C). DSA is not indicated for perimesencephalic SAH unless CTA is insufficient or there is disagreement about the perimesencephalic pattern |
| Grading, initial assessment | None | Grade the patient clinically on Hunt–Hess or WFNS scale (class 1, level of evidence B). Urgently evaluate and treat (class 1, level of evidence B) | Grade the patient using a system based on Glasgow Coma Scale, such as the PAASH (class 3, level C) |
| Hospital and system of care | Treat SAH patients at high-volume centers that have specialty neurointensive care units, neurointensivists, vascular neurosurgeons, and interventional neuroradiologists (moderate-quality evidence, strong recommendation). Monitor patient in a place with multidisciplinary expertise, especially during the risk of DCI (moderate-quality evidence, strong recommendation) | Consider transfer and treatment at high-volume centers (>35 aneurysmal SAH cases/year, class 1, level of evidence B). Monitor complication rates and credential treating physicians (class 2a, level of evidence C) | Monitor patient in intensive care at least until aneurysm repaired |
| Ruptured aneurysm repair | Early aneurysm repair (high-quality evidence, strong recommendation) | Repair as early as possible (class 1, level of evidence B). Repair ruptured aneurysm completely if possible (class 1, level of evidence C). Endovascular coiling is preferred for suitable aneurysms (class 1, level of evidence B). Vascular imaging after aneurysm repair to identify remnants or recurrence (class 1, level of evidence B) | Early treatment (within 72 hours of onset), regardless of grade (class 3, level C). Endovascular coiling preferred for aneurysms suitable for clipping or coiling (class 1, level A) |

| | | | |
|---|---|---|---|
| | aneurysm repair (<72 hours) may be considered (low-quality evidence, weak recommendation). Avoid delayed (>48 hours after SAH) or prolonged (>3 days) antifibrinolytic therapy (high-quality evidence, strong recommendation). Avoid antifibrinolytics in patients with risk factors for venous thromboembolism (moderate-quality evidence, strong recommendation). Treat extreme blood pressure elevations before aneurysm repair (low-quality evidence, strong recommendation) | aneurysm repair (class 1, level of evidence B). Systolic blood pressure <160 mmHg is reasonable (class 2a, level of evidence C). Short course (<72 hours) of antifibrinolytic drug for unavoidable delayed aneurysm treatment, no medical contraindication and significant risk of rebleeding (class 2a, level of evidence B) | before aneurysm repair and after repair; only treat extreme blood pressure elevations (good clinical practice, class 4, level C). No medical treatment that improves outcome by reducing rebleeding (class 1, level A). Further investigation of hemostatic agents indicated (class 2, level C) |
| Hydrocephalus | None | Insert ventricular or lumbar drain to manage acute symptomatic hydrocephalus (class 1, level of evidence B). Treat chronic hydrocephalus with permanent CSF diversion (class 1, level of evidence C). Weaning ventricular drain over >24 hours does not reduce risk of permanent hydrocephalus (class 3, level of evidence B). Fenestration of the lamina terminalis not routinely recommended (class 3, level of evidence B) | Insert ventricular drain for hydrocephalus and third/fourth ventricles filled with blood (good clinical practice). Lumbar puncture can be considered if the third/fourth ventricles are not filled with blood (class 4, level C). Treat chronic hydrocephalus with permanent CSF diversion (good clinical practice) |
| Seizures | Phenytoin is not recommended (low-quality evidence, strong recommendation). Other anticonvulsants can be considered (very-low-quality evidence, weak recommendation). If anticonvulsants are used, short treatment <7 days is recommended (low-quality evidence, weak recommendation). Treat patients who have a seizure with anticonvulsants for some time (low-quality evidence, weak recommendation). Continuous EEG monitor of patients who are poor-grade and fail to improve or who have neurologic deterioration (low-quality evidence, strong recommendation) | Prophylactic anticonvulsants may be considered acutely (class 2b, level of evidence B). Long-term anticonvulsants generally only for patients with risk factors for seizures (class 2b, level of evidence B) | Administer anticonvulsants in patients who have seizures (good clinical practice). No evidence for prophylactic anticonvulsant drugs (class 4, level C) |
| Cardiopulmonary complications | Assess baseline cardiac function (enzymes, echocardiography, low-quality evidence, strong recommendation) | None | None |
| Glucose | Keep serum glucose <200 mg/dL (moderate-quality evidence, strong recommendation). Avoid glucose <80 mg/dL (high-quality | Careful glucose control, avoid hypoglycemia (class 2b, level of evidence B) | Keep blood glucose <180 mg/dL (10 mmol/L, good clinical practice) |

*Continued*

*Table 12.7*
Continued

| Management | Neurocritical Care Society (Diringer et al., 2011) | American Heart Association (Connolly et al., 2012) | European Guidelines (Steiner et al., 2013) |
|---|---|---|---|
| | evidence, strong recommendation). If microdialysis is used, adjust serum glucose to avoid very low cerebral glucose (very-low-quality evidence, weak recommendation) | | |
| Fever | Monitor temperature and exclude infection as cause of fever (high-quality evidence, strong recommendation). Control fever especially during risk of DCI (low-quality evidence, strong recommendation). Use pharmacologic agents first to maintain normothermia (moderate-quality evidence, strong recommendation).<br><br>Use cooling devices if pharmacologic agents fail to control fever (high-quality evidence, strong recommendation). Treat shivering (high-quality evidence, strong recommendation) | Maintain normothermia acutely (class 2a, level of evidence B) | Fever should be treated medically and physically (good clinical practice) |
| Anemia and transfusion targets | Minimize blood loss (low-quality evidence, strong recommendation). Transfuse if hemoglobin < 8–10 g/dL (moderate-quality evidence, strong recommendation). Higher hemoglobin may be better for patients with DCI, but whether transfusion is useful is unknown (no evidence, strong recommendation) | Transfuse for anemia but the optimal hemoglobin concentration is unknown (class 2b, level of evidence B) | None |
| Endocrine function | Consider hypothalamic dysfunction in patients unresponsive to vasopressors (moderate-quality evidence, weak recommendation). Do not administer corticosteroids (high-quality evidence, weak recommendation) | None | No evidence that steroids are effective in patients with SAH (class 4, level C) |
| Venous thromboembolism | All SAH patients should have measures to reduce risk of venous thromboembolism (high-quality evidence, strong recommendation). Sequential compression devices recommended in all patients (high-quality evidence, strong recommendation). No | Heparin-induced thrombocytopenia and deep-vein thrombosis should be detected early and treated, but methods for screening are ill defined (class 1, level of evidence B) | Pneumatic devices and/or compression stockings before aneurysm repair (class 2, level B). Low-molecular-weight heparin can be started 12 hours after surgical treatment and immediately after coiling (class 2, level B) |

| | | | |
|---|---|---|---|
| | prophylactic low-molecular-weight or unfractionated heparin before surgery (low-quality evidence, strong recommendation). Can start unfractionated heparin 24 hours after surgery (moderate-quality evidence, strong recommendation). Withhold pharmacologic prophylaxis 24 hours and after intracranial procedures (moderate-quality evidence, strong recommendation). Screen patients given antifibrinolytics (moderate-quality evidence, strong recommendation) | | |
| Nimodipine | Administer 60 mg every 4 hours for 21 days (high-quality evidence, strong recommendation) | Oral nimodipine should be administered to all patients (class 1, level of evidence A) | Oral nimodipine, 60 mg every 4 hours (class 1, level A). If oral administration is not possible, the drug should be given intravenously (good clinical practice) |
| Other prophylaxis for DCI | None | Prophylactic hypervolemia or balloon angioplasty not recommended (class 3, level of evidence B) | None |
| Volume status and hyponatremia | Monitor volume status (moderate-quality evidence, weak recommendation). Fluid management should not be based on central venous pressure measurements alone and these or pulmonary artery catheters should not be placed for sole purpose of assessing volume (moderate-quality evidence, strong recommendation). Target euvolemia (avoid excessive fluid intake), especially if pulmonary edema or adult respiratory distress syndrome (moderate- to high-quality evidence, strong recommendation). Prophylactic hypervolemic therapy should not be used (high-quality evidence, strong recommendation). Fludrocortisone or hydrocortisone can be considered for persistent negative fluid balance (moderate-quality evidence, weak recommendation). Do not use fluid restriction for hyponatremia (weak-quality evidence, strong recommendation), treat with hypertonic saline (very-low-quality evidence, strong recommendation) | Target euvolemia and normal circulating blood volume (class 1, level of evidence B). Fludrocortisone and hypertonic saline are reasonable for preventing and correcting hyponatremia (class 2a, level of evidence B) | Maintain euvolemia |

Continued

*Table 12.7*

Continued

| Management | Neurocritical Care Society (Diringer et al., 2011) | American Heart Association (Connolly et al., 2012) | European Guidelines (Steiner et al., 2013) |
|---|---|---|---|
| Statins | Continue statins in patients who were taking them before SAH (low-quality evidence, strong recommendation). Consider starting statins if patient not on one, pending outcome of ongoing trials (moderate-quality evidence, weak recommendation) | None | They are under study |
| Monitoring for DCI | Monitor patients at risk for DCI, preferably in intensive care unit (very-low-quality evidence, strong recommendation). Image vascular anatomy or perfusion or transcranial Doppler in good-grade patients who are suspected of developing DCI (strong-quality evidence, strong recommendation). Use a strategy for monitoring and detection of DCI; multiple modalities are acceptable (low- to high-quality evidence, weak to strong recommendation) | Transcranial Doppler monitoring is reasonable (class 2a, level of evidence B). Perfusion CT or MRI can be used to identify cerebral ischemia (class 2a, level of evidence B) | None |
| Triggers for intervention | No triggers can be recommended; monitoring and treatment addressed in other sections | None | None |
| Hemodynamic management of DCI | Induce hypertension (moderate-quality evidence, strong recommendation) in a stepwise fashion (poor-quality evidence, strong recommendation), with no specific inotropes/vasopressors recommended (moderate-quality evidence, strong recommendation) | Induction of hypertension is recommended (class 1, level of evidence B) | Keep mean arterial pressure > 90 mmHg (good clinical practice). There is no evidence that induced hypertension or hypervolemia improves outcome in patients with DCI (class 4, level C) |
| Endovascular management of DCI | Prophylactic cerebral angioplasty should not be used (high-quality evidence, strong recommendation). Intra-arterial vasodilators and/or angioplasty may be considered, for ischemic symptoms refractory to medical management (moderate-quality evidence, strong recommendation) | Balloon or pharmacologic angioplasty is reasonable for DCI without response to induced hypertension (class 2a, level of evidence B) | |
| Long-term care, rehabilitation, neuropsychologic evaluation | | Refer patient for cognitive, behavioral, and psychosocial assessments after discharge (class 2a, level of evidence B) | |

| | |
|---|---|
| Risk factors for SAH and prevention of SAH | Treat hypertension to reduce risk of SAH (class 1, level of evidence B). Avoid tobacco and alcohol misuse (class 1, level of evidence B). Vegetables may reduce risk of SAH (class 2b, level of evidence B) | Hypertension considered a risk factor for SAH and possibly aneurysm formation. Cigarette smoking is most important modifiable aneurysm formation, growth and rupture factor and should be avoided. Avoid alcohol abuse and binge drinking as risk factor for SAH (class 3, level C) |
| Unruptured aneurysms | Consider size and location of aneurysm, patient health and age and aneurysm morphology and hemodynamics when contemplating aneurysm repair (class 2b, level of evidence B). Reasonable to screen patients with at least one first-degree relative with aneurysmal SAH or aneurysmal SAH themselves (class 2b, level of evidence B) | Screening not advised if only one first-degree relative affected. If two or more first-degree relatives affected, then consider screening (class 3, level C) |

CTA, computed tomographic angiography; DSA, digital subtraction angiography; SAH, subarachnoid hemorrhage; CT, computed tomography; MRI, magnetic resonance imaging; MRA, magnetic resonance angiography; WFNS, World Federation of Neurologic Surgeons; PAASH, Prognosis on Admission of Aneurysmal SAH; CPP, cerebral perfusion pressure; CSF, cerebrospinal fluid; EEG, electroencephalogram; DCI, delayed cerebral ischemia.

quality of life and have depression, anxiety, and fatigue (Al-Khindi et al., 2010). Patients who have had SAH have a risk of another SAH 15 times that of the general population (Rinkel and Algra, 2011). Their long-term standardized mortality ratio is 1.5, in excess of the general population, and mostly related to cardiovascular and cerebrovascular disease (Huhtakangas et al., 2015).

Studies of biomarkers in SAH have been reviewed (Hong et al., 2014). One review noted that blood C-reactive protein, selectin, thrombin–antithrombin complex, creatine kinase B, and malondialdehyde had reasonable sensitivity and specificity for differentiating favorable from unfavorable outcome (Hong et al., 2014). Another review concluded that promising blood biomarkers for predicting outcome were tumor necrosis factor-$\alpha$, soluble tumor necrosis factor receptor 1, interleukin-1 receptor antagonist, and neurofilament, and that ET-1, interleukin-6, fibrinopeptide A, thrombin–antithrombin complex, and membrane-bound tissue factor were potential CSF biomarkers for DCI (Lad et al., 2012). No studies included more than a few hundred patients or were externally validated.

## NEUROREHABILITATION

In clinical practice, collecting a formal assessment of outcome is uncommon. However, multiple national and international guidelines recommend determining functional and cognitive outcome using various scales because it facilitates decision making about whether patients can return to work, drive, and whether they may benefit from rehabilitation therapies (Bowen and Patchick, 2014).

Several studies including an RCT showed early mobilization starting within days of aneurysm repair after SAH seems to be safe, although effects on in-hospital complications and long-term outcome are unclear (Olkowski et al., 2013; Karic et al., 2016).

Gillespie et al. (2015) performed a systematic review of Cochrane systematic reviews and RCTs of cognitive rehabilitation (for attention deficits, memory deficits, spatial neglect, perceptual disorders, motor apraxia, and executive dysfunction) for stroke. Most studies did not specifically address SAH. They concluded that, despite 44 RCTs including 1500 patients, there was very little strong evidence to show cognitive rehabilitation had any long-term beneficial effects. On the other hand, many studies had method limitations and lack of benefit could not be ruled out until further RCTs were done taking into account, among other factors, age, stroke subtype, type of therapy offered, and intensity of therapy and effect of therapies on mood, quality of life, and activities of daily living.

## REFERENCES

Abruzzo T, Moran C, Blackham KA et al. (2012). Invasive interventional management of post-hemorrhagic cerebral vasospasm in patients with aneurysmal subarachnoid hemorrhage. J Neurointerv Surg 4: 169–177.

Agid R, Andersson T, Almqvist H et al. (2010). Negative CT angiography findings in patients with spontaneous subarachnoid hemorrhage: when is digital subtraction angiography still needed? AJNR Am J Neuroradiol 31: 696–705.

Alen JF, Lagares A, Lobato RD et al. (2003). Comparison between perimesencephalic nonaneurysmal subarachnoid hemorrhage and subarachnoid hemorrhage caused by posterior circulation aneurysms. J Neurosurg 98: 529–535.

Algra AM, Klijn CJ, Helmerhorst FM et al. (2012). Female risk factors for subarachnoid hemorrhage: a systematic review. Neurology 79: 1230–1236.

Al-Khindi T, Macdonald RL, Schweizer TA (2010). Cognitive and functional outcome after aneurysmal subarachnoid hemorrhage. Stroke 41: e519–e536.

Amin-Hanjani S, Ogilvy CS, Barker FG (2004). Does intracisternal thrombolysis prevent vasospasm after aneurysmal subarachnoid hemorrhage? A meta-analysis. Neurosurgery 54: 326–334.

Anderson C, Ni MC, Scott D et al. (2003). Triggers of subarachnoid hemorrhage: role of physical exertion, smoking, and alcohol in the Australasian Cooperative Research on Subarachnoid Hemorrhage Study (ACROSS). Stroke 34: 1771–1776.

Andreasen TH, Bartek Jr J, Andresen M et al. (2013). Modifiable risk factors for aneurysmal subarachnoid hemorrhage. Stroke 44: 3607–3612.

Arora S, Swadron SP, Dissanayake V (2010). Evaluating the sensitivity of visual xanthochromia in patients with subarachnoid hemorrhage. J Emerg Med 39: 13–16.

Backes D, Rinkel GJ, Kemperman H et al. (2012). Time-dependent test characteristics of head computed tomography in patients suspected of nontraumatic subarachnoid hemorrhage. Stroke 43: 2115–2119.

Backes D, Vergouwen MD, Tiel Groenestege AT et al. (2015). PHASES score for prediction of intracranial aneurysm growth. Stroke 46: 1221–1226.

Backes D, Rinkel GJ, Laban KG et al. (2016). Patient- and aneurysm-specific risk factors for intracranial aneurysm growth: a systematic review and meta-analysis. Stroke 47: 951–957.

Baharoglu MI, Germans MR, Rinkel GJ et al. (2013). Antifibrinolytic therapy for aneurysmal subarachnoid haemorrhage. Cochrane Database Syst Rev 8. CD001245.

Bakker NA, Groen RJ, Foumani M et al. (2014). Repeat digital subtraction angiography after a negative baseline assessment in nonperimesencephalic subarachnoid hemorrhage: a pooled data meta-analysis. J Neurosurg 120: 99–103.

Barth M, Capelle HH, Weidauer S et al. (2007). Effect of nicardipine prolonged-release implants on cerebral vasospasm and clinical outcome after severe aneurysmal subarachnoid hemorrhage: a prospective, randomized, double-blind phase IIa study. Stroke 38: 330–336.

Beck J, Rohde S, Berkefeld J et al. (2006). Size and location of ruptured and unruptured intracranial aneurysms measured by 3-dimensional rotational angiography. Surg Neurol 65: 18–25.

Beseoglu K, Holtkamp K, Steiger HJ et al. (2013). Fatal aneurysmal subarachnoid haemorrhage: causes of 30-day in-hospital case fatalities in a large single-centre historical patient cohort. Clin Neurol Neurosurg 115: 77–81.

Boogaarts HD, van Amerongen MJ, de Vries J et al. (2014). Caseload as a factor for outcome in aneurysmal subarachnoid hemorrhage: a systematic review and meta-analysis. J Neurosurg 120: 605–611.

Bowen A, Patchick E (2014). Cognitive rehabilitation and recovery after stroke. In: TA Schweizer, RL Macdonald (Eds.), The Behavioral Consequences of Stroke, Springer Science+Business Media, New York.

Broderick JP, Brown Jr RD, Sauerbeck L et al. (2009). Greater rupture risk for familial as compared to sporadic unruptured intracranial aneurysms. Stroke 40: 1952–1957.

Brown Jr RD, Broderick JP (2014). Unruptured intracranial aneurysms: epidemiology, natural history, management options, and familial screening. Lancet Neurol 13: 393–404.

Bruder N, Rabinstein A (2011). Cardiovascular and pulmonary complications of aneurysmal subarachnoid hemorrhage. Neurocrit Care 15: 257–269.

Brunell A, Ridefelt P, Zelano J (2013). Differential diagnostic yield of lumbar puncture in investigation of suspected subarachnoid haemorrhage: a retrospective study. J Neurol 260: 1631–1636.

Budohoski KP, Guilfoyle M, Helmy A et al. (2014). The pathophysiology and treatment of delayed cerebral ischaemia following subarachnoid haemorrhage. J Neurol Neurosurg Psychiatry 85: 1343–1353.

Button KS, Ioannidis JP, Mokrysz C et al. (2013). Power failure: why small sample size undermines the reliability of neuroscience. Nat Rev Neurosci 14: 365–376.

Carrera E, Schmidt JM, Oddo M et al. (2009). Transcranial Doppler for predicting delayed cerebral ischemia after subarachnoid hemorrhage. Neurosurgery 65: 316–323.

Centers for Disease Control and Prevention (2016). Mortality data. Available online at http://www.cdc.gov/nchs/deaths.htm. (accessed August 18, 2016).

Chen S, Li Q, Wu H et al. (2014). The harmful effects of subarachnoid hemorrhage on extracerebral organs. Biomed Res Int 2014: 858496.

Chou CH, Reed SD, Allsbrook JS et al. (2010). Costs of vasospasm in patients with aneurysmal subarachnoid hemorrhage. Neurosurgery 67: 345–352.

Claassen J, Bernardini GL, Kreiter K et al. (2001). Effect of cisternal and ventricular blood on risk of delayed cerebral ischemia after subarachnoid hemorrhage: the Fisher scale revisited. Stroke 32: 2012–2020.

Connolly Jr ES, Rabinstein AA, Carhuapoma JR et al. (2012). Guidelines for the management of aneurysmal subarachnoid hemorrhage: a guideline for healthcare professionals from the American Heart Association/American Stroke Association. Stroke 43: 1711–1737.

Crowley RW, Medel R, Dumont AS et al. (2011). Angiographic vasospasm is strongly correlated with cerebral infarction after subarachnoid hemorrhage. Stroke 42: 919–923.

Dankbaar JW, Slooter AJ, Rinkel GJ et al. (2010). Effect of different components of triple-H therapy on cerebral perfusion in patients with aneurysmal subarachnoid haemorrhage: a systematic review. Crit Care 14: R23.

Darby JM, Yonas H, Marks EC et al. (1994). Acute cerebral blood flow response to dopamine-induced hypertension after subarachnoid hemorrhage. J Neurosurg 80: 857–864.

de Oliveira Manoel AL, Mansur A, Sampaio GS et al. (in press). Functional outcome after poor-grade subarachnoid hemorrhage: a single center study and systematic literature review. Neurocritical Care.

de Rooij NK, Linn FH, van der Plas JA et al. (2007). Incidence of subarachnoid haemorrhage: a systematic review with emphasis on region, age, gender and time trends. J Neurol Neurosurg Psychiatry 78: 1365–1372.

de Steenhuijsen Piters WA, Algra A, van den Broek MF et al. (2013). Seasonal and meteorological determinants of aneurysmal subarachnoid hemorrhage: a systematic review and meta-analysis. J Neurol 260: 614–619.

Deane M, Pigott T, Dearing P (1996). The value of the Short Form 36 score in the outcome assessment of subarachnoid haemorrhage. Br J Neurosurg 10: 187–191.

Degen LA, Dorhout Mees SM, Algra A et al. (2011). Interobserver variability of grading scales for aneurysmal subarachnoid hemorrhage. Stroke 42: 1546–1549.

Dey M, Stadnik A, Riad F et al. (2015). Bleeding and infection with external ventricular drainage: a systematic review in comparison with adjudicated adverse events in the ongoing Clot Lysis Evaluating Accelerated Resolution of Intraventricular Hemorrhage Phase III (CLEAR-III IVH) trial. Neurosurgery 76: 291–300.

Dhar S, Tremmel M, Mocco J et al. (2008). Morphology parameters for intracranial aneurysm rupture risk assessment. Neurosurgery 63: 185–196.

Dhar R, Scalfani MT, Zazulia AR et al. (2012). Comparison of induced hypertension, fluid bolus, and blood transfusion to augment cerebral oxygen delivery after subarachnoid hemorrhage. J Neurosurg 116: 648–656.

Diringer MN, Bleck TP, Hemphill III CJ et al. (2011). Critical care management of patients following aneurysmal subarachnoid hemorrhage: recommendations from the Neurocritical Care Society's Multidisciplinary Consensus Conference. Neurocrit Care 15: 211–240.

Dorhout Mees SM, Rinkel GJ, Feigin VL et al. (2007). Calcium antagonists for aneurysmal subarachnoid haemorrhage. Cochrane Database Syst Rev. CD000277.

Dorsch NWC, King MT (1994). A review of cerebral vasospasm in aneurysmal subarachnoid hemorrhage. Part 1: Incidence and effects. J Clin Neurosci 1: 19–26.

Drake CG, Hunt WE, Sano K et al. (1988). Report of World Federation of Neurological Surgeons committee on a universal subarachnoid hemorrhage grading scale. J Neurosurg 68: 985–986.

Dreier JP (2011). The role of spreading depression, spreading depolarization and spreading ischemia in neurological disease. Nat Med 17: 439–447.

Dreier JP, Major S, Manning A et al. (2009). Cortical spreading ischaemia is a novel process involved in ischaemic damage in patients with aneurysmal subarachnoid haemorrhage. Brain 132: 1866–1881.

Dupont S, Rabinstein AA (2013). CT evaluation of lateral ventricular dilatation after subarachnoid hemorrhage: baseline bicaudate index values [correction of balues]. Neurol Res 35: 103–106.

Edlow JA, Caplan LR (2000). Avoiding pitfalls in the diagnosis of subarachnoid hemorrhage [see comments]. N Engl J Med 342: 29–36.

Eide PK, Bentsen G, Sorteberg AG et al. (2011). A randomized and blinded single-center trial comparing the effect of intracranial pressure and intracranial pressure wave amplitude-guided intensive care management on early clinical state and 12-month outcome in patients with aneurysmal subarachnoid hemorrhage. Neurosurgery 69: 1105–1115.

Etminan N, Vergouwen MD, Ilodigwe D et al. (2011). Effect of pharmaceutical treatment on vasospasm, delayed cerebral ischemia, and clinical outcome in patients with aneurysmal subarachnoid hemorrhage: a systematic review and meta-analysis. J Cereb Blood Flow Metab 31: 1443–1451.

Etminan N, Beseoglu K, Eicker SO et al. (2013a). Prospective, randomized, open-label phase II trial on concomitant intraventricular fibrinolysis and low-frequency rotation after severe subarachnoid hemorrhage. Stroke 44: 2162–2168.

Etminan N, Beseoglu K, Heiroth HJ et al. (2013b). Early perfusion computerized tomography imaging as a radiographic surrogate for delayed cerebral ischemia and functional outcome after subarachnoid hemorrhage. Stroke 44: 1260–1266.

Etminan N, Vergouwen MD, Macdonald RL (2013c). Angiographic vasospasm versus cerebral infarction as outcome measures after aneurysmal subarachnoid hemorrhage. Acta Neurochir Suppl 115: 33–40.

Etminan N, Beseoglu K, Barrow DL et al. (2014a). Multidisciplinary consensus on assessment of unruptured intracranial aneurysms: proposal of an international research group. Stroke 45: 1523–1530.

Etminan N, Dreier R, Buchholz BA et al. (2014b). Age of collagen in intracranial saccular aneurysms. Stroke 45: 1757–1763.

Feigin VL, Rinkel GJ, Lawes CM et al. (2005). Risk factors for subarachnoid hemorrhage: an updated systematic review of epidemiological studies. Stroke 36: 2773–2780.

Fisher CM, Kistler JP, Davis JM (1980). Relation of cerebral vasospasm to subarachnoid hemorrhage visualized by computerized tomographic scanning. Neurosurgery 6: 1–9.

Flaherty ML, Haverbusch M, Kissela B et al. (2005). Perimesencephalic subarachnoid hemorrhage: incidence, risk factors, and outcome. J Stroke Cerebrovasc Dis 14: 267–271.

Francis SE, Tu J, Qian Y et al. (2013). A combination of genetic, molecular and haemodynamic risk factors contributes to the formation, enlargement and rupture of brain aneurysms. J Clin Neurosci 20: 912–918.

Friedrich V, Flores R, Muller A et al. (2010). Escape of intra-luminal platelets into brain parenchyma after subarachnoid hemorrhage. Neuroscience 165: 968–975.

Friedrich B, Muller F, Feiler S et al. (2012). Experimental subarachnoid hemorrhage causes early and long-lasting microarterial constriction and microthrombosis: an in-vivo microscopy study. J Cereb Blood Flow Metab 32: 447–455.

Frontera JA, Claassen J, Schmidt JM et al. (2006). Prediction of symptomatic vasospasm after subarachnoid hemorrhage: the modified Fisher scale. Neurosurgery 59: 21–27.

Fujii Y, Takeuchi S, Sasaki O et al. (1996). Ultra-early rebleeding in spontaneous subarachnoid hemorrhage. J Neurosurg 84: 35–42.

Fujii M, Yan J, Rolland WB et al. (2013). Early brain injury, an evolving frontier in subarachnoid hemorrhage research. Transl. Stroke Res 4: 432–446.

Gathier CS, Dankbaar JW, van der Jagt M et al. (2015). Effects of induced hypertension on cerebral perfusion in delayed cerebral ischemia after aneurysmal subarachnoid hemorrhage: a randomized clinical trial. Stroke 46: 3277–3281.

Germans MR, Post R, Coert BA et al. (2013). Ultra-early tranexamic acid after subarachnoid hemorrhage (ULTRA): study protocol for a randomized controlled trial. Trials 14: 143.

Germanwala AV, Huang J, Tamargo RJ (2010). Hydrocephalus after aneurysmal subarachnoid hemorrhage. Neurosurg Clin N Am 21: 263–270.

Gigante P, Hwang BY, Appelboom G et al. (2010). External ventricular drainage following aneurysmal subarachnoid haemorrhage. Br J Neurosurg 24: 625–632.

Giller CA, Giller AM, Landreneau F (1998). Detection of emboli after surgery for intracerebral aneurysms. Neurosurgery 42: 490–493.

Gillespie DC, Bowen A, Chung CS et al. (2015). Rehabilitation for post-stroke cognitive impairment: an overview of recommendations arising from systematic reviews of current evidence. Clin Rehabil 29: 120–128.

Gress DR (2011). Monitoring of volume status after subarachnoid hemorrhage. Neurocrit Care 15: 270–274.

Greving JP, Wermer MJ, Brown Jr RD et al. (2014). Development of the PHASES score for prediction of risk of rupture of intracranial aneurysms: a pooled analysis of six prospective cohort studies. Lancet Neurol 13: 59–66.

Guresir E, Schuss P, Vatter H et al. (2009). Decompressive craniectomy in subarachnoid hemorrhage. Neurosurg Focus 26: E4.

Hanggi D (2011). Monitoring and detection of vasospasm II: EEG and invasive monitoring. Neurocrit Care 15: 318–323.

Hanggi D, Eicker S, Beseoglu K et al. (2009). Dose-related efficacy of a continuous intracisternal nimodipine treatment on cerebral vasospasm in the rat double subarachnoid hemorrhage model. Neurosurgery 64: 1155–1159.

Hanggi D, Etminan N, Macdonald RL et al. (2015). NEWTON: nimodipine microparticles to enhance recovery while reducing toxicity after subarachnoid hemorrhage. Neurocrit Care 23: 274–284.

Harada K, Fukuyama K, Shirouzu T et al. (2013). Prevalence of unruptured intracranial aneurysms in healthy asymptomatic Japanese adults: differences in gender and age. Acta Neurochir (Wien) 155: 2037–2043.

Hasan DM, Chalouhi N, Jabbour P et al. (2013). Evidence that acetylsalicylic acid attenuates inflammation in the walls of human cerebral aneurysms: preliminary results. J Am Heart Assoc 2: e000019.

Heuer GG, Smith MJ, Elliott JP et al. (2004). Relationship between intracranial pressure and other clinical variables in patients with aneurysmal subarachnoid hemorrhage. J Neurosurg 101: 408–416.

Hijdra A, Brouwers PJ, Vermeulen M et al. (1990). Grading the amount of blood on computed tomograms after subarachnoid hemorrhage. Stroke 21: 1156–1161.

Hong CM, Tosun C, Kurland DB et al. (2014). Biomarkers as outcome predictors in subarachnoid hemorrhage – a systematic review. Biomarkers 19: 95–108.

Hop JW, Rinkel GJ, Algra A et al. (1999). Initial loss of consciousness and risk of delayed cerebral ischemia after aneurysmal subarachnoid hemorrhage. Stroke 30: 2268–2271.

Horikoshi T, Akiyama I, Yamagata Z et al. (2002). Retrospective analysis of the prevalence of asymptomatic cerebral aneurysm in 4518 patients undergoing magnetic resonance angiography – when does cerebral aneurysm develop? Neurol Med Chir (Tokyo) 42: 105–112.

Hudson JS, Hoyne DS, Hasan DM (2013). Inflammation and human cerebral aneurysms: current and future treatment prospects. Future Neurol 8.

Huhtakangas J, Lehto H, Seppa K et al. (2015). Long-term excess mortality after aneurysmal subarachnoid hemorrhage: patients with multiple aneurysms at risk. Stroke 46: 1813–1818.

Hunt WE, Hess RM (1968). Surgical risk as related to time of intervention in the repair of intracranial aneurysms. J Neurosurg 28: 14–20.

Huttunen T, von und zu Fraunberg M, Koivisto T et al. (2011). Long-term excess mortality of 244 familial and 1502 sporadic one-year survivors of aneurysmal subarachnoid hemorrhage compared with a matched Eastern Finnish catchment population. Neurosurgery 68: 20–27.

Ibrahim GM, Fallah A, Macdonald RL (2013). Clinical, laboratory, and radiographic predictors of the occurrence of seizures following aneurysmal subarachnoid hemorrhage. J Neurosurg 119: 347–352.

Ingall TJ, Asplund K, Mähönen M et al. (2000). A multinational comparison of subarachnoid hemorrhage epidemiology in the WHO MONICA stroke study. Stroke 31: 1054–1061.

Jahromi BS, Aihara Y, Ai J et al. (2008). Voltage-gated $K^+$ channel dysfunction in myocytes from a dog model of subarachnoid hemorrhage. J Cereb Blood Flow Metab 28: 797–811.

Jaja BN, Cusimano MD, Etminan N et al. (2013). Clinical prediction models for aneurysmal subarachnoid hemorrhage: a systematic review. Neurocrit Care 18: 143–153.

Jaja BN, Attalla D, Macdonald RL et al. (2014). The subarachnoid hemorrhage international trialists (SAHIT) repository: advancing clinical research in subarachnoid hemorrhage. Neurocrit Care 21: 551–559.

Juvela S (2002). Risk factors for aneurysmal subarachnoid hemorrhage. Stroke 33: 2152–2153.

Juvela S, Poussa K, Porras M (2001). Factors affecting formation and growth of intracranial aneurysms: a long-term follow-up study. Stroke 32: 485–491.

Karic T, Roe C, Nordenmark TH et al. (2016). Effect of early mobilization and rehabilitation on complications in aneurysmal subarachnoid hemorrhage. J Neurosurg: 1–9.

Kasuya H, Onda H, Takeshita M et al. (2002). Efficacy and safety of nicardipine prolonged-release implants for preventing vasospasm in humans. Stroke 33: 1011–1015.

Kaufmann TJ, Huston III J, Mandrekar JN et al. (2007). Complications of diagnostic cerebral angiography: evaluation of 19,826 consecutive patients. Radiology 243: 812–819.

Kemp III WJ, Fulkerson DH, Payner TD et al. (2013). Risk of hemorrhage from de novo cerebral aneurysms. J Neurosurg 118: 58–62.

Kojima M, Nagasawa S, Lee YE et al. (1998). Asymptomatic familial cerebral aneurysms. Neurosurgery 43: 776–781.

Kolias AG, Kirkpatrick PJ, Hutchinson PJ (2013). Decompressive craniectomy: past, present and future. Nat Rev Neurol 9: 405–415.

Komotar RJ, Schmidt JM, Starke RM et al. (2009). Resuscitation and critical care of poor-grade subarachnoid hemorrhage. Neurosurgery 64: 397–410.

Korja M, Kaprio J (2016). Controversies in epidemiology of intracranial aneurysms and SAH. Nat Rev Neurol 12: 50–55.

Korja M, Silventoinen K, McCarron P et al. (2010). Genetic epidemiology of spontaneous subarachnoid hemorrhage: Nordic Twin Study. Stroke 41: 2458–2462.

Korja M, Silventoinen K, Laatikainen T et al. (2013). Cause-specific mortality of 1-year survivors of subarachnoid hemorrhage. Neurology 80: 481–486.

Korja M, Lehto H, Juvela S (2014). Lifelong rupture risk of intracranial aneurysms depends on risk factors: a prospective Finnish cohort study. Stroke 45: 1958–1963.

Kowalski RG, Claassen J, Kreiter KT et al. (2004). Initial misdiagnosis and outcome after subarachnoid hemorrhage. JAMA 291: 866–869.

Kulcsar Z, Ugron A, Marosfoi M et al. (2011). Hemodynamics of cerebral aneurysm initiation: the role of wall shear stress and spatial wall shear stress gradient. AJNR Am J Neuroradiol 32: 587–594.

Kurki MI, Gaal EI, Kettunen J et al. (2014). High risk population isolate reveals low frequency variants predisposing to intracranial aneurysms. PLoS Genet 10: e1004134.

Lad SP, Hegen H, Gupta G et al. (2012). Proteomic biomarker discovery in cerebrospinal fluid for cerebral vasospasm following subarachnoid hemorrhage. J Stroke Cerebrovasc Dis 21: 30–41.

Lai L, Morgan MK (2013). Predictors of in-hospital shunt-dependent hydrocephalus following rupture of cerebral aneurysms. J Clin Neurosci 20: 1134–1138.

Lall RR, Eddleman CS, Bendok BR et al. (2009). Unruptured intracranial aneurysms and the assessment of rupture risk based on anatomical and morphological factors: sifting through the sands of data. Neurosurg Focus 26: E2.

Lannes M, Teitelbaum J, Del Pilar CM et al. (2012). Milrinone and homeostasis to treat cerebral vasospasm associated with subarachnoid hemorrhage: the Montreal Neurological Hospital protocol. Neurocrit Care 16: 354–362.

Lanterna LA, Ruigrok Y, Alexander S et al. (2007). Meta-analysis of APOE genotype and subarachnoid hemorrhage: clinical outcome and delayed ischemia. Neurology 69: 766–775.

Lanzino G, D'Urso PI, Suarez J (2011). Seizures and anticonvulsants after aneurysmal subarachnoid hemorrhage. Neurocrit Care 15: 247–256.

Larsen CC, Astrup J (2013). Rebleeding after aneurysmal subarachnoid hemorrhage: a literature review. World Neurosurg 79: 307–312.

Li H, Pan R, Wang H et al. (2013a). Clipping versus coiling for ruptured intracranial aneurysms: a systematic review and meta-analysis. Stroke 44: 29–37.

Li MH, Chen SW, Li YD et al. (2013b). Prevalence of unruptured cerebral aneurysms in Chinese adults aged 35 to 75 years: a cross-sectional study. Ann Intern Med 159: 514–521.

Lindbohm JV, Kaprio J, Korja M (in press). Cholesterol as a risk factor for subarachnoid hemorrhage: a systematic review. PlosOne.

Liu GJ, Luo J, Zhang LP et al. (2011). Meta-analysis of the effectiveness and safety of prophylactic use of nimodipine in patients with an aneurysmal subarachnoid haemorrhage. CNS Neurol Disord Drug Targets 10: 834–844.

Liu GJ, Wang ZJ, Wang YF et al. (2012). Systematic assessment and meta-analysis of the efficacy and safety of fasudil in the treatment of cerebral vasospasm in patients with subarachnoid hemorrhage. Eur J Clin Pharmacol 68: 131–139.

Liu Q-G, Guo X, Song Z-B et al. (2013). Comparison of 64-slice CT angiography with 3D digital subtraction angiography in the diagnosis of intracranial aneurysms: a meta-analysis [Chinese]. Chinese Journal of Contemporary Neurology and Neurosurgery 13. March.

Lovelock CE, Rinkel GJ, Rothwell PM (2010). Time trends in outcome of subarachnoid hemorrhage: population-based study and systematic review. Neurology 74: 1494–1501.

Lu J, Ji N, Yang Z et al. (2012). Prognosis and treatment of acute hydrocephalus following aneurysmal subarachnoid haemorrhage. J Clin Neurosci 19: 669–672.

Lummel N, Bernau C, Thon N et al. (2015). Prevalence of superficial siderosis following singular, acute aneurysmal subarachnoid hemorrhage. Neuroradiology 57: 349–356.

Macdonald RL (2014). Delayed neurological deterioration after subarachnoid haemorrhage. Nat Rev Neurol 10: 44–58.

Macdonald RL, Schweizer TA (2016). Spontaneous subarachnoid haemorrhage. Lancet (in press).

Macdonald RL, Weir BK (1991). A review of hemoglobin and the pathogenesis of cerebral vasospasm. Stroke 22: 971–982.

Macdonald RL, Kassell NF, Mayer S et al. (2008). Clazosentan to overcome neurological ischemia and infarction occurring after subarachnoid hemorrhage (CONSCIOUS-1): randomized, double-blind, placebo-controlled phase 2 dose-finding trial. Stroke 39: 3015–3021.

Mahaney KB, Chalouhi N, Viljoen S et al. (2013). Risk of hemorrhagic complication associated with ventriculoperitoneal shunt placement in aneurysmal subarachnoid hemorrhage patients on dual antiplatelet therapy. J Neurosurg 119: 937–942.

Mak CH, Lu YY, Wong GK (2013). Review and recommendations on management of refractory raised intracranial pressure in aneurysmal subarachnoid hemorrhage. Vasc Health Risk Manag 9: 353–359.

Manavalan P, Richardson D, Rayford R et al. (1997). ECG and cardiac enzymes changes associated with subarachnoid hemorrhage. J Ark Med Soc 93: 592–593.

Matz PG, Fujimura M, Lewen A et al. (2001). Increased cytochrome c-mediated DNA fragmentation and cell death in manganese-superoxide dismutase-deficient mice after exposure to subarachnoid hemolysate. Stroke 32: 506–515.

Molyneux AJ, Kerr RS, Birks J et al. (2009). Risk of recurrent subarachnoid haemorrhage, death, or dependence and standardised mortality ratios after clipping or coiling of an intracranial aneurysm in the International Subarachnoid Aneurysm Trial (ISAT): long-term follow-up. Lancet Neurol 8: 427–433.

Morita A, Kirino T, Hashi K et al. (2012). The natural course of unruptured cerebral aneurysms in a Japanese cohort. N Engl J Med 366: 2474–2482.

Naidech AM, Kreiter KT, Janjua N et al. (2005). Cardiac troponin elevation, cardiovascular morbidity, and outcome after subarachnoid hemorrhage. Circulation 112: 2851–2856.

Nasreddine ZS, Phillips NA, Bedirian V et al. (2005). The Montreal Cognitive Assessment, MoCA: a brief screening tool for mild cognitive impairment. J Am Geriatr Soc 53: 695–699.

Nieuwkamp DJ, Setz LE, Algra A et al. (2009). Changes in case fatality of aneurysmal subarachnoid haemorrhage over time, according to age, sex, and region: a meta-analysis. Lancet Neurol 8: 635–642.

Niu PP, Yang G, Xing YQ et al. (2014). Effect of cilostazol in patients with aneurysmal subarachnoid hemorrhage: a systematic review and meta-analysis. J Neurol Sci 336: 146–151.

Ogawa T, Inugami A, Fujita H et al. (1995). MR diagnosis of subacute and chronic subarachnoid hemorr: comparison with CT. AJR Am J Roentgenol 165: 1257–1262.

Ohman J, Heiskanen O (1989). Timing of operation for ruptured supratentorial aneurysms: a prospective randomized study. J Neurosurg 70: 55–60.

Olkowski BF, Devine MA, Slotnick LE et al. (2013). Safety and feasibility of an early mobilization program for patients with aneurysmal subarachnoid hemorrhage. Phys Ther 93: 208–215.

Ostergaard L, Aamand R, Karabegovic S et al. (2013). The role of the microcirculation in delayed cerebral ischemia and chronic degenerative changes after subarachnoid hemorrhage. J Cereb Blood Flow Metab 33: 1825–1837.

Oudshoorn SC, Rinkel GJ, Molyneux AJ et al. (2014). Aneurysm treatment <24 versus 24-72 h after subarachnoid hemorrhage. Neurocrit Care 21: 4–13.

Pakarinen S (1967). Incidence, aetiology, and prognosis of primary subarachnoid hemorrhage. Acta Neurol Scand 43 (Suppl 29): 1–128.

Park KW, Metais C, Dai HB et al. (2001). Microvascular endothelial dysfunction and its mechanism in a rat model of subarachnoid hemorrhage. Anesth Analg 92: 990–996.

Peerless SJ (1979). Pre- and postoperative management of cerebral aneurysms. Clin Neurosurg 26: 209–231.

Perrone RD, Malek AM, Watnick T (2015). Vascular complications in autosomal dominant polycystic kidney disease. Nat Rev Nephrol 11: 589–598.

Perry JJ, Stiell IG, Sivilotti ML et al. (2011). Sensitivity of computed tomography performed within six hours of onset of headache for diagnosis of subarachnoid haemorrhage: prospective cohort study. BMJ 343: d4277.

Perry JJ, Stiell IG, Sivilotti ML et al. (2013). Clinical decision rules to rule out subarachnoid hemorrhage for acute headache. JAMA 310: 1248–1255.

Peymani A, Adams HH, Cremers LG et al. (2015). Genetic determinants of unruptured intracranial aneurysms in the general population. Stroke 46: 2961–2964.

Pierot L, Portefaix C, Rodriguez-Regent C et al. (2013). Role of MRA in the detection of intracranial aneurysm in the acute phase of subarachnoid hemorrhage. J Neuroradiol 40: 204–210.

Pluta RM, Oldfield EH (2007). Analysis of nitric oxide (NO) in cerebral vasospasm after aneursymal bleeding. Rev Recent Clin Trials 2: 59–67.

Raabe A, Beck J, Keller M et al. (2005). Relative importance of hypertension compared with hypervolemia for increasing cerebral oxygenation in patients with cerebral vasospasm after subarachnoid hemorrhage. J Neurosurg 103: 974–981.

Ranieri VM, Rubenfeld GD, Thompson BT et al. (2012). Acute respiratory distress syndrome: the Berlin definition. JAMA 307: 2526–2533.

Rankin J (1957). Cerebral vascular accidents in patients over the age of 60. I. General considerations. Scott Med J 2: 127–136.

Rasmussen R, Wetterslev J, Stavngaard T et al. (2015). Effects of prostacyclin on cerebral blood flow and vasospasm after subarachnoid hemorrhage: randomized, pilot trial. Stroke 46: 37–41.

Rawal S, Barnett C, John-Baptiste A et al. (2015). Effectiveness of diagnostic strategies in suspected delayed cerebral ischemia: a decision analysis. Stroke 46: 77–83.

Refai D, Botros JA, Strom RG et al. (2008). Spontaneous isolated convexity subarachnoid hemorrhage: presentation, radiological findings, differential diagnosis, and clinical course. J Neurosurg 109: 1034–1041.

Reilly C, Amidei C, Tolentino J et al. (2004). Clot volume and clearance rate as independent predictors of vasospasm after aneurysmal subarachnoid hemorrhage. J Neurosurg 101: 255–261.

Rinkel GJ (2008). Natural history, epidemiology and screening of unruptured intracranial aneurysms. Rev Neurol (Paris) 164: 781–786.

Rinkel GJ, Algra A (2011). Long-term outcomes of patients with aneurysmal subarachnoid haemorrhage. Lancet Neurol 10: 349–356.

Roman RJ, Renic M, Dunn KM et al. (2006). Evidence that 20-HETE contributes to the development of acute and delayed cerebral vasospasm. Neurol Res 28: 738–749.

Roos YB, Levi M, Carroll TA et al. (2001). Nimodipine increases fibrinolytic activity in patients with aneurysmal subarachnoid hemorrhage. Stroke 32: 1860–1862.

Rosengart AJ, Huo JD, Tolentino J et al. (2007). Outcome in patients with subarachnoid hemorrhage treated with antiepileptic drugs. J Neurosurg 107: 253–260.

Ruigrok YM, Rinkel GJ, Buskens E et al. (2000). Perimesencephalic hemorrhage and CT angiography: a decision analysis. Stroke 31: 2976–2983.

Sakowitz OW, Santos E, Nagel A et al. (2013). Clusters of spreading depolarizations are associated with disturbed cerebral metabolism in patients with aneurysmal subarachnoid hemorrhage. Stroke 44: 220–223.

Schievink WI, Torres VE, Piepgras DG et al. (1992). Saccular intracranial aneurysms in autosomal dominant polycystic kidney disease. J Am Soc Nephrol 3: 88–95.

Schweizer TA, Al-Khindi T, Macdonald RL (2012). Diffusion tensor imaging as a surrogate marker for outcome after perimesencephalic subarachnoid hemorrhage. Clin Neurol Neurosurg 114: 798–800.

Shah KH, Edlow JA (2002). Distinguishing traumatic lumbar puncture from true subarachnoid hemorrhage. J Emerg Med 23: 67–74.

Shojima M, Oshima M, Takagi K et al. (2004). Magnitude and role of wall shear stress on cerebral aneurysm: computational fluid dynamic study of 20 middle cerebral artery aneurysms. Stroke 35: 2500–2505.

Spetzler RF, McDougall CG, Albuquerque FC et al. (2013). The Barrow Ruptured Aneurysm Trial: 3-year results. J Neurosurg 119: 146–157.

Stein SC, Browne KD, Chen XH et al. (2006). Thromboembolism and delayed cerebral ischemia after subarachnoid hemorrhage: an autopsy study. Neurosurgery 59: 781–787.

Steiner T, Juvela S, Unterberg A et al. (2013). European stroke organization guidelines for the management of intracranial aneurysms and subarachnoid haemorrhage. Cerebrovasc Dis 35: 93–112.

Stoltenburg-Didinger G, Schwarz K (1987). Brain lesions secondary to subarachniod hemorrhage due to ruptured aneurysms. In: J Cervos-Navarro, R Ferszt (Eds.), Stroke and Microcirculation. Raven Press, New York.

Suzuki H (2015). What is early brain injury? Transl Stroke Res 6: 1–3.

Taylor CL, Yuan Z, Selman WR et al. (1995). Cerebral arterial aneurysm formation and rupture in 20,767 elderly patients: hypertension and other risk factors. J Neurosurg 83: 812–819.

Teasdale GM, Wardlaw JM, White PM et al. (2005). The familial risk of subarachnoid haemorrhage. Brain 128: 1677–1685.

Treggiari MM (2011). Hemodynamic management of subarachnoid hemorrhage. Neurocrit Care 15: 329–335.

Turowski B, Hanggi D, Beck A et al. (2007). New angiographic measurement tool for analysis of small cerebral vessels: application to a subarachnoid haemorrhage model in the rat. Neuroradiology 49: 129–137.

Uhl E, Lehmberg J, Steiger HJ et al. (2003). Intraoperative detection of early microvasospasm in patients with subarachnoid hemorrhage by using orthogonal polarization spectral imaging. Neurosurgery 52: 1307–1315.

van Donkelaar CE, Bakker NA, Veeger NJ et al. (2015). Predictive factors for rebleeding after aneurysmal subarachnoid hemorrhage: rebleeding aneurysmal subarachnoid hemorrhage study. Stroke 46: 2100–2106.

van Gijn J, Hijdra A, Wijdicks EF et al. (1985). Acute hydrocephalus after aneurysmal subarachnoid hemorrhage. J Neurosurg 63: 355–362.

van Gijn J, Kerr RS, Rinkel GJ (2007). Subarachnoid haemorrhage. Lancet 369: 306–318.

van Heuven AW, Dorhout Mees SM, Algra A et al. (2008). Validation of a prognostic subarachnoid hemorrhage grading scale derived directly from the Glasgow Coma Scale. Stroke 39: 1347–1348.

Vatter H, Konczalla J, Seifert V (2011). Endothelin related pathophysiology in cerebral vasospasm: what happens to the cerebral vessels? Acta Neurochir Suppl 110: 177–180.

Vergouwen MD, Vermeulen M, de Haan RJ et al. (2007). Dihydropyridine calcium antagonists increase fibrinolytic activity: a systematic review. J Cereb Blood Flow Metab 27: 1293–1308.

Vergouwen MD, Vermeulen M, van Gijn J et al. (2010). Definition of delayed cerebral ischemia after aneurysmal subarachnoid hemorrhage as an outcome event in clinical trials and observational studies: proposal of a multidisciplinary research group. Stroke 41: 2391–2395.

Vergouwen MD, Etminan N, Ilodigwe D et al. (2011a). Lower incidence of cerebral infarction correlates with improved functional outcome after aneurysmal subarachnoid hemorrhage. J Cereb Blood Flow Metab 31: 1545–1553.

Vergouwen MD, Ilodigwe D, Macdonald RL (2011b). Cerebral infarction after subarachnoid hemorrhage contributes to poor outcome by vasospasm-dependent and -independent effects. Stroke 42: 924–929.

Vlak MH, Algra A, Brandenburg R et al. (2011a). Prevalence of unruptured intracranial aneurysms, with emphasis on sex, age, comorbidity, country, and time period: a systematic review and meta-analysis. Lancet Neurol 10: 626–636.

Vlak MH, Rinkel GJ, Greebe P et al. (2011b). Trigger factors and their attributable risk for rupture of intracranial aneurysms: a case-crossover study. Stroke 42: 1878–1882.

Vlak MH, Rinkel GJ, Greebe P et al. (2013a). Independent risk factors for intracranial aneurysms and their joint effect: a case-control study. Stroke 44: 984–987.

Vlak MH, Rinkel GJ, Greebe P et al. (2013b). Risk of rupture of an intracranial aneurysm based on patient characteristics: a case-control study. Stroke 44: 1256–1259.

Voldby B, Enevoldsen EM (1982). Intracranial pressure changes following aneurysm rupture. Part 1: clinical and angiographic correlations. J Neurosurg 56: 186–196.

Wartenberg KE, Schmidt JM, Claassen J et al. (2006). Impact of medical complications on outcome after subarachnoid hemorrhage. Crit Care Med 34: 617–623.

Washington CW, Zipfel GJ (2011). Detection and monitoring of vasospasm and delayed cerebral ischemia: a review and assessment of the literature. Neurocrit Care 15: 312–317.

Weidauer S, Vatter H, Beck J et al. (2008). Focal laminar cortical infarcts following aneurysmal subarachnoid haemorrhage. Neuroradiology 50: 1–8.

Weir B (1987). Aneurysms Affecting the Nervous System. Williams & Wilkins, Baltimore.

Weir B (2002). Unruptured intracranial aneurysms: a review. J Neurosurg 96: 3–42.

Weir B, Grace M, Hansen J et al. (1978). Time course of vasospasm in man. J Neurosurg 48: 173–178.

Weir B, Disney L, Karrison T (2002). Sizes of ruptured and unruptured aneurysms in relation to their sites and the ages of patients. J Neurosurg 96: 64–70.

Wermer MJ, van der Schaaf I, Algra A et al. (2007). Risk of rupture of unruptured intracranial aneurysms in relation to patient and aneurysm characteristics: an updated meta-analysis. Stroke 38: 1404–1410.

Westerlaan HE, van Dijk JM, Jansen-van der Weide M et al. (2011). Intracranial aneurysms in patients with subarachnoid hemorrhage: CT angiography as a primary examination tool for diagnosis – systematic review and meta-analysis. Radiology 258: 134–145.

Wheelock B, Weir B, Watts R et al. (1983). Timing of surgery for intracerebral hematomas due to aneurysm rupture. J Neurosurg 58: 476–481.

Wiebers DO, Whisnant JP, Huston III J et al. (2003). Unruptured intracranial aneurysms: natural history, clinical outcome, and risks of surgical and endovascular treatment. Lancet 362: 103–110.

Wilson JT, Pettigrew LE, Teasdale GM (1998). Structured interviews for the Glasgow Outcome Scale and the extended Glasgow Outcome Scale: guidelines for their use. J Neurotrauma 15: 573–585.

Wintermark M, Ko NU, Smith WS et al. (2006). Vasospasm after subarachnoid hemorrhage: utility of perfusion CT and CT angiography on diagnosis and management. AJNR Am J Neuroradiol 27: 26–34.

Wittsack HJ, Wohlschlager AM, Ritzl EK et al. (2008). CT-perfusion imaging of the human brain: advanced deconvolution analysis using circulant singular value decomposition. Comput Med Imaging Graph 32: 67–77.

Woitzik J, Dreier JP, Hecht N et al. (2012). Delayed cerebral ischemia and spreading depolarization in absence of angiographic vasospasm after subarachnoid hemorrhage. J Cereb Blood Flow Metab 32: 203–212.

Xie A, Aihara Y, Bouryi VA et al. (2007). Novel mechanism of endothelin-1-induced vasospasm after subarachnoid hemorrhage. J Cereb Blood Flow Metab 27: 1692–1701.

Yasuno K, Bakircioglu M, Low SK et al. (2011). Common variant near the endothelin receptor type A (EDNRA) gene is associated with intracranial aneurysm risk. Proc Natl Acad Sci U S A 108: 19707–19712.

*Handbook of Clinical Neurology*, Vol. 140 (3rd series)
*Critical Care Neurology, Part I*
E.F.M. Wijdicks and A.H. Kramer, Editors
http://dx.doi.org/10.1016/B978-0-444-63600-3.00013-1

Chapter 13

# Management of acute neuromuscular disorders

E.F.M. WIJDICKS*

*Division of Critical Care Neurology, Mayo Clinic and Neurosciences Intensive Care Unit, Mayo Clinic Campus, Saint Marys Hospital, Rochester, MN, USA*

## Abstract

Imminent neuromuscular respiratory failure is recognized by shortness of breath, restlessness, and tachycardia and is often followed by tachypnea, constantly interrupting speech, asynchronous breathing and sometimes paradoxical breathing and use of scalene and sternocleidomastoid muscles. Once a patient presents with such a constellation of signs, there are some difficult decisions to be made and include assessment of the severity of respiratory failure and in particular when to intubate. Failure of the patient to manage secretions as a result of oropharyngeal weakness rather than neuromuscular respiratory weakness may be another reason for acute intubation. Any patient with rapidly worsening weakness on presentation will need admission and observation in an intensive care unit. This chapter summarizes the pathophysiology of acute neuromuscular respiratory failure, its clinical recognition and respiratory management and outcome expectations.

Acutely progressing neuromuscular disorders are often admitted to neurology wards first, and a fraction of these patients require acute respiratory care and mechanical ventilation. Decisions in patients who are inconspicuously unstable, remain difficult. Neurocritical care requires a solid foundation of knowledge in the care of neuromuscular respiratory failure or, rather, diagnosis and management are best reserved for neurointensivists. We are often reminded of the potential unexpected turn for the worse and need for emergency intubation in patients with myasthenia gravis (MG) and Guillain–Barré syndrome (GBS) (Wijdicks et al., 2003; Alshekhlee et al., 2008).

Neuromuscular disorders are rarely acute and are mostly managed in out-of-hospital settings. However, when patients are affected with an acute and severe manifestation, treatment of acute neuromuscular disorders in the intensive care unit (ICU) poses major management challenges. Fortunately, only a few acute neuromuscular diseases are seen in neurology practices and, more commonly, in the emergency department. These are GBS, acute MG, and amyotrophic lateral sclerosis (ALS).

Rarely, one may encounter acute vasculitic neuropathies, acute myopathy syndromes, West Nile myelitis, or even tick paralysis (Schaumburg and Herskovitz, 2000; Burakgazi and Hoke, 2010).

Acquired, rapidly evolving neuromuscular disease involves the respiratory system directly as a result of loss of mechanics, often three mechanisms – weakness of the respiratory bellow, inability to protect an open airway, as a result of abnormal oropharyngeal function causing pooling and aspiration of secretions, and a poor cough due to weak abdominal muscles – are at work, and this critical condition necessitates transfer of the patient to the ICU. It should also be recognized that some "acute" weakness may actually be more "acutely noticed" weakness, particularly with motor neuron disease. Patients with progressive ALS may be admitted to in a medical ICU with respiratory failure before being diagnosed. In developing countries, tetanus and botulism remain prevalent.

This chapter mainly provides insights into the mechanics of acute neuromuscular weakness. The diaphragm is important for inspiration and the abdominal muscles are

*Correspondence to: Eelco F.M. Wijdicks, Department of Neurology, Mayo Clinic, 200 First Street SW, Rochester MN 55905, USA. E-mail: wijde@mayo.edu

necessary for a strong cough (Bolton et al., 2004). Management also includes specific therapies, monitoring, treatment of dysautonomia (Burns et al., 2001), and management of systemic complications (Greenland and Griggs, 1980; Lawn and Wijdicks, 1999; Henderson et al., 2003). The main focus is on recognition of the entity and stabilization of the worsening, weak, and dyspneic patient with a new neurologic disease.

## EPIDEMIOLOGY

Most tertiary centers with neurointensive care programs would admit 5–10 patients a year with acute neuromuscular failure. In myasthenia gravis (MG), this would be labeled a "crisis," but this moniker probably applies to all patients admitted suddenly (Chaudhuri and Behan, 2009). Some experts in neuromuscular disease have argued the word "crisis" may be too histrionic and too alarmist for patients and families, but there can be no question that everything about a patient with worsening MG is problematic, unexpected, and truly dangerous. Some patients are admitted as a result of systemic complications (e.g., pulmonary embolus from prolonged immobilization or infections associated with immunosuppression). Complications of intravenous immunoglobulin (IVIG) infusion or plasma exchange are very uncommon but could also prompt a transfer.

In a recent study (Cabrera Serrano and Rabinstein, 2010) at Mayo Clinic, 85 patients with acute neuromuscular failure were seen in 7 years; and MG, Guillain–Barré syndrome (GBS), myopathies, and amyotrophic lateral sclerosis (ALS) were causes of respiratory failure. The causes to consider are shown in Table 13.1. Highly unusual causes are shown in Table 13.2.

GBS is an acute, self-limiting, inflammatory, demyelinating polyneuropathy. The annual incidence has remained fairly constant at 1 per 100 000 (McGrogan et al., 2009; Fokke et al., 2014; van den Berg et al., 2014; Winer, 2014). GBS is commonly precipitated by

*Table 13.1*

**Causes of acute neuromuscular respiratory failure**

Guillain–Barré syndrome
Myasthenia gravis
West Nile myelopathy
Organophosphate or sarin poisoning
Paraneoplastic neuropathy
Motor neuron disease
Endocrine myopathies
Hypophosphatemia
Hypokalemia
Mitochondrial myopathies
Acid maltase deficiencies

*Table 13.2*

**Rare causes of acute weakness and respiratory failure**

Tick paralysis (children)
Botulism
Organophosphate poisoning
Fish poisoning (tetrodotoxin)
Snake bite
Vasculitis
Hypophosphatemia
Hypokalemia/hyperkalemia
Hypermagnesemia
Acute porphyria

an infection, often a relatively trivial viral respiratory infection. Certain pathogens predominate as triggers in GBS, mainly influenza, *Campylobacter jejuni*, cytomegalovirus, Epstein–Barr virus, and *Mycoplasma pneumoniae*. Zika virus is the most recently identified trigger (Broutet et al., 2016). Other, less robust associations exist with vaccinations, surgery, and lymphoma. No preceding illness can be identified in one-third of patients (Re et al., 2000; van der Meche and van Doorn, 2000; Hadden et al., 2001; van Doorn et al., 2008; Kwong et al., 2013).

MG is an autoimmune disease of defective neurotransmission leading to fatigable muscle weakness. The annual incidence is 0.5–5 cases per 100, 000. The pathogenesis can be briefly summarized as an antibody reaction at the antigen epitopes of the acetylcholine receptor, eventually leading to destruction and simplification of the junctional fold and widening synaptic cleft. Onset may be at any age but tends to be earlier in females (mean 28 years) than in males (mean 42 years). MG results in either transient or persistent focal or generalized fatigability or weakness.

## PATHOPHYSIOLOGY

The immunopathogenesis of GBS has remained elusive. Some studies have suggested that complement activation triggers myelin destruction. Complement cascade activation is mediated by the binding of antibodies to the Schwann cells and results in vesicular myelin degeneration. The axon may be a target as well, often after *C. jejuni* infection (Yuki, 2007), or may be involved in more severe cases of GBS ("the innocent bystander" theory). The proclivity of motor axonal involvement has led to the designation of acute motor axonal neuropathy. Another acronym (acute motor-sensory axonal neuropathy or AMSAM) can also be grouped under a more general term axonal GBS. The target molecule in purely demyelinating disease is yet unknown. Despite this differentiation into subtype, treatment is similar. Prognosis differs with a more protracted course in axonal forms. Lack of demyelinization but presence of macrophages within the periaxonal spaces of myelinated fibers in these patients is highly suggestive of direct macrophage invasion. A competing explanation involves antibodies to ganglioside epitopes or myelin proteins (Griffin et al., 1996; Hafer-Macko et al., 1996; Hughes et al., 1999; Hughes and Cornblath, 2005; Kuwabara and Yuki, 2013).

MG occurs as a result of antibodies targeting postsynaptic acetylcholine receptors scattered throughout motor endplates of skeletal muscles. The immunocomplexes causing injury and complement activation cause loss of synaptic membranes, with unfolding and reduction of surface area contact. Antibodies can be directed against voltage-gated calcium channels in the presynaptic area of the motor endplate, as is seen in Eaton–Lambert syndrome. This syndrome is seldom severe enough to warrant neurosciences intensive care unit (ICU)admission, and often only when there is bulbar involvement.

## CLINICAL FEATURES

The diagnosis of GBS is often straightforward. Severe back pain and limb paresthesias, starting in the ankles and wrists, with a "tight band" sensation are typical presenting symptoms. The paresthesias gradually scatter over the limbs and move proximally. Although paresthesias are often the presenting symptom, sensory modalities remain normal or only mildly impaired. Weakness begins in the more proximal muscles, causing difficulty with climbing stairs and getting out of a chair, and is notable 1 or 2 days after the onset of paresthesias. Symmetric weak muscles are accompanied by depressed or absent deep tendon reflexes. Legs are usually involved more than arms and create the clinical impression of an ascending paralysis. Facial and oropharyngeal muscles are affected in 50% of cases, and weakness of these muscle groups may be the initial manifestation. Patients may have staccato speech (ability to speak only short sentences) and show small tidal volume respiration with increased rate. Respiratory failure, if it occurs, commonly appears within 1 week of the onset of paresthesias. Depending on the definition, dysautonomia occurs in up to 70% of patients in the ICU, manifesting as arrhythmias, tachycardia, diaphoresis, labile blood pressure, urinary retention, or ileus (Ropper et al., 1988, 1991; Ropper and Wijdicks, 1990).

Myasthenic crisis is arbitrarily defined as MG complicated by respiratory failure requiring mechanical ventilation, or delayed extubation for more than 24 hours in an already intubated myasthenic patient (Thomas et al., 1997; Seneviratne et al., 2008; Kalita et al., 2014). Myasthenic crises may also involve a serious overdose of

cholinergic drugs. These effects can be best remembered by the acronym SLUDGE – salivation, lacrimation, urination, defecation, gastrointestinal upset, and emesis.

Myasthenic crisis associated with respiratory failure is seen in 10–60% of MG patients (and thus is a hit-or-miss situation), but it is not uncommon for it to occur within the first 12 months of disease onset (Jani-Acsadi and Lisak, 2007).

The need for ventilatory assistance usually follows onset of weakness of diaphragmatic or accessory respiratory muscles, but mechanical ventilation also may become necessary because of airway compromise from oropharyngeal muscle weakness, stridor related to vocal cord weakness (rare), or the inability to clear secretions. Large series have reported that a third of patients may have recurrent myasthenic crisis, pointing towards some individual predisposition. Precipitating causes include any mundane viral or bacterial infection aspiration with worsening weakness of oropharyngeal muscles and reduction of pyridostigmine dose, or initiation of a high dose of corticosteroids. Other precipitating factors are surgical procedures (particularly extensive thoracic or abdominal surgeries), pregnancy, or exposure to drugs with neuromuscular blocking action, such as aminoglycosides. No precipitating factor can be identified for myasthenic crisis in 30% of patients, except for an acknowledged period of emotional stress.

## NEUROMUSCULAR RESPIRATORY FAILURE

There are several caveats that should be known: (1) it is difficult to be completely certain whether the patient is ventilating well and not struggling; (2) normal blood gases may precede respiratory arrest; (3) pulmonary function tests can be unreliable, not only due to poor patient effort, but also poor coaching; (4) failure to manage secretions, and not so much overt respiratory weakness, may be the most common reason for acute intubation; and (5) the degree of limb weakness does not always coincide with involvement of the diaphragm.

Generally, there are some very difficult decisions to be made, including assessment of the severity of respiratory failure, triage of the patient, how to instruct the nursing staff to recognize worsening, and what set of tests to order that could assist not only in the diagnosis, but also in anticipating serious problems down the line. Patients with acute neuromuscular respiratory failure are often misjudged, and every year patients "code on the floor," often at night. In some instances, after careful review, warning signs were present that could have prompted better triage, preferably to a monitored setting (Galtrey et al., 2012).

How do we best understand acute neuromuscular respiratory failure? During respiration, lungs can expand and recoil in two ways: by downward and upward movement of the diaphragm that lengthens and shortens the chest cavity, and by elevation and depression of the ribs to increase and decrease the anteroposterior diameter of the chest. Normal quiet breathing is largely accomplished by contraction of the diaphragm. In general, the diaphragm is responsible for approximately two-thirds of the ventilatory effort to generate inspiration. Accessory inspiratory muscles, including the external intercostals, scalenes, and sternocleidomastoid muscles, may supplement respiration. Expiration is mostly due to recoil of the thoracic cage, but abdominal wall muscles are also necessary to generate forced expiration and are responsible for coughing. Moving air into the lungs is dependent on respiratory load (the sum of resistance to inspiratory flow, the elastance of the chest wall and lungs, and the positive pressure at peak expiration) (Fig. 13.1). When inspiratory muscles contract, a negative force overcomes this respiratory load, resulting in inward movement of air. With weakness, the respiratory load can only be partly overcome, leading to less air flow and collapse of lung regions. The neuromuscular respiratory failure thus follows a predictable pattern: failure of diaphragm and intercostal muscles, followed by compensatory use of accessory muscles, but eventually resulting in hypoventilation and atelectasis, further leading to shunting and hypoxia. Whether long-standing poor mechanics lead to microatelectasis is unclear, but it seems to be much less of an issue in patients with chronic neuromuscular disorders (Derenne et al., 1978a, b, c; Griggs et al., 1981; Wijdicks, 2002, 2014; Laghi and Tobin, 2003; Walgaard et al., 2010).

Respiratory muscle weakness leads to low-tidal-volume ("shallow") breathing and poor gas exchange, in turn leading to tachypnea and later hypercapnia. These patients also have increased dead-space ventilation associated with their elevated respiratory drive. The rapid breathing is the result of signals to the respiratory center from the abnormal and weak respiratory muscle. Usually the arterial $P_{CO_2}$ will decrease due to this rapid breathing, but when respiratory muscle strength is reduced by more than 25%, $P_{CO_2}$ may increase.

Paradoxic breathing, also known as thoracoabdominal asynchrony, occurs with severe respiratory weakness (Fig. 13.2). Normally, the abdomen and chest expand and contract in a synchronized fashion. During inspiration, a downward movement of the diaphragm pushes the abdominal contents down and out, while the rib margins are also lifted and moved out, causing both the chest and abdomen to rise.

Respiratory failure in GBS can be assessed clinically as with any other case of acute neuromuscular respiratory failure, but relevant additional tests include forced maximal inspiratory and expiratory pressures and vital capacity (VC). These tests may not be readily available, but they do have good predictive value. Several studies have found that VC and the proximal to distal compound muscle action potential ratio of the common peroneal nerve are independent predictors of the need for mechanical ventilation. Others found that the time between onset of weakness and hospital admission, the presence of facial weakness or oropharyngeal dysfunction, and the severity of limb weakness assessed using the Medical Research Council Subscore predicted respiratory failure and the need for endotracheal intubation. This confirms the clinical impression that difficulty clearing secretions in patients with a rapid onset, defined as occurring within

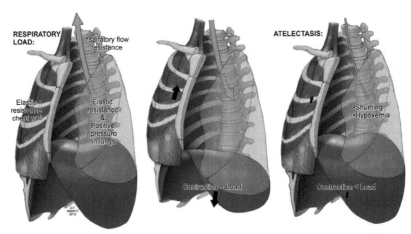

**Fig. 13.1.** Inspiratory load determined by several factors and mechanisms of atelectasis. Used with the permission of Mayo foundation for Medical Education and Research. All rights reserved.

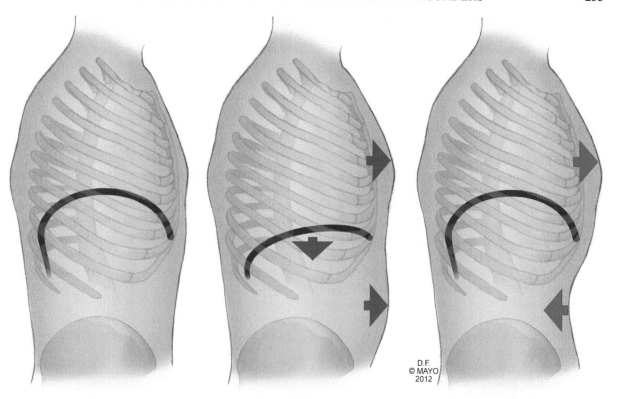

**Fig. 13.2.** Schematic drawing of diaphragm movement and chest movement. (Blue arrows represent normal respiratory movement; red arrows represent diaphagm standstill and 'paradoxical' movement (chest out, abdomen in). Used with the permission of Mayo foundation for Medical Education and Research. All rights reserved.

3 days of onset, may indicate high risk of respiratory failure.

Respiratory failure in MG is more difficult to recognize. Patients may have been overdosed with cholinesterase inhibitors and may have excessive salivation and sweating, abdominal cramps, and urinary urgency. Most recently, MG associated with muscle specific tyrosine kinase (MuSK) antibodies has been reported to have more prominent oculobulbar weakness, although they develop more generalized weakness eventually. Patients with MuSK antibody-positive MG do not respond as well to acetylcholine esterase inhibitors.

As a general rule, imminent neuromuscular respiratory failure is typically recognized by restlessness, tachycardia with a rate of > 100 beats/minute, tachypnea with a respiratory rate of > 20 breaths/minute, use of sternocleidomastoid or scalene muscles, hesitant or constantly interrupted speech, asynchronous and sometimes paradoxic breathing, and the presence of forehead sweating. It should be pointed out that patients will continue to have a sensation of breathlessness even in the presence of a normal arterial blood gas. When $Pa_{CO_2}$ rises, patients will experience further "air hunger," which is a result of increase in respiratory drive and hypercapnic stimulation of chemoreceptors. The sensation of hypoxemia,

however, can be different and patients will develop a sensation of "rapid breathing." Patients often have an unpleasant and frightening feeling while struggling to breathe that is an indicator that intubation is necessary.

## DIAGNOSTIC TESTS

Bedside pulmonary function tests can be useful in certain conditions (GBS, ALS), and very unreliable in others (MG). Patients with diaphragmatic weakness show a fall in the VC when the patient is supine, but it must be more than 25% from baseline to be considered abnormal. Conversely, a normal supine VC makes inspiratory muscle weakness highly unlikely. The maximal inspiratory pressure (MIP) has the advantage that recoil of the chest wall contributes to the value. A high MIP (>−80 cmH$_2$O), particularly in combination with VC, makes neuromuscular respiratory failure unlikely.

In more slowly progressive neurologic disorders, these pulmonary function tests are also important to follow the course of disease. For example, a normal MIP in ALS suggests that the patient may be spared mechanical ventilation in 6 months. A maximal expiratory pressure (MEP) >60 cmH$_2$O predicts the ability to cough in patients with neuromuscular disease, and in one study in ALS, an MEP > 70 cmH$_2$O also correlated with a > 50% predictive value of tracheostomy-free survival. This, again, emphasizes the importance of MEP and the ability to cough effectively to reduce the chance of mucus plugging, and as a result, pneumonia.

Pulse oximetry is important in any patient with neuromuscular respiratory disease, but obviously it does not identify CO$_2$ retention. Rapid and shallow breathing leads to chronic hypercapnia in patients with neuromuscular disease. With rapid, shallow breathing, the total volume is markedly decreased, the inspiratory time shortened, and VC truncated, resulting in hypercarbia. An overnight pulse oximeter is an essential monitor because nocturnal hypoventilation indicates respiratory muscle weakness in the appropriate setting.

Arterial blood gas measurement may or may not be informative. It may show mixed hypoxemic and hypercapnic respiratory failure in a patient with obvious respiratory distress. However, in more subtle presentations, the arterial blood gas can be deceptive. A normal arterial blood gas may be seen in markedly fatigued patients. Normally, one would expect a reduced $Pa$CO$_2$ in a tachypneic patient. A normal arterial $P$CO$_2$ in a tachypneic patient therefore is a sign of impending fatigue, because the patient cannot "blow off CO$_2$." Thus hypercapnia is a late feature in acute neuromuscular failure. In other words, poor bellows lead to poor ventilation due to alveolar collapse, resulting in hypoxemia. There is a "normal" $Pa$CO$_2$, only to rise when the system completely fails.

Cerebrospinal fluid analysis in GBS typically shows high protein with a normal white blood cell count (the classic albuminocytologic dissociation). A white blood cell count > 10 cells per microliter is unusual, and may be seen, although more commonly in associated disorders such as Lyme disease, sarcoidosis, and human immunodeficiency virus infections. Blood tests to consider include a toxicology screen for poisoning and a full metabolic screen (i.e., porphyria) in suspected GBS.

Electrophysiologic studies are more useful for diagnosis and less useful for prognostication. The typical finding is demyelination, seen as conduction block or increased conduction velocities. Specific tests for proximal nerve involvement seen early in the disease course include recording of F waves and nerve signal abnormalities like dispersion or dropout in signal. Prolonged F waves may be the only finding if the patient is tested early on. Needle electromyography may be normal in the first 2 weeks. Recovery often starts after the second week. Progression over 8 weeks more likely suggests the diagnosis is chronic inflammatory demyelinating polyneuropathy.

In MG, it is important to test for serum antibodies (acetylcholine receptor, MuSK, voltage-gated calcium channels). Neurophysiologic studies such as electromyogram, single-fiber electromyogram for orbicularis oculi nerve conduction for conduction block and F waves, and repetitive motor nerve testing of limb and facial muscles and imaging of the spine may be needed.

## HOSPITAL COURSE

Below follow a few general remarks on further treatment of the primary neurologic disorder. Treatment for GBS and MG is plasma exchange or IVIG, but treatment for MG also involves corticosteroids (Fergusson et al., 2005; Stangel and Pul, 2006). Improvement is seen in approximately three-quarters of patients. Plasma exchange may involve five to seven exchanges of 2–3 liters each, usually every other day. In MG, plasma exchange markedly reduces autoantibodies, and there is clinical improvement both in patients with acetylcholine receptor antibodies as well as patients with anti-MuSK antibodies. In more resistant patients with anti-MuSK antibodies, rituximab has been prescribed.

Specific treatment for GBS or MG may cause complications. Acute treatment with IVIG is associated with acute renal failure due to high sucrose load and may lead to a marked rise in creatinine, even up to a point that dialysis is temporarily initiated (sucrose-light IVIG may be considered, e.g., Gamunex).

Finally, it is important to recognize also that acute neuromuscular disease has autonomic effects and there are potential systemic complications. Many patients with severe GBS will have dysautonomia that is manifested by cardiac arrhythmias and wide blood pressure swings (Emmons et al., 1975).

Mechanical ventilation can be prolonged in GBS, short-term in MG and permanent in ALS or other major muscular disorders. Any patient with GBS or MG ventilated for a prolonged period of time will need a plan for weaning from the ventilator. Generally, weaning from mechanical ventilation should be guided by improvement in strength and normalization of values on serial pulmonary function tests. In GBS, diaphragmatic weakness may reverse before extremity weakness; thus, the timing of weaning should not be gauged solely by recovery of extremity muscle strength. There are several conditions that need to be considered before even attempting to wean the patient from the ventilator. In MG, one important priority is to have satisfactory treatment of the myasthenic symptoms. In addition, the patient should have no major pulmonary problem and no evidence of atelectasis, pleural effusion, or marked difficulty handling secretion. Secretion volume, whether the patient is comfortable with a T-piece trial, and a completely normal chest X-ray, together have a good predictive value for successful extubation in any patient with acute neuromuscular respiratory failure. Pulmonary function tests can predict, in some sense, weaning but are far from reliable. The MEP reflects the ability to cough up secretions, and thus abdominal musculature strength, and might be the best predictor of successful weaning.

In MG, an optimal dose of pyridostigmine needs to be found and patients cannot be liberated from the ventilator without adequate treatment, despite multiple IVIG courses or plasma exchange courses. Weaning trials may begin when VC exceeds 15 mL/kg, MIP exceeds $-30$ cm $H_2O$, and oxygen saturation is adequate with inspired oxygen concentrations ($Fio_2$) of 40% or less. It is important to reintroduce cholinesterase inhibitors before extubation trials are initiated.

Methods of weaning from mechanical ventilation may vary. Patients can be switched to continuous positive airway pressure with pressure support ventilation and the level decreased 1–3 cm $H_2O$ each day. In GBS, weaning should be undertaken as early as possible because of the number of significant complications related to prolonged intubation. After intubation, however, respiratory function parameters often continue to fall. Reducing intermittent mandatory ventilation rate or reducing pressure support level can be used as weaning approaches, at the discretion of the treating physician. However, one should anticipate weeks on the ventilator. MIP exceeding $-50$ cm $H_2O$ and VC improvement by 4 mL/kg from preintubation to pre-extubation are associated with successful extubation.

## NEUROREHABILITATION

The quality of life after MG is largely determined by the severity of muscle weakness, which may include weakness of neck muscles and constant head drop, dysphagia and chewing problems, ptosis, diplopia, and a speech impediment. Quality of life is also influenced by the secondary effects of immunosuppressive therapy. This may include recurrent infections, osteoporosis, cataracts, as well as other comorbid disorders. Outcome is thus dependent on choice of treatment and its long-term side-effects.

Timely diagnosis and appropriate treatment with IVIG or plasma exchange for patients with bulbar and respiratory muscle weakness have helped to reduce the seriousness of the clinical course and total time of hospital stay from myasthenic crisis, but still care of a patient with MG may be prolonged and very complicated. Hospital stay after a myasthenic crisis in an elderly patient complicated by aspiration may easily be up to 4 weeks. The prognosis of MG may also be dependent on the presence of acute diaphragmatic failure and on timely therapy, with higher mortality in patients in whom plasma exchange was delayed for more than 2 days after presentation.

Thymectomy improves on outcome. Results from a recent clinical trial showed that patients with thymectomy had significantly greater clinical improvement at three years compared with those treated with prednisone alone (Wolfe et al., 2016). This was not surprising because transsternal thymectomy was considered effective by many physicians, who have seen the procedure increase the likelihood of remission. The trial also noted that there were still considerable number of patients on steroids after surgery.

Generally speaking, onset of MG in middle age has less severe manifestations, but lower probability of full remission and higher mortality when compared with early-onset myasthenia. A worse outcome can be expected in patients with malignant thymoma, but only if the tumor has breached the capsule and caused metastasis.

In GBS, once the patient is mechanically ventilated, a prolonged ICU stay is anticipated, with a high number of patients requiring a tracheostomy despite early administration of IVIG or plasma exchange treatment. Still, most mechanically ventilated patients (about 75%) eventually regain the ability to walk independently, in some cases up to 2 years after onset of GBS. Upper-limb paralysis at peak disability predicts a lesser ability to ambulate in the future. Nonetheless, because patients may show ongoing clinically significant improvement beyond 1–2 years, aggressive rehabilitation is warranted. It remains, however, difficult to predict who will stand up from a wheelchair and who will remain in a wheelchair forever. Fortunately, most patients after a bout of GBS will regain the ability to walk. Mortality in GBS has been estimated at 3%, but doubles in long-term mechanically ventilated patients and may even approach 10–20% in patients with very significant comorbidity. Better ICU care and respiratory rehabilitation have greatly improved these percentages, but pre-existing illness (in particular, prior chronic obstructive pulmonary disease) and the fragility of advanced age remain major disadvantages. Patients may succumb from an otherwise trivial pneumonitis progressing to sepsis.

## CONCLUSION

Acute neuromuscular respiratory failure requires neurointensivist expertise. There are well-defined criteria to come to the diagnosis. Long-term management, which may include tracheostomy and mechanical ventilation, is mainstream neurocritical care. Patients with both these interventions will typically leave the unit in a disabled state, but recover well in the months ahead.

## References

Alshekhlee A, Hussain Z, Sultan B et al. (2008). Guillain–Barré syndrome: incidence and mortality rates in US hospitals. Neurology 70: 1608–1613.

Bolton CF, Chen R, Wijdicks EFM et al. (2004). Neurology of Breathing. Butterworth-Heinemann, Philadelphia.

Broutet N, Krauer F, Riesen M et al. (2016). Zika Virus as a Cause of Neurologic Disorders. N Engl J Med 374 (16): 1506–1509.

Burakgazi AZ, Hoke A (2010). Respiratory muscle weakness in peripheral neuropathies. Journal of the Peripheral Nervous System : JPNS 15: 307–313.

Burns TM, Lawn ND, Low PA et al. (2001). Adynamic ileus in severe Guillain–Barré syndrome. Muscle & Nerve 24: 963–965.

Cabrera Serrano M, Rabinstein AA (2010). Causes and outcomes of acute neuromuscular respiratory failure. Archives of Neurology 67: 1089–1094.

Chaudhuri A, Behan PO (2009). Myasthenic crisis. QJM : Monthly Journal of the Association of Physicians 102: 97–107.

Derenne JP, Macklem PT, Roussos C (1978a). The respiratory muscles: mechanics, control, and pathophysiology. The American Review of Respiratory Disease 118: 119–133.

Derenne JP, Macklem PT, Roussos C (1978b). The respiratory muscles: mechanics, control, and pathophysiology. Part 2. The American Review of Respiratory Disease 118: 373–390.

Derenne JP, Macklem PT, Roussos C (1978c). The respiratory muscles: mechanics, control, and pathophysiology. Part III. The American Review of Respiratory Disease 118: 581–601.

Emmons PR, Blume WT, Dushane JW (1975). Cardiac monitoring and demand pacemaker in Guillain–Barré syndrome. Archives of Neurology 32: 59–61.

Fergusson D, Hutton B, Sharma M et al. (2005). Use of intravenous immunoglobulin for treatment of neurologic conditions: a systematic review. Transfusion 45: 1640–1657.

Fokke C, van den Berg B, Drenthen J et al. (2014). Diagnosis of Guillain–Barré syndrome and validation of Brighton criteria. Brain : A Journal of Neurology 137: 33–43.

Galtrey CM, Faulkner M, Wren DR (2012). How it feels to experience three different causes of respiratory failure. Practical Neurology 12: 49–54.

Greenland P, Griggs RC (1980). Arrhythmic complications in the Guillain–Barré syndrome. Archives of Internal Medicine 140: 1053–1055.

Griffin JW, Li CY, Ho TW et al. (1996). Pathology of the motor-sensory axonal Guillain–Barré syndrome. Annals of Neurology 39: 17–28.

Griggs RC, Donohoe KM, Utell MJ et al. (1981). Evaluation of pulmonary function in neuromuscular disease. Archives of Neurology 38: 9–12.

Hadden RD, Karch H, Hartung HP et al. (2001). Preceding infections, immune factors, and outcome in Guillain–Barré syndrome. Neurology 56: 758–765.

Hafer-Macko CE, Sheikh KA, Li CY et al. (1996). Immune attack on the Schwann cell surface in acute inflammatory demyelinating polyneuropathy. Annals of Neurology 39: 625–635.

Henderson RD, Lawn ND, Fletcher DD et al. (2003). The morbidity of Guillain–Barré syndrome admitted to the intensive care unit. Neurology 60: 17–21.

Hughes RA, Cornblath DR (2005). Guillain–Barré syndrome. Lancet 366: 1653–1666.

Hughes RA, Hadden RD, Gregson NA et al. (1999). Pathogenesis of Guillain–Barré syndrome. Journal of Neuroimmunology 100: 74–97.

Jani-Acsadi A, Lisak RP (2007). Myasthenic crisis: guidelines for prevention and treatment. Journal of the Neurological Sciences 261: 127–133.

Kalita J, Kohat AK, Misra UK (2014). Predictors of outcome of myasthenic crisis. Neurological Sciences : Official Journal of the Italian Neurological Society and of the Italian Society of Clinical Neurophysiology 35: 1109–1114.

Kuwabara S, Yuki N (2013). Axonal Guillain–Barré syndrome: concepts and controversies. The Lancet. Neurology 12: 1180–1188.

Kwong JC, Vasa PP, Campitelli MA et al. (2013). Risk of Guillain–Barré syndrome after seasonal influenza vaccination and influenza health-care encounters: a self-controlled study. The Lancet. Infectious Diseases 13: 769–776.

Laghi F, Tobin MJ (2003). Disorders of the respiratory muscles. American Journal of Respiratory and Critical Care Medicine 168: 10–48.

Lawn ND, Wijdicks EF (1999). Fatal Guillain–Barré syndrome. Neurology 52: 635–638.

McGrogan A, Madle GC, Seaman HE et al. (2009). The epidemiology of Guillain–Barré syndrome worldwide. A systematic literature review. Neuroepidemiology 32: 150–163.

Re D, Schwenk A, Hegener P et al. (2000). Guillain–Barré syndrome in a patient with non-Hodgkin's lymphoma. Ann Oncol 11: 217–220.

Ropper AH, Wijdicks EF (1990). Blood pressure fluctuations in the dysautonomia of Guillain–Barré syndrome. Archives of Neurology 47: 706–708.

Ropper AE, Albert JW, Addison R (1988). Limited relapse in Guillain–Barré syndrome after plasma exchange. Archives of Neurology 45: 314–315.

Ropper AH, Wijdicks EFM, Truax BT (1991). Guillain–Barré Syndrome. F. A. Davis, Philadelphia.

Schaumburg HH, Herskovitz S (2000). The weak child – a cautionary tale. The New England Journal of Medicine 342: 127–129.

Seneviratne J, Mandrekar J, Wijdicks EF et al. (2008). Noninvasive ventilation in myasthenic crisis. Archives of Neurology 65: 54–58.

Stangel M, Pul R (2006). Basic principles of intravenous immunoglobulin (IVIg) treatment. Journal of Neurology 253 (Suppl 5): V18–V24.

Thomas CE, Mayer SA, Gungor Y et al. (1997). Myasthenic crisis: clinical features, mortality, complications, and risk factors for prolonged intubation. Neurology 48: 1253–1260.

van den Berg B, Walgaard C, Drenthen J et al. (2014). Guillain–Barré syndrome: pathogenesis, diagnosis, treatment and prognosis. Nature Reviews. Neurology 10: 469–482.

van der Meche FG, van Doorn PA (2000). Guillain–Barré syndrome. Current Treatment Options in Neurology 2: 507–516.

van Doorn PA, Ruts L, Jacobs BC (2008). Clinical features, pathogenesis, and treatment of Guillain–Barré syndrome. The Lancet. Neurology 7: 939–950.

Walgaard C, Lingsma HF, Ruts L et al. (2010). Prediction of respiratory insufficiency in Guillain–Barré syndrome. Annals of Neurology 67: 781–787.

Wijdicks EFM (2002). Short of breath, short of air, short of mechanics. Practical Neurology 2: 208–213.

Wijdicks EFM (2014). Core Principles of Acute Neurology (Volumes 1–4), Oxford University Press, Oxford.

Wijdicks EFM, Henderson RD, McClelland RL (2003). Emergency intubation for respiratory failure in Guillain–Barré syndrome. Archives of Neurology 60: 947–948.

Winer JB (2014). An update in Guillain–Barré syndrome. Autoimmune Diseases 2014: 793024.

Wolfe GI, Kaminski HJ, Aban IB et al. (2016). Randomized Trial of Thymectomy in Myasthenia Gravis. N Engl J Med 375: 511–522.

Yuki N (2007). Campylobacter sialyltransferase gene polymorphism directs clinical features of Guillain–Barré syndrome. Journal of Neurochemistry 103 (Suppl 1): 150–158.

*Handbook of Clinical Neurology*, Vol. 140 (3rd series)
*Critical Care Neurology, Part I*
E.F.M. Wijdicks and A.H. Kramer, Editors
http://dx.doi.org/10.1016/B978-0-444-63600-3.00014-3

Chapter 14

# Critical care management of traumatic brain injury

D.K. MENON* AND A. ERCOLE

*Division of Anaesthesia, University of Cambridge and Neurosciences/Trauma Critical Care Unit, Addenbrooke's Hospital, Cambridge, UK*

## Abstract

Traumatic brain injury (TBI) is a growing global problem, which is responsible for a substantial burden of disability and death, and which generates substantial healthcare costs. High-quality intensive care can save lives and improve the quality of outcome. TBI is extremely heterogeneous in terms of clinical presentation, pathophysiology, and outcome. Current approaches to the critical care management of TBI are not under-pinned by high-quality evidence, and many of the current therapies in use have not shown benefit in randomized control trials. However, observational studies have informed the development of authoritative international guidelines, and the use of multimodality monitoring may facilitate rational approaches to optimizing acute physiology, allowing clinicians to optimize the balance between benefit and risk from these interventions in individual patients. Such approaches, along with the emerging impact of advanced neuroimaging, genomics, and protein biomarkers, could lead to the development of precision medicine approaches to the intensive care management of TBI.

## INTRODUCTION

Traumatic brain injury (TBI) is an important cause for admission to intensive care units (ICUs) in general, and to neurocritical care units in particular. National population-based figures for ICU caseload (as opposed to more specific stratification into mild, moderate, or severe TBI) are difficult to find, but the UK Intensive Care National Audit and Research Centre (ICNARC, 2015) reported that in 2014–2015, approximately 2% of all ICU admissions and about 10% of admissions to neurocritical care units were due to TBI. These patients are at high risk of death or poor neurologic outcome. Mortality in a 3200-patient cohort study from this popu-lation base (Harrison et al., 2013) was 18% at ICU discharge, rising to 26% at 6 months. Independent sur-vival by 6 months was only achieved in 39% of patients. Other global data suggest similar outcome figures in hospitalized patients, though data from large, unselected case series based on ICU populations (rather than specific data on moderate or severe TBI) are not widely available. However, a comparative analysis of UK and

US data suggested that TBI patients admitted to critical care services in the USA may have a less severe overall distribution of severity, with about half not being mechanically ventilated at admission from the emer-gency room (Wunsch et al., 2011). This is unsurprising, given that the USA has about twice the number of ICU beds in a population-based analysis, and it would be reasonable to infer that the absolute caseload from TBI may be higher in US ICUs, but TBI severity may be lower, and crude outcomes better. However, the wider TBI data suggest a similar large burden of case mix adjusted mortality and morbidity.

This burden of mortality and residual disability demands a comprehensive therapeutic response. How-ever, despite substantial efforts and investment by the pharmaceutical industry, we still do not have a specific neuroprotective therapy that is effective in clinical TBI, and we may need to look elsewhere to improve out-comes (Menon and Maas, 2015). Little can be done about the extent of primary injury to the brain when patients present to ICUs following head trauma, but the detrimen-tal contribution to outcome from secondary neuronal

*Correspondence to: Professor David K. Menon, Box 93, Addenbrooke's Hospital, Cambridge CB2 2QQ, UK. Tel: +44-1223-217889, Fax: +44-1223-217887, E-mail: dkm13@cam.ac.uk

injury can be substantial. Much of such secondary injury, and (at least currently) all of the avoidable secondary injury, is triggered by physiologic insults to the injured brain, which can be substantially mitigated by good neurocritical care. While accumulating evidence from case series and historic comparisons suggest that the overall process of protocol-driven neurocritical care may make a difference in this setting (English et al., 2013), this benefit has been more difficult to demonstrate in formal randomized controlled trials of specific interventions. Given this context, this chapter not only summarizes the clinical evidence available, but also seeks to provide a basis for rational clinical management based on knowledge of pathophysiology where the paucity of trial evidence makes definitive formal recommendations impossible.

## EPIDEMIOLOGY

There have been several attempts to provide a robust and objective definition of TBI. Most recently, an interagency working party defined TBI as "an alteration in brain function or other evidence of brain pathology caused by an external force" (Menon et al., 2010). This statement highlighted potential diagnostic confounders, and sought to rely on a combination of injury narrative, symptoms, neuroimaging, and wider context to establish a diagnosis. Despite these efforts, good data on TBI epidemiology are hard to find. Pooling of available age-adjusted incidence rates for the general population revealed that the reported incidence of TBI varies considerably, ranging from 59.6 to 811.0 per 100 000 (Roozenbeek et al., 2013). Figures for population-based ICU admissions with TBI are even scarcer, due to difficulties in defining the population denominator in most studies.

Notwithstanding difficulties with epidemiologic definition and categorization, it is clear that TBI is an important cause of mortality and morbidity across the world, and that its global impact is rising. Despite the predicted incidence of dementia over the coming decades, it is salutary to note that TBI is estimated to remain, by far, the most important cause of neurodisability up to 2030 (WHO, 2006). However, the epidemiologic pattern of TBI is changing globally (Roozenbeek et al., 2013). In high-income countries such as the USA, there is growing concern about the long-term impact of mild TBI and concussion, but such patients are unlikely to present to critical care units. However, increasing road usage in low- and middle-income countries, unaccompanied by appropriate traffic education and road safety measures, has increased the incidence of moderate and severe TBI. High-income countries have seen a marked increase in TBI, predominantly due to falls, in older patients. The availability of better

prehospital facilities means that many patients with severe extracranial trauma are now surviving, and though associated intracranial injury may not be dominant in these subjects, the physiologic compromise of severe critical illness means that many of these patients may have late disability associated with lesser severities of TBI. Finally, there is increasing concern that patients who sustain even a single moderate or severe TBI are at risk of increased mortality for decades after the ictus (McMillan et al., 2014; Greenwald et al., 2015; Puljula et al., 2016). Furthermore, survivors may carry a substantial burden of chronic (and possibly progressive) disability (Masel, 2015), and a minority may experience progressive cognitive and/or neurologic deterioration (McMillan et al., 2012), as well as an increased risk of late neurodegenerative disease (Shively et al., 2012; Smith et al., 2013). These issues are relevant to our current and future care of TBI in critical care settings.

## CLINICAL NEUROPATHOLOGY AND PATHOPHYSIOLOGY

Acute neuropathology following TBI (Blumbergs et al., 2008) determines early treatment, and can characterize acute pathophysiology. Acute neuropathology has conventionally been categorized as either focal or diffuse (Table 14.1). At later stages, the pathologic changes seen in survivors can explain disability and deficits (Adams et al., 1999, 2011; Maxwell et al., 2004). Finally, the associations of TBI with late neurodegeneration, including Alzheimer's disease and chronic traumatic encephalopathy, have been primarily recognized by neuropathologic studies (Smith et al., 2013; Daneshvar et al., 2015).

### Focal pathology

Epidural hematomas (EDHs) account for ~10% of cases of intracranial hemorrhage in TBI, and are associated in the majority of cases with skull fractures (classically of the middle meningeal artery, associated with fractures of the squamous temporal plate). An EDH may be

*Table 14.1*

**Focal and nonfocal pathology in traumatic brain injury**

| Focal pathology | Nonfocal pathology |
| --- | --- |
| Extradural hematoma (EDH) | Global ischemia |
| Subdural hematoma (SDH) | Traumatic axonal |
| Traumatic intracerebral hematoma (TICH) | injury |
| | Diffuse brain swelling |
| Contusions | Posttraumatic |
| | hydrocephalus |

associated with minimal or no underlying brain injury, and since bleeding into the extradural space needs to strip the dura from the inner table of the skull, hematoma accumulation may be slow, and patients may initially appear well and later deteriorate – often termed a "lucid interval" in patients who "talk and die" (Reilly et al., 1975). While this picture has been classically associated with EDH, more recent reports suggest other pathologic substrates, including bifrontal contusions, coagulopathy, or anticoagulant medication (Goldschlager et al., 2007; Peterson and Chesnut, 2011; Kim et al., 2013). Classically, subdural hematomas (SDHs) commonly arise from rupture of bridging veins, and are often associated with underlying brain injury. However, bleeding into the subdural space may develop with minimal brain trauma in elderly patients on anticoagulants. Traumatic intracerebral hemorrhage (TICH) is commonly associated with superficial contusions, or may be deep-seated (e.g., in the basal ganglia) as a consequence of shearing forces. Superficial contusions commonly occur as a consequence of *coup* or *contrecoup* impacts, most commonly in the frontal and temporal lobes, where the moving brain impacts the irregular inner surface of the skull. Where such hemorrhagic contusions are in continuity with an overlying SDH, the term "burst lobe" is sometimes applied. Intracranial hemorrhages represent the most common indication for surgical intervention following TBI, and can produce mass effect either because of their volume, or (particularly with SDH or TICH), due to the perilesional edema that commonly develops. Such mass effect may be delayed, particularly with bifrontal contusions, or can develop suddenly following a delay with temporal lesions, as an expanding contusion or hemorrhage that was originally confined to the temporal fossa enlarges and produces a more generalized effect. Contusion expansion is associated with microvascular failure, and may have a stereotyped molecular narrative, in which the sulfonylurea receptor (Sur 1) may play an important part (Simard et al., 2012).

## Nonfocal (diffuse) pathology

The phrase "diffuse pathology" is a misnomer, since all three classic forms of this pathology are more likely to be multifocal, rather than diffuse. Ischemia is common in the first 24 hours after TBI, and focal infarcts are frequent (~90%) in fatal TBI, either in watershed perfusion zones, or less commonly as a consequence of blunt vascular injury (Graham et al., 1978, 1989). Less commonly, true global ischemia may occur, often triggered by a long period of refractory intracranial hypertension or systemic hypotension. Traumatic axonal injury (TAI) (Hill et al., 2016) arises as a consequence of acceleration–deceleration rotational forces and affects white-matter bundles in the brain, classically involving the dorsolateral brainstem, corpus callosum, and the corona radiata, most often in the frontal and temporal regions. When extensive, it is commonly referred to as diffuse axonal injury (DAI). Axons can also be injured at the interface of gray and white matter, at the point at which they enter the cortical mantle. While some axons can be physically sheared at the time of initial impact (primary axotomy), TAI can be more subtle and result in beading or undulation of axons with cytoskeletal damage, and matures due to metabolic or functional derangements in energy production or axonal transport, with late axonal breakdown (secondary axotomy). The maturation of TAI processes may take hours to days, and the activation of neuroinflammation that accompanies TBI may result in ongoing white-matter loss over months to years.

The clinical impact of TAI is variable, and mild TAI may simply result in a period of loss of consciousness. However, extensive DAI probably provides the substrate for the worst outcomes seen in TBI. TAI is commonly accompanied by injury to the small vessels that accompany white-matter bundles. While the resulting microhemorrhages were simply viewed as a convenient biomarker of TAI, there has been recent interest in traumatic vascular injury as an important pathology in its own right (Kenney et al., 2016), although the relationship of radiologically or pathologically detectable TBI to abnormal vascular function in TBI is as yet unclear.

## Genetic modulation of disease course and outcome in TBI

Only 35% of the variance in outcome can be explained by available prognostic models (see later section). It is likely that at least part of the residual variance in disease course and outcome could be explained by genetic variability in the host response, both in the acute and the postacute phases.

Mitochondrial DNA haplotype K, which is overrepresented amongst centenarians and underrepresented in neurodegenerative disease, is associated with better global outcomes (Bulstrode et al., 2014), and carriers of haplotypes K, I, and J are less disabled following TBI (Conley et al., 2014). Intronic variations in the antiapoptotic proto-oncogene BCL2 are associated with poor outcome in severe TBI (Hoh et al., 2010). Polymorphisms in genes coding for several cytokines have been shown to modulate TBI outcome, including tumor necrosis factor-α (TNF-α) (Waters et al., 2013), interleukin-1β (IL-1β) (Uzan et al., 2005), and IL-1Ra (Hadjigeorgiou et al., 2005). Heterozygotes at a single-nucleotide polymorphism in IL-1β also showed substantially higher risk of posttraumatic sei-zure development (over 36-month follow-up) in one cohort (Diamond et al., 2014).

In the postacute phase, outcome has been shown to be associated with polymorphisms in genes coding for brain-derived neurotrophic factor, though some results are conflicting (Krueger et al., 2011; McAllister et al., 2012; Barbey et al., 2014). Polymorphisms in a range of neurotransmitter-related genes also modulate out-come. These include the GRIN2A gene, which codes for an NMDAR subunit (Raymont et al., 2008), genes responsible for dopamine signaling (e.g., Val158Met polymorphism in the gene coding for catechol-*O*-methyltransferase, or the ANKK1 gene modulating expression of the DRD2 dopamine receptor) (Lipsky et al., 2005; McAllister et al., 2008; Willmott et al., 2013; Yue et al., 2015; Winkler et al., 2016), and seroto-nin transport protein, 5-HTTLPR (Failla et al., 2013). The most extensively studied gene in the field of TBI is the cholesterol transport protein, apolipoprotein E, which has three well-characterized alleles (ε2, 3, and 4). Possession of the ε4 allele is known to increase the risk of late-onset Alzheimer's disease, and has been shown in several studies to worsen outcome or the trajectory of recovery from TBI (Teasdale et al., 1997, 2005; Ponsford et al., 2011; Lawrence et al., 2015). Possession of this allele also increases the risk of late dementia follow-ing TBI. This risk is modulated by age and TBI severity (see Shively et al., 2012, for review), but the combination of an ε4 allele and a history of severe TBI may increase late dementia risk 10-fold. While all of these effects have been attributed to late modulation of cognitive outcome, genetic variations may also modulate pathophysiology in the acute phase. For example, neurotransmitter dynam-ics are known to play a part in secondary neuronal injury, and ε4 inhibits neurite outgrowth and increases release of proinflammatory mediators (IL-6, nitric oxide) from stimulated microglia (Vitek et al., 2009).

## Molecular mechanisms of injury

The molecular mechanisms of injury in TBI resemble those seen in other acute insults such as ischemia, and have been reviewed elsewhere (Kochanek et al., 2015; Krishnamurthy and Laskowitz, 2015). Briefly, second-ary injury mechanisms include excitotoxicity and calcium influx, oxidative injury (through lipid peroxida-tion, protein nitrosylation, and DNA damage), cellular and humoral inflammatory mediators, and energy failure, which result in secondary neuronal loss through a range of cell death modes (necrosis, apoptosis, necroptosis, paraptosis, parthanosis, autophagy, and phagoptosis of injured but viable cells by activated microglia).

## Brain swelling, dysautoregulation, and energy failure

Brain swelling in TBI is classically attributed to cyto-toxic edema, vasogenic edema, or vascular congestion, which have time-varying profiles after TBI (Fig. 14.1).

Original support for the role of vascular congestion in causing brain swelling (Kelly et al., 1996) was chal-lenged by the increasing use of diffusion-weighted mag-netic resonance imaging (MRI) in this context over the last 15 years, which led to an increased focus on cyto-toxic edema (Kawamata et al., 2000; Kucinski et al., 2002; Marmarou et al., 2006; Pasco et al., 2006), but on its own, this process only results in a translocation of water from the interstitial space to the cellular com-partment, and no increase in overall brain volume (Donkin and Vink, 2010). More recent publications have renewed interest in microvascular injury (Logsdon et al., 2015), vasogenic edema (resulting from altered blood–brain barrier (BBB) permeability (Price et al., 2015)), and the cerebral venous compartment (Chen et al., 2015) as important causes of brain swelling.

Cytotoxic edema may arise from either reduced energy supply or increased energy demand. Systemic hypoxia and hypotension are important causes of inade-quate oxygen and substrate delivery, and powerful mod-ulators of outcome (Chesnut et al., 1993; Jones et al., 1994; Manley et al., 2001). However, even if systemic

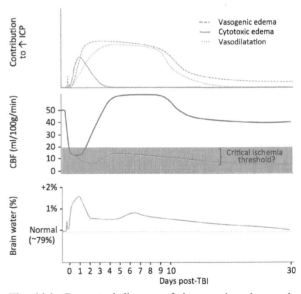

**Fig. 14.1.** Conceptual diagram of time-varying changes in physiology in traumatic brain injury (TBI) (top panel) and their contribution to increases in brain water (lower panel), and to intracranial hypertension (middle panel). The depicted changes in physiology are based on a consensus from human and experimental research data. ICP, intracranial pressure; CBF, cerebral blood flow.

physiology is well maintained, classic ischemia can be seen, commonly within the first 24 hours after TBI (Bouma et al., 1991, 1992; Coles et al., 2004), and often in relation to contusions and SDHs. Additional contributors to impaired energy generation (Fig. 14.2) include tissue hypoxia arising from impaired oxygen diffusion, microvascular ischemia (Menon et al., 2004), or mitochondrial dysfunction causing metabolic crisis (Verweij et al., 2000; Vespa et al., 2005). Mitochondrial dysfunction may be due to mechanical disruption of mitochondria, or due to competitive inhibition in the respiratory chain by elevated levels of nitric oxide (Brown, 2000). These different models of energy failure have similar consequences in terms of metabolic markers, with elevation of tissue lactate and lactate/pyruvate ratio detectable by clinical microdialysis. However, the multimodality monitoring or imaging of cerebral blood flow (CBF), oxygen extraction fraction, and tissue oxygen may reveal variations in pathophysiology, which could be treated with different therapeutic approaches.

Increased energy demand may be the consequence of seizures, which may be nonconvulsive and only detectable by electroencephalography (EEG) (Ronne-Engstrom and Winkler, 2006; Olivecrona et al., 2009; Vespa et al., 2010) or fever (Sacho et al., 2010; Li and Jiang, 2012; Bao et al., 2014). Recent interest has focused on the role of cortical spreading depression (CSD; Fig. 14.3), which causes profound depolarization of cortical tissue, and is associated with worse outcomes (Hartings et al., 2011a). Most literature on CSD has focused on electrocorticographic (ECoG) detection, but there is increasing evidence that scalp surface EEG may provide clues to its presence (Hartings et al., 2014). Restoration of membrane potential following CSD is hugely energy demanding, and may be associated with prolonged tissue hypoxia (Takano et al., 2007). While the classic literature has focused on oxygen deficiency in the context of reduced substrate delivery, there is increasing appreciation that metabolic crisis may also arise from inadequate glucose delivery, or an inability to use glucose. Even low-normal blood sugars (e.g., in the context of tight glycemic control) may result in low brain tissue glucose (Oddo et al., 2008; Meierhans et al., 2010), especially in abnormal tissue (Magnoni et al., 2012), and low brain glucose is an independent driver of CSD (Parkin et al., 2005) and of poor outcome (Vespa et al., 2003).

Vasogenic edema, arising from breakdown of the BBB (Shlosberg et al., 2010; Alves, 2014), is commonly seen in perilesional regions, and in some patients may result in generalized brain swelling. In animal models, BBB breakdown is a biphasic process, with an initial transient leak occurring soon after impact, and a subsequent secondary phase hours to days after TBI. This

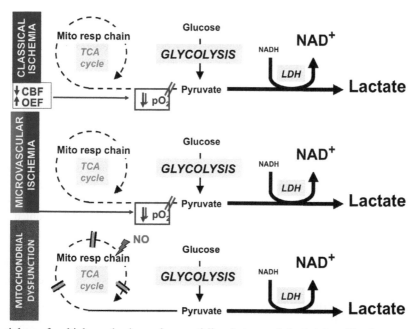

**Fig. 14.2.** Pathophysiology of multiple mechanisms of energy failure in traumatic brain injury. The downstream metabolic effects (elevations in lactate and lactate/pyruvate ratio) are common to all three, but a reduced cerebral blood flow (CBF), high oxygen extraction fraction (OEF), and a low brain tissue $po_2$ ($P_{bt}O_2$) characterize classic ischemia, while microvascular ischemia only shows the reductions in $P_{bt}O_2$. Neither OEF nor $P_{bt}O_2$ is abnormal in mitochondrial failure, although low $P_{bt}O_2$ may unmask functional mitochondrial abnormalities due to high levels of nitric oxide (NO), which competes with oxygen at the mitochondrial respiratory chain. TCA, tricarboxylic acid; LDH, lactate dehydrogenase.

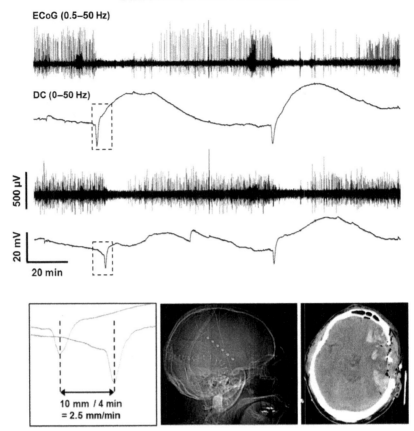

**Fig. 14.3.** Electrocorticographic (ECoG) recordings from a 61-year-old male following a traumatic brain injury (TBI) from a motorcycle accident. The patient underwent decompressive surgery after enlargement of left frontal and temporal contusions that resulted in a drop in Glasgow Coma Scale from 14 to 11. At surgery, an electrode strip was placed on the left superior temporal gyrus. A total of 89 spreading depolarizations were observed in 5 days of ECoG monitoring. The upper and middle panel show bandpass-filtered (0.5–50 Hz) ECoG and direct current (DC) signal from two adjacent electrodes, 10 mm apart, in a cortical strip array, from a patient 26 hours after TBI. The onset of the cortical spreading depolarization episode (denoted by reduction in ECoG activity coupled with negative wave in DC potential) has different start times in the two electrodes. Superimposition of the two DC signals (bottom panel, left) shows a propagation rate of 2.5 mm/min between the two electrodes. The images on the middle and right in the lower panel show a lateral image of the skull showing the location of the ECoG strip, and the postoperative computed tomography (CT) appearances on X-ray CT. The patient eventually had an outcome graded as lower severe disability on the extended Glasgow Outcome Scale. (Data and images courtesy of Dr. Jed Hartings, University of Cincinnati.)

sequence is less clearly recognizable in clinical TBI. The mechanisms responsible for BBB leak include oxidant injury and inflammation (see below), and recent interest has focused on the role of the sulfonylurea receptor in generating microvascular failure and BBB breakdown (Simard et al., 2012). Low-grade BBB leak may persist for decades after TBI (Hay et al., 2015).

## Abnormalities in vasomotor tone and reactivity

Classically, CBF has been reported to exhibit a triphasic behavior (Martin et al., 1997) following TBI (Fig. 14.1), with early reductions in blood flow within the first 12–24 hours postinjury (Bouma et al., 1991, 1992). Physiologic imaging with positron emission tomography (PET)

demonstrates that this is more prominent in the vicinity of contusions and underlying SDHs, and that, in many cases, these CBF reductions represent true ischemia rather than appropriately coupled hypoperfusion in regions of low metabolic demand (Coles et al., 2004). At later points, CBF increases and may reach supranormal levels (Kelly et al., 1996; Coles et al., 2007). Again, PET imaging shows that at least some of this is true hyperemia (i.e., CBF in excess of demand). Such abnormal vasomotor tone may be responsible for brain swelling by causing pathologic vasodilatation. While a subsequent phase of late CBF reduction due to vasospasm is sometimes seen, the incidence is unclear, though some groups suggest that this may be an underestimated contributor to pathophysiology (Romner et al., 1996; Lee et al., 1997; Oertel et al., 2005).

These time-varying hemodynamic responses also define potential windows for treatment that address each of the underlying processes. However, patients vary enormously, and different mechanisms responsible for intracranial hypertension may operate concurrently even within a single individual at different time points. However, the discussion above provides a conceptual framework for selection of initial "best-guess" therapies in individuals, which can be refined in the light of data from multimodality monitoring.

TBI patients commonly show loss of vascular reactivity to perfusion pressure, and, less commonly, to changes in $Pa_{CO_2}$ (Newell et al., 1997; Lee et al., 2001). Both these derangements are indicators of worse prognosis. However, in patients in whom autoregulation is preserved, the autoregulatory range of cerebral perfusion pressure (CPP) over which CBF is maintained may be reduced and/or shifted from the normally accepted 50–150-mmHg range. This altered range of autoregulation can be identified using bedside monitoring of ICP and CPP, and there is increasing evidence that maintenance of CPP at or close to the optimal range for autoregulation (often termed CPPopt) (Steiner et al., 2002; Aries et al., 2012) is associated with improved outcomes (see later).

## CLINICAL PRESENTATION

TBI presentation can be highly varied and may coexist with a diverse range of extracranial pathology. Severity has traditionally been classified in terms of postresuscitation Glasgow Coma Scale (GCS) (Teasdale and Jennett, 1974), with severe TBI being defined as GCS ≤ 8. Although the GCS has stood the test of time (Teasdale et al., 2014), it has some shortcomings in practice. Alternatives have been proposed to overcome some of these difficulties. For example, the Full Outline of UnResponsiveness (FOUR) score (Wijdicks et al., 2005) has advantages in terms of incorporating pupillary reflexes (an important outcome predictor after TBI) and other brainstem reflexes. The respiratory pattern is also used as a scoring variable, but may be less informative of neurological state if the $Pa_{CO_2}$ is low in the fully mechanically ventilated patient, since spontaneous ventilatory drive may be suppressed. Adjustment of the ventilator is needed to asses for ventilatory drive of the patient. The FOUR score has been shown to perform comparably to the GCS in TBI (Sadaka et al., 2012; Okasha et al., 2014; Kasprowicz et al., 2016; Nyam et al., 2017).

Nevertheless, the use of any coma score in the definition of TBI severity is questionable; it is well known that many very different intracranial injuries with diverse outcomes may lead to the same GCS (Saatman et al., 2008). If one studies patients in the ultra-early prehospital setting, brief periods of unconsciousness are common

even after more trivial head injuries. Furthermore, with the increasing availability of advanced prehospital intervention, the resuscitation of, for example, a hypoxic and hypovolemic patient may occur simultaneously with intubation, so that a true postresuscitation GCS is never obtained. Finally, some patients who are fully conscious at the scene may still go on to die as a result of their injuries (Reilly et al., 1975), which demonstrates that the primary injury itself does not entirely account for mortality.

Hypotension (generally as a result of extracranial hemorrhage) and hypoxia (as a result of aspiration, pulmonary injury, or airway obstruction) frequently coexist in the early phase of TBI (Stocchetti et al., 1996). Both of these factors have been repeatedly shown to be key independent determinants of survival (Chesnut et al., 1993; Fearnside et al., 1993; Hill et al., 1993; Murray et al., 2007; Krishnamoorthy et al., 2015), likely in a dose-dependent and perhaps synergistic way (Manley et al., 2001; McHugh et al., 2007). The precise threshold for harmful early hypotension is not known, but there is evidence injury may occur substantially above the thresholds used in previous studies, where hypotension has been considered as systolic blood pressures below 90 mmHg (Butcher et al., 2007).

Both hypoxia and hypotension are potentially remediable/preventable in the ultra-early phase, and advances in prehospital trauma care are changing the presentation of TBI to hospitals. These factors are also determinants of survival in trauma patients irrespective of TBI. The CRASH-2 study demonstrated a survival benefit for early administration of tranexamic acid in bleeding trauma patients (CRASH-2 trial collaborators et al., 2010). A nested study within CRASH-2 (Perel et al., 2012) examining the subgroup of patients with mild, moderate, or severe TBI and abnormal computed tomographic (CT) brain findings found a trend towards reduction in hemorrhage growth, fewer ischemic lesions, and fewer deaths when tranexamic acid was administered, although none of these were statistically significant. These findings have formed the basis for CRASH-3, a trial of tranexamic acid in TBI with intracranial hemorrhage (Dewan et al., 2012).

The incidence of intracranial hypertension at the time of presentation to hospital and in the prehospital phase is unknown, but likely to be low, except in patients with surgical intracranial space-occupying lesions. Seizures are also commonly reported by bystanders and prehospital teams, although again, the true incidence is unknown. It is not clear how often various abnormality movements, such as posturing, are mistaken for seizures. Furthermore it is not known what fraction of events can be attributed to the brain injury or are instead a result of hypoxia from transient airway obstruction or caused by hypotension, and therefore it is difficult to exactly specify the prognostic significance of this finding.

## IMAGING

Neuroimaging is used for diagnosis, therapy selection (especially for surgical interventions), and prognostication. CT and MRI both have their specific place, but their relative roles are currently in some flux.

At presentation, especially with more severe grades of TBI, imaging is used to detect and quantify injury, identify treatable lesions, and guide surgical interventions. Multidetector CT remains the technique of choice in this context, allowing rapid integrated examination of the head and cervical spine (Parizel et al., 2005), and detection and evaluation of surgically treatable lesions, both by quantifying lesion volume, and its impact in terms of space occupation (by identifying the extent of midline shift, and sulcal and cisternal effacement). The detection of intracranial hematomas which do not require evacuation may prompt intracranial pressure (ICP) monitoring, or trigger serial CT for detecting hematoma or contusion expansion, or for identifying development of hydrocephalus (most commonly with subarachnoid or intraventricular hemorrhage). Current surgical guidelines recommend surgery based primarily on CT findings, with craniotomy recommended for subdural or extradural hematomas larger than 30 mL or associated midline shift exceeding 5 mm; and for parenchymal hematomas exceeding 20 mL in noneloquent cortex (see Bullock et al., 2006, and subsequent articles in the same supplement).

Over the past decade, substantial improvements in CT technology have enhanced its role (Rostami et al., 2014). Additional data available from fast multidetector CT include CT angiography (to exclude vascular injury), and increasing use of mobile CT scanners reduces the risks of transport in unstable patients (Carlson and Yonas, 2012; Agrawal et al., 2016). While CT perfusion studies can provide parametric images of CBF, cerebral blood volume, and mean transit time alongside CT angiography and structural imaging, this technique is still primarily confined to research studies.

CT as a sole technique does not characterize TBI completely (Fig. 14.4), particularly with reference to posterior fossa lesions, TAI, and early ischemia, and MRI provides complementary information in this context (Altmeyer et al., 2016). Conventional structural MRI can provide better characterization of parenchymal abnormalities, especially in the posterior fossa, and increases the sensitivity for detection of TAI (Mannion et al., 2007). The microvascular shearing associated with TAI may be visible as microhemorrhages on CT, but the sensitivity and interobserver variability of this finding are poor (Harrison et al., 2013). CT has some prognostic content, perhaps best characterized by the Marshall grading system or Rotterdam CT Score (Maas et al., 2005),

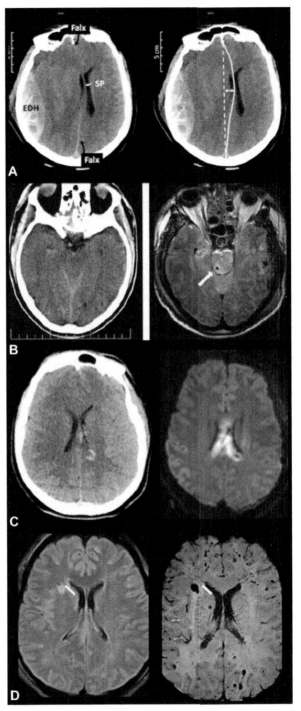

**Fig. 14.4.** Imaging in traumatic brain injury. (**A**) Computed tomography (CT) remains the imaging modality of choice for the demonstration of surgical lesions, such as this extradural hematoma (EDH), and demonstration of their space-occupying impact in terms of midline shift of the falx cerebri and septum pellucidum (SP). (**B**) However, CT is poor at imaging the posterior fossa – see the brainstem lesion that is not seen on CT (left) but clearly demonstrated by magnetic resonance imaging (MRI: right). Also note the detail of microstructural abnormality in the medial right temporal contusion on MRI,

but is imperfect at predicting outcomes in patients with moderate and severe TBI, 20% of whom have normal or near-normal admission CT appearances, but who may still have poor outcomes because of undetected DAI. Conversely, rapid surgical evacuation combined with high-quality intensive care can deliver good outcomes in patients with very abnormal initial CT scans, including those with large intracranial hematomas. MRI may provide increased prognostic capacity in this setting, over and above that provided by clinical and laboratory features and CT (Moen et al., 2014).

Diffusion-weighted MRI can directly image axonal shearing and map such injury (Newcombe et al., 2007), but an additional strength of MR in detecting acute TAI lies in its exquisite sensitivity for detecting microhemorrhages that accompany axonal lesions, especially with a new generation of T2*-sensitive sequences. Different MR sequences show specific patterns of lesion evolution, and while fluid-attenuated inversion recovery (FLAIR) and diffusion-weighted imaging may predict outcome early in the acute phase, they appear to lose conspicuity over time, and may underestimate the extent of injury at 3 months (Moen et al., 2012). Susceptibility-weighted imaging sequences, on the other hand, show good lesion detectability at 3 months, only fading by 12 months postinjury. Persistent neurologic symptoms may be the result of subtle microstructural alterations, such as TAI, which are often demonstrated at autopsy, but have remained undetected by conventional antemortem imaging in the past.

Logistic and clinical considerations, however, limit use of MRI, particularly in the acute setting. The need to exclude contraindications to MRI in the comatose patient, the requirement to change to dedicated MR-compatible monitoring, and the longer duration of MR studies mean that the use of MR in the acute setting is less common than its capabilities might suggest. As a consequence, the most common clinical (as opposed to research) indication for MR studies in TBI in the ICU is to explain clinical progress that is worse than expected based on the CT and to evaluate prognosis in patients who fail to emerge from coma following cessation of sedation (Galanaud et al., 2012; Stevens et al., 2014).

---

which is not seen on CT. (C) Diffusion-weighted MRI (on the right) can show traumatic axonal injury (here in the corpus callosum) with greater sensitivity than CT (on the left). (D) Susceptibility-weighted imaging (right) shows petechial hemorrhages associated with traumatic axonal injury in peripheral white matter more conspicuously and with greater sensitivity than conventional MR sequences such as fluid-attenuated inversion recovery (left).

## BIOMARKERS

There has been substantial recent interest in the use of protein biomarkers in blood, and to a lesser extent in cerebrospinal fluid (CSF), to aid in the diagnosis, monitoring, and prognostic assessment of TBI (Kawata et al., 2016; Kulbe and Geddes, 2016). The key proteins that are currently in clinical use or evaluation are listed in Table 14.2, but only one of these (S100-B) is part of a consensus guideline pathway, where it has been used to stratify patients with mild TBI for CT imaging at presentation (Unden et al., 2015).

At first sight, a diagnostic TBI marker may appear to have limited relevance in the ICU setting, since the severity of TBI which predicates critical care would be easily detectable. Indeed, the major application of diagnostic biomarkers has been in the emergency room, in diagnosing mild TBI, or assessing the need for neuroimaging (Kulbe and Geddes, 2016). However, such data may also be critically relevant for the intubated patient admitted with multiple trauma, where the CT scan is not impressive, but the presence of extracranial injuries precludes reversal of sedation and full neurologic assessment. In such a context, increases in blood levels of protein biomarkers could trigger repeat neuroimaging after an interval, placement of ICP monitoring, and more rigorous attention to cardiorespiratory targets.

Many of these diagnostic biomarkers have also been used for monitoring progress with severe TBI in the critical care setting. Perhaps the best-characterized biomarkers in this context are S100-B, glial fibrillary acidic protein (GFAP), and neuron-specific enolase, measured in blood or CSF, which have been shown to correlate with secondary insults such as lesion expansion and brain hypoxia. However, the available literature suggests that such late elevations may document the occurrence of secondary insults, rather than warn of their impending likelihood. This does not detract from the prognostic impact of such serial measurement (perhaps using area-under-the-curve approaches to quantifying injury). However, this makes it difficult to understand how integration of protein biomarker measurement into a management algorithm could refine or expedite interventions aimed at preventing or mitigating these events. While not in common clinical use, the measurement of mediators that drive tissue injury may hold more promise in the future. Elevations in IL-8, TNF-α, or complement fractions may provide warning of activation of an injury process before it has time to fully impact on tissue fate, or by stratifying patients for therapy with specific biologic modulators.

Finally, levels of single biomarkers, or combinations of biomarkers, have been used to refine assessment of prognosis in TBI. There is reasonable evidence that

*Table 14.2*

**Protein biomarkers in traumatic brain injury**

| Biomarker | Source | Phase | Type | Limitations |
|---|---|---|---|---|
| S100-B | Blood | Acute | Glial/blood–brain barrier change | Not central nervous system-specific |
| Neuron-specific enolase | Blood | Acute | Neuronal | Present in red blood cells, elevated with hemolysis |
| Glial fibrillary acidic protein | Blood | Acute | Glial | |
| UCH-L1 | Blood | Acute | Neuronal | Raised in gut neoplasia |
| αII-Spectrin breakdown products | Blood | Acute | Axonal | Under investigation |
| Neurofilament proteins | Cerebrospinal fluid | Acute/subacute | Axonal | Under investigation |
| Tau, phospho-tau, amyloid β | Cerebrospinal fluid (blood) | Acute/chronic | Neurodegeneration | Under investigation |
| Cytokines | Blood, cerebrospinal fluid, microdialysate | Subacute/chronic | Innate immune response | Under investigation. Not central nervous system-specific |
| Autoantibodies | Blood | Chronic | Adaptive immune response | Under investigation. Clinical relevance unclear |

Summarized from several publications (Pelinka et al., 2004; Vos et al., 2004; Honda et al., 2010; Bohmer et al., 2011; Mondello et al., 2011, 2012; Papa et al., 2012; Stein et al., 2012; Okonkwo et al., 2013; Diaz-Arrastia et al., 2014; Korley et al., 2016).

measurements of S100-B, GFAP, and UCH-L1 could provide prognostic information, and that the combination of GFAP and UCH-L1 may perform better than a single biomarker. Perhaps even more relevant, there is now emerging evidence that the addition of biomarker data to well-established clinical outcome prediction schemes can provide added value, and refine prognostication.

## BEDSIDE NEURODIAGNOSTICS AND MONITORING

The fundamental basis for assessment of patients with TBI, whenever possible, remains the clinical examination (Riker et al., 2014). Both the GCS and the FOUR score provide well-validated schemes for following disease evolution and resolution, particularly in nonsedated patients. Even in sedated patients, attention to brainstem reflexes and clinical signs can add value to the assessment (Sharshar et al., 2014). However, in some patients, the clinical examination may be inadequate and additional monitoring may be needed to provide early warning of the development and mechanisms of physiologic deterioration (Oddo et al., 2016).

A fundamental goal of neurointensive care is to ensure that oxygen and metabolic substrate delivery is appropriate to prevent neuronal injury. Reduction in CBF in response to rising ICP is perhaps the best-known mechanism by which supply can be threatened and motivates the

widespread use of ICP measurement and CPP-guided therapy, and has formed the basis of widely adopted international guidelines (Brain Trauma Foundation, American Association of Neurological Surgeons, Congress of Neurological Surgeons, 2007a). Measurement of ICP alone, however, is a somewhat blunt instrument (Hutchinson et al., 2013). It does not allow the clinician to determine whether a physiologic threshold has been reached at which oxygen supply, for example, has become inadequate; this may depend on many factors. Furthermore, in reality there are many other pathologic states that may cause supply–demand imbalance apart from perfusion embarrassment due to raised ICP/low CPP. A recent randomized controlled trial of ICP monitoring directed treatment failed to show a survival benefit (Chesnut et al., 2012). However, a recent consensus-based interpretation of this study highlighted our inability to identify critical thresholds for harm from intracranial hypertension, calibrate the dose of intracranial hypertension for individual patients (Vik et al., 2008), and personalize interventions on this basis (Chesnut et al., 2015). For example (see earlier section on pathophysiology), impaired oxygen diffusion, mitochondrial dysfunction or high cerebral metabolic rate of oxygen from inadequate sedation or seizures may all lead to failure of aerobic metabolism when this is already precarious. Ideally we would make a full diagnosis of the dominant mechanism(s) for energy failure in a particular patient and at a particular time. This would allow precision therapeutic strategies (National Research Council Committee on A Framework for Developing a New Taxonomy of Disease, 2011) and minimize harm from the inevitable side-effects of choosing treatments that are less appropriate under the specific circumstances.

A multimodality approach integrating data from a variety of implantable sensors is needed to formulate a full picture of dominant pathobiology in real time (Le Roux et al., 2014; Hutchinson et al., 2015). Such bedside technology works in real time, allowing the physician to assess the response to therapies. However multimodality sensing is necessarily insensitive to focal pathology distant to the site of the probe.

The availability of routine CT imaging provides invaluable information on structural pathology. More advanced imaging technologies exist that can provide detailed comprehensive spatial assessment of CBF, substrate delivery, connectivity, and functional or metabolic abnormalities (see earlier section) (Amyot et al., 2015). Whilst imaging is invaluable and sensitive to focal pathology (unlike bedside techniques), logistical constraints and concerns about radiation burden with repeated imaging mean that it can provide only snapshots. In reality the clinician must combine all these techniques for the most comprehensive assessment of cerebral pathology.

## BEDSIDE MULTIMODALITY MONITORING

Invasive ICP monitoring is widely employed in the management of severe TBI in intensive care (Chesnut et al., 2015). A variety of technologies exist, amongst which direct CSF pressure measurement via an external ventricular drain is the most accurate method and has the additional advantage of permitting CSF drainage to reduce ICP. Intraparenchymal pressure transducers based on miniature resistive or fiberoptic strain gauge technologies are a popular alternative, as they have a lower infection risk than external ventricular drains, are simpler to introduce, and are sufficiently small that they may be introduced through a burrhole, either alone or in combination with other multimodality sensors through a multiple-lumen bolt (Hutchinson et al., 2000) (Fig. 14.5).

Brain oxygenation (Oddo et al., 2014) can be assessed by the measurement of tissue oxygen tension ($P_{bt}O_2$) either electrochemically (Licox, Integra Lifesciences, Plainsboro, NJ, USA)) or by the oxygen-dependent fluorescence quenching (Neurovent-PTO, Raumedic, Helmbrechts, Germany). $P_{bt}O_2$ is a spatial average of oxygen partial pressure and is determined by the balance between oxygen supply and consumption, but also by diffusion, which may be impaired after TBI (Rosenthal et al., 2008).

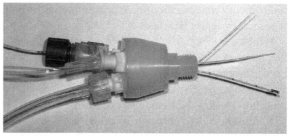

**Fig. 14.5.** "Triple bolt" for introducing invasive multimodality monitoring. The bolt is placed via a frontal burrhole (noneloquent and generally nondominant brain to minimize the functional consequences of hemorrhagic complication). Emerging on the right hand side are (top to bottom): Licox $P_{bt}O_2$ probe, microdialysis, and Codman intraparenchymal intracranial pressure probe.

Cerebral microdialysis (Hutchinson et al., 2015) is less well established, but is nonetheless employed clinically in a number of neuroscience critical care centers. A crystalloid perfusate is passed through a coaxial intraparenchymal catheter (Fig. 14.6) with a semipermeable membrane so that the effluent reflects brain chemistry. Flow rates are a tradeoff between reliable chemical recovery and providing sufficient effluent for analysis on a clinically meaningful timescale. Typically, hourly measurements are made using an automated bedside colorimetric assay. Typical clinical catheters have a cutoff of 20 kDa, and are suitable for the recovery of a range of small molecules. The lactate:pyruvate ratio (LPR) and brain tissue glucose have received most application clinically. LPR is an assay for anaerobic glucose utilization, and this has been demonstrated to have prognostic significance (Timofeev et al., 2011). Brain tissue glucose is sensitive to ischemia/hyperemia, and the balance between supply and hyper-/hypometabolism and low

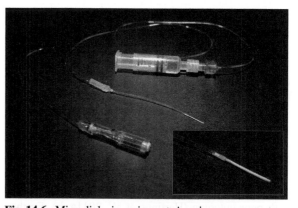

**Fig. 14.6.** Microdialysis equipment. A syringe pump creates a flow of crystalloid solution through the coaxial semipermeable probe (inset). At typical flow rates of 0.3 μL/min, good recovery can be obtained and hourly sampling of effluent is possible using a system of removable vials.

brain glucose concentrations may be an important driver of secondary injury (Rostami et al., 2014).

Whilst complications from invasive monitoring are rare, they can occasionally be devastating. This has motivated attempts to find noninvasive alternatives. Noninvasive ICP measurements based on a variety of techniques are being developed and may be promising.

Noninvasive determination of cerebral oxygenation (Oddo et al., 2014) is possible by near-infrared spectroscopy (NIRS). Biologic tissue transmits near-infrared light well. By placing optodes on the scalp and determining the transmission at different wavelengths and distances, it is possible to estimate the hemoglobin oxygen saturation (as well as hemoglobin concentration and other chromophore concentrations depending on the design of the equipment). Since much of the blood volume in the brain is venous, NIRS is thought to be largely (but not exclusively) sensitive to oxygen extraction and therefore can be used to determine critical oxygen supply/demand mismatch. However contamination of the signal from extracranial blood can complicate NIRS interpretation, particularly in adults (the optical path must traverse the scalp, for example).

Patients with TBI are at high risk of seizures, including in the early stages postinjury. Continuous EEG (cEEG) has demonstrated a high prevalence (up to one-third: Ronne-Engstrom and Winkler, 2006) of nonconvulsive seizures (NCS), particularly in patients with penetrating injuries, depressed skull fractures, or large hematomas. On balance, it is uncertain whether prophylactic treatment with antiepileptic medicines is beneficial; practices vary accordingly. Nevertheless persistent seizures are predictive of poor outcome (Vespa et al., 2010) and seizure activity is undesirable because of its deleterious effects on metabolic rate and ICP (Vespa, 2016), which are plausible mechanisms for secondary injury. Thus cEEG has become an important monitoring strategy in neurocritical care for detecting NCS and ensuring the adequacy of sedation (Claassen et al., 2014).

More recently there has been growing research interest in the use of invasive ECoG or depth electrode to detect cortical spreading depolarizations in TBI (Strong et al., 2002; Fabricius et al., 2006). These are slow-moving mass depolarizations of neurons that are associated with massive ionic and osmotic fluxes and energy crisis in metabolically precarious tissue (Hinzman et al., 2016). Spreading depolarizations have been repeatedly identified after TBI (Hartings et al., 2011a) and shown to have an independent association with poor outcome (Hartings et al., 2011a, b). Further work to understand the significance of this phenomenon in TBI is required. Nevertheless, the occurrence of spreading depolarizations may be modulated by sedative drugs; for example, ketamine markedly reduces their incidence (Hertle et al., 2012a) and if this proves to be a useful intervention, then ECoG (or a robust noninvasive cEEG correlate (Hartings et al., 2014)) may become an important monitoring modality in the future.

Often, combinations of parameters convey useful physiologic significance beyond the parameters alone. The simplest is the derived parameter CPP that is calculated automatically from mean arterial pressure (MAP) and ICP, and displayed by most monitors. Another more complex derived parameter that is showing promise as a clinically useful marker of autoregulation is the pressure–reactivity index (PRx). PRx is calculated as the correlation coefficient between a 10-second moving window of MAP and ICP. Autoregulation often fails after severe TBI, so that increases in MAP cause an increase in cerebral blood volume and therefore ICP, rather than the reflex vasoconstriction expected in health. Thus, the correlation between MAP and ICP becomes positive and PRx > 0 indicates impaired autoregulation (Fig. 14.7). PRx may be automatically calculated in real time by a computer and has clinical significance. Positive PRx has been shown to be an independent predictor of mortality (Sorrentino et al., 2011), and PRx-derived patient-specific thresholds for CPP show a stronger association with outcome than average population values (Lazaridis et al., 2014).

Furthermore, over longer periods of time, PRx often shows a U-shaped relationship with CPP (Fig. 14.8), reflecting the autoregulatory range (Steiner et al., 2002). This leads to the concept of the optimal CPP (CPPopt), which is the CPP for which PRx is lowest, and therefore for which autoregulation is best preserved. In retrospective observational studies, patients managed below their CPPopt had a higher mortality, whereas those above had worse than expected disability (Aries et al., 2012). High-level evidence for the use of autoregulation as a clinical parameter is lacking, but the optimization of autoregulation may prove to be one further method by which clinicians could seek to personalize CPP targets and balance the harm from either hypo- or hyperperfusion.

The use of multimodality monitoring is supported by a number of guidelines and international consensus statements (Brain Trauma Foundation, American Association of Neurological Surgeons, Congress of Neurological Surgeons, 2007a; Le Roux et al., 2014). Without clear randomized prospective data, normal ranges and treatment thresholds are derived from observational data studying a variety of outcomes and correlates of tissue injury (Table 14.3). It is misleading to base treatment on any individual parameter: often the concordance or discordance between measurements from different modalities may be just as significant in building up a picture of the dominant physiology. Localized measurements (such as $P_{bt}O_2$ or microdialysis) must be assessed in the knowledge of the probe location, since

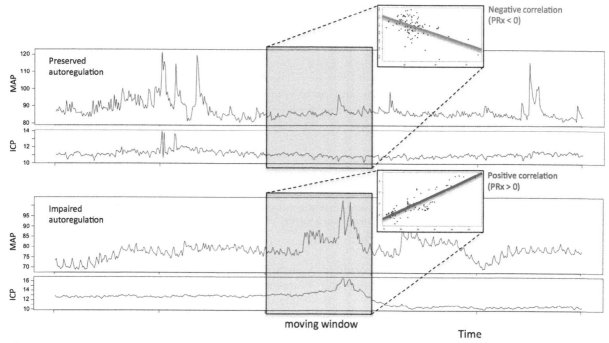

**Fig. 14.7.** Pressure–reactivity index (PRx) is calculated as the correlation coefficient for a 10-second moving window of mean arterial pressure (MAP) and intracranial pressure (ICP) signals. The upper panel shows a patient in whom autoregulation is preserved and PRx is negative or near zero. In the lower trace, the ICP is pressure-passive as autoregulation is impaired. This is revealed by a PRx > 0.

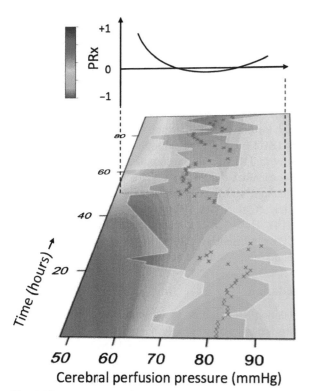

**Fig. 14.8.** Pressure–reactivity index (PRx) often displays a U-shaped relationship with cerebral perfusion pressure (CPP) over time, reflecting the autoregulatory range. The CPP for which PRx is lowest (CPP$_{opt}$) is the CPP for which autoregulation is best preserved.

abnormal values in pericontusional tissue or "healthy" brain will have very different interpretations, and trigger different interventions.

## HOSPITAL COURSE AND MANAGEMENT

Current intensive care management of severe TBI is based on maintaining physiology so as to minimize secondary insults that may occur, especially over the first few days. Secondary injury may arise as a result of systemic (hypotension, hypoxemia, hypocapnia, hypo- or hyperthermia, or metabolic) disturbances or intracranial causes (intracranial hypertension, ischemia, hyperemia, edema, or hemorrhage) (Chesnut et al., 1993; Jones et al., 1994; Signorini et al., 1999; Macmillan et al., 2001; Manley et al., 2001; Sarrafzadeh et al., 2001; Jeremitsky et al., 2003; Chi et al., 2006; Brenner et al., 2012). The clinical trajectory of TBI varies enormously between patients, as may the impact of comorbidity or extracranial injuries, such that a holistic and individualized approach is essential.

Central to neurocritical care is the control of ICP and maintenance of CPP. A variety of strategies are available for the nonsurgical management of raised ICP. All are associated with at least some degree of harmful side-effects and a stepwise escalation of therapeutic intensity is prudent. Guidelines have been published (Brain Trauma Foundation, Surgeons, American Association of Neurological Surgeons, Congress of

*Table 14.3*

**Normal ranges and treatment thresholds for common mulitimodality monitoring variables**

| | | Threshold for injury/treatment | |
|---|---|---|---|
| Parameter | "Normal" range (intensive care unit patients) | Less stringent | More stringent |
| Intracranial pressure | <15 mmHg | 20–25 mmHg | 20 mmHg |
| $P_{bt}O_2$ | ~30 mmHg | 15–25 mmHg | <15 mmHg |
| Lactate:pyruvate ratio | <25 | >25 | >40 |
| Brain tissue glucose | 1–2 mmol/L | <0.8 mmol/L | <0.2 mmol/L |

"Normal" ranges derived from patients with probes placed in structurally normal brain, and no evidence of acute brain injury. Prospective intervention data are not available, so treatment thresholds are inferred from observational heterogeneous outcome data (Le Roux et al., 2014; Rostami, 2014; Hutchinson et al., 2015). The two sets of injury thresholds reflect varying severity of physiologic derangement, with more aggressive therapies possibly justified only for more severe abnormalities.

Neurological Surgeons, 2007e) and a protocolized approach is helpful to facilitate timely escalation and de-escalation of therapy.

### Ventilatory strategies

Endotracheal intubation and mechanical ventilation are important to protect the airway in TBI patients with reduced consciousness and may be indicated by the presence of extracranial injury, but are also critical to ensure optimal arterial oxygen and $CO_2$ tension. Carbon dioxide is a potent cerebral vasodilator, and hypercapnia may cause increases in ICP if intracranial compliance is limited. Conversely, hypocapnic vasoconstriction may result in substantial ICP reductions when ICP is very high and/or intracranial compliance is low (Steiner et al., 2005). However, when intracranial hypertension is modest, the effects on CPP are overwhelmed by the associated arteriolar vasoconstriction, which can lead to dangerous ischemia (Muizelaar et al., 1991; Coles et al., 2002, 2007). Resetting of extravascular pH with prolonged ventilation in TBI patients may mean that the hypocapnia-associated reduction in ICP is transient, but the detrimental CBF reductions that it causes may persist (Steiner et al., 2004). Consequently, unless the increase in ICP is high enough to present a greater hazard than the cerebral hypoperfusion caused by hyperventilation (as during a plateau wave, for example), ventilation should target levels of $Paco_2$ that are at the low end of normal. Apart from brief use in emergent settings, more extreme hyperventilation ($Paco_2$ below 30 mmHg) should only be undertaken with monitoring of $P_{bt}O_2$ or jugular bulb saturation. Hypoxia needs to be scrupulously avoided (arterial oxygen saturations > 95%), both because of direct hypoxic injury, but also to avoid hypoxic cerebral vasodilatation (and consequent ICP

increases), which may occur at oxygenation levels that are acceptable in critically ill patients without neurologic injury (Gupta et al., 1997). There is increasing interest in using normobaric hyperoxia to elevate $P_{bt}O_2$ and reduce elevations in lactate and LPR (Beynon et al., 2012). Increases in $Pao_2$ can, in the short term, improve oxygen metabolism (Nortje et al., 2008) and reduce cytotoxic edema (Veenith et al., 2014) in at-risk regions in TBI, and there have been recent phase II trials of both normobaric (Taher et al., 2016) and hyperbaric (Rockswold et al., 2013) hyperoxia suggesting benefit in TBI. However, there is also emerging concern about the potential harm caused by hyperoxia in TBI (Rincon et al., 2014), and widespread use of this intervention should await demonstration of benefit from a substantive randomized clinical trial. Patients who require prolonged endotracheal intubation and ventilation usually undergo tracheostomy. While there are no randomized clinical trials (RCTs) addressing the optimal timing of tracheostomy in TBI patients, accumulating non-RCT evidence suggests that early (< 8 days) tracheostomy may reduce infection, and accelerate weaning and ICU discharge (Rizk et al., 2011; Wang et al., 2012; Alali et al., 2014). However, secondary brain injury from raised ICP or transient alterations in gas exchange during the tracheostomy must be carefully avoided.

### Sedation

Sedation is often used in the acute phase of severe TBI. This is particularly the case in intubated patients in whom sedation improves tolerance of endotracheal intubation, promotes compliance with mechanical ventilation, and avoids ICP rises associated with coughing. In addition, sedative agents can intrinsically reduce ICP by reducing cerebral metabolic rate; a combination of hypnotic and opioid infusions has the additional benefit of suppressing cough and gag reflexes, and controlling pain, which is helpful for ICP control (Oddo et al., 2016). A suggested algorithm for rational use of sedatives is shown in Figure 14.9. The first-line sedative agent is typically propofol or a benzodiazepine, each of which has advantages and disadvantages. Propofol is more expensive, and tends to cause more hypotension. Though formal comparisons suggest that ICP control is similar with both agents overall (Sanchez-Izquierdo-Riera et al., 1998), midazolam may be less effective at controlling refractory intracranial hypertension, and tachyphylaxis to the drug may require increasing doses, with resulting accumulation of metabolites and delayed emergence from sedation (Shafer, 1998). However, despite this better control of intracranial hypertension, the use of high doses of propofol (>4–5 mg/kg/h) for prolonged periods runs the risk of propofol infusion syndrome (PRIS) (Cremer et al., 2001). Accumulating evidence suggests that the profile of PRIS may be changing, and that the syndrome may be observed at lower doses in older patients (Krajcova et al., 2015), presumably due to slower elimination – a

concern that may also apply to patients who are hypothermic (Dengler et al., 2015). Alternative sedative agents include ketamine, which may have particular benefits in reducing spreading depolarization (Hertle et al., 2012b), and dexmedetomidine, which may produce a better sedation profile, but at the risk of greater hypotension (Pajoumand et al., 2016).

A range of opioids has been used to supplement sedation in this setting, but recent interest has focused on remifentanil, the metabolism of which is context-insensitive, and which may allow rapid emergence from sedation for neurologic assessment (Karabinis et al., 2004). However, the agent is not appropriate for prolonged sedation during periods of intracranial hypertension, when the stability afforded by long-acting opioids may be beneficial. Agitation is common during the period of emergence from coma, and is commonly treated with butyrophenones, benzodiazepines, clonidine, or dexmedetomidine. There is continuing concern about the long-term effects of these agents, possibly through

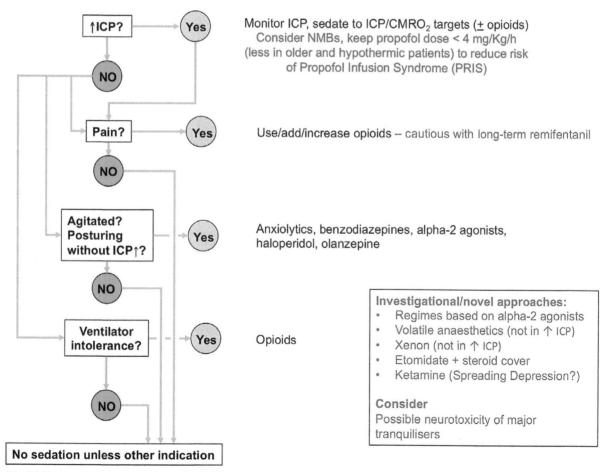

**Fig. 14.9.** A suggested scheme for optimal sedation in patients with traumatic brain injury. ICP, intracranial pressure; $CMRO_2$, cerebral metabolic rate of oxygen; NMBs, neuromuscular blocking drugs.

inhibition of plasticity (see later). While their use is unavoidable in many patients, attempts should be made to reduce their use if possible.

## ICP and CPP targets

ICP monitoring allows intracranial compliance and CPP to be targeted. It is typical for intracranial hypertension to rise over the first several days, plateau, and then slowly resolve. High levels of ICP are associated with mortality (Balestreri et al., 2006), and even brief (> 5 minutes) episodes of intracranial hypertension are associated with worse outcome (Stein et al., 2011). Consequently, intracranial hypertension is a prominent target in TBI guidelines. However, there continues to be lack of certainty about what thresholds of ICP justify therapies that have intrinsic toxicities (see later), and the definition of the critical "dose" of intracranial hypertension remains an important, but elusive, goal (Chesnut et al., 2015).

Similarly, the choice of CPP targets in TBI is not based on high-quality evidence. The original Brain Trauma Foundation (BTF) guidelines (Brain Trauma Foundation, American Association of Neurological Surgeons, The Joint Section on Neurotrauma and Critical Care, 2000) recognized the limited evidence in this area, but suggested a CPP threshold of 70 mmHg as a treatment option. However, there was recognition of alternative models of CPP management, such as the Lund protocol (Grande, 2006). A landmark paper by Robertson and colleagues (1999) suggested that the cerebral hemodynamic benefits of CPP elevation were substantially offset by cardiopulmonary complications associated with fluid loading and vasoactive drugs used for rigorous CPP maintenance. These findings led to a revision of CPP targets in a subsequent version of the BTF guidelines (Brain Trauma Foundation, American Association of Neurological Surgeons, Congress of Neurological Surgeons, 2007b), which advised against aggressive interventions to maintain CPP above 70 mmHg. More recent discussions recognize that optimal CPP (and ICP) targets may vary between patients, and at different stages of the disease trajectory in the same patient (Hutchinson et al., 2013). Multimodality monitoring may allow context-dependent refinement of physiologic targets (Sorrentino et al., 2012; Lazaridis et al., 2014).

## Blood glucose targets

Admission hyperglycemia (blood glucose > 180 mg/dL) has been repeatedly associated with worse outcomes in TBI (Van Beek et al., 2007), but tight glycemic control may trigger critically low brain glucose levels (Oddo et al., 2008; Meierhans et al., 2010), especially in injured regions (Magnoni et al., 2012), as well as cerebral energy crisis (Oddo et al., 2008), increased risk of spreading depression (Parkin et al., 2005), and poor outcome (Vespa et al., 2003). Concerns have been further heightened by an increasing recognition that tight glycemic control in TBI is associated with increased risk of hypoglycemia (Finfer et al., 2015), and current advice focuses on the avoidance of hyperglycemia without aiming for tight glycemic control (Kramer et al., 2012). It is worth reflecting, however, that intensive glycemic control that avoided hypoglycemia was associated (in a single-center study) with improved outcomes (Van den Berghe et al., 2005), and that safer approaches to tight glycemic control might allow the adoption of time-varying individualized blood glucose targets (Meier et al., 2008), perhaps guided by microdialysis monitoring of brain glucose levels.

## Temperature management

Decisions about temperature management in TBI address three main issues: the use of therapeutic hypothermia as a universal neuroprotective intervention, use of hypothermia as a treatment for intracranial hypertension, and the avoidance of hyperthermia (fever control). Despite substantial supportive evidence from case series and single-center trials, multicenter trials (Clifton et al., 2001, 2011) failed to show benefit of universal cooling to 32–34°C, and a recent systematic review (Saxena et al., 2014) could find no evidence to support less intensive hypothermia in TBI. Therapeutic hypothermia is known to effectively reduce ICP, but the recent Eurotherm3235 Trial (Andrews et al., 2015) showed no benefit from titrated cooling to maintain ICP less than 20 mmHg. Recent interest has focused on the use of targeted temperature management to avoid fever in TBI, and two recent studies suggest that this strategy may be superior to induced hypothermia (Maekawa et al., 2015; Hifumi et al., 2016). Current practice, based on limited evidence, focuses on treating significant elevations in temperature (above a threshold of 38.0–38.5°C), and the continued use of hypothermia for ICP control, but with higher ICP thresholds (typically 25–30 mmHg; O'Leary et al., 2016).

## Seizure prophylaxis

Guidelines recommend the use of 7 days of antiepileptic drug (AED) therapy to reduce early seizures after TBI (Chang and Lowenstein, 2003; Brain Trauma Foundation, American Association of Neurological Surgeons, Congress of Neurological Surgeons, 2007d) in patients with risk factors (GCS score <10; cortical contusion; depressed skull fracture, SDH; EDH; intracerebral hematoma; penetrating head wound). There is no role for using early AED therapy to prevent late posttraumatic seizures. Levetiracetam may have a better safety profile compared to phenytoin, which has been the traditional AED in use in this context (Xu et al., 2016). The detection and treatment of NCS (see earlier section) may be facilitated by continuous EEG monitoring.

## Osmotic therapy

Infusions of hyperosmotic agents are effective in controlling cerebral edema. Hypertonic saline is effective (Lazaridis et al., 2013), and may be preferred over mannitol, as it expands intravascular volume, and (unlike mannitol) is not associated with a subsequent diuresis which may lead to hypovolemia and hypotension. These attributes may explain why recent meta-analyses suggest that hypertonic saline may be more effective in ICP management (Kamel et al., 2011; Li et al., 2015). There appears to be no benefit from using hyperosmotic solutions prophylactically to prevent ICP elevations after TBI (Ryu et al., 2013).

## Routine ICU interventions

Current guidelines recommend the early initiation of enteral nutrition, aiming to achieve full caloric supplementation by 7 days post-TBI (Brain Trauma Foundation, American Association of Neurological Surgeons, Congress of Neurological Surgeons, 2007c). Stress ulcer prophylaxis with $H_2$-receptor antagonists or a proton pump inhibitor is commonly used, at least until full enteral feeding is established. Coagulopathy is common in TBI, as is the incidence of venous thromboembolic disease; both issues are discussed in a later section. Electrolyte abnormalities are common in TBI – osmotic diuretics and cold diuresis may result in electrolyte loss. It is common to encounter both hypernatremia (due to hyperosmotic therapy, relative free-water restriction, or diabetes insipidus) and hyponatremia (due to the syndrome of inappropriate antidiuretic hormone secretion, cerebral salt wasting, or inappropriate use of hypotonic fluids). Therapy in the acute phase should aim to correct these abnormalities, while avoiding any hyponatremia (which may increase cerebral edema) or hypovolemia (which may make CPP targets difficult to achieve).

## "SECOND-LINE" AND RESCUE THERAPIES

A number of strategies are available which, although potentially harmful, may be effective in controlling otherwise refractory intracranial hypertension. Brief periods of hyperventilation can be effective for reducing ICP and the risks of vasoconstriction and ischemia may be mitigated by simultaneously monitoring $P_{bt}o_2$ or jugular venous oxygen saturation. However this procedure is only transiently effective until CSF chemistry adjusts and is at best suitable for use only as an emergency temporizing measure. The routine early use of aggressive cooling (core temperatures 32–34°C) is associated with worse outcome (Andrews et al., 2015). Hypothermia is associated with cardiovascular instability, coagulopathy, immunosuppression, and electrolyte shifts, which are highly undesirable. However, as a rescue therapy, it is nevertheless effective in reducing ICP and should be considered. Where hypothermia is employed, rewarming must be very slow.

Similarly, whilst early decompressive craniectomy for relatively moderate intracranial hypertension has been shown not to improve outcome after TBI (Cooper et al., 2011), it is effective in controlling otherwise refractory intracranial hypertension. The Randomized Evaluation of Surgery with Craniectomy for Uncontrollable Elevation of Intra-Cranial Pressure (RESCUEicp) trial has studied decompressive craniectomy as a rescue therapy for persistent ICP > 25 mmHg, and can result in increased survival at 6 months, with improved functional outcome at 12 months, but at the expense of increased numbers of survivors with severe disability (Hutchinson et al., 2016).

A final rescue strategy that may be employed for medical management of refractory ICP elevation is metabolic suppression through deep sedation to the point of a near isoelectric EEG. This may be achieved using barbiturates, which are known to suppress metabolism, reduce excitotoxicity, and inhibit lipid peroxidation. Again, prophylactic or early use in preference to osmotherapy is known to be ineffective and potentially harmful. At the high doses required, barbiturates are associated with hemodynamic instability and hypotension, which offset ICP-lowering effects (Roberts and Sydenham, 2012), as well as respiratory complications, hypokalemia, and hepatic and renal impairment. Their long elimination times are also undesirable. Again, however, barbiturates are effective in lowering ICP (Majdan et al., 2013) and should nevertheless be considered as a rescue therapy.

## ICP AND CPP MANAGEMENT PROTOCOLS

The rational use of the many available treatment options for ICP and CPP control is facilitated by the use of protocols. The algorithm in use in Cambridge is shown as an example (Fig. 14.10). Although other centers may use protocols that differ in detail, the broad principles remain the same, with establishment of both systemic and brain-specific monitoring. Consideration should be given to clinically significant lesions that may be evacuated (e.g., subdural or extradural hematomas causing mass effect). Any change in intracranial physiology or increasing difficulty in controlling ICP should trigger a search for new or evolving pathology that may be amenable to surgical intervention. Drainage of CSF via a ventriculostomy should ideally be an early

## Traumatic Brain Injury ICP/CPP Algorithm

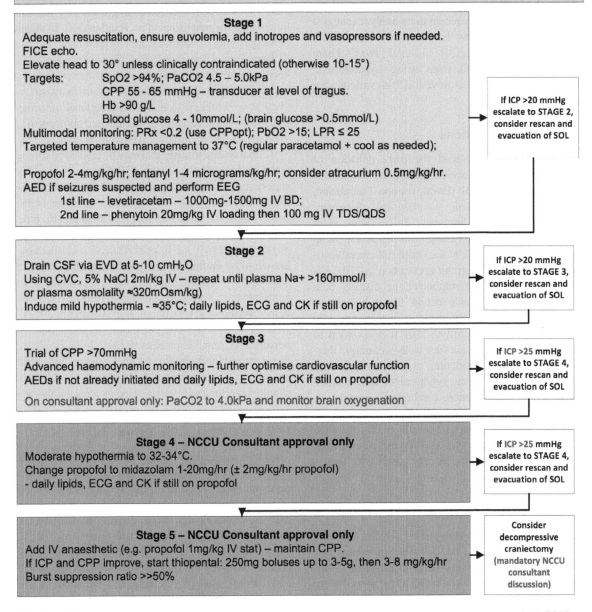

Patients with traumatic brain injury (TBI) admitted to the NCCU are managed according to this protocol. Each step of the protocol must be preceded by thorough checking of the position and accuracy of all intracranial monitoring. Surgical referral for evacuation of significant space occupying lesion(s) (SOL) is mandatory before escalating medical treatment. Consider EVD insertion before escalating medical treatment.

All patients managed according to this protocol must have the following within 4 hours of admission to NCCU:
1) invasive arterial (transducer at the tragus) and central venous catheter
2) ICP monitoring
3) Cerebral microdialysis catheter and PbO2 probe
4) ICM+

Initial target of CPP of 65mmHg (CPP >55mmHg may be acceptable). Autoregulation parameters and brain biochemistry are used to individualise targets.

**Stage 1**
Adequate resuscitation, ensure euvolemia, add inotropes and vasopressors if needed.
FICE echo.
Elevate head to 30° unless clinically contraindicated (otherwise 10-15°)
Targets: SpO2 >94%; PaCO2 4.5 – 5.0kPa
CPP 55 - 65 mmHg – transducer at level of tragus.
Hb >90 g/L
Blood glucose 4 - 10mmol/L; (brain glucose >0.5mmol/L)
Multimodal monitoring: PRx <0.2 (use CPPopt); PbO2 >15; LPR ≤ 25
Targeted temperature management to 37°C (regular paracetamol + cool as needed);

Propofol 2-4mg/kg/hr; fentanyl 1-4 micrograms/kg/hr; consider atracurium 0.5mg/kg/hr.
AED if seizures suspected and perform EEG
1st line – levetiracetam – 1000mg-1500mg IV BD;
2nd line – phenytoin 20mg/kg IV loading then 100 mg IV TDS/QDS

*If ICP >20 mmHg escalate to STAGE 2, consider rescan and evacuation of SOL*

**Stage 2**
Drain CSF via EVD at 5-10 cmH2O
Using CVC, 5% NaCl 2ml/kg IV – repeat until plasma Na+ >160mmol/l or plasma osmolality ≈320mOsm/kg)
Induce mild hypothermia - ≈35°C; daily lipids, ECG and CK if still on propofol

*If ICP >20 mmHg escalate to STAGE 3, consider rescan and evacuation of SOL*

**Stage 3**
Trial of CPP >70mmHg
Advanced haemodynamic monitoring – further optimise cardiovascular function
AEDs if not already initiated and daily lipids, ECG and CK if still on propofol

On consultant approval only: PaCO2 to 4.0kPa and monitor brain oxygenation

*If ICP >25 mmHg escalate to STAGE 4, consider rescan and evacuation of SOL*

**Stage 4 – NCCU Consultant approval only**
Moderate hypothermia to 32-34°C.
Change propofol to midazolam 1-20mg/hr (± 2mg/kg/hr propofol)
- daily lipids, ECG and CK if still on propofol

*If ICP >25 mmHg escalate to STAGE 4, consider rescan and evacuation of SOL*

**Stage 5 – NCCU Consultant approval only**
Add IV anaesthetic (e.g. propofol 1mg/kg IV stat) – maintain CPP.
If ICP and CPP improve, start thiopental: 250mg boluses up to 3-5g, then 3-8 mg/kg/hr
Burst suppression ratio >>50%

*Consider decompressive craniectomy (mandatory NCCU consultant discussion)*

Version 19                                                                 June 2016

**Fig. 14.10.** Cambridge traumatic brain injury (TBI) intracranial pressure (ICP)/cerebral perfusion pressure (CPP) management algorithm. NCCU, neurosciences critical care unit; EVD, external ventricular drain; FICE, focused intensive care echo; PRx, pressure–reactivity index; CPPopt, optimal range for autoregulation; LPR, lactate:pyruvate ratio; EEG, electroencephalogram; CSF, cerebrospinal fluid; CVC, central venous catheter; ECG, electrocardiogram; CK, creatine kinase; AEDs, antiepileptic drugs.

intervention for intracranial hypertension, but must, in any case, be contemplated before escalation of medical therapies or before surgical decompression.

## CLINICAL TRIALS AND GUIDELINES

A clinically effective pharmacologic neuroprotective intervention continues to elude us (Janowitz and Menon, 2010; Menon and Maas, 2015; Bragge et al., 2016). The last few years have seen further negative neuroprotection trials of erythropoietin and hypothermia, and shown no benefit from higher transfusion thresholds in TBI. Given the limited class I evidence available, clinical protocols and guidelines have been largely based on expert consensus, both for monitoring (Le Roux et al., 2014) and for treatment. The 2007 BTF guidelines for in-hospital management of TBI provided a pragmatic synthesis of the (often relatively poor-quality) available evidence on TBI management (Brain Trauma Foundation, American Association of Neurological Surgeons, Congress of Neurological Surgeons, 2007a).

These guidelines probably provided the most commonly used evidence base for critical care management of TBI. A more recent revision (Brain Trauma Foundation, American Association of Neurological Surgeons, Congress of Neurological Surgeons, 2016) provides conclusions more stringently based on high-quality evidence, with a reduced number of recommendations, which include a treatment threshold of 22 mmHg for ICP, and a CPP target of between 60 and 70 mmHg, with choice of target depending on individual autoregulatory status. This revision highlights the paucity of high-quality evidence to guide therapy. However, it provides little guidance on what might be seen as best practice, even in the absence of high quality evidence.

Retrospective analyses (Patel et al., 2005; Brown et al., 2010; Tepas et al., 2013) suggest that mortality, functional outcome, and cost-effectiveness are improved by transferring TBI patients to specialist trauma or neurosurgical centers, and possibly by transfer to high-volume centers (seeing greater than 40 cases of severe TBI per quarter: Tepas et al., 2013). In addition, many studies suggest that intensive protocol-driven therapy (typically based on BTF guidelines, and including ICP monitoring) results in lower mortality and better outcomes (Bulger et al., 2002; Elf et al., 2002; Patel et al., 2002; Fakhry et al., 2004; Fuller et al., 2011; Alali et al., 2013). In addition, a large prospective study of TBI patients requiring intensive care, which corrected for key known covariates, showed that transfer to specialist centers was cost-effective, even for patients who did not require an acute operative neurosurgical intervention (Harrison et al., 2013). While these data drive current practice in many countries, these analyses cannot account for unmeasured confounders, and evidence of

such benefit is inconsistent: at least one study (Cremer et al., 2005) and two recent meta-analyses (Su et al., 2014; Yuan et al., 2015) suggest no overall benefit from aggressive, ICP-guided management. Indeed, the BEST-TRIP trial (which represents the only class I evidence in this context) suggests that clinical care based on imaging and serial clinical examination, at least in low- and middle-income countries, is not inferior to a strategy based on ICP-guided management (Chesnut et al., 2012). The case has been made for repeating this study in centers from high-income countries (Chesnut et al., 2015).

New approaches have emerged for optimizing this translational process. At one end of this pathway there has been a drive to use experimental medicine approaches in the clinical laboratory of the neurointensive care unit (Janowitz and Menon, 2010), so as to optimize our understanding of pathophysiology, document its modulation by both existing and novel interventions, and find ways to stratify patients into groups that are more likely to respond to a given intervention. At the other end of the translational pathway there has been increasing interest in using precision medicine and comparative effectiveness research (Maas et al., 2012) to advance research and clinical care in TBI – these themes are the focus of a large international initiative (http:/intbir.nih.gov/).

## COMPLEX CLINICAL DECISIONS
### Hemostatic abnormalities after TBI

TBI is associated with both hemostatic deficits and hypercoagulopathy (Laroche et al., 2012; Maegele, 2013), with up to 60% of patients showing abnormal values in severe TBI (Hoyt, 2004). Risk factors include injury severity, age, and prehospital hypotension (Wafaisade et al., 2010a, b). Many patients have delayed worsening of hemostasis (Lustenberger et al., 2010; Greuters et al., 2011). Admission coagulopathy is associated with a 10-fold increase in mortality and a 30-fold increase in poor outcome in TBI (Harhangi et al., 2008; Wafaisade et al., 2010a; Greuters et al., 2011). Platelet count below 175 000/μL increases the risk of ICH progression, and counts less than 100 000/μL independently predict mortality. Antiplatelet agents or anticoagulants modulate outcome (Batchelor and Grayson, 2012a, b; Grandhi et al., 2015). Preinjury warfarin (Batchelor and Grayson, 2012a) increases the risk of poor outcome, but the reported impact of antiplatelet agents is inconsistent (Batchelor and Grayson, 2013; Fabbri et al., 2013; Joseph et al., 2014). In addition, selective serotonin reuptake inhibitors may have significant effects on hemostasis (Hackam and Mrkobrada, 2012), but their impact on TBI course and outcome is poorly investigated. Finally, the newer target-specific oral anticoagulants (also termed newer oral anticoagulants) confer new (and as yet poorly quantified) risks to patients with TBI (Miller et al., 2014). Much of the literature on hemostatic abnormalities in TBI has focused on conventional laboratory assays, but these may correlate poorly with bleeding risk and need for hemostatic correction. "Global" hemostatic tests, such as viscoelastic assays (TEG and ROTEM), and thrombin generation tests, may provide more integrated information regarding hemostatic potential, dynamic hemostasis, and clot stability, and may hence be more clinically relevant (Schochl et al., 2011). Recent consensus recommendations address viscoelastic thresholds for treatment in trauma (Inaba et al., 2015) (Fig. 14.2), and, if validated in TBI, could contribute to precision medicine approaches to managing coagulopathy in TBI.

Current treatment strategies for managing hemostatic defects in TBI follow those for general trauma, except for avoiding permissive hypotension, and targeting higher platelet counts ($>100 \times 10^9$/L) in the acute phase. The use of early empiric use of fresh frozen plasma and platelets has not been shown to be beneficial in TBI (Etemadrezaie et al., 2007; Anglin et al., 2013). While blood components continue to be commonly used to correct coagulation abnormalities, there is increasing interest in the use of factor concentrates (Narayan et al., 2008; Spahn et al., 2013; Yanamadala et al., 2014) and hemostatic drugs such as desmopressin and tranexamic acid (TXA). A subgroup analysis in the CRASH-2 trial suggested that TXA may reduce hemorrhage growth (Perel et al., 2012). The restriction of benefit to administration of TXA within 3 hours after injury in the overall trauma population in CRASH 2 (CRASH-2 collaborators et al., 2011) has not been as yet confirmed or refuted in TBI, but may be resolved by the currently recruiting CRASH-3 study (Dewan et al., 2012).

## When to start thromboprophylaxis

The association between trauma and venous thromboembolism is well established. Pharmacologic thromboprophylaxis appears to be safe among TBI patients with stabilized or improved hemorrhagic patterns (Shen et al., 2015). However, additional evidence is needed regarding effectiveness of the intervention, and better clarification of preferred agents, dose, and timing. With no evidence of intracranial bleeding, many clinicians would consider starting low-molecular-weight heparin prophylaxis within 48–72 hours of injury, but this would be delayed by up to 2 weeks with intracranial bleeding (Jamjoom and Jamjoom, 2013). Pharmacologic thromboprophylaxis is associated with a 13-fold increase in odds of further hemorrhage progression for those patients whose follow-up cranial computed tomography

within 1 day of admission showed ICH progression (Levy et al., 2010). Stratification scores for the identification of TBI patients with low, moderate, or high risk for spontaneous cerebral bleeding may help to allow early thromboprophylaxis while maintaining a good risk–benefit ratio (Schaible and Thal, 2013).

## The elderly patient

Older individuals in high-income countries are at high risk of TBI (Faul et al., 2010; EuroSafe, 2013; Feigin et al., 2013). Limited data from low- and middle-income countries (Hyder et al., 2007) do not show this, but demographic projections and urbanization suggest that TBI in the elderly is likely to become a growing global problem. Overall, the median age of patients likely to be cared for in critical care units and included in observational studies has doubled since the 1980s (Fig. 1.4), and the percentage of patients $\geq 50$ years of age increased threefold (Roozenbeek et al., 2013).

While this substantial rise in the incidence of TBI in older patients is partly attributable to an aging population, it is also due to the increased health and mobility of older patients, and increased case ascertainment due to the commoner use of protocol-driven CT imaging. These patients have a high need for hospitalization (50%) and a high mortality (with injury-related mortality doubling in EU statistics from 1990 to 2010, from 38% in 1990 to 49% in 2010; EuroSafe, 2013).

Some of this increased morbidity may be due to reduced physiologic reserve and frailty, with cardiovascular and other comorbidities impacting outcome in this age group. In addition, the therapies used for common comorbidities, such as anticoagulant and antiplatelet therapy, increase the risk of intracranial hemorrhage following TBI. Pre-existing neurodegenerative and cerebrovascular disease may also limit cognitive reserve and limit the scope for recovery. These differences have prompted some reassessment of TBI severity in older subjects (Kehoe et al., 2015) and lead to lower thresholds for referral to specialist care (Caterino et al., 2011). However, the broader picture is more worrisome. Patients over the age of 65 years are rarely recruited to RCTs. Further, there is substantial nihilism in the management of older patients with TBI, who experience less aggressive therapy, delayed CT imaging, lower likelihood of transfer to specialist neurosurgical facilities, and care by more junior medical staff (Kirkman et al., 2013). Treatment-limiting decisions may be more frequently justified in this group, but initial active therapy, coupled with reassessment of progress and response to therapy, provides some opportunities for rational stratification. In carefully selected subsets, aggressive therapy, including decompressive craniectomy, may deliver good outcomes

(De Bonis et al., 2011) in between 39% and 50% of older patients (Stocchetti et al., 2012) and better long-term life satisfaction after severe TBI (Anke et al., 2015).

## Monitoring the nonassessable patient

Where patients present with clear signs of a space-occupying lesion, or other evidence of raised ICP on neuroimaging, most centers would seek to place an ICP monitor to guide sedation and management of cerebral edema. When the CT is unimpressive or borderline in a patient who has been sedated and intubated prior to imaging, many centers would seek to hold sedative drugs for a brief period to assess neurologic status, and proceed to sedation withdrawal and extubation if the patient was neurologically appropriate. However, this strategy may not be possible in patients in whom significant extracranial injury or physiologic instability precludes sedation reduction. In such situations, the options are to either place an ICP monitor, or be guided by serial imaging. Both strategies are used, and the decision in any individual case needs to balance the small but definite risks of ICP placement against the possibility that near-normal imaging may coexist with intracranial hypertension, and certainly cannot detect episodic ICP elevations.

## Balancing second-tier therapies

The evidence base for clinical practice in TBI is limited in general. This paucity of evidence becomes particularly acute in the context of the 10–20% of patients with intracranial hypertension refractory to first-line therapies (Stocchetti et al., 2008), since commonly used second-tier therapies (hypothermia, decompressive craniectomy, and metabolic suppression) are all associated with significant side-effects. Decision making in this context is further complicated by the results of the Decompressive Craniectomy in Diffuse Traumatic Brain Injury (DECRA) (Cooper et al., 2011) and Eurotherm3235 trials (Andrews et al., 2015), which suggest lack of benefit or even harm from the use of decompressive craniectomy and harm from induced hypothermia. However, it is important to note that both trials tested the two therapies early in the management algorithm for intracranial hypertension, rather than for refractory intracranial hypertension unresponsive to standard therapies. This is a critical issue, since the calculus balancing risk and benefit may be very different in this context (O'Leary et al., 2016): while the threshold for harm or mortality is not clear, there is little doubt that marked and sustained ICP elevation (well above the normal treatment threshold of 20 mmHg) is a strong driver of mortality (Balestreri et al., 2006). A recently completed study of decompressive craniectomy as a rescue therapy for refractory intracranial hypertension, however, suggests a mortality benefit at six months, which translates into improved functional outcome (measured as independent survival at home or better) by 12 months. However this was also associated with an increase in severely disabled survivors (Hutchinson et al. 2016). However, there is no currently active trial that examines the use of induced hypothermia in a similar context. Until such data become available, it is difficult to provide recommendations on using or withholding any one of these three therapies in patients in whom refractory intracranial hypertension represents a significant hazard to life.

## When to transfuse

Adequate hemoglobin concentration is essential for oxygen delivery. However, transfusion is associated with a number of risks in the critically ill, including increased rates of infection, thromboembolism, and death. Whilst a restrictive transfusion threshold of 7 g/dL is widely regarded as safe in most critically ill patients (Hebert et al., 1999), including those after cardiac surgery (Hajjar et al., 2010), there have been concerns that this level may be insufficient for those patients with TBI where oxygen delivery may be critical.

Outcome differences have not been demonstrated between restrictive and liberal transfusion strategies after TBI in randomized controlled trials (McIntyre et al., 2006; Robertson et al., 2014) and liberal transfusion has been associated with increased incidence of adverse events (Robertson et al., 2014). Observational studies have also signaled that transfusion may be associated with worse long-term outcome (Warner et al., 2010; Elterman et al., 2013; Leal-Noval et al., 2016). There is also some evidence to suggest that higher transfusion thresholds of 10 g/dL may predispose to progression or development of intracerebral hematomas (Vedantam et al., 2016), implicating a mechanism involving microvascular damage from transfused blood.

At the same time, higher hemoglobin concentrations are associated with improved cardiovascular stability. Furthermore, there is evidence for a detrimental influence of anemia on cerebral oxygenation. Transfusion acutely improves brain tissue oxygenation (Smith et al., 2005; Zygun et al., 2009), although this does not have a measurable effect on cerebral metabolism (Zygun et al., 2009). Increased rates of brain tissue hypoxia have been detected with transfusion thresholds of 7 g/dL compared to 10 g/dL (Yamal et al., 2015), and this was associated with an increased risk of early death, but a reduced risk of late death.

Given the lack of definitive evidence, a reasonable approach would be to individualize transfusion thresholds according to the prevailing physiology as measured by multimodality monitoring.

# Managing multiple trauma in the context of TBI

TBI commonly coexists with extracranial trauma, particularly after high-energy mechanisms such as road traffic collisions or falls from height. Severe extracranial injury may have a significant impact on TBI.

There have been significant advances in trauma management over the last decade or so. There has been a trend towards permissive hypotension in the ultra-early phase of management, motivated by concerns regarding the development of coagulopathy (Morrison et al., 2011). However, this must be balanced against the known dangers of arterial hypotension in severe TBI and thus is probably not appropriate for most of these patients. At the same time there has been a move towards damage control surgery to control early hemorrhage. The use of early whole-body CT has been demonstrated to confer a survival benefit after major trauma (Huber-Wagner et al., 2009) and improvements in imaging technology have increased speed and availability to such an extent that even relatively unstable patients can be scanned. This is immensely helpful, not only for planning surgery, but also for identifying the extent of TBI before damage control and therefore personalizing physiologic targets very early, hopefully limiting harm from unnecessarily aggressive resuscitation.

There is no good evidence to guide the timing of orthopedic interventions, and the expert view on timing for such surgery has been organized under the rubrics of early total care (early definitive fixation) (Bone et al., 1989), damage control orthopedics (which focuses on the stabilization of injuries, usually with external fixation (Pape et al., 2009)), and (most recently) early appropriate care (which allocates management strategies based on physiologic stability, response to resuscitation, and other risk factors) (Vallier et al., 2013). While the last of these three strategies would seem to be most rational, in effect, the presence of moderate or severe TBI (Pape et al., 2009), especially with the need for cranial surgery (Vallier et al., 2013), places patients in a high-risk category, or excludes them from these schemes. Definitive management of fractured extremities is generally not an emergency. However, fractures are painful and may have a deleterious influence on ICP, as well as convey an increased risk of fat embolus, acute lung injury, and ongoing hemorrhage until the fracture is fixed. Conversely, the increased blood loss and hemodynamic instability associated with more definitive procedures may increase the risk of low CPP and/or high ICP. These decisions are best individualized, based on physiologic stability, intracranial compliance, and logistic feasibility. Occasionally there may be a window of opportunity for fixation in the first few days postinjury, as intracranial compliance may be preserved before cerebral edema develops, while external fixation may be feasible in patients who are too unstable to undergo definitive fixation. Pelvic fractures can pose particular problems due to their propensity for bleeding, associated risk of venous thromboembolism, and restriction on patient positioning. Combined with early CT angiography, endovascular embolization of bleeding pelvic vessels has made minimally invasive hemorrhage control possible. At the same time, temporary inferior vena cava filters are increasingly used to prevent venous thromboembolism in patients with multiple injuries, but in whom prophylactic anticoagulation is not possible due to the nature of their TBI.

Spinal injuries often coexist with TBI, and a proportion of such cases also have spinal cord involvement. Like the brain, the spinal cord is also sensitive to secondary injury from a fall in perfusion pressure; hypotension must therefore be avoided, and there is some evidence to support maintenance of an elevated systemic arterial pressure to optimize cord perfusion (Vale et al., 1997; Hawryluk et al., 2015). Surgical decompression should ideally not be delayed (Fehlings et al., 2012), but TBI or other injuries may make this difficult. Where possible, early fixation of concurrent spinal injuries is helpful in limiting pulmonary complications and may improve outcome (O'Boynick et al., 2014).

Pulmonary injuries pose a significant challenge in the presence of TBI. Acute respiratory distress syndrome occurs in over 20% of severe TBI patients (Aisiku et al., 2016), as a result of direct pulmonary trauma, aspiration pneumonitis or later infection, or as a complication of resuscitation. Although this patient group has been little studied, the mortality benefit of low-tidal-volume mechanical ventilation with permissive hypercapnia to avoid volutrauma/barotrauma is generally accepted (The Acute Respiratory Distress Syndrome Network, 2000), but may be difficult to achieve in patients in whom intracranial compliance is poor and hypercapnia leads to substantial rises in ICP. The use of fluids and vasoactive agents for CPP management along with second-tier therapies such as hypothermia and barbiturates may further aggravate respiratory failure, particularly in patients with myocardial injury.

The need to avoid secondary neurologic injury due to hypoxemia demands meticulous intensive care management. Extracorporeal membrane oxygenation has been successfully used in TBI patients, but anticoagulation risks hematoma expansion/hemorrhage. Less invasive technologies for extracorporeal carbon dioxide elimination have advanced significantly in recent years and may also have a role in limiting the impact of mechanical ventilation in such complex patients (Munoz-Bendix et al., 2015).

# NEUROREHABILITATION

Debate exists regarding the optimal timing for rehabilitation interventions. Some centers advocate early in-hospital initiation (Andelic et al., 2014), but most rehabilitation centers will only accept patients when they are "trainable" (i.e., after return of consciousness and once they are out of post-traumatic amnesia). There is a strong case to be made for embedding the rehabilitation ethos into acute care of TBI, from the point of admission. During the acute TBI phase, interventions need to focus on maximizing preservation of neurologic function, avoiding secondary complications, and maintaining musculoskeletal function to provide a basis for subsequent rehabilitation. The more direct rehabilitation-related interventions become relevant as patients begin to improve. Key interventions in this context address ensuring adequate delivery of nutrition (usually enterally), limiting the duration of neuromuscular blockade to avoid muscle wasting, timely treatment of infections, and minimization of sedatives and other medication (such as first-generation AEDs) that have been associated with worse rehabilitation outcomes. The last of these issues may demand careful clinical judgment, since drugs may be needed to control agitation and ensure patient safety. Agitation is common during the process of recovery from TBI, may adversely affect engagement with rehabilitation, and may be associated with worse outcomes (Bogner et al., 2001; Lequerica et al., 2007). Many agents, including benzodiazepines, butyrophenones, atypical antipsychotics, beta-blockers, and antiepileptic agents have been used to treat this condition, but none is uniformly successful (Fugate et al., 1997; Levy et al., 2005; Fleminger et al., 2006). Experimental data suggest that some of these agents may impede recovery (Kline et al., 2008) and rehabilitative learning (Hoffman et al., 2008) after TBI. While these data have not been convincingly replicated in humans, and use of these agents is often unavoidable in behavioral emergencies, a careful analysis of the risk–benefit ratio is warranted in each patient.

Prompt attention to extracranial injuries can facilitate mobilization and physiotherapy. Physiotherapy, first with passive movements and later with active exercises, may help minimize spasticity and fixed joint deformities. Particularly resistant spasticity may benefit from local injections of botulinum toxin. In patients with severe TBI and a compromised level of consciousness or airway incompetence, or in those with severe extracranial injuries, early tracheostomy may accelerate liberation from ventilator support. Paroxysmal sympathetic hyperactivity is not uncommon in severe TBI, especially in patients with extensive TAI, and the careful selection and titration of medication (including, for example, beta-blockers, clonidine, gabapentin) aimed at minimizing sympathetic storms may allow rapid reduction of sedative medication. Injections of botulinum toxin into the parotid glands may be beneficial in patients in whom hypersalivation is a particular problem.

An additional issue of direct relevance to intensivists is the use of drugs to accelerate emergence from coma (Mura et al., 2014); the only well-conducted positive randomized clinical trial involves administration of amantadine (Giacino et al., 2012). Notwithstanding use of such agents, it is important to emphasize that early targeted rehabilitative therapies may be important in achieving the best possible outcome in this setting (Seel et al., 2013).

TBI may begin as an acute condition, but eventually becomes a chronic disease, with an ongoing burden of excess mortality persisting decades after the initial injury, and persistent disability that continues to affect quality of life. Besides physical disability, TBI survivors suffer from pervasive cognitive deficits (particularly in mental energy, memory, attention, and learning), mental health sequelae (including depression and posttraumatic stress disorder), and impaired self-regulatory behavior (increased impulsivity, poor decision making, and impulsive-aggressive behavior). TBI is also an important risk factor for late posttraumatic epilepsy, with a reported incidence of 0.2–14% for nonpenetrating TBI (Ding et al., 2016) and a substantially increased risk following penetrating TBI (odds ratio 18.77, confidence interval 9.21–38.23) (Pugh et al., 2015). These problems hamper community and vocational integration and quality of life (Andelic et al., 2009; Corrigan et al., 2014), and may trigger institutional placement. TBI survivors may also suffer sleep disorders, neuroendocrine dysregulation, bowel and bladder incontinence, and late (sometimes progressive) abnormalities in metabolic regulation.

TBI may also be a progressive disease. A 13-year longitudinal study (McMillan et al., 2011) showed high rates of disability (50%) and death during follow-up (40%), with substantial change in the level of disability and dependency during follow-up, with about 50% of survivors experiencing reclassification on the Glasgow Outcome Scale – Extended (GOSE). Half of these involved an improvement in functional level, but the rest worsened between 7 and 14 years post-TBI. The GOSE initially increases and peaks approximately 10 years postinjury, and then decreases (Pretz and Dams-O'Connor, 2013). There is also now a clear recognition that TBI is an important risk factor for late neurodegeneration (Shively et al., 2012; DeKosky et al., 2013; Smith et al., 2013), underpinned by a polypathology (Washington et al., 2016) that involves deposition of protein aggregates (such as amyloid and hyperphosphorylated tau), and neuroinflammation. One major challenge for neurointensive care in the future may be the characterization of such late consequences of TBI, and their modulation by therapies that we deliver in the ICU.

*Table 14.4*

Outcome schemes for traumatic brain injury (TBI)

| Glasgow Outcome Scale (GOS) | Dichotomized outcome | Glasgow Outcome Scale – Extended (GOSE) | Outcome description | Societal consequence |
|---|---|---|---|---|
| Good outcome | Favorable outcome | Upper good outcome | Resumed normal life, no symptoms | Resumed pre-TBI life |
| | | Lower good outcome | Resumed normal life, some symptoms | |
| Moderate disability | | Upper moderate disability | Limited in one or more life roles | Independent, and able to participate, but resumption of pre-TBI life not possible |
| | | Lower moderate disability | Unable to participate in one or more life roles | |
| Severe disability | Unfavorable outcome | Upper severe disability | Dependent, needs some help | Recovered consciousness and awareness, but not independent |
| | | Lower severe disability | Dependent, needs frequent help | |
| Vegetative state | | Vegetative state | Unconscious/unaware | Survival; no recovery of consciousness/awareness |
| Death | | Death | Cardiac arrest due to terminal extubation or brain death | Potential for organ donation |

## OUTCOME

Given the burden of disability arising from TBI, it follows that simple estimates of mortality would seriously underestimate the impact of TBI, and any useful risk prediction model needs to provide estimates of poor neurologic outcome other than mortality. Functional outcome from TBI is typically characterized using the five-level GOS (Jennett and Bond, 1975) or the eight-level GOSE (Jennett et al., 1981). In using both these schemes, several previous publications have dichotomized the scores into favorable and unfavorable outcomes, with severe disability, vegetative state (VS), and death included in the latter (Table 14.4).

There is a growing appreciation that such global instruments are crude metrics of outcome and disability, with substantial fine variation within outcome categories. Thus, for example, a patient in a lower "good outcome" category may be able to cope with activities of daily living, but continue to have significant cognitive deficits, often affecting working memory, executive function, and self-regulation of impulsive behaviors, which may only be detected by formal cognitive testing. In addition, many patients experience psychiatric and psychologic problems, with depression being seen in over a third of severe TBI survivors. At the other end of the scale, there has been substantial refinement in characterization of patients with prolonged disorders of consciousness (Giacino and Kalmar, 2005; Giacino et al., 2014; Turner-Stokes, 2014). The threshold between VS and severe disability is now recognized to

include discrete behavioral levels as VS patients emerge into a minimally conscious state (MCS, which is sometimes further subdivided as MCS+ and MCS−), and then make the transition from MCS to full consciousness through a transitional state. Further, these clinician reported outcomes take no account of patients' views, and there is an increasing recognition of the need to apply patient-reported outcome measures such as the Quality of Life after Brain Injury (Qolibri) scale (von Steinbuchel et al., 2010).

## OUTCOME PREDICTION

Accurate prediction of prognosis in TBI is important for several purposes (Lingsma et al., 2010; Maas et al., 2015). These include calibrating the expectations of patients and families, planning clinical care, accurate risk-adjusted comparative audit of clinical performance of institutions, and for efficient clinical trial design using novel techniques (such as sliding dichotomy and proportional odds approaches) (Roozenbeek et al., 2011). Unfortunately, classic risk adjustment programs commonly used in general critical care do not perform optimally in TBI (Hyam et al., 2006). The key clinical features at presentation that determine outcome in TBI are well documented, and include age, GCS score, and CT appearance. However, given the complex interactions of injury and host variables in driving outcome, a clear need exists for a prognostic scheme that integrates these factors. In 2006, a systematic review (Perel et al., 2006) concluded that most predictive models were inadequately validated, poorly presented, and based on small single-center samples that excluded patients from low-income countries (where TBI is most common). In the last decade, two groups have used large study datasets to provide more accurate prognostic models in TBI: the International Mission on Prognosis and Analysis of Clinical Trials in TBI (IMPACT) and Medical Research Council Corticosteroid Randomization after Significant Head Injury (MRC CRASH) trial (MRC Crash Trial Collaborators, 2008; Steyerberg et al., 2008). The IMPACT authors collected data from 9205 patients with TBI enrolled in eight randomized clinical trials and three large observational studies. CRASH, the largest clinical trial ever conducted in TBI, collected data in over 10 000 patients with TBI.

The CRASH dataset of patients was used to develop separate sets of risk prediction models (MRC Crash Trial Collaborators, 2008) for high-income countries, and for low-/middle-income countries. Within each of these categories, the models allow prediction either with or without knowledge of CT appearances. The models have been made publicly available on a web-based calculator, which allows entry of clinical and imaging data to produce an estimated risk of death or disability with confidence intervals for each estimate (http://crash2.lshtm.ac.uk/Risk%20calculator/index.html). The models perform reasonably well, and the high-income countries model was externally validated against a large number of patients from the IMPACT database.

The IMPACT model (Steyerberg et al., 2008) predicts mortality and GOS at 6 months after injury, and was externally validated in 6681 patients from the MRC CRASH trial population. The strongest predictors of outcome were age, GCS motor score, pupil reactivity, and admission CT scan. Model performance was significantly improved by the inclusion of secondary insults (hypotension and hypoxia), and laboratory variables (blood glucose and hemoglobin). External validation against patients from the CRASH database showed reasonable performance, which improved when validation was undertaken against a subset of CRASH patients from high-income countries. Like the CRASH prediction methodology, the IMPACT model is available online, thus allowing access for risk prediction in individual subjects (http://www.tbi-impact.org/). The IMPACT model has been validated in multiple settings, and shows good discrimination of favorable and unfavorable outcomes (Maas et al., 2015), but sometimes poor calibration in new patient populations (Harrison et al., 2013), which can be substantially improved by recalibration in these contexts (Harrison et al., 2015).

Despite these advances, it is sobering to reflect that the current covariates in prognostic schemes account only for about one-third of the variance observed in TBI outcome. Advanced neuroimaging (including MRI), protein biomarkers, and genetic variation could add to the prognostic accuracy of schemes that only include simple clinical variables. Proof of such incremental benefit is now emerging, and future versions of these established prognostic schemes may integrate data from these sources.

## ACKNOWLEDGMENTS

DKM and AE are supported by a European Union Framework Program 7 grant (CENTER-TBI; agreement no. 602150). DKM is supported by funding from the National Institute for Health Research (NIHR) UK through a Senior Investigator Award, and the Cambridge NIHR Biomedical Research Centre.

We would like to acknowledge the immense help provided by Joanne Outtrim and Jemma Andrews in organizing this manuscript, and Dr. Jed Hartings for providing the image in Figure 14.3. The Cambridge Neurosciences Critical Care Unit (NCCU) ICP/CPP protocol has been developed jointly by the NCCU and the Neurosurgical Unit at Addenbrooke's Hospital; the algorithm in Figure 14.10 includes input from Dr. Ronan O'Leary and Dr. Andrea Lavinio (NCCU), and David de Monteverdi-Robb (Pharmacy Department).

## REFERENCES

Adams JH, Jennett B, McLellan DR et al. (1999). The neuropathology of the vegetative state after head injury. J Clin Pathol 52: 804–806.

Adams JH, Jennett B, Murray LS et al. (2011). Neuropathological findings in disabled survivors of a head injury. J Neurotrauma 28: 701–709.

Agrawal D, Saini R, Singh PK et al. (2016). Bedside computed tomography in traumatic brain injury: experience of 10 000 consecutive cases in neurosurgery at a level 1 trauma center in India. Neurol India 64: 62–65.

Aisiku IP, Yamal JM, Doshi P et al. (2016). The incidence of ARDS and associated mortality in severe TBI using the Berlin definition. J Trauma Acute Care Surg 80: 308–312.

Alali AS, Fowler RA, Mainprize TG et al. (2013). Intracranial pressure monitoring in severe traumatic brain injury: results from the American College of Surgeons Trauma Quality Improvement Program. J Neurotrauma 30: 1737–1746.

Alali AS, Scales DC, Fowler RA et al. (2014). Tracheostomy timing in traumatic brain injury: a propensity-matched cohort study. J Trauma Acute Care Surg 76: 70–76. discussion 76–78.

Altmeyer W, Steven A, Gutierrez J (2016). Use of magnetic resonance in the evaluation of cranial trauma. Magn Reson Imaging Clin N Am 24: 305–323.

Alves JL (2014). Blood–brain barrier and traumatic brain injury. J Neurosci Res 92: 141–147.

Amyot F, Arciniegas DB, Brazaitis MP et al. (2015). A review of the effectiveness of neuroimaging modalities for the detection of traumatic brain injury. J Neurotrauma 32: 1693–1721.

Andelic N, Hammergren N, Bautz-Holter E et al. (2009). Functional outcome and health-related quality of life 10 years after moderate-to-severe traumatic brain injury. Acta Neurol Scand 120: 16–23.

Andelic N, Ye J, Tornas S et al. (2014). Cost-effectiveness analysis of an early-initiated, continuous chain of rehabilitation after severe traumatic brain injury. J Neurotrauma 31: 1313–1320.

Andrews PJD, Sinclair HL, Rodriguez A et al. (2015). Hypothermia for intracranial hypertension after traumatic brain injury. N Engl J Med 373: 2403–2412.

Anglin CO, Spence JS, Warner MA et al. (2013). Effects of platelet and plasma transfusion on outcome in traumatic brain injury patients with moderate bleeding diatheses. J Neurosurg 118: 676–686.

Anke A, Andelic N, Skandsen T et al. (2015). Functional recovery and life satisfaction in the first year after severe traumatic brain injury: a prospective multicenter study of a Norwegian national cohort. J Head Trauma Rehabil 30: E38–E49.

Aries MJ, Czosnyka M, Budohoski KP et al. (2012). Continuous determination of optimal cerebral perfusion pressure in traumatic brain injury. Crit Care Med 40: 2456–2463.

Balestreri M, Czosnyka M, Hutchinson P et al. (2006). Impact of intracranial pressure and cerebral perfusion pressure on severe disability and mortality after head injury. Neurocrit Care 4: 8–13.

Bao L, Chen D, Ding L et al. (2014). Fever burden is an independent predictor for prognosis of traumatic brain injury. PLoS One 9: e90956.

Barbey AK, Colom R, Paul E et al. (2014). Preservation of general intelligence following traumatic brain injury: contributions of the Met66 brain-derived neurotrophic factor. PLoS One 9: e88733.

Batchelor JS, Grayson A (2012a). A meta-analysis to determine the effect of anticoagulation on mortality in patients with blunt head trauma. Br J Neurosurg 26: 525–530.

Batchelor JS, Grayson A (2012b). A meta-analysis to determine the effect on survival of platelet transfusions in patients with either spontaneous or traumatic antiplatelet medication-associated intracranial haemorrhage. BMJ Open 2: e000588.

Batchelor JS, Grayson A (2013). A meta-analysis to determine the effect of preinjury antiplatelet agents on mortality in patients with blunt head trauma. Br J Neurosurg 27: 12–18.

Blumbergs PC, Reilly P, Vink R (2008). Trauma. In: S Love, D Louis, DW Ellison (Eds.), Greenfield's Neuropathology, 8th edn. Taylor & Francis, London.

Bogner JA, Corrigan JD, Fugate L et al. (2001). Role of agitation in prediction of outcomes after traumatic brain injury. Am J Phys Med Rehabil 80: 636–644.

Bohmer AE, Oses JP, Schmidt AP et al. (2011). Neuron-specific enolase, S100B, and glial fibrillary acidic protein levels as outcome predictors in patients with severe traumatic brain injury. Neurosurgery 68: 1624–1630. discussion 1630–1621.

Bone LB, Johnson KD, Weigelt J et al. (1989). Early versus delayed stabilization of femoral fractures. A prospective randomized study. J Bone Joint Surg Am 71: 336–340.

Bouma GJ, Muizelaar JP, Choi SC et al. (1991). Cerebral circulation and metabolism after severe traumatic brain injury: the elusive role of ischemia. J Neurosurg 75: 685–693.

Bouma GJ, Muizelaar JP, Stringer WA et al. (1992). Ultra-early evaluation of regional cerebral blood flow in severely head-injured patients using xenon-enhanced computerized tomography. J Neurosurg 77: 360–368.

Bragge P, Synnot A, Maas AI et al. (2016). A state-of-the-science overview of randomized controlled trials evaluating acute management of moderate-to-severe traumatic brain injury. J Neurotrauma 33: 1461–1478.

Brain Trauma Foundation, American Association of Neurological Surgeons, Congress of Neurological Surgeons (2007a). Guidelines for the management of severe traumatic brain injury. J Neurotrauma 24 (Suppl 1): S1–S106.

Brain Trauma Foundation, American Association of Neurological Surgeons, Congress of Neurological Surgeons (2007b). Guidelines for the management of severe traumatic brain injury. IX. Cerebral perfusion thresholds. J Neurotrauma 24 (Suppl 1): S59–S64.

Brain Trauma Foundation, American Association of Neurological Surgeons, Congress of Neurological Surgeons (2007c). Guidelines for the management of severe traumatic brain injury. XII. Nutrition. J Neurotrauma 24 (Suppl 1): S77–S82.

Brain Trauma Foundation, American Association of Neurological Surgeons, Congress of Neurological Surgeons (2007d). Guidelines for the management of severe traumatic brain injury. XIII. Antiseizure prophylaxis. J Neurotrauma 24 (Suppl 1): S83–S86.

Brain Trauma Foundation, Surgeons, American Association of Neurological Surgeons, Congress of Neurological Surgeons (2007e). Guidelines for the management of severe traumatic brain injury. J Neurotrauma 24 (Suppl 1): S1–S106.

Brain Trauma Foundation, American Association of Neurological Surgeons, The Joint Section on Neurotrauma and Critical Care (2000). Guidelines for cerebral perfusion pressure. J Neurotrauma 17: 507–511.

Brain Trauma Foundation, American Association of Neurological Surgeons, Congress of Neurological Surgeons (2016). https://braintrauma.org/uploads/03/12/Guidelines_for_Management_of_Severe_TBI_4th_Edition.pdf (last accessed 18th October 2016).

Brenner M, Stein DM, Hu PF et al. (2012). Traditional systolic blood pressure targets underestimate hypotension-induced secondary brain injury. J Trauma Acute Care Surg 72: 1135–1139.

Brown GC (2000). Nitric oxide as a competitive inhibitor of oxygen consumption in the mitochondrial respiratory chain. Acta Physiol Scand 168: 667–674.

Brown JB, Stassen NA, Cheng JD et al. (2010). Trauma center designation correlates with functional independence after severe but not moderate traumatic brain injury. J Trauma 69: 263–269.

Bulger EM, Nathens AB, Rivara FP et al. (2002). Management of severe head injury: institutional variations in care and effect on outcome. Crit Care Med 30: 1870–1876.

Bullock MR, Chesnut R, Ghajar J et al. (2006). Surgical management of acute subdural hematomas. Neurosurgery 58: S16–S24. discussion Si-iv.

Bulstrode H, Nicoll JA, Hudson G et al. (2014). Mitochondrial DNA and traumatic brain injury. Ann Neurol 75: 186–195.

Butcher I, Maas AI, Lu J et al. (2007). Prognostic value of admission blood pressure in traumatic brain injury: results from the IMPACT study. J Neurotrauma 24: 294–302.

Carlson AP, Yonas H (2012). Portable head computed tomography scanner – technology and applications: experience with 3421 scans. J Neuroimaging 22: 408–415.

Caterino JM, Raubenolt A, Cudnik MT (2011). Modification of Glasgow Coma Scale criteria for injured elders. Acad Emerg Med 18: 1014–1021.

Chang BS, Lowenstein DH (2003). Practice parameter: antiepileptic drug prophylaxis in severe traumatic brain injury: report of the Quality Standards Subcommittee of the American Academy of Neurology. Neurology 60: 10–16.

Chen S, Chen Y, Xu L et al. (2015). Venous system in acute brain injury: mechanisms of pathophysiological change and function. Exp Neurol 272: 4–10.

Chesnut RM, Marshall LF, Klauber MR et al. (1993). The role of secondary brain injury in determining outcome from severe head injury. J Trauma 34: 216–222.

Chesnut RM, Temkin N, Carney N et al. (2012). A trial of intracranial-pressure monitoring in traumatic brain injury. N Engl J Med 367: 2471–2481.

Chesnut RM, Bleck TP, Citerio G et al. (2015). A consensus-based interpretation of the benchmark evidence from South American trials: treatment of intracranial pressure trial. J Neurotrauma 32: 1722–1724.

Chi JH, Knudson MM, Vassar MJ et al. (2006). Prehospital hypoxia affects outcome in patients with traumatic brain injury: a prospective multicenter study. J Trauma 61: 1134–1141.

Claassen J, Vespa P, Participants in the International Multidisciplinary Consensus Conference on Multimodality Monitoring (2014). Electrophysiologic monitoring in acute brain injury. Neurocrit Care 21 (Suppl 2): S129–S147.

Clifton GL, Miller ER, Choi SC et al. (2001). Lack of effect of induction of hypothermia after acute brain injury. N Engl J Med 344: 556–563.

Clifton GL, Valadka A, Zygun D et al. (2011). Very early hypothermia induction in patients with severe brain injury (the National Acute Brain Injury Study: Hypothermia II): a randomised trial. Lancet Neurol 10: 131–139.

Coles JP, Minhas PS, Fryer TD et al. (2002). Effect of hyperventilation on cerebral blood flow in traumatic head injury: clinical relevance and monitoring correlates. Crit Care Med 30: 1950–1959.

Coles JP, Fryer TD, Smielewski P et al. (2004). Incidence and mechanisms of cerebral ischemia in early clinical head injury. Journal of Cerebral Blood Flow & Metabolism 24: 202–211.

Coles JP, Fryer TD, Coleman MR et al. (2007). Hyperventilation following head injury: effect on ischemic burden and cerebral oxidative metabolism. Crit Care Med 35: 568–578.

Conley YP, Okonkwo DO, Deslouches S et al. (2014). Mitochondrial polymorphisms impact outcomes after severe traumatic brain injury. J Neurotrauma 31: 34–41.

Cooper DJ, Rosenfeld JV, Murray L et al. (2011). Decompressive craniectomy in diffuse traumatic brain injury. N Engl J Med 364: 1493–1502.

Corrigan JD, Cuthbert JP, Harrison-Felix C et al. (2014). US population estimates of health and social outcomes 5 years after rehabilitation for traumatic brain injury. J Head Trauma Rehabil 29: E1–E9.

MRC Crash Trial Collaborators, Perel P, Arango M et al. (2008). Predicting outcome after traumatic brain injury: practical prognostic models based on large cohort of international patients. BMJ 336: 425–429.

CRASH-2 collaborators, Roberts I, Shakur H et al. (2011). The importance of early treatment with tranexamic acid in bleeding trauma patients: an exploratory analysis of the CRASH-2 randomised controlled trial. Lancet 377: 1096–1101. 1101 e1091-1092.

CRASH-2 trial collaborators, Shakur H, Roberts I et al. (2010). Effects of tranexamic acid on death, vascular occlusive events, and blood transfusion in trauma patients with significant haemorrhage (CRASH-2): a randomised, placebo-controlled trial. Lancet 376: 23–32.

Cremer OL, Moons KG, Bouman EA et al. (2001). Long-term propofol infusion and cardiac failure in adult head-injured patients. Lancet 357: 117–118.

Cremer OL, van Dijk GW, van Wensen E et al. (2005). Effect of intracranial pressure monitoring and targeted intensive care on functional outcome after severe head injury. Crit Care Med 33: 2207–2213.

Daneshvar DH, Goldstein LE, Kiernan PT et al. (2015). Post-traumatic neurodegeneration and chronic traumatic encephalopathy. Mol Cell Neurosci 66: 81–90.

De Bonis P, Pompucci A, Mangiola A et al. (2011). Decompressive craniectomy for elderly patients with traumatic brain injury: it's probably not worth the while. J Neurotrauma 28: 2043–2048.

DeKosky ST, Blennow K, Ikonomovic MD et al. (2013). Acute and chronic traumatic encephalopathies: pathogenesis and biomarkers. Nat Rev Neurol 9: 192–200.

Dengler B, Garvin R, Seifi A (2015). Can therapeutic hypothermia trigger propofol-related infusion syndrome? J Crit Care 30: 823–824.

Dewan Y, Komolafe EO, Mejia-Mantilla JH et al. (2012). CRASH-3 – tranexamic acid for the treatment of significant traumatic brain injury: study protocol for an international randomized, double-blind, placebo-controlled trial. Trials 13: 87.

Diamond ML, Ritter AC, Failla MD et al. (2014). IL-1β associations with posttraumatic epilepsy development: a genetics and biomarker cohort study. Epilepsia 55 (7): 1109–1119.

Diaz-Arrastia R, Wang KK, Papa L et al. (2014). Acute biomarkers of traumatic brain injury: relationship between plasma levels of ubiquitin C-terminal hydrolase-L1 and glial fibrillary acidic protein. J Neurotrauma 31: 19–25.

Ding K, Gupta PK, Diaz-Arrastia R (2016). Frontiers in neuroscience epilepsy after traumatic brain injury. In: D Laskowitz, G Grant (Eds.), Translational Research in Traumatic Brain Injury. CRC Press/Taylor and Francis, Boca Raton, FL.

Donkin JJ, Vink R (2010). Mechanisms of cerebral edema in traumatic brain injury: therapeutic developments. Curr Opin Neurol 23: 293–299.

Elf K, Nilsson P, Enblad P (2002). Outcome after traumatic brain injury improved by an organized secondary insult program and standardized neurointensive care. Crit Care Med 30: 2129–2134.

Elterman J, Brasel K, Brown S et al. (2013). Transfusion of red blood cells in patients with a prehospital Glasgow Coma Scale score of 8 or less and no evidence of shock is associated with worse outcomes. J Trauma Acute Care Surg 75: 8–14. discussion 14.

English SW, Turgeon AF, Owen E et al. (2013). Protocol management of severe traumatic brain injury in intensive care units: a systematic review. Neurocrit Care 18: 131–142.

Etemadrezaie H, Baharvahdat H, Shariati Z et al. (2007). The effect of fresh frozen plasma in severe closed head injury. Clin Neurol Neurosurg 109: 166–171.

EuroSafe (2013). Injuries in the European Union: report on injury statistics 2008–2010, EuroSafe, Amsterdam.

Fabbri A, Servadei F, Marchesini G et al. (2013). Antiplatelet therapy and the outcome of subjects with intracranial injury: the Italian SIMEU study. Crit Care 17: R53.

Fabricius M, Fuhr S, Bhatia R et al. (2006). Cortical spreading depression and peri-infarct depolarization in acutely injured human cerebral cortex. Brain 129: 778–790.

Failla MD, Burkhardt JN, Miller MA et al. (2013). Variants of SLC6A4 in depression risk following severe TBI. Brain Inj 27: 696–706.

Fakhry SM, Trask AL, Waller MA et al. (2004). Management of brain-injured patients by an evidence-based medicine protocol improves outcomes and decreases hospital charges. J Trauma 56: 492–499. discussion 499–500.

Faul M, Xu L, Wald M et al. (2010). Traumatic brain injury in the United States: emergency department visits hospitalizations and deaths 2002–2006, Centers for Disease Control and Prevention, National Center for Injury Prevention and Control, Atlanta, GA.

Fearnside MR, Cook RJ, McDougall P et al. (1993). The Westmead Head Injury Project outcome in severe head injury. A comparative analysis of pre-hospital, clinical and CT variables. Br J Neurosurg 7: 267–279.

Fehlings MG, Vaccaro A, Wilson JR et al. (2012). Early versus delayed decompression for traumatic cervical spinal cord injury: results of the Surgical Timing in Acute Spinal Cord Injury Study (STASCIS). PLoS One 7e32037.

Feigin VL, Theadom A, Barker-Collo S et al. (2013). Incidence of traumatic brain injury in New Zealand: a population-based study. Lancet Neurol 12: 53–64.

Finfer S, Chittock D, Li Y et al. (2015). Intensive versus conventional glucose control in critically ill patients with traumatic brain injury: long-term follow-up of a subgroup of patients from the NICE-SUGAR study. Intensive Care Med 41: 1037–1047.

Fleminger S, Greenwood RJ, Oliver DL (2006). Pharmacological management for agitation and aggression in people with acquired brain injury. Cochrane Database Syst Rev Cd003299.

Fugate LP, Spacek LA, Kresty LA et al. (1997). Measurement and treatment of agitation following traumatic brain injury: II. A survey of the Brain Injury Special Interest Group of the American Academy of Physical Medicine and Rehabilitation. Arch Phys Med Rehabil 78: 924–928.

Fuller G, Bouamra O, Woodford M et al. (2011). The effect of specialist neurosciences care on outcome in adult severe head injury: a cohort study. J Neurosurg Anesthesiol 23: 198–205.

Galanaud D, Perlbarg V, Gupta R et al. (2012). Assessment of white matter injury and outcome in severe brain trauma: a prospective multicenter cohort. Anesthesiology 117: 1300–1310.

Giacino JT, Kalmar K (2005). Diagnostic and prognostic guidelines for the vegetative and minimally conscious states. Neuropsychol Rehabil 15: 166–174.

Giacino JT, Whyte J, Bagiella E et al. (2012). Placebo-controlled trial of amantadine for severe traumatic brain injury. N Engl J Med 366: 819–826.

Giacino JT, Fins JJ, Laureys S et al. (2014). Disorders of consciousness after acquired brain injury: the state of the science. Nat Rev Neurol 10: 99–114.

Goldschlager T, Rosenfeld JV, Winter CD (2007). 'Talk and die' patients presenting to a major trauma centre over a 10 year period: a critical review. J Clin Neurosci 14: 618–623. discussion 624.

Graham DI, Adams JH, Doyle D (1978). Ischaemic brain damage in fatal non-missile head injuries. J Neurol Sci 39: 213–234.

Graham DI, Ford I, Adams JH et al. (1989). Ischaemic brain damage is still common in fatal non-missile head injury. J Neurol Neurosurg Psychiatry 52: 346–350.

Grande PO (2006). The "Lund concept" for the treatment of severe head trauma – physiological principles and clinical application. Intensive Care Med 32: 1475–1484.

Grandhi R, Harrison G, Voronovich Z et al. (2015). Preinjury warfarin, but not antiplatelet medications, increases mortality in elderly traumatic brain injury patients. J Trauma Acute Care Surg 78: 614–621.

Greenwald BD, Hammond FM, Harrison-Felix C et al. (2015). Mortality following traumatic brain injury among individuals unable to follow commands at the time of rehabilitation admission: a National Institute on Disability and Rehabilitation Research traumatic brain injury model systems study. J Neurotrauma 32: 1883–1892.

Greuters S, van den Berg A, Franschman G et al. (2011). Acute and delayed mild coagulopathy are related to outcome in patients with isolated traumatic brain injury. Crit Care 15: R2.

Gupta AK, Menon DK, Czosnyka M et al. (1997). Thresholds for hypoxic cerebral vasodilation in volunteers. Anesth Analg. 85 (4): 817–820.

Hackam DG, Mrkobrada M (2012). Selective serotonin reuptake inhibitors and brain hemorrhage: a meta-analysis. Neurology 79: 1862–1865.

Hadjigeorgiou GM, Paterakis K, Dardiotis E et al. (2005). IL-1RN and IL-1B gene polymorphisms and cerebral hemorrhagic events after traumatic brain injury. Neurology 65: 1077–1082.

Hajjar LA, Vincent JL, Galas FR et al. (2010). Transfusion requirements after cardiac surgery: the TRACS randomized controlled trial. JAMA 304: 1559–1567.

Harhangi BS, Kompanje EJ, Leebeek FW et al. (2008). Coagulation disorders after traumatic brain injury. Acta Neurochir (Wien) 150: 165–175. discussion 175.

Harrison DA, Prabhu G, Grieve R et al. (2013). Risk Adjustment In Neurocritical care (RAIN) – prospective validation of risk prediction models for adult patients with acute traumatic brain injury to use to evaluate the optimum location and comparative costs of neurocritical care: a cohort study. Health Technol Assess 17: vii–viii. 1–350.

Harrison DA, Griggs KA, Prabhu G et al. (2015). External validation and recalibration of risk prediction models for acute traumatic brain injury among critically ill adult patients in the United Kingdom. J Neurotrauma 32: 1522–1537.

Hartings JA, Bullock MR, Okonkwo DO et al. (2011a). Spreading depolarisations and outcome after traumatic brain injury: a prospective observational study. Lancet Neurol 10: 1058–1064.

Hartings JA, Watanabe T, Bullock MR et al. (2011b). Spreading depolarizations have prolonged direct current shifts and are associated with poor outcome in brain trauma. Brain 134: 1529–1540.

Hartings JA, Wilson JA, Hinzman JM et al. (2014). Spreading depression in continuous electroencephalography of brain trauma. Ann Neurol 76: 681–694.

Hawryluk G, Whetstone W, Saigal R et al. (2015). Mean arterial blood pressure correlates with neurological recovery after human spinal cord injury: analysis of high frequency physiologic data. J Neurotrauma 32: 1958–1967.

Hay JR, Johnson VE, Young AM et al. (2015). Blood–brain barrier disruption is an early event that may persist for many years after traumatic brain injury in humans. J Neuropathol Exp Neurol 74: 1147–1157.

Hebert PC, Wells G, Blajchman MA et al. (1999). A multicenter, randomized, controlled clinical trial of transfusion requirements in critical care. Transfusion Requirements in Critical Care Investigators, Canadian Critical Care Trials Group. N Engl J Med 340: 409–417.

Hertle DN, Dreier JP, Woitzik J et al. (2012a). Effect of analgesics and sedatives on the occurrence of spreading depolarizations accompanying acute brain injury. Brain 135: 2390–2398.

Hertle DN, Dreier JP, Woitzik J et al. (2012b). Effect of analgesics and sedatives on the occurrence of spreading depolarizations accompanying acute brain injury. Brain 135: 2390–2398.

Hifumi T, Kuroda Y, Kawakita K et al. (2016). Fever control management is preferable to mild therapeutic hypothermia in traumatic brain injury patients with Abbreviated Injury Scale 3-4: a multi-center, randomized controlled trial. J Neurotrauma 33: 1047–1053.

Hill DA, Abraham KJ, West RH (1993). Factors affecting outcome in the resuscitation of severely injured patients. Aust N Z J Surg 63: 604–609.

Hill CS, Coleman MP, Menon DK (2016). Traumatic axonal injury: mechanisms and translational opportunities. Trends Neurosci 39: 311–324.

Hinzman JM, Wilson JA, Mazzeo AT et al. (2016). Excitotoxicity and metabolic crisis are associated with spreading depolarizations in severe traumatic brain injury patients. J Neurotrauma (epub ahead of print).

Hoffman AN, Cheng JP, Zafonte RD et al. (2008). Administration of haloperidol and risperidone after neurobehavioral testing hinders the recovery of traumatic brain injury-induced deficits. Life Sci 83: 602–607.

Hoh NZ, Wagner AK, Alexander SA et al. (2010). BCL2 genotypes: functional and neurobehavioral outcomes after severe traumatic brain injury. J Neurotrauma 27: 1413–1427.

Honda M, Tsuruta R, Kaneko T et al. (2010). Serum glial fibrillary acidic protein is a highly specific biomarker for traumatic brain injury in humans compared with S-100B and neuron-specific enolase. J Trauma 69: 104–109.

Hoyt DB (2004). A clinical review of bleeding dilemmas in trauma. Semin Hematol 41: 40–43.

Huber-Wagner S, Lefering R, Qvick LM et al. (2009). Effect of whole-body CT during trauma resuscitation on survival: a retrospective, multicentre study. Lancet 373: 1455–1461.

Hutchinson PJ, Hutchinson DB, Barr RH et al. (2000). A new cranial access device for cerebral monitoring. Br J Neurosurg 14: 46–48.

Hutchinson PJ, Kolias AG, Czosnyka M et al. (2013). Intracranial pressure monitoring in severe traumatic brain injury. BMJ 346: f1000.

Hutchinson PJ, Jalloh I, Helmy A et al. (2015). Consensus statement from the 2014 International Microdialysis Forum. Intensive Care Med 41: 1517–1528.

Hutchinson PJ, Kolias AG, Timofeev IS et al. (2016). Trial of Decompressive craniectomy for traumatic intracranial hypertension. N Engl J Med 375: 1119–1130.

Hyam JA, Welch CA, Harrison DA et al. (2006). Case mix, outcomes and comparison of risk prediction models for admissions to adult, general and specialist critical care units for head injury: a secondary analysis of the ICNARC Case Mix Programme Database. Crit Care 10 (Suppl 2): S2.

Hyder AA, Wunderlich CA, Puvanachandra P et al. (2007). The impact of traumatic brain injuries: a global perspective. NeuroRehabilitation 22: 341–353.

ICNARC (2015). Annual Quality Report 2013/14 for adult, neurocritical (neuro, combined ICU/neuro) care, Intensive Care National Audit and Research Centre, London.

Inaba K, Rizoli S, Veigas PV et al. (2015). 2014 Consensus conference on viscoelastic test-based transfusion guidelines for early trauma resuscitation: report of the panel. J Trauma Acute Care Surg 78: 1220–1229.

Jamjoom AA, Jamjoom AB (2013). Safety and efficacy of early pharmacological thromboprophylaxis in traumatic brain injury: systematic review and meta-analysis. J Neurotrauma 30: 503–511.

Janowitz T, Menon DK (2010). Exploring new routes for neuroprotective drug development in traumatic brain injury. Sci Transl Med 2: 27rv21.

Jennett B, Bond M (1975). Assessment of outcome after severe brain damage. Lancet 1: 480–484.

Jennett B, Snoek J, Bond MR et al. (1981). Disability after severe head injury: observations on the use of the Glasgow Outcome Scale. J Neurol Neurosurg Psychiatry 44: 285–293.

Jeremitsky E, Omert L, Dunham CM et al. (2003). Harbingers of poor outcome the day after severe brain injury: hypothermia, hypoxia, and hypoperfusion. J Trauma 54: 312–319.

Jones PA, Andrews PJ, Midgley S et al. (1994). Measuring the burden of secondary insults in head-injured patients during intensive care. J Neurosurg Anesthesiol 6: 4–14.

Joseph B, Pandit V, Aziz H et al. (2014). Clinical outcomes in traumatic brain injury patients on preinjury clopidogrel: a prospective analysis. J Trauma Acute Care Surg 76: 817–820.

Kamel H, Navi BB, Nakagawa K et al. (2011). Hypertonic saline versus mannitol for the treatment of elevated intracranial pressure: a meta-analysis of randomized clinical trials. Crit Care Med 39: 554–559.

Karabinis A, Mandragos K, Stergiopoulos S et al. (2004). Safety and efficacy of analgesia-based sedation with remifentanil versus standard hypnotic-based regimens in intensive care unit patients with brain injuries: a randomised, controlled trial [ISRCTN50308308]. Crit Care 8: R268–R280.

Kasprowicz M, Burzynska M, Melcer T et al. (2016). A comparison of the Full Outline of UnResponsiveness (FOUR) score and Glasgow Coma Score (GCS) in predictive modelling in traumatic brain injury. Br J Neurosurg 30: 211–220.

Kawamata T, Katayama Y, Aoyama N et al. (2000). Heterogeneous mechanisms of early edema formation in cerebral contusion: diffusion MRI and ADC mapping study. Acta Neurochir Suppl 76: 9–12.

Kawata K, Liu CY, Merkel SF et al. (2016). Blood biomarkers for brain injury: what are we measuring? Neurosci Biobehav Rev 68: 460–473.

Kehoe A, Rennie S, Smith JE (2015). Glasgow Coma Scale is unreliable for the prediction of severe head injury in elderly trauma patients. Emerg Med J 32: 613–615.

Kelly DF, Kordestani RK, Martin NA et al. (1996). Hyperemia following traumatic brain injury: relationship to intracranial hypertension and outcome. J Neurosurg 85: 762–771.

Kenney K, Amyot F, Haber M et al. (2016). Cerebral vascular injury in traumatic brain injury. Exp Neurol 275 (Pt 3): 353–366.

Kim J, Kemp S, Kullas K et al. (2013). Injury patterns in patients who "talk and die". J Clin Neurosci 20: 1697–1701.

Kirkman MA, Jenks T, Bouamra O et al. (2013). Increased mortality associated with cerebral contusions following trauma in the elderly: bad patients or bad management? J Neurotrauma 30: 1385–1390.

Kline AE, Hoffman AN, Cheng JP et al. (2008). Chronic administration of antipsychotics impede behavioral recovery after experimental traumatic brain injury. Neurosci Lett 448: 263–267.

Kochanek PM, Jackson TC, Ferguson NM et al. (2015). Emerging therapies in traumatic brain injury. Semin Neurol 35: 83–100.

Korley FK, Diaz-Arrastia R, Wu AH et al. (2016). Circulating brain-derived neurotrophic factor has diagnostic and prognostic value in traumatic brain injury. J Neurotrauma 33: 215–225.

Krajcova A, Waldauf P, Andel M et al. (2015). Propofol infusion syndrome: a structured review of experimental studies and 153 published case reports. Crit Care 19: 398.

Kramer AH, Roberts DJ, Zygun DA (2012). Optimal glycemic control in neurocritical care patients: a systematic review and meta-analysis. Crit Care 16: R203.

Krishnamoorthy V, Vavilala MS, Mills B et al. (2015). Demographic and clinical risk factors associated with hospital mortality after isolated severe traumatic brain injury: a cohort study. J Intensive Care 3: 46.

Krishnamurthy K, Laskowitz DT (2015). Cellular and molecular mechanisms of secondary neuronal injury following traumatic brain injury. Translational Research in Traumatic Brain Injury. CRC Press, Boca Raton, FL.

Krueger F, Pardini M, Huey ED et al. (2011). The role of the Met66 brain-derived neurotrophic factor allele in the recovery of executive functioning after combat-related traumatic brain injury. J Neurosci 31: 598–606.

Kucinski T, Vaterlein O, Glauche V et al. (2002). Correlation of apparent diffusion coefficient and computed tomography density in acute ischemic stroke. Stroke 33: 1786–1791.

Kulbe JR, Geddes JW (2016). Current status of fluid biomarkers in mild traumatic brain injury. Exp Neurol 275 (Pt 3): 334–352.

Laroche M, Kutcher ME, Huang MC et al. (2012). Coagulopathy after traumatic brain injury. Neurosurgery 70: 1334–1345.

Lawrence DW, Comper P, Hutchison MG et al. (2015). The role of apolipoprotein E epsilon (epsilon)-4 allele on outcome following traumatic brain injury: a systematic review. Brain Inj 29: 1018–1031.

Lazaridis C, Neyens R, Bodle J et al. (2013). High-osmolarity saline in neurocritical care: systematic review and meta-analysis. Crit Care Med 41: 1353–1360.

Lazaridis C, DeSantis SM, Smielewski P et al. (2014). Patient-specific thresholds of intracranial pressure in severe traumatic brain injury. J Neurosurg 120: 893–900.

Le Roux P, Menon DK, Citerio G et al. (2014). The International Multidisciplinary Consensus Conference on Multimodality Monitoring in Neurocritical Care: a list of recommendations and additional conclusions: a statement for healthcare professionals from the Neurocritical Care Society and the European Society of Intensive Care Medicine. Neurocrit Care 21 (Suppl 2): S282–S296.

Leal-Noval SR, Munoz-Serrano A, Arellano-Orden V et al. (2016). Effects of red blood cell transfusion on long-term disability of patients with traumatic brain injury. Neurocrit Care 24: 371–380.

Lee JH, Martin NA, Alsina G et al. (1997). Hemodynamically significant cerebral vasospasm and outcome after head injury: a prospective study. J Neurosurg 87: 221–233.

Lee JH, Kelly DF, Oertel M et al. (2001). Carbon dioxide reactivity, pressure autoregulation, and metabolic suppression reactivity after head injury: a transcranial Doppler study. J Neurosurg 95: 222–232.

Lequerica AH, Rapport LJ, Loeher K et al. (2007). Agitation in acquired brain injury: impact on acute rehabilitation therapies. J Head Trauma Rehabil 22: 177–183.

Levy M, Berson A, Cook T et al. (2005). Treatment of agitation following traumatic brain injury: a review of the literature. NeuroRehabilitation 20: 279–306.

Levy AS, Salottolo K, Bar-Or R et al. (2010). Pharmacologic thromboprophylaxis is a risk factor for hemorrhage progression in a subset of patients with traumatic brain injury. J Trauma 68: 886–894.

Li J, Jiang JY (2012). Chinese Head Trauma Data Bank: effect of hyperthermia on the outcome of acute head trauma patients. J Neurotrauma 29: 96–100.

Li M, Chen T, Chen SD et al. (2015). Comparison of equimolar doses of mannitol and hypertonic saline for the treatment of elevated intracranial pressure after traumatic brain injury: a systematic review and meta-analysis. Medicine (Baltimore) 94. e736.

Lingsma HF, Roozenbeek B, Steyerberg EW et al. (2010). Early prognosis in traumatic brain injury: from prophecies to predictions. Lancet Neurol 9: 543–554.

Lipsky RH, Sparling MB, Ryan LM et al. (2005). Association of COMT Val158Met genotype with executive functioning following traumatic brain injury. J Neuropsychiatry Clin Neurosci 17: 465–471.

Logsdon AF, Lucke-Wold BP, Turner RC et al. (2015). Role of microvascular disruption in brain damage from traumatic brain injury. Compr Physiol 5: 1147–1160.

Lustenberger T, Talving P, Kobayashi L et al. (2010). Time course of coagulopathy in isolated severe traumatic brain injury. Injury 41: 924–928.

Maas AI, Hukkelhoven CW, Marshall LF et al. (2005). Prediction of outcome in traumatic brain injury with computed tomographic characteristics: a comparison between the computed tomographic classification and combinations of computed tomographic predictors. Neurosurgery 57: 1173–1182. discussion 1173–1182.

Maas AI, Menon DK, Lingsma HF et al. (2012). Re-orientation of clinical research in traumatic brain injury: report of an international workshop on comparative effectiveness research. J Neurotrauma 29: 32–46.

Maas AI, Lingsma HF, Roozenbeek B (2015). Predicting outcome after traumatic brain injury. Handb Clin Neurol 128: 455–474.

Macmillan CS, Andrews PJ, Easton VJ (2001). Increased jugular bulb saturation is associated with poor outcome in traumatic brain injury. J Neurol Neurosurg Psychiatry 70: 101–104.

Maegele M (2013). Coagulopathy after traumatic brain injury: incidence, pathogenesis, and treatment options. Transfusion 53 (Suppl 1): 28s–37s.

Maekawa T, Yamashita S, Nagao S et al. (2015). Prolonged mild therapeutic hypothermia versus fever control with tight hemodynamic monitoring and slow rewarming in patients with severe traumatic brain injury: a randomized controlled trial. J Neurotrauma 32: 422–429.

Magnoni S, Tedesco C, Carbonara M et al. (2012). Relationship between systemic glucose and cerebral glucose is preserved in patients with severe traumatic brain injury, but glucose delivery to the brain may become limited when oxidative metabolism is impaired: implications for glycemic control. Crit Care Med 40: 1785–1791.

Majdan M, Mauritz W, Wilbacher I et al. (2013). Barbiturates use and its effects in patients with severe traumatic brain injury in five European countries. J Neurotrauma 30: 23–29.

Manley G, Knudson MM, Morabito D et al. (2001). Hypotension, hypoxia, and head injury: frequency, duration, and consequences. Arch Surg 136: 1118–1123.

Mannion RJ, Cross J, Bradley P et al. (2007). Mechanism-based MRI classification of traumatic brainstem injury and its relationship to outcome. J Neurotrauma 24: 128–135.

Marmarou A, Signoretti S, Fatouros PP et al. (2006). Predominance of cellular edema in traumatic brain swelling in patients with severe head injuries. J Neurosurg 104: 720–730.

Martin NA, Patwardhan RV, Alexander MJ et al. (1997). Characterization of cerebral hemodynamic phases following severe head trauma: hypoperfusion, hyperemia, and vasospasm. J Neurosurg 87: 9–19.

Masel BE (2015). The chronic consequences of neurotrauma. J Neurotrauma 32: 1833.

Maxwell WL, Pennington K, MacKinnon MA et al. (2004). Differential responses in three thalamic nuclei in moderately disabled, severely disabled and vegetative patients after blunt head injury. Brain 127: 2470–2478.

McAllister TW, Flashman LA, Harker Rhodes C et al. (2008). Single nucleotide polymorphisms in ANKK1 and the dopamine D2 receptor gene affect cognitive outcome shortly after traumatic brain injury: a replication and extension study. Brain Inj 22: 705–714.

McAllister TW, Tyler AL, Flashman LA et al. (2012). Polymorphisms in the brain-derived neurotrophic factor gene influence memory and processing speed one month after brain injury. J Neurotrauma 29: 1111–1118.

McHugh GS, Engel DC, Butcher I et al. (2007). Prognostic value of secondary insults in traumatic brain injury: results from the IMPACT study. J Neurotrauma 24: 287–293.

McIntyre LA, Fergusson DA, Hutchison JS et al. (2006). Effect of a liberal versus restrictive transfusion strategy on mortality in patients with moderate to severe head injury. Neurocrit Care 5: 4–9.

McMillan TM, Teasdale GM, Weir CJ et al. (2011). Death after head injury: the 13 year outcome of a case control study. J Neurol Neurosurg Psychiatry 82: 931–935.

McMillan TM, Teasdale GM, Stewart E (2012). Disability in young people and adults after head injury: 12–14 year follow-up of a prospective cohort. J Neurol Neurosurg Psychiatry 83: 1086–1091.

McMillan TM, Weir CJ, Wainman-Lefley J (2014). Mortality and morbidity 15 years after hospital admission with mild head injury: a prospective case-controlled population study. J Neurol Neurosurg Psychiatry 85: 1214–1220.

Meier R, Bechir M, Ludwig S et al. (2008). Differential temporal profile of lowered blood glucose levels (3.5 to 6.5 mmol/l versus 5 to 8 mmol/l) in patients with severe traumatic brain injury. Crit Care 12: R98.

Meierhans R, Bechir M, Ludwig S et al. (2010). Brain metabolism is significantly impaired at blood glucose below 6 mM and brain glucose below 1 mM in patients with severe traumatic brain injury. Crit Care 14: R13.

Menon DK, Maas AI (2015). Traumatic brain injury in 2014. Progress, failures and new approaches for TBI research. Nat Rev Neurol 11: 71–72.

Menon DK, Coles JP, Gupta AK et al. (2004). Diffusion limited oxygen delivery following head injury. Crit Care Med 32: 1384–1390.

Menon DK, Schwab K, Wright DW et al. (2010). Position statement: definition of traumatic brain injury. Arch Phys Med Rehabil 91: 1637–1640.

Miller MP, Trujillo TC, Nordenholz KE (2014). Practical considerations in emergency management of bleeding in the setting of target-specific oral anticoagulants. Am J Emerg Med 32: 375–382.

Moen KG, Skandsen T, Folvik M et al. (2012). A longitudinal MRI study of traumatic axonal injury in patients with moderate and severe traumatic brain injury. J Neurol Neurosurg Psychiatry 83: 1193–1200.

Moen KG, Brezova V, Skandsen T et al. (2014). Traumatic axonal injury: the prognostic value of lesion load in corpus callosum, brain stem, and thalamus in different magnetic resonance imaging sequences. J Neurotrauma 31: 1486–1496.

Mondello S, Papa L, Buki A et al. (2011). Neuronal and glial markers are differently associated with computed tomography findings and outcome in patients with severe traumatic brain injury: a case control study. Crit Care 15: R156.

Mondello S, Jeromin A, Buki A et al. (2012). Glial neuronal ratio: a novel index for differentiating injury type in patients with severe traumatic brain injury. J Neurotrauma 29: 1096–1104.

Morrison CA, Carrick MM, Norman MA et al. (2011). Hypotensive resuscitation strategy reduces transfusion requirements and severe postoperative coagulopathy in trauma patients with hemorrhagic shock: preliminary results of a randomized controlled trial. J Trauma 70: 652–663.

Muizelaar JP, Marmarou A, Ward JD et al. (1991). Adverse effects of prolonged hyperventilation in patients with severe head injury: a randomized clinical trial. J Neurosurg 75: 731–739.

Munoz-Bendix C, Beseoglu K, Kram R (2015). Extracorporeal decarboxylation in patients with severe traumatic brain injury and ARDS enables effective control of intracranial pressure. Crit Care 19: 381.

Mura E, Pistoia F, Sara M et al. (2014). Pharmacological modulation of the state of awareness in patients with disorders of consciousness: an overview. Curr Pharm Des 20: 4121–4139.

Murray GD, Butcher I, McHugh GS et al. (2007). Multivariable prognostic analysis in traumatic brain injury: results from the IMPACT study. J Neurotrauma 24: 329–337.

Narayan RK, Maas AI, Marshall LF et al. (2008). Recombinant factor VIIA in traumatic intracerebral hemorrhage: results of a dose-escalation clinical trial. Neurosurgery 62: 776–786. discussion 786–778.

National Research Council Committee on A Framework for Developing a New Taxonomy of Disease (2011). The National Academies Collection: Reports funded by National Institutes of Health. Toward Precision Medicine: Building a Knowledge Network for Biomedical Research and a New Taxonomy of Disease. National Academies Press (US) National Academy of Sciences, Washington (DC).

Newcombe VF, Williams GB, Nortje J et al. (2007). Analysis of acute traumatic axonal injury using diffusion tensor imaging. Br J Neurosurg 21: 340–348.

Newell DW, Aaslid R, Stooss R et al. (1997). Evaluation of hemodynamic responses in head injury patients with transcranial Doppler monitoring. Acta Neurochir (Wien) 139: 804–817.

Nortje J, Coles JP, Timofeev I et al. (2008). Effect of hyperoxia on regional oxygenation and metabolism after severe traumatic brain injury: preliminary findings. Crit Care Med. 36 (1): 273–281.

Nyam TTE, Ao KH, Hung SY et al. (2017). FOUR Score predicts early outcome in patients after traumatic brain Injury. Neurocrit Care, in press.

O'Boynick CP, Kurd MF, Darden 2nd BV et al. (2014). Timing of surgery in thoracolumbar trauma: is early intervention safe? Neurosurg Focus 37: E7.

Oddo M, Schmidt JM, Carrera E et al. (2008). Impact of tight glycemic control on cerebral glucose metabolism after severe brain injury: a microdialysis study. Crit Care Med 36: 3233–3238.

Oddo M, Bosel J, Participants in the International Multidisciplinary Consensus Conference on Multimodality Monitoring (2014). Monitoring of brain and systemic oxygenation in neurocritical care patients. Neurocrit Care 21 (Suppl 2): S103–S120.

Oddo M, Crippa IA, Mehta S et al. (2016). Optimizing sedation in patients with acute brain injury. Crit Care 20: 128.

Oertel M, Boscardin WJ, Obrist WD et al. (2005). Posttraumatic vasospasm: the epidemiology, severity, and time course of an underestimated phenomenon: a prospective study performed in 299 patients. J Neurosurg 103: 812–824.

Okasha AS, Fayed AM, Saleh AS (2014). The FOUR score predicts mortality, endotracheal intubation and ICU length of stay after traumatic brain injury. Neurocrit Care 21: 496–504.

Okonkwo DO, Yue JK, Puccio AM et al. (2013). GFAP-BDP as an acute diagnostic marker in traumatic brain injury: results from the prospective transforming research and clinical knowledge in traumatic brain injury study. J Neurotrauma 30: 1490–1497.

O'Leary R, Hutchinson PJ, Menon D (2016). Hypothermia for Intracranial Hypertension after Traumatic Brain Injury. N Engl J Med 374: 1383–1384.

Olivecrona M, Zetterlund B, Rodling-Wahlstrom M et al. (2009). Absence of electroencephalographic seizure activity in patients treated for head injury with an intracranial pressure-targeted therapy. J Neurosurg 110: 300–305.

Pajoumand M, Kufera JA, Bonds BW et al. (2016). Dexmedetomidine as an adjunct for sedation in patients with traumatic brain injury. J Trauma Acute Care Surg 81: 345–351.

Papa L, Lewis LM, Falk JL et al. (2012). Elevated levels of serum glial fibrillary acidic protein breakdown products in mild and moderate traumatic brain injury are associated with intracranial lesions and neurosurgical intervention. Ann Emerg Med 59: 471–483.

Pape HC, Tornetta 3rd P, Tarkin I et al. (2009). Timing of fracture fixation in multitrauma patients: the role of early total care and damage control surgery. J Am Acad Orthop Surg 17: 541–549.

Parizel PM, Van Goethem JW, Ozsarlak O et al. (2005). New developments in the neuroradiological diagnosis of craniocerebral trauma. Eur Radiol 15: 569–581.

Parkin M, Hopwood S, Jones DA et al. (2005). Dynamic changes in brain glucose and lactate in pericontusional areas of the human cerebral cortex, monitored with rapid sampling on-line microdialysis: relationship with depolarisation-like events. J Cereb Blood Flow Metab 25: 402–413.

Pasco A, Ter Minassian A, Chapon C et al. (2006). Dynamics of cerebral edema and the apparent diffusion coefficient of water changes in patients with severe traumatic brain injury. A prospective MRI study. Eur Radiol 16: 1501–1508.

Patel HC, Menon DK, Tebbs S et al. (2002). Specialist neurocritical care and outcome from head injury. Intensive Care Med 28: 547–553.

Patel HC, Bouamra O, Woodford M et al. (2005). Trends in head injury outcome from 1989 to 2003 and the effect of neurosurgical care: an observational study. Lancet 366: 1538–1544.

Pelinka LE, Kroepfl A, Leixnering M et al. (2004). GFAP versus S100B in serum after traumatic brain injury: relationship to brain damage and outcome. J Neurotrauma 21: 1553–1561.

Perel P, Edwards P, Wentz R et al. (2006). Systematic review of prognostic models in traumatic brain injury. BMC Med Inform Decis Mak 6: 38.

Perel P, Al-Shahi Salman R, Kawahara T et al. (2012). CRASH-2 (Clinical Randomisation of an Antifibrinolytic in Significant Haemorrhage) intracranial bleeding study: the effect of tranexamic acid in traumatic brain injury – a nested randomised, placebo-controlled trial. Health Technol Assess 16: iii–xii. 1–54.

Peterson EC, Chesnut RM (2011). Talk and die revisited: bifrontal contusions and late deterioration. J Trauma 71: 1588–1592.

Ponsford J, McLaren A, Schonberger M et al. (2011). The association between apolipoprotein E and traumatic brain injury severity and functional outcome in a rehabilitation sample. J Neurotrauma 28: 1683–1692.

Pretz CR, Dams-O'Connor K (2013). Longitudinal description of the Glasgow Outcome Scale-Extended for individuals in the traumatic brain injury model systems national database: a National Institute on Disability and Rehabilitation Research traumatic brain injury model systems study. Arch Phys Med Rehabil 94: 2486–2493.

Price L, Wilson C, Grant G (2015). Blood–brain barrier pathophysiology following traumatic brain injury. Translational Research in Traumatic Brain Injury. CRC Press, Boca Raton, FL.

Pugh MJ, Orman JA, Jaramillo CA et al. (2015). The prevalence of epilepsy and association with traumatic brain injury in veterans of the Afghanistan and Iraq wars. J Head Trauma Rehabil 30: 29–37.

Puljula J, Vaaramo K, Tetri S et al. (2016). Risk for all-cause and traumatic death in head trauma subjects: a prospective population-based case-control follow-up study. Ann Surg 263: 1235–1239.

Raymont V, Greathouse A, Reding K et al. (2008). Demographic, structural and genetic predictors of late cognitive decline after penetrating head injury. Brain 131: 543–558.

Reilly PL, Graham DI, Adams JH et al. (1975). Patients with head injury who talk and die. Lancet 2: 375–377.

Riker RR, Fugate JEParticipants in the International Multidisciplinary Consensus Conference on Multimodality Monitoring (2014). Clinical monitoring scales in acute brain injury: assessment of coma, pain, agitation, and delirium. Neurocrit Care 21 (Suppl 2): S27–S37.

Rincon F, Kang J, Vibbert M et al. (2014). Significance of arterial hyperoxia and relationship with case fatality in traumatic brain injury: a multicentre cohort study. J Neurol Neurosurg Psychiatry 85 (7): 799–805.

Rizk EB, Patel AS, Stetter CM et al. (2011). Impact of tracheostomy timing on outcome after severe head injury. Neurocrit Care 15: 481–489.

Roberts I, Sydenham E (2012). Barbiturates for acute traumatic brain injury. Cochrane Database Syst Rev 12: Cd000033.

Robertson CS, Valadka AB, Hannay HJ et al. (1999). Prevention of secondary ischemic insults after severe head injury. Crit Care Med 27: 2086–2095.

Robertson CS, Hannay HJ, Yamal JM et al. (2014). Effect of erythropoietin and transfusion threshold on neurological recovery after traumatic brain injury: a randomized clinical trial. JAMA 312: 36–47.

Rockswold SB, Rockswold GL, Zaun DA et al. (2013). A prospective, randomized Phase II clinical trial to evaluate the effect of combined hyperbaric and normobaric hyperoxia on cerebral metabolism, intracranial pressure, oxygen toxicity, and clinical outcome in severe traumatic brain injury. J Neurosurg. 118 (6): 1317–1328.

Romner B, Bellner J, Kongstad P et al. (1996). Elevated transcranial Doppler flow velocities after severe head injury: cerebral vasospasm or hyperemia? J Neurosurg 85: 90–97.

Ronne-Engstrom E, Winkler T (2006). Continuous EEG monitoring in patients with traumatic brain injury reveals a high incidence of epileptiform activity. Acta Neurol Scand 114: 47–53.

Roozenbeek B, Lingsma HF, Perel P et al. (2011). The added value of ordinal analysis in clinical trials: an example in traumatic brain injury. Crit Care 15: R127.

Roozenbeek B, Maas AI, Menon DK (2013). Changing patterns in the epidemiology of traumatic brain injury. Nat Rev Neurol 9: 231–236.

Rosenthal G, Hemphill 3rd JC, Sorani M et al. (2008). Brain tissue oxygen tension is more indicative of oxygen diffusion than oxygen delivery and metabolism in patients with traumatic brain injury. Crit Care Med 36: 1917–1924.

Rostami E (2014). Glucose and the injured brain-monitored in the neurointensive care unit. Front Neurol 5: 91.

Rostami E, Engquist H, Enblad P (2014). Imaging of cerebral blood flow in patients with severe traumatic brain injury in the neurointensive care. Front Neurol 5: 114.

Ryu JH, Walcott BP, Kahle KT et al. (2013). Induced and sustained hypernatremia for the prevention and treatment of cerebral edema following brain injury. Neurocrit Care 19: 222–231.

Saatman KE, Duhaime AC, Bullock R et al. (2008). Classification of traumatic brain injury for targeted therapies. J Neurotrauma 25: 719–738.

Sacho RH, Vail A, Rainey T et al. (2010). The effect of spontaneous alterations in brain temperature on outcome: a prospective observational cohort study in patients with severe traumatic brain injury. J Neurotrauma 27: 2157–2164.

Sadaka F, Patel D, Lakshmanan R (2012). The FOUR score predicts outcome in patients after traumatic brain injury. Neurocrit Care 16: 95–101.

Sanchez-Izquierdo-Riera JA, Caballero-Cubedo RE, Perez-Vela JL et al. (1998). Propofol versus midazolam: safety and efficacy for sedating the severe trauma patient. Anesth Analg 86: 1219–1224.

Sarrafzadeh AS, Peltonen EE, Kaisers U et al. (2001). Secondary insults in severe head injury – do multiply injured patients do worse? Crit Care Med 29: 1116–1123.

Saxena M, Andrews PJ, Cheng A et al. (2014). Modest cooling therapies (35 masculineC to 37.5 masculineC) for traumatic brain injury. Cochrane Database Syst Rev: Cd006811.

Schaible EV, Thal SC (2013). Anticoagulation in patients with traumatic brain injury. Curr Opin Anaesthesiol 26: 529–534.

Schochl H, Solomon C, Traintinger S et al. (2011). Thromboelastometric (ROTEM) findings in patients suffering from isolated severe traumatic brain injury. J Neurotrauma 28: 2033–2041.

Seel RT, Douglas J, Dennison AC et al. (2013). Specialized early treatment for persons with disorders of consciousness: program components and outcomes. Arch Phys Med Rehabil 94: 1908–1923.

Shafer A (1998). Complications of sedation with midazolam in the intensive care unit and a comparison with other sedative regimens. Crit Care Med 26: 947–956.

Sharshar T, Citerio G, Andrews PJ et al. (2014). Neurological examination of critically ill patients: a pragmatic approach. Report of an ESICM expert panel. Intensive Care Med 40: 484–495.

Shen X, Dutcher SK, Palmer J et al. (2015). A systematic review of the benefits and risks of anticoagulation following traumatic brain injury. J Head Trauma Rehabil 30: E29–E37.

Shively S, Scher AI, Perl DP et al. (2012). Dementia resulting from traumatic brain injury: what is the pathology? Arch Neurol 69: 1245–1251.

Shlosberg D, Benifla M, Kaufer D et al. (2010). Blood–brain barrier breakdown as a therapeutic target in traumatic brain injury. Nat Rev Neurol 6: 393–403.

Signorini DF, Andrews PJ, Jones PA et al. (1999). Adding insult to injury: the prognostic value of early secondary insults for survival after traumatic brain injury. J Neurol Neurosurg Psychiatry 66: 26–31.

Simard JM, Woo SK, Schwartzbauer GT et al. (2012). Sulfonylurea receptor 1 in central nervous system injury: a focused review. J Cereb Blood Flow Metab 32: 1699–1717.

Smith MJ, Stiefel MF, Magge S et al. (2005). Packed red blood cell transfusion increases local cerebral oxygenation. Crit Care Med 33: 1104–1108.

Smith DH, Johnson VE, Stewart W (2013). Chronic neuropathologies of single and repetitive TBI: substrates of dementia? Nat Rev Neurol 9: 211–221.

Sorrentino E, Budohoski KP, Kasprowicz M et al. (2011). Critical thresholds for transcranial Doppler indices of cerebral autoregulation in traumatic brain injury. Neurocrit Care 14: 188–193.

Sorrentino E, Diedler J, Kasprowicz M et al. (2012). Critical thresholds for cerebrovascular reactivity after traumatic brain injury. Neurocrit Care 16: 258–266.

Spahn DR, Bouillon B, Cerny V et al. (2013). Management of bleeding and coagulopathy following major trauma: an updated European guideline. Crit Care 17: R76.

Stein DM, Hu PF, Brenner M et al. (2011). Brief episodes of intracranial hypertension and cerebral hypoperfusion are associated with poor functional outcome after severe traumatic brain injury. J Trauma 71: 364–373. discussion 373–364.

Stein DM, Lindell AL, Murdock KR et al. (2012). Use of serum biomarkers to predict cerebral hypoxia after severe traumatic brain injury. J Neurotrauma 29: 1140–1149.

Steiner LA, Czosnyka M, Piechnik SK et al. (2002). Continuous monitoring of cerebrovascular pressure reactivity allows determination of optimal cerebral perfusion pressure in patients with traumatic brain injury. Crit Care Med 30: 733–738.

Steiner LA, Balestreri M, Johnston AJ et al. (2004). Sustained moderate reductions in arterial $CO_2$ after brain trauma time-course of cerebral blood flow velocity and intracranial pressure. Intensive Care Med. 30 (12): 2180–2187.

Steiner LA, Balestreri M, Johnston AJ et al. (2005). Predicting the response of intracranial pressure to moderate hyperventilation. Acta Neurochir (Wien). 147 (5): 477–483; discussion 483.

Stevens RD, Hannawi Y, Puybasset L (2014). MRI for coma emergence and recovery. Curr Opin Crit Care 20: 168–173.

Steyerberg EW, Mushkudiani N, Perel P et al. (2008). Predicting outcome after traumatic brain injury: development and international validation of prognostic scores based on admission characteristics. PLoS Med 5: e165. discussion e165.

Stocchetti N, Furlan A, Volta F (1996). Hypoxemia and arterial hypotension at the accident scene in head injury. J Trauma 40: 764–767.

Stocchetti N, Zanaboni C, Colombo A et al. (2008). Refractory intracranial hypertension and "second-tier" therapies in traumatic brain injury. Intensive Care Med 34: 461–467.

Stocchetti N, Paterno R, Citerio G et al. (2012). Traumatic brain injury in an aging population. J Neurotrauma 29: 1119–1125.

Strong AJ, Fabricius M, Boutelle MG et al. (2002). Spreading and synchronous depressions of cortical activity in acutely injured human brain. Stroke 33: 2738–2743.

Su SH, Wang F, Hai J et al. (2014). The effects of intracranial pressure monitoring in patients with traumatic brain injury. PLoS One 9: e87432.

Taher A, Pilehvari Z, Poorolajal J et al. (2016). Effects of Normobaric Hyperoxia in Traumatic Brain Injury: A Randomized Controlled Clinical Trial. Trauma Mon. 21 (1): e26772.

Takano T, Tian GF, Peng W et al. (2007). Cortical spreading depression causes and coincides with tissue hypoxia. Nat Neurosci 10: 754–762.

Teasdale G, Jennett B (1974). Assessment of coma and impaired consciousness. A practical scale. Lancet 2: 81–84.

Teasdale GM, Nicoll JA, Murray G et al. (1997). Association of apolipoprotein E polymorphism with outcome after head injury. Lancet 350: 1069–1071.

Teasdale GM, Murray GD, Nicoll JA (2005). The association between APOE epsilon4, age and outcome after head injury: a prospective cohort study. Brain 128: 2556–2561.

Teasdale G, Maas A, Lecky F et al. (2014). The Glasgow Coma Scale at 40 years: standing the test of time. Lancet Neurol 13: 844–854.

Tepas JJ, Pracht EE, Orban BL et al. (2013). High-volume trauma centers have better outcomes treating traumatic brain injury. J Trauma Acute Care Surg 74: 143–147. discussion 147–148.

The Acute Respiratory Distress Syndrome Network (2000). Ventilation with lower tidal volumes as compared with traditional tidal volumes for acute lung injury and the acute respiratory distress syndrome. N Engl J Med 342: 1301–1308.

Timofeev I, Carpenter KL, Nortje J et al. (2011). Cerebral extracellular chemistry and outcome following traumatic brain injury: a microdialysis study of 223 patients. Brain 134: 484–494.

Turner-Stokes L (2014). Prolonged disorders of consciousness: new national clinical guidelines from the Royal College of Physicians, London. Clin Med (Lond) 14: 4–5.

Unden L, Calcagnile O, Unden J et al. (2015). Validation of the Scandinavian guidelines for initial management of minimal, mild and moderate traumatic brain injury in adults. BMC Med 13: 292.

Uzan M, Tanriverdi T, Baykara O et al. (2005). Association between interleukin-1 beta (IL-1beta) gene polymorphism and outcome after head injury: an early report. Acta Neurochir (Wien) 147: 715–720. discussion 720.

Vale FL, Burns J, Jackson AB et al. (1997). Combined medical and surgical treatment after acute spinal cord injury: results of a prospective pilot study to assess the merits of aggressive medical resuscitation and blood pressure management. J Neurosurg 87: 239–246.

Vallier HA, Wang X, Moore TA et al. (2013). Timing of orthopaedic surgery in multiple trauma patients: development of a protocol for early appropriate care. J Orthop Trauma 27: 543–551.

Van Beek JG, Mushkudiani NA, Steyerberg EW et al. (2007). Prognostic value of admission laboratory parameters in traumatic brain injury: results from the IMPACT study. J Neurotrauma 24: 315–328.

Van den Berghe G, Schoonheydt K, Becx P et al. (2005). Insulin therapy protects the central and peripheral nervous system of intensive care patients. Neurology 64: 1348–1353.

Vedantam A, Yamal JM, Rubin ML et al. (2016). Progressive hemorrhagic injury after severe traumatic brain injury: effect of hemoglobin transfusion thresholds. J Neurosurg 1–6.

Veenith TV, Carter EL, Grossac J et al. (2014). Use of diffusion tensor imaging to assess the impact of normobaric hyperoxia within at-risk pericontusional tissue after traumatic brain injury. J Cereb Blood Flow Metab. 34 (10): 1622–1627.

Verweij BH, Muizelaar JP, Vinas FC et al. (2000). Impaired cerebral mitochondrial function after traumatic brain injury in humans. J Neurosurg 93: 815–820.

Vespa PM (2016). Brain hypoxia and ischemia after traumatic brain injury: is oxygen the right metabolic target? JAMA Neurol 73: 504–505.

Vespa PM, McArthur D, O'Phelan K et al. (2003). Persistently low extracellular glucose correlates with poor outcome 6 months after human traumatic brain injury despite a lack of increased lactate: a microdialysis study. J Cereb Blood Flow Metab 23: 865–877.

Vespa P, Bergsneider M, Hattori N et al. (2005). Metabolic crisis without brain ischemia is common after traumatic brain injury: a combined microdialysis and positron emission tomography study. J Cereb Blood Flow Metab 25: 763–774.

Vespa PM, McArthur DL, Xu Y et al. (2010). Nonconvulsive seizures after traumatic brain injury are associated with hippocampal atrophy. Neurology 75: 792–798.

Vik A, Nag T, Fredriksli OA et al. (2008). Relationship of "dose" of intracranial hypertension to outcome in severe traumatic brain injury. J Neurosurg 109: 678–684.

Vitek MP, Brown CM, Colton CA (2009). APOE genotype-specific differences in the innate immune response. Neurobiol Aging 30: 1350–1360.

von Steinbuchel N, Wilson L, Gibbons H et al. (2010). Quality of Life after Brain Injury (QOLIBRI): scale validity and correlates of quality of life. J Neurotrauma 27: 1157–1165.

Vos PE, Lamers KJ, Hendriks JC et al. (2004). Glial and neuronal proteins in serum predict outcome after severe traumatic brain injury. Neurology 62: 1303–1310.

Wafaisade A, Lefering R, Tjardes T et al. (2010a). Acute coagulopathy in isolated blunt traumatic brain injury. Neurocrit Care 12: 211–219.

Wafaisade A, Wutzler S, Lefering R et al. (2010b). Drivers of acute coagulopathy after severe trauma: a multivariate analysis of 1987 patients. Emerg Med J 27: 934–939.

Wang HK, Lu K, Liliang PC et al. (2012). The impact of tracheostomy timing in patients with severe head injury: an observational cohort study. Injury 43: 1432–1436.

Warner MA, O'Keeffe T, Bhavsar P et al. (2010). Transfusions and long-term functional outcomes in traumatic brain injury. J Neurosurg 113: 539–546.

Washington PM, Villapol S, Burns MP (2016). Polypathology and dementia after brain trauma: does brain injury trigger distinct neurodegenerative diseases, or should they be classified together as traumatic encephalopathy? Exp Neurol 275 (Pt 3): 381–388.

Waters RJ, Murray GD, Teasdale GM et al. (2013). Cytokine gene polymorphisms and outcome after traumatic brain injury. J Neurotrauma 30: 1710–1716.

WHO (2006). Neurological disorders: public health challenges, Switzerland, World Health Organization, Geneva.

Wijdicks EF, Bamlet WR, Maramattom BV et al. (2005). Validation of a new coma scale: the FOUR score. Ann Neurol 58: 585–593.

Willmott C, Ponsford J, McAllister TW et al. (2013). Effect of COMT Val158Met genotype on attention and response to methylphenidate following traumatic brain injury. Brain Inj 27: 1281–1286.

Winkler EA, Yue JK, McAllister TW et al. (2016). COMT Val 158 Met polymorphism is associated with nonverbal cognition following mild traumatic brain injury. Neurogenetics 17: 31–41.

Wunsch H, Angus DC, Harrison DA et al. (2011). Comparison of medical admissions to intensive care units in the United States and United Kingdom. Am J Respir Crit Care Med 183: 1666–1673.

Xu JC, Shen J, Shao WZ et al. (2016). The safety and efficacy of levetiracetam versus phenytoin for seizure prophylaxis after traumatic brain injury: a systematic review and meta-analysis. Brain Inj 1–8.

Yamal JM, Rubin ML, Benoit JS et al. (2015). Effect of hemoglobin transfusion threshold on cerebral hemodynamics and oxygenation. J Neurotrauma 32: 1239–1245.

Yanamadala V, Walcott BP, Fecci PE et al. (2014). Reversal of warfarin associated coagulopathy with 4-factor prothrombin complex concentrate in traumatic brain injury and intracranial hemorrhage. J Clin Neurosci 21: 1881–1884.

Yuan Q, Wu X, Sun Y et al. (2015). Impact of intracranial pressure monitoring on mortality in patients with traumatic brain injury: a systematic review and meta-analysis. J Neurosurg 122: 574–587.

Yue JK, Pronger AM, Ferguson AR et al. (2015). Association of a common genetic variant within ANKK1 with six-month cognitive performance after traumatic brain injury. Neurogenetics 16: 169–180.

Zygun DA, Nortje J, Hutchinson PJ et al. (2009). The effect of red blood cell transfusion on cerebral oxygenation and metabolism after severe traumatic brain injury. Crit Care Med 37: 1074–1078.

*Handbook of Clinical Neurology*, Vol. 140 (3rd series)
*Critical Care Neurology, Part I*
E.F.M. Wijdicks and A.H. Kramer, Editors
http://dx.doi.org/10.1016/B978-0-444-63600-3.00015-5

Chapter 15

# Management of acute traumatic spinal cord injuries

C.D. SHANK, B.C. WALTERS, AND M.N. HADLEY*

*Department of Neurosurgery, University of Alabama, Birmingham, AL, USA*

## Abstract

Acute traumatic spinal cord injury (SCI) is a devastating disease process affecting tens of thousands of people across the USA each year. Despite the increase in primary prevention measures, such as educational programs, motor vehicle speed limits, automobile running lights, and safety technology that includes automobile passive restraint systems and airbags, SCIs continue to carry substantial permanent morbidity and mortality. Medical measures implemented following the initial injury are designed to limit secondary insult to the spinal cord and to stabilize the spinal column in an attempt to decrease devastating sequelae.

This chapter is an overview of the contemporary management of an acute traumatic SCI patient from the time of injury through the stay in the intensive care unit. We discuss initial triage, immobilization, and transportation of the patient by emergency medical services personnel to a definitive treatment facility. Upon arrival at the emergency department, we review initial trauma protocols and the evidence-based recommendations for radiographic evaluation of the patient's vertebral column. Finally, we outline closed cervical spine reduction and various aggressive medical therapies aimed at improving neurologic outcome.

## EPIDEMIOLOGY

Each year, accidents rank among the most common causes of death in the USA. While early trauma-associated mortality is overwhelmingly due to exsanguination, cardiovascular collapse, and respiratory insufficiency, neurologic injury, including spinal cord injury (SCI), continues to be a common cause of disability and late trauma-associated mortality (American College of Surgeons, 2012).

There are approximately 14 000 traumatic SCIs annually in the USA. While the rate of traumatic SCI differs based on geography and time of year, the demographics of this group in large part mirror that of the general trauma population. Patients who sustain traumatic SCIs tend to be young and predominantly male. Indeed, males have a traumatic SCI rate up to 20 times higher than that of age-matched females. Within this subpopulation, motor vehicle accidents represent the single most

common mechanism. While all levels of the spinal column are at risk of injury, especially in the absence of appropriate restraints, the cervical spine is the most commonly affected region. Unfortunately, cervical spinal injuries have the highest rate of associated cord injury and of associated morbidity and mortality (Hadley et al., 2002; Hadley and Walters, 2013; Vollmer et al., 2011).

Over the preceding decades and in large part due to the aging population, there has been an increase in geriatric SCIs. In contrast to the younger trauma population, there does not appear to be a difference in the relative rate of injury in elderly men versus women. The mechanism of injury differs based on age. Within this elderly subpopulation, falls are implicated in the vast majority of cases. The presence of underlying cervical spondylosis and spinal stenosis may potentiate a significant SCI even in the absence of bony or ligamentous disruption. The cervical spine continues to be the most commonly

---

*Correspondence to: Mark N. Hadley, M.D., 510 20th Street South, FOT 1030, Birmingham AL 35294-3410, USA. Tel: +1-205-934-1439, Fax: +1-205-975-6081, E-mail: mhadley@uabmc.edu

affected region, and while the overall rate of traumatic SCI is significantly lower in this elderly subpopulation than in younger persons, their advanced age and medical comorbidities result in an overall higher mortality (Vollmer et al., 2011).

Despite the advent of motor vehicle passive restraint systems and other primary prevention techniques, SCI continues to result in substantial morbidity and mortality. With the introduction of contemporary spinal instrumentation, there has been considerable advancement in the surgical treatment of spinal fractures, spinal instability, and SCI. Simultaneously, over the past half-century, there has been a substantial improvement in the nonsurgical care of SCI patients in the prehospital, emergency room, and intensive care unit (ICU) settings.

Improvements in SCI care (and outcomes) have been in large part due to the propagation of evidence-based guidelines, the formation of organized trauma networks, timeliness of transport to treatment institutions, and improvements in critical care medicine (Tator et al., 1984, 1993; Burney et al., 1989). Improved emergency medical response systems have resulted in more rapid recovery and triage of patients at the scene of the accident. Patients with potential SCIs are more efficiently transported to appropriate treatment centers, and their evaluation and stabilization are carried out in a timely, organized, and methodical manner. Many centers now have specialty-specific ICUs, including those specifically designed for care of patients with acute traumatic SCI. These ICUs are staffed with critical care specialists, neurosurgeons, and neurologists who have specific training in contemporary SCI management. This chapter is a contemporary overview of the nonsurgical care of the acute traumatic SCI patient for the neurointensivist (Table 15.1).

## Table 15.1

**Ten key steps in the management of a patient with acute traumatic spinal cord injury (SCI)**

1. Resuscitate, immobilize at scene
2. Rapid transport to nearest definitive SCI care facility
3. ABCs, MAP management (85 mmHg)
4. No steroids
5. Image (CT study of choice)
6. Promptly realign cervical spine (closed vs. open reduction)
7. Immobilize
8. Maintain MAP perfusion parameters
9. MRI for mass lesion, extent of cord injury
10. Operative decompression early – may delay for stabilization only

ABCs, airway, breathing, circulation; MAP, mean arterial pressure; CT, computed tomography; MRI, magnetic resonance imaging.

# CLINICAL PRESENTATION AND PREHOSPITAL MANAGEMENT

## Field triage and spine clearance

The critical care of the patient with a potential acute traumatic SCI should begin at the scene of the accident, long before the patient arrives in the emergency room. Because up to 25% of SCIs occur after the initial incident, the early management of patients with known or suspected SCIs involves initial resuscitation, rapid triage, and spinal immobilization as judged necessary by first responders (Geisler et al., 1966; Hachen, 1974a; Burney et al., 1989; Prasad et al., 1999). Spinal immobilization is intended to prevent further pathologic motion of potentially unstable vertebral segments in an attempt to prevent further spinal cord or root compression and to minimize the ultimate neurologic deficit.

The primary concern of contemporary first responders in patients with suspected SCI is safe extraction from the site of the accident, initial resuscitation, and rapid determination of the likelihood of SCI (Kossuth, 1965; Farrington, 1968; Rimel et al., 1981; Moylan, 1985; Toscano, 1988). Contemporary initial assessment of patients with acute SCI has been studied in great detail. Class I medical evidence exists in support of trained emergency medical services (EMS) personnel utilizing specific spinal injury protocols to determine the need for immobilization (Kossuth, 1965; Farrington, 1968; San Mateo County, 1991; Brown et al., 1998; Stroh and Braude, 2001; Burton et al., 2006).

All EMS personnel now go through extensive training to recognize and immobilize patients with the potential for SCI. While EMS policies may differ, many services utilize some variation of the spine immobilization protocol described in Table 15.2 (San Mateo County, 1991). Well-trained EMS personnel and accurate implementation of defined, reliable, and validated spinal clearance protocols have resulted in improvement in the initial neurologic status of acute SCI patients on arrival to the emergency departments of definitive acute SCI treatment facilities (Gunby, 1981; Green et al., 1987).

## Table 15.2

**Emergency medical services cervical spine clearance criteria**

No spinal pain or tenderness
No significant multiple-system trauma
No significant head or facial trauma
No extremity neurologic deficit
No loss of consciousness
No altered mental status
No known or suspected intoxication
No significant distracting injury

## Complications of spinal immobilization

Despite its obvious potential benefits, spinal immobilization is not without risk (Liew and Hill, 1994). Even correct immobilization may be associated with increased pain in an awake trauma patient (Cordell et al., 1995) and may be difficult to implement in some patients with combined head and neck injuries. Appropriate spinal immobilization takes time to apply and could potentially delay transport.

Several authors have evaluated the potential morbidity (and mortality) associated with spinal immobilization (Podolsky et al., 1983; Linares et al., 1987; Bauer and Kowalski, 1988; Mawson et al., 1988; Schafermeyer et al., 1991; Hewitt, 1994; Blaylock, 1996; Davies et al., 1996; Black et al., 1998; Kolb et al., 1999; Totten and Sugarman, 1999; Thumbikat et al., 2007).

When left in place too long, spinal immobilization may result in pressure ulcers. (Linares et al., 1987; Mawson et al., 1988; Hewitt, 1994; Blaylock, 1996; Black et al., 1998). Entire spinal column and body restraints may limit respiratory function and be associated with higher rates of aspiration. Respiratory indices, including vital capacity, are reduced by spinal immobilization methods in both adults and children. (Bauer and Kowalski, 1988; Schafermeyer et al., 1991; Totten and Sugarman, 1999).

Use of hard cervical collars has been associated with elevations in intracranial pressure (ICP). Davies et al. (1996) reported a mean increase in ICP of 4.5 mmHg when utilizing properly fitted cervical collars. Kolb et al. (1999) subsequently reported a similar increase in ICP utilizing a different rigid cervical collar, but questioned the clinical importance of this degree of elevation.

Patients with associated medical comorbidities may be at particularly increased risk of spine immobilization-related morbidity, including those with ankylosing spondylitis (Podolsky et al., 1983; Thumbikat et al., 2007).

Patients with penetrating neck trauma are at increased risk with the use of cervical immobilization devices. Haut et al. (2010) reported that patients who were immobilized for penetrating neck trauma were twice as likely to die compared to those who were not immobilized. It was argued that the time necessary to properly immobilize such patients might delay their resuscitation and contribute to increased morbidity or mortality. The overwhelming number of penetrating neck injuries do not result in spinal instability, therefore, routine cervical spine immobilization in patients with significant penetrating neck trauma is not recommended.

Because spinal immobilization may cause complications, robust medical evidence supports the concept that it should not be utilized in trauma patients who are cleared by trained EMS personnel using vetted spinal clearance protocols, or in those who have known contraindications to immobilization (Theodore et al., 2013b).

## Methods of spinal immobilization

Acute trauma patients who do not meet the criteria for clearance of the cervical spine in the field and who do not have a specific contraindication are placed in full spinal precautions. At present, no single immobilization device has been found to be superior. Cline et al. (1985) published on the historic use of a soft collar and rolled-up blankets compared to several newer immobilization methods, and found that none were superior to the short-board method. De Lorenzo, evaluated a more rigid immobilization technique using a hard collar (De Lorenzo, 1996). Podolsky et al. (1983) corroborated the superiority of hard foam and plastic collars compared to soft collars for immobilization. McCabe and Nolan (1986) found that a polyethylene-1 collar provides the most restriction in flexion only. Rosen et al. (1992) compared four different cervical collars and reported that vacuum split collars were the most effective in restricting neck range of motion. Finally, Del Rossi et al. (2004) evaluated several cervical collars utilizing a cadaveric model. They found that manual inline stabilization, rather than cervical collar type, remained the most effective cervical immobilization.

While no single device has been found to be superior for spinal immobilization after spinal column trauma, the American College of Surgeons Advanced Trauma Life Support guidelines (2012) recommend a rigid backboard in conjunction with a hard cervical collar and tape or straps to immobilize the entire patient. These methods are recommended over the historic, long-standing practice of sandbag immobilization of the head and neck, since heavy sandbags may shift or slide against the patient's neck during transport, despite attempted long board immobilization (American College of Surgeons, 2012; Theodore et al., 2013b).

## Transportation of the patient

Comprehensive SCI care cannot be provided at the scene of the accident. After extraction, initial resuscitation, triage, and immobilization, EMS personnel are charged with rapid and safe transport of the patient to a treatment facility equipped to treat acute SCI. Transport options over long distances include traditional ground ambulance, as well as helicopter and fixed-wing aircraft. Several authors have compared the mode and timing of transportation of acute SCI patients and their potential effect on outcomes. The consensus from these studies is that the exact method of transportation is less important than ensuring rapid and safe transport to the nearest facility capable of definitive SCI care (Hachen, 1974a, b, 1977; Tator et al., 1984, 1993; Boyd et al., 1989; Burney et al., 1989).

A corollary to the call for rapid transport of patients to definitive treatment facilities is the argument for the creation of designated acute traumatic SCI centers. DeVivo et al. (2002) compared SCI patients transferred early for definitive care to those transferred to their center later for rehabilitation purposes, and reported improved neurologic outcomes, a significant reduction in the length of acute hospital stay, as well as a significant decrease in pressure ulcer rates in those patients transferred early. Opponents of centralized treatment argue that specialized SCI treatment centers are, in general, self-designated as such. At present there is no governing body to regulate such designations. At the heart of the debate is the tenuous and elusive definition of a "definitive treatment center" and whether that center is operationally consistent 24 hours a day, 365 days a year. Rapid transfer of acute traumatic SCI patients to definitive treatment centers is supported by multiple class III studies, and currently represents a level III recommendation by the American Association of Neurological Surgeons (AANS) and the Congress of Neurological Surgeons (CNS) (Theodore et al., 2013a).

## HOSPITAL COURSE AND MANAGEMENT

### Initial hospital evaluation

Upon arrival to the acute SCI treatment facility, the patient is evaluated by emergency medicine, trauma surgery, and neurointensive care personnel. In accordance with established Advanced Trauma Life Support guidelines, the evaluation of trauma patients includes primary and secondary surveys, with adjunctive radiographic evaluation as deemed necessary, all carried out while maintaining spinal precautions. After attention to "ABC" stability, the team proceeds with a rapid assessment of neurologic status.

After determination of the patient's gross neurologic status (Table 15.3), attention is turned to the spinal

*Table 15.3*

**Initial neurological exam for patients with potential acute traumatic spinal cord injury**

| Initial neurologic exam |
| --- |
| Level and content of consciousness |
| Brainstem reflexes |
| Gross extremity movement |
| Gross sensation and potential sensory level |

evaluation. While maintaining inline cervical stabilization, as well as utilizing a log-roll maneuver to protect the thoracic and lumbar spinal segments, the patient's entire spinal column is assessed. Because of the noted complications associated with its prolonged use, the backboard is typically removed at this time.

The initial trauma evaluation provides insufficient information to ascertain the level and severity of a spinal column and/or SCI. Several assessment tools have been developed to classify the severity of SCI as well as the patient's functional neurologic status. These tools are designed to provide rapid, accurate, and reproducible measures for determining the presence and severity of SCI, as well as potential change in neurologic function over time (Hadley et al., 2013). The most valid, reliable, and widely used tools continue to be the American Spinal Injury Association (ASIA) scoring system and the ASIA Impairment Scale (AIS) (ASIA/IMSOP, 2000).

Trained trauma, emergency department, critical care, rehabilitation medicine, neurology, or neurosurgery practitioners typically carry out determination of the ASIA score and AIS grade. Practitioners should carefully perform the following: a detailed motor exam, including strength testing for each major muscle group in isolation; a light-touch modality sensory exam; and assessment for sacral root involvement by assessing rectal tone. The ASIA scale form (Fig. 15.1A) allows for rapid visualization of the level and severity of acute SCI, and can then be used for longitudinal assessment of improvement over time. The components of the neurologic exam using the ASIA scale are then compiled and an AIS score is derived (Fig. 15.1B). The ability to perform an accurate examination on an acute SCI patient can be influenced by confounding factors, such as level of consciousness, age, intoxication, and associated injuries (Burns et al., 2003).

Historically, a variety of neurologic assessment scales have been used to describe patients with acute traumatic SCI. The inconsistency and variety of these scales hampered both interprovider communication and research. Since 1996, the ASIA scale and AIS have become the most widely used descriptors of a patient's neurologic condition following acute SCI. Several authors have evaluated the reliability and validity of the 1996 and updated 2000 ASIA scale as a neurologic assessment tool. These multiple class I medical evidence studies support the use of the ASIA scale as the most valid and reliable means of determining neurologic loss following acute SCI (Kirshblum et al., 2002; Savic et al., 2007).

### Initial radiographic analysis

Immediately after initial evaluation and resuscitation of the acute SCI patient, a thoughtful approach to radiographic evaluation of the spine is needed. Appropriate

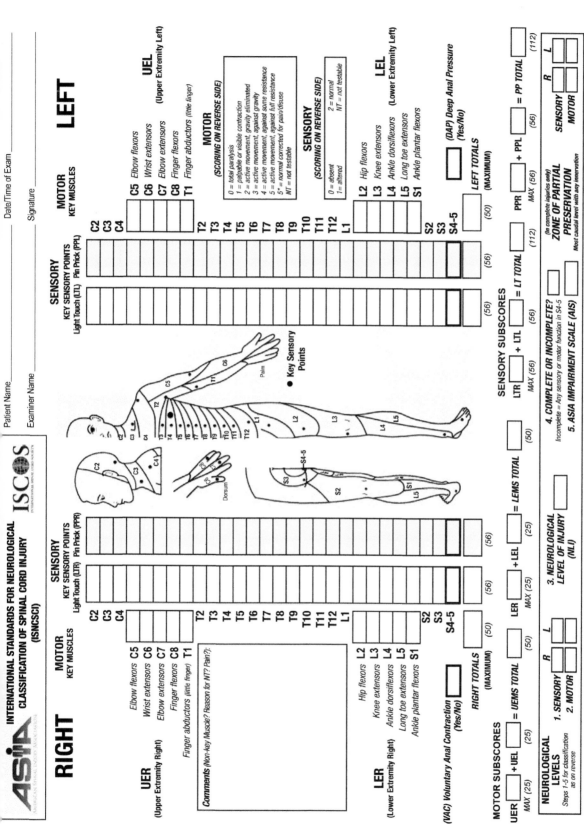

**Fig. 15.1 (A).** American Spinal Injury Association (ASIA) scale form.

## Muscle Function Grading

**0** = total paralysis

**1** = palpable or visible contraction

**2** = active movement, full range of motion (ROM) with gravity eliminated

**3** = active movement, full ROM against gravity

**4** = active movement, full ROM against gravity and moderate resistance in a muscle specific position

**5** = (normal) active movement, full ROM against gravity and full resistance in a functional muscle position expected from an otherwise unimpaired person

**5*** = (normal) active movement, full ROM against gravity and sufficient resistance to be considered normal if identified inhibiting factors (i.e. pain, disuse) were not present

**NT** = not testable (i.e. due to immobilization, severe pain such that the patient cannot be graded, amputation of limb, or contracture of > 50% of the normal ROM)

## Sensory Grading

**0** = Absent

**1** = Altered, either decreased/impaired sensation or hypersensitivity

**2** = Normal

**NT** = Not testable

## When to Test Non-Key Muscles:

In a patient with an apparent AIS B classification, non-key muscle functions more than 3 levels below the motor level on each side should be tested to most accurately classify the injury (differentiate between AIS B and C).

| Movement | Root level |
|---|---|
| Shoulder: Flexion, extension, abduction, adduction, internal and external rotation<br>Elbow: Supination | C5 |
| Elbow: Pronation<br>Wrist: Flexion | C6 |
| Finger: Flexion at proximal joint, extension.<br>Thumb: Flexion, extension and abduction in plane of thumb | C7 |
| Finger: Flexion at MCP joint<br>Thumb: Opposition, adduction and abduction perpendicular to palm | C8 |
| Finger: Abduction of the index finger | T1 |
| Hip: Adduction | L2 |
| Hip: External rotation | L3 |
| Hip: Extension, abduction, internal rotation<br>Knee: Flexion<br>Ankle: Inversion and eversion<br>Toe: MP and IP extension | L4 |
| Hallux and Toe: DIP and PIP flexion and abduction | L5 |
| Hallux: Adduction | S1 |

## ASIA Impairment Scale (AIS)

**A = Complete.** No sensory or motor function is preserved in the sacral segments S4-5.

**B = Sensory Incomplete.** Sensory but not motor function is preserved below the neurological level and includes the sacral segments S4-5 (light touch or pin prick at S4-5 or deep anal pressure) AND no motor function is preserved more than three levels below the motor level on either side of the body.

**C = Motor Incomplete.** Motor function is preserved at the most caudal sacral segments for voluntary anal contraction (VAC) OR the patient meets the criteria for sensory incomplete status (sensory function preserved at the most caudal sacral segments (S4-S5) by LT, PP or DAP), and has some sparing of motor function more than three levels below the ipsilateral motor level on either side of the body.

(This includes key or non-key muscle functions to determine motor incomplete status.) For AIS C – less than half of key muscle functions below the single NLI have a muscle grade ≥ 3.

**D = Motor Incomplete.** Motor incomplete status as defined above, with at least half (half or more) of key muscle functions below the single NLI having a muscle grade ≥ 3.

**E = Normal.** If sensation and motor function as tested with the ISNCSCI are graded as normal in all segments, and the patient had prior deficits, then the AIS grade is E. Someone without an initial SCI does not receive an AIS grade.

**Using ND:** To document the sensory, motor and NLI levels, the ASIA Impairment Scale grade, and/or the zone of partial preservation (ZPP) when they are unable to be determined based on the examination results.

## Steps in Classification

The following order is recommended for determining the classification of individuals with SCI.

**1. Determine sensory levels for right and left sides.**
The sensory level is the most caudal, intact dermatome for both pin prick and light touch sensation.

**2. Determine motor levels for right and left sides.**
Defined by the lowest key muscle function that has a grade of at least 3 (on supine testing), providing the key muscle functions represented by segments above that level are judged to be intact (graded as a 5).
Note: in regions where there is no myotome to test, the motor level is presumed to be the same as the sensory level, if testable motor function above that level is also normal.

**3. Determine the neurological level of injury (NLI)**
This refers to the most caudal segment of the cord with intact sensation and antigravity (3 or more) muscle function strength, provided that there is normal (intact) sensory and motor function rostrally respectively.
The NLI is the most cephalad of the sensory and motor levels determined in steps 1 and 2.

**4. Determine whether the injury is Complete or Incomplete.**
(i.e. absence or presence of sacral sparing)
If voluntary anal contraction = **No** AND all S4-5 sensory scores = **0** AND deep anal pressure = **No**, then injury is **Complete**. Otherwise, injury is **Incomplete**.

**5. Determine ASIA Impairment Scale (AIS) Grade:**

Is injury Complete?   If YES, AIS=A and can record ZPP (lowest dermatome or myotome on each side with some preservation)

NO ↓

Is injury Motor Complete?   If YES, AIS=B

NO ↓   (No=voluntary anal contraction OR motor function more than three levels below the motor level on a given side, if the patient has sensory incomplete classification)

Are at least half (half or more) of the key muscles below the neurological level of injury graded 3 or better?

NO ↓   YES ↓

AIS=C   AIS=D

If sensation and motor function is normal in all segments, **AIS=E**
Note: AIS E is used in follow-up testing when an individual with a documented SCI has recovered normal function. If at initial testing no deficits are found, the individual is neurologically intact; the ASIA Impairment Scale does not apply.

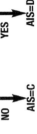

AMERICAN SPINAL INJURY ASSOCIATION

**INTERNATIONAL STANDARDS FOR NEUROLOGICAL CLASSIFICATION OF SPINAL CORD INJURY**

ISCOS
INTERNATIONAL SPINAL CORD SOCIETY

**Fig. 15.1 (B)** ASIA impairment scale

imaging provides key information to practitioners regarding the nature and severity of the spinal injury, the need for continued immobilization, and the need for more definitive treatment. Because of the expense and significant radiation exposure associated with cervical spine imaging, practitioners must carefully ascertain who warrants radiographic investigation. Accordingly, patients with potential spinal injuries may be categorized into three groups: the awake and asymptomatic group, the awake and symptomatic group, and the group that is obtunded or cannot be evaluated for some other reason.

Several large studies have evaluated the need for radiographic workup of awake and asymptomatic trauma patients. Hoffman et al. (2000) evaluated more than 34 000 blunt cervical trauma patients, 4300 of whom were asymptomatic. Patients meeting all of the specific criteria outlined in Table 15.4 were considered at low risk for cervical spine injury. This decision-making tool, known as the National Emergency X-Radiography Utilization (NEXUS) criteria, had 99% sensitivity for the identification of a cervical spine injury.

Steell et al. (2001) evaluated almost 9000 awake and asymptomatic trauma patients across Canada. Their goal was to convert more than 20 clinical findings into a decision analysis tree and reduce the amount of unnecessary imaging in the trauma population. The resulting Canadian C-spine Rule (CCR) had 100% sensitivity for the presence of a significant cervical spine injury. Steell et al. (2003) subsequently compared the NEXUS criteria with the CCR; nearly 400 physicians evaluated more than 8000 patients using both criteria. The CCR was found to be more sensitive than the NEXUS criteria for detecting significant cervical spine injury in adult trauma patients.

Anderson et al. (2010) assessed existing medical evidence for radiographic evaluation in asymptomatic trauma patients. From 1966 to 2004 there were 14 class I studies, which used criteria similar to the CCR and NEXUS studies. The combined sensitivity of such

### Table 15.4

**Criteria for clinical clearance of cervical immobilization device in an awake and asymptomatic patient**

Criteria for collar clearance in the awake and asymptomatic patient

No midline cervical tenderness
No focal neurologic deficit
Normal alertness and mentation
No intoxicants or confounders
No distracting injury

criteria was found to be 98% (Anderson et al., 2010). Given such overwhelming evidence, trauma patients who are awake and without neck pain, neurologic deficit, signs of intoxication, or other distracting injury need not undergo radiographic evaluation and should have cervical collars and spinal immobilization discontinued (Ryken et al., 2013a). This represents a level I recommendation.

Patients who do not meet the NEXUS or CCR criteria have a higher likelihood of harboring a spine injury. Several studies have compared plain radiography to computed tomography (CT) to evaluate the spinal column. Mathen et al. (2007) prospectively evaluated more than 600 symptomatic trauma patients with plain radiographs and CT imaging. CT scans had 100% sensitivity and 99.5% specificity to discover cervical spine fractures. In comparison, the sensitivity of plain radiographs was only 45%. This represents class I medical evidence in support of CT imaging as the radiographic assessment modality of choice following acute spinal trauma. Bailitz et al. (2009) prospectively evaluated more than 1500 trauma patients in a blinded fashion. The sensitivities for the discovery of spinal fractures with plain film and CT imaging were 36% and 100%, respectively.

The Eastern Association for the Surgery of Trauma group reviewed more than 50 studies comparing plain radiographs to CT imaging in trauma patients, and concluded that CT had supplanted plain radiography as the diagnostic imaging of choice for the assessment of spinal fractures in acute trauma patients (Como et al., 2009). Given the class I evidence presented above, CT imaging is the initial modality of choice to assess the spinal column in awake and symptomatic trauma patients. If high-quality CT imaging is unavailable, cervical spine X-rays through T1, including anteroposterior, lateral, and odontoid views, is a secondary option (Ryken et al., 2013a).

Some controversy exists about cervical spine clearance in awake patients with normal CT imaging and persistent neck pain. There has been conflicting evidence regarding the use of dynamic imaging (flexion/extension X-rays) under these circumstances (Davis et al., 2001; Pollack et al., 2001; Insko et al., 2002). Pollack et al. (2001) evaluated dynamic imaging in the acute management of more than 800 trauma patients, and only 2 patients had hypermobility injuries detected with dynamic imaging, suggesting there is relatively little benefit in routinely using dynamic plain radiography. In contrast, Insko et al. (2002) retrospectively evaluated more than 100 trauma patients who had dynamic cervical imaging as part of their initial radiographic workup. While a sizable proportion of patients were unable to complete adequate dynamic imaging due to limited neck range of motion, 7% who underwent imaging had significant ligamentous injury. These authors argue for complete dynamic studies in all trauma patients with per-sistent neck pain, even with normal CT studies. In patients who cannot complete dynamic imaging due to neck pain or limited range of motion, they recommend magnetic resonance imaging (MRI) to evaluate for liga-mentous injury (class III evidence).

The role of MRI in patients with persistent neck pain and negative imaging has also been the topic of academic debate. Duane et al. (2010) assessed more than 22 000 trauma patients and evaluated 49 patients with negative CT imaging, but persistent neck pain with dynamic plain radiography and MRI. Eight patients were found to have ligamentous injury on MRI, none of which were visual-ized as hypermobility or subluxation on dynamic imaging. This is the only study directly comparing dynamic imag-ing and MRI, such that the authors concluded that MRI should supplant dynamic imaging in trauma patients with persistent neck pain despite negative initial CT workup.

Schuster et al. (2005) prospectively evaluated the role of MRI in trauma patients with persistent neck pain despite negative initial imaging. Ninety-three patients underwent MRI. Although several patients were found to have varying degrees of degenerative disease, all were negative for clin-ically significant injury. These authors argue against the use of MRI in trauma patients with normal initial CT imaging and a normal motor exam (class III evidence).

Because of the lack of class I or class II evidence for further imaging in patients with negative CT scans but persistent neck pain, and because of the evidentiary dis-agreement regarding the need for dynamic or MRI in this subpopulation, current guidelines for collar clear-ance of the cervical spine and cervical orthosis removal in this setting are considered level III recommendations and are outlined in Table 15.5 (Ryken et al., 2013a).

The final trauma patient group in question is those who are obtunded or cannot be evaluated for other rea-sons. The initial evaluation proceeds according to the awake but symptomatic algorithm, with CT imaging.

*Table 15.5*

**Management options for cervical immobilization in awake but symptomatic patients with potential acute traumatic spinal cord injury**

| Criteria for collar clearance in the awake but symptomatic patient |
| --- |
| Continue cervical immobilization until asymptomatic |
| Discontinue cervical immobilization following normal and adequate dynamic flexion/extension radiographs |
| Discontinue cervical immobilization following a normal magnetic resonance imaging obtained within 48 hours of injury |
| Discontinue cervical immobilization at the discretion of the treating physician |

However, the controversy arises with respect to clearing the cervical spine and removing the cervical collar. Unlike its use in awake and cooperative patients who can actively flex and extend their neck, the use of dynamic imaging in the obtunded patient is more contentious and carries rare but potentially significant morbidity.

Hennessy et al. (2010) prospectively evaluated more than 400 obtunded trauma patients over a 4-year period, all of whom underwent both CT and dynamic plain radi-ography of the cervical spine. Only 1 patient had an injury found only on dynamic imaging. Based on their analysis, the authors argued against the routine use of dynamic radiography in the setting of normal CT imag-ing. Padayachee et al. (2006) corroborated this conclu-sion in their analysis of 276 patients. Dynamic imaging failed to identify any significant injury not seen on CT or neutral lateral cervical radiographs.

The use of dynamic imaging in awake patients is pred-icated on their ability to actively participate in the exam and the neck motion required for the study. Patients will presumably halt neck motion due to pain prior to incur-ring potential neurologic injury. Active participation is obviously not possible in the obtunded patient and thus dynamic imaging requires passive flexion and extension of the neck. Despite its exceedingly rare incidence, dev-astating neurologic deficits may be induced through pas-sive range of motion in the obtunded patient who might have ligamentous instability. Davis et al. (2001) evalu-ated dynamic imaging in 300 obtunded trauma patients and reported on 1 patient who developed quadriplegia that was thought to have been attributable to the test.

Several authors have argued for the use of MRI to rule out ligamentous injury. However, as with the awake and symptomatic population, there is conflicting evidence regarding its utility. Muchow et al. (2008) performed a meta-analysis assessing the use of MRI in the setting of negative CT imaging in obtunded trauma patients. The combined analysis of more than 450 patients revealed 97 injuries that were not identified on initial radiographs or CT imaging. With more than 20% of inju-ries identified only on MRI, the authors concluded that MRI evaluation is high-yield. Schoenfeld and col-leagues' (2010) meta-analysis of 11 studies corroborated this claim; significant ligamentous injury was identified in 47% of patients. Ninety-six patients (6%) had a change in management due to the MRI findings.

In contrast, Tomycz et al. (2008) retrospectively reviewed nearly 700 obtunded patients who had both CT and MRI over a 3-year period. MRI was exceedingly unlikely to identify an injury previously not identi-fied on high-quality CT imaging. Horn et al. (2004) reached the same conclusion in a separate retrospective analysis. Schoenwaelder et al. (2009) reported that CT imaging had a negative predictive value of 82% for

*Table 15.6*

**Management options for cervical immobilization in obtunded or otherwise unevaluable patients with potential acute traumatic spinal cord injury**

Criteria for collar clearance in the obtunded or unevaluable patient

Continue cervical immobilization until asymptomatic
Discontinue cervical immobilization following normal magnetic resonance imaging obtained within 48 hours of injury
Discontinue cervical immobilization at the discretion of the treating physician

discoligamentous injury and 100% negative predictive value for an unstable injury. They concluded that high-quality CT with sagittal reformats successfully excluded unstable injuries, rendering MRI unnecessary. More recently, Patel et al. (2015) performed an updated systematic review and reported no neurologic decline after clearance of the cervical spine with negative CT imaging only. Of note, MRI evaluation has the potential to delay extubation and lengthen hospital stay. Even when MRI signal change is observed in the soft tissues of the neck, the clinical significance is not always clear.

In summary, there is considerable evidentiary ambiguity regarding the use of dynamic imaging, MRI, and cervical spine clearance in obtunded patients. Current guidelines for cervical spine clearance and use of further imaging modalities in this subpopulation are based on only class III evidence (Table 15.6) (Ryken et al., 2013a).

## Closed cervical spine reduction

A variety of directional forces may cause spinal fractures and resulting SCI. Axial loading, flexion, extension, and distraction are the most common forces that result in injury to cervical vertebrae and compromise the spinal canal. A combination of flexion and distraction may yield a fracture-dislocation-type injury. Such injuries disrupt one or both facet joints, resulting in their subluxation or translation, and often result in SCI through reduction of the canal diameter and direct compression of the spinal cord. While fracture-dislocation injuries carry a high rate of SCI, they are amenable to early closed reduction. Closed reduction is designed to restore bony alignment and canal diameter, as well as decompress the spinal cord. It is recommended that it occur as early as possible once the spinal dislocation is identified on initial radiographic analysis (Fig. 15.2).

Closed cervical reduction of a fracture-dislocation injury was first reported by Walton in 1893. The use of tongs to perform cranial-cervical traction and reduction of a cervical fracture-dislocation deformity was later

described by Crutchfield (1954). Since that time, numerous authors have evaluated the efficacy and safety of closed cervical spine reduction utilizing manual manipulation, Gardner-Wells tongs traction (Fig. 15.3), and halo ring traction (Fig. 15.4) for both awake and anesthetized patients (Key, 1975; Maiman et al., 1986; Hadley et al., 1992; Shapiro, 1993).

In 1961, Evans evaluated 17 patients with cervical fracture-dislocation injuries treated with manual manipulation under anesthesia (MUA). They reported a 100% reduction rate, and noted that 13 of the 17 patients had improved neurologic exams following reduction. Despite the small sample size, the authors concluded that reduction under anesthesia is safe and effective.

Building on the protocol established by Evans, Burke and Berryman (1971) published their algorithm for closed cervical reduction in 41 patients with traumatic fracture injuries, which was successful in 37. Preanesthetic reduction was attempted in each patient. If unsuccessful, the patient was then anesthetized and traction reapplied. If reduction was still unsuccessful, manual manipulation was attempted. Twenty-one patients had their injuries successfully reduced using preanesthetic traction alone. An additional 11 patients underwent successful reduction using postanesthetic traction. Five additional patients' injuries were successfully reduced using manual MUA. The authors reported two cases of neurologic deterioration: one case was the result of overdistraction, the other occurred because of an unrecognized rostral injury. Despite this morbidity, the authors concluded that both cervical traction and MUA are safe if the proper diagnosis is made and strict attention is paid to the intraprocedural radiographs.

Utilizing a similar protocol in a series of 216 patients, Shrosbree (1979) reported successful reduction in 74% and 64% of patients with unilateral and bilateral facet disruption, respectively. Those patients who were successfully reduced were more likely to improve neurologically.

Throughout the 1980s and 1990s, there was increasing use of tong or halo ring-assisted cranial-cervical traction, with many authors citing the more precise and controlled nature of reduction compared to manual manipulation. Numerous investigators reported safe and highly effective reduction using device-assisted traction (Sonntag, 1981; Kleyn, 1984; Maiman et al., 1986; Star et al., 1990; Hadley et al., 1992). In combination, these studies suggest that more than 70% of patients with cervical fracture–dislocation injuries can be successfully reduced. Neurologic improvement occurred in 53–80% of patients whose injuries were reduced. Cumulatively, only one of nearly 270 patients who underwent attempted closed reduction had a worsened, ascending SCI, and two had permanent root injuries.

Despite the general preference for controlled, progressive craniocervical traction over MUA in the late 20th

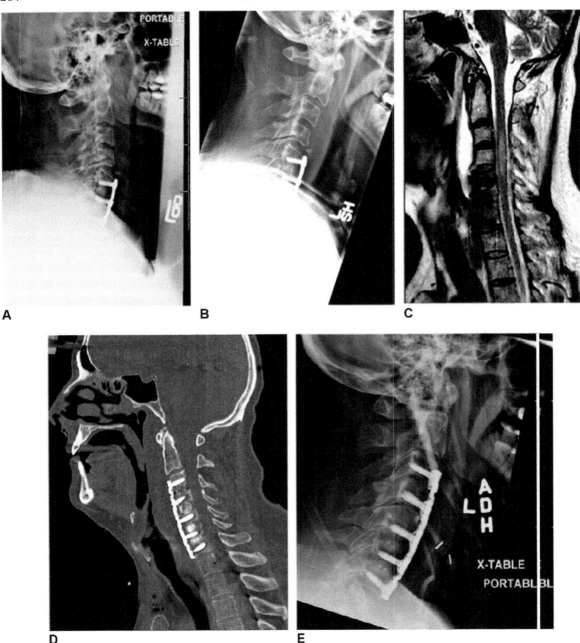

**Fig. 15.2.** Successful closed reduction of cervical fracture-dislocation. (**A**) A prereduction lateral cervical X-ray of a cervical fracture-dislocation injury adjacent to a prior anterior cervical fusion construct in a patient with an American Spinal Injury Association (ASIA) C acute traumatic spinal cord injury (SCI). Note the C4–C5 fracture subluxation above the prior C5–C7 anterior cervical discectomy and fusion construct. (**B**) A postreduction lateral cervical X-ray. Successful reduction was accomplished through rapid and controlled use of the halo ring. Realignment was achieved with 35 pounds of craniocervical traction within 45 minutes of arrival to the intensive care unit. (**C**) After reduction was accomplished and the cervical spine was secured using the halo vest, a noncontrast magnetic resonance imaging of the cervical spine was obtained, which revealed no compressive pathology and thus no need for urgent open surgical intervention. (**D**) After medical stabilization, the patient underwent reoperative transcervical exposure and extension of his anterior construct from C3 to C7 to stabilize the C4–C5 fracture injury, as seen in the postoperative computed tomography image. (**E**) A 3-month postdischarge clinic follow-up cervical X-ray reveals the intact construct and good alignment.

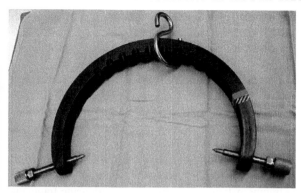

**Fig. 15.3.** Gardner-Wells tongs. From Thompson and Zlololow (2012).

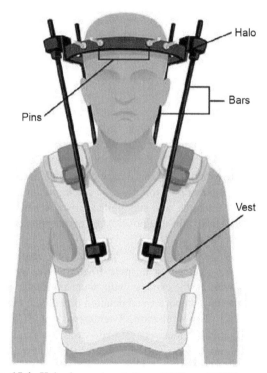

**Fig. 15.4.** Halo ring and vest. From Williams (2013).

century, only one study directly compared the two methods of reduction. Lee et al. (1994) published a series of more than 200 patients who were reduced using either rapid progressive craniocervical traction or MUA. The two groups were generally similar, except that the traction group had, on average, more significant delay to treatment. Successful fracture injury reduction was reported in 73% and 88% of patients in the MUA group and traction group, respectively, with some of the traction group failure being attributed to delays in treatment. There were 6 patients who experienced neurologic deterioration (reduction in ASIA score)

following MUA. Only 1 patient developed neurologic deterioration with the use of controlled, progressive craniocervical traction. The authors concluded that, while both reduction strategies are generally safe, controlled cervical traction appeared more effective and safer than MUA.

To date there has been no comparative analysis comparing Gardner-Wells tongs (two-point cranial fixation) and the halo ring (four-point cranial fixation) in conjunction with craniocervical traction. While Gardner-Wells tongs are easier to apply, they lack the ability to use positional, directed traction to reduce the fracture injury. Once reduced, they cannot be used to immobilize the realigned spinal column. In contrast, the halo is effective with positional, directed traction (flexion/extension), and is easily incorporated into the halo immobilization vest for rigid fixation of the cervical spine following injury reduction.

Most authors reported greater concern for the timing of closed reduction, rather than the specific cranial fixation device used. O'Conner et al. (2003) evaluated 21 patients with cervical fracture-dislocation and reported that reduction was successful in none of the 5 patients treated more than 5 days after injury. Cowan and McGillicuddy (2008) correlated the time interval to reduction with both ease of injury reduction and improvement in neurologic function.

While each of these studies utilized a slightly different protocol, the composite efficacy of closed cervical fracture reduction is roughly 80%. The composite risk of transient neurologic deficit with closed craniocervical traction is 2–4%, and the risk of a permanent neurologic deficit is <1% (Gelb et al., 2013). Because of its relatively high efficacy and safety, rapid closed reduction of fracture-dislocation injuries is recommended when carried out by experienced personnel in properly equipped centers. For these reasons, early transport of patients to specialized centers equipped for such interventions represents a level III recommendation by the AANS and CNS (Brunette and Rockswold, 1987; Lee et al., 1994; Greg Anderson et al., 2004; Cowan and McGillicuddy, 2008).

One area of contention regarding closed reduction is when to obtain MRI. Despite the very low rate of closed reduction-associated neurologic deficit, the desire to eliminate all associated morbidity has led some authors to argue for obtaining a pre-reduction MRI. They cite concern for ruptured disc material ventral to the spinal cord that might potentially herniate and exacerbate cord compression, thus potentiating neurologic deficit. In theory, a pre-reduction MRI establishes the presence or absence of a significant disc herniation or compressive epidural hematoma. However, obtaining a pre-reduction MRI requires transport of the patient with an unstable cervical spine to and from the MRI suite and delays decompression of the spinal cord via closed traction.

Several authors have examined the utility of pre-reduction MRI in awake, cooperative patients with acute cervical spine fracture-dislocation injuries and have reported a 46–100% incidence of disc injury or hernia-tion (Vaccaro et al., 1992; Doran et al., 1993; Rizzolo et al., 1994). However, despite the high incidence of disc pathology, no patient suffered a referable neurologic def-icit following successful closed reduction (Grant et al., 1999). Interestingly, Daursaut et al. (2006) reported res-olution of all disc pathology visualized on pretraction reduction MRI in patients successfully treated with closed reduction. Thus, there does not appear to be any benefit of pre-reduction MRI in the awake, evaluable patient, and delay in closed fracture reduction may result in worse neurologic outcome (Brunette and Rockswold, 1987; Greg Anderson et al., 2004). Conversely, the absence of a reliable neurologic exam in the obtunded patient may increase the potential for morbidity associ-ated with closed reduction. In this setting, a pre-reduction MRI is recommended (Gelb et al., 2013).

Unlike closed reduction, disc-related neurologic dete-rioration has been reported following open reduction of fracture-dislocation injuries in those patients who failed initial attempts at closed reduction, such that a preoper-ative MRI is also recommended in this situation. Further-more, the presence or absence of disc pathology in patients with irreducible injuries may alter surgical plan-ning and impact the decision for either dorsal or ventral open reduction with internal fixation and fusion (Gelb et al., 2013).

## Respiratory management

Patients who suffer an acute SCI often have signifi-cant associated cardiopulmonary dysfunction. Respira-tory insufficiency, hypotension, cardiac dysrhythmias, and other complications are more prevalent in patients with more severe AIS grade injuries and those with a higher anatomic level of injury (Lehmann et al., 1987; Grossman et al., 2012). Monitoring of SCI patients utiliz-ing tools such as electrocardiography, arterial and central venous catheters, and capnometers allows for the rapid detection of potential cardiopulmonary complications.

Due to the nature of their injury, acute traumatic SCI patients are at risk for developing catastrophic airway loss, resulting in hypoxemia, hypotension, neurologic deterioration, or potentially death. Patients with high cer-vical SCIs are at particularly high risk and require urgent airway assessment and management (Hassid et al., 2008). Immediate airway management in the acute trau-matic SCI patient includes establishing a definitive air-way to allow for adequate ventilation and oxygenation

in the setting of compromised respiratory mechanics sec-ondary to the neurologic injury. While no class I or class II medical studies exist on this subject, the possibility of significant neurologic consequences with airway manip-ulation in the unstable SCI patient has prompted several authors to evaluate the safety and efficacy of different intubation techniques (Grande et al., 1988; Shatney et al., 1995; American College of Surgeons, 2012; Hindman et al., 2015, 2016).

The American College of Surgeons has published guidelines on defining and establishing a definitive airway in trauma patients, including those with acute traumatic SCI (American College of Surgeons, 2012). They argue that orotracheal intubation while maintaining manual inline cervical immobilization is both a safe and effective method for establishing a definitive airway. Advanced techniques such as video laryngoscopy and fiberoptic intubation may be utilized when available and deemed necessary.

Grande et al. (1988) reported on the safe and effective nature of oral intubation in more than 3000 trauma patients at Maryland Shock Trauma. They reported that, while approximately 1% of those patients were found to have cervical spine fractures, none had worsened neurologic function following standard laryngoscopy and orotracheal intubation. Additionally, they remark that blind nasal intu-bation may result in increased rates of hypoxia, increased chances of intracranial injury in the setting of skull base and facial fractures, and suboptimal airway control due to endotracheal tube malpositioning or damage during intubation.

In 1995, Shatney et al. prospectively evaluated 81 patients with cervical spine fractures but without SCI, as well as 69 patients with acute traumatic SCI. A trauma surgeon performed detailed neurologic exams before and after intubation. Twenty-two non-SCI and 26 SCI patients underwent standard orotracheal intuba-tion, with no patients suffering neurologic deterioration as a result of intubation.

The widespread concern for further mechanical dis-ruption of the cervical spine in patients with fractures led Hindman et al. (2015) to evaluate the force of intuba-tion in cadavers. Specifically, they intubated 14 cadavers with and without cervical spine fractures (type II odon-toid fracture) using force-sensing laryngoscopes and standard orotracheal intubation practices, with the goal of evaluating C1–C2 segmental motion. They reported that the biomechanics of cervical spine motion at seg-ments C1–C5 was similar to live humans. Standard oro-tracheal intubation did not appear to exceed physiologic values associated with significant hyperextension and cord injury during intubation and the degree of exten-sion/subluxation did not differ between the intact and injured groups. The same group also evaluated C3–C4 segmental motion in 14 cadavers with iatrogenic flexion-distraction injuries (Hindman et al., 2016). The results corroborated their initial study: the degree of extension and anteroposterior subluxation did not differ between the intact and injured groups.

Respiratory complications are common following acute SCI (Ledsome and Sharp, 1981; Hassid et al., 2008; Berney et al., 2011). While multisystem trauma may result in thoracic injury with any level of SCI, neurogenic respiratory failure is most common in patients with SCIs above the C5 level due to complete or partial paralysis of the phrenic nerve. However, respiratory failure may also occur with lower injury levels because of poor cough and loss of tone of the intercostal musculature. Careful laryngoscopy and orotracheal intubation are rapid, safe, and effective methods for establishing definitive airway control in patients with unstable cervical spine fractures when combined with standard inline cervical stabilization. Rapid and definitive airway control is of paramount importance in acute traumatic SCI patients due to both ventilation compromise and reduced pulmonary function secondary to neurologic injury.

Multiple studies have demonstrated a significant reduction in pulmonary function following SCI, which may not be apparent in the early hours postinjury, but may develop as patients develop increasing atelectasis and, in some cases, become hypercarbic. Ledsome and Sharp (1981) evaluated pulmonary function tests in 16 complete (ASIA A) cervical SCI patients over a 5-month period following their injury. They found a reduction in forced vital capacity (FVC) following acute SCI, particularly in patients with injuries at or above the C4 level. These patients had a higher rate of requiring mechanical ventilator support. Over time, all patients demonstrated some improvement in their FVC. Of those patients who did not require mechanical ventilation, some of whom appeared to be breathing adequately, most were found to be consistently hypoxemic. While this was easily treated with oxygen supplementation, the presence of hypoxemia in the setting of acute SCI is a major risk factor for secondary insult and worsening of neurologic function.

Berney et al. (2011) evaluated more than 100 SCI patients with respect to pulmonary function after implementation of a new pulmonary care decision-making pathway. They noted decreased FVC, increased airway secretions, and compromised gas exchange, particularly in patients with high cervical injuries; these variables were predictive of the need for endotracheal intubation and mechanical ventilation.

In patients who fail mechanical ventilation wean, attention must be turned to chronic airway management. While there are no class I or II studies evaluating its use in acute traumatic SCI patients, several authors have reported clinical predictors and timing parameters for tracheostomy in

this patient population (Harrop et al., 2004; O'Keeffe et al., 2004; Romero et al., 2009; Berney et al., 2011; Leelapattana et al., 2012; Babu et al., 2013).

Harrop et al. (2004) retrospectively evaluated 156 ASIA A SCI patients over a 6-year period in an effort to identify predictors of tracheostomy requirement. Of these patients, 107 ultimately required tracheostomy due to failed mechanical ventilation wean. The authors identified age, level of injury, pre-existing medical comorbidity, pre-existing lung disease, and presence of pneumonia as statistically significant predictors of tracheostomy requirement. Berney et al. (2011) corroborated these predictors in their systematic review. Their 21-study review of over 1200 patients reported both completeness and level of injury as significant predictors of tracheostomy requirement. Leelapattana et al. (2012) reported that approximately 75% of cervical SCI patients require intubation and mechanical intubation and that up to 67% of intubated patients with cervical SCI ultimately require tracheostomy. They identified completeness of injury, high injury severity scores, and persistent $PA_{O_2}/F_{I_{O_2}} < 300$ as predictors of tracheostomy requirement.

O'Keeffe et al. (2004) broached the subject of tracheostomy timing following anterior cervical surgery in patients with cervical fractures and/or SCI. While they remarked that ideal timing requires further study, they reported safe tracheostomy insertion 6–10 days following anterior cervical surgery. In an effort to elucidate the ideal timing for tracheostomy after SCI, Romero et al. (2009) retrospectively evaluated the clinical course of more than 150 patients. Patients receiving early tracheostomy (before 7 days postinjury) had shorter ICU lengths of stay and decreased laryngotracheal complications. Babu et al. (2013) corroborated this argument with a retrospective review of 5 years of data on patients who underwent both anterior cervical surgery and tracheostomy placement. Their analysis revealed late tracheostomy placement as a predictor of overall complication rate.

While no prospective, randomized trials regarding tracheostomy use and timing in acute traumatic SCI patients exist to date, multiple authors present a reasonable and consistent argument for the early use of tracheostomy in SCI patients who are likely to require prolonged intubation (for example, high-cervical-level injuries or patients with significant chest/pulmonary trauma). Even patients who have recently undergone anterior cervical surgery may safely undergo tracheostomy placement with an acceptably low cross-contamination rate (Babu et al., 2013).

## HEMODYNAMIC MANAGEMENT

Hypotension may develop following SCI due to a variety of factors, including volume loss due to multisystem trauma and neurogenic shock, with vasodilatation and bradycardia. While there are no prospective studies evaluating the effect of hypotension on SCI, its presence is thought to contribute to secondary neurologic injury.

To minimize the potential for exacerbation of SCI, avoidance of hypotension (systolic blood pressure < 90 mmHg) is essential. Further, to ensure adequate spinal perfusion, maintenance of mean arterial blood pressure (MAP) > 85 mmHg has been recommended, albeit based on very limited data (Ryken et al., 2013b). Initial volume augmentation is carried out with intravenous crystalloid. If patients remain below the MAP target, vasopressors are initiated. Norepinephrine, phenylephrine, and dopamine are all reasonable choices. Dopamine may be particularly useful among patients with bradycardia, although its use may also result in a greater risk of tachyarrhythmias, particularly in older patients (Inoue et al., 2014; Ready et al., 2015). At present, while no randomized study has determined the ideal time period for MAP management, multiple observational studies have led to the recommendation of blood pressure augmentation for at least 7 days following acute SCI (Levi et al., 1996; Vale et al., 1997; Casha and Christie, 2011; Hawryluk et al., 2015).

Wolf et al. (1991) published a series of more than 50 acute SCI patients managed with an aggressive regimen, including an MAP goal > 85 mmHg. They reported neurologic improvement in more than 20% of complete SCI patients and in more than 60% of patients with incomplete injuries, and cited MAP augmentation as a possible reason for this degree of neurologic improvement.

Levi et al. (1993) evaluated 50 patients with acute cervical SCI. Monitoring cardiac function and systemic vascular resistance, vasopressors were utilized to maintain MAP >90 mmHg. The authors reported a relatively high rate of neurologic improvement in patients whose systemic vascular resistance was raised with the use of vasopressors for MAP management.

In 1997, Vale et al. corroborated the argument for MAP management in their study of 77 patients. They found that 100% of patients with complete and 70% of incomplete SCI patients were hypotensive on arrival. Patients were monitored in the ICU and MAP maintained at > 85 mmHg for at least 1 week. Despite variability in neurologic improvement at 1 year, there was measurable improvement in all ASIA A injury groups. Three of 15 ASIA A cervical SCI and 88% of incomplete SCI patients regained ambulatory capacity at 1-year follow-up. The authors conclude that neurologic outcome in their series of patients with acute SCI may have been optimized by early, aggressive resuscitation and blood pressure management, and was in addition to and distinct from any potential benefit provided by surgery. Their work offers class III evidence in support of blood pressure augmentation for 7 days following acute SCI.

Casha and Christie (2011) performed a systematic review of hemodynamic management following acute traumatic SCI. They found that patients monitored in an ICU setting and those who underwent MAP augmentation had more substantial improvement in neurologic function over time.

Hawryluk et al. (2015) recently analyzed MAP records in the first 7 days in 100 acute SCI patients. Using minute-by-minute MAP records, they found a correlation between the percent time spent above the MAP target (85 mmHg in accordance with the SCI guidelines) and the degree of recovery in the initial 7 days postinjury. In addition, they found that patients who spent a higher percentage of time below the MAP threshold were more likely to experience a motor decline over the treatment period.

Autonomic instability secondary to acute traumatic SCI can cause refractory bradycardia. Compared to the topic of blood pressure management in this population, there is a paucity of research on the management of symptomatic bradycardia. While several authors have evaluated the incidence and pathophysiology behind SCI-related bradycardia (Hector et al., 2013; Bartholdy et al., 2014), very few authors have described a treatment paradigm.

In 2011, Moerman et al. retrospectively evaluated their management of 106 patients with acute traumatic cervical SCI. They found an incidence of bradycardia of 14% (15 of 106 patients). Nearly half (47%) of these patients underwent cardiac pacemaker placement. Of those who received this intervention, the rates of cardiovascular instability, major bradycardia episodes, and intervention with atropine were significantly reduced.

In summary, acute traumatic SCI is associated with a high incidence of cardiopulmonary complications. Hypoxemia and hypotension may exacerbate the existing cord injury. Several studies reported a lower incidence of systemic complications, earlier treatment if they did occur, and improved neurologic status when acute SCI patients are initially managed in an ICU (Zäch et al., 1976; Hachen, 1977; McMichan et al., 1980; Tator et al., 1984; Casha and Christie, 2011). While the optimal duration of cardiopulmonary monitoring in an ICU is debatable, the first 5–7 days following injury appear to be the most crucial with respect to the occurrence of complications (Piepmeier et al., 1985). Additional studies are needed to determine the optimal MAP treatment threshold and the ideal length of time for hemodynamic augmentation.

## Pharmacologic therapy

The goal of neuroprotective strategies is to reduce the primary insult and minimize the secondary injury cascade that occurs after acute neural injury. There has been considerable basic and clinical science research on neuroprotection in acute SCI. While a number of pharmacologic agents have been studied in randomized controlled trials, methylprednisolone (MP) has received the most scrutiny.

The National Acute Spinal Cord Injury Studies (NASCIS I, II, and III) evaluated the potential protective benefit of MP given at varying doses and times following acute SCI (Bracken et al., 1984, 1990, 1998). While NASCIS I and III were negative with respect to all endpoints, many practitioners continue to utilize MP in the acute SCI setting, citing the results of the NASCIS II trial, which reported a measurable benefit in ASIA score when MP was given within an 8-hour window.

However, the NASCIS II trial was actually negative with respect to all preplanned endpoints outlined in the initial protocol. The arbitrary 8-hour window (and its associated purported benefit) was discovered in *post hoc* analysis, which included only 66 MP-treated patients out of 291 originally randomized, and utilized only right body motor scores. There was considerable omission of data due to patients being lost to follow-up, inconsistency in reported benefit (motor, sensory, both, or neither), and lack of clinically relevant functional outcomes. It stands to reason mathematically that if the overall result was negative, and the 8-hour subpopulation experienced a slightly positive effect, then the patients who received MP outside of this 8-hour window must have experienced a slightly negative effect. Examination of the morbidity and mortality data reported in both NASCIS II and III yields just such a result. The treatment groups in both NASCIS II and III studies had higher rates of pneumonia, sepsis, respiratory failure, and death (Bracken et al., 1992, 1998). Because the positive result of NASCIS II was only in a *post hoc* analysis, as well as the negative result from NASCIS I and III, and the trend towards increased mortality in the treatment groups, MP is not recommended in the treatment of human patients with acute SCI (Hurlbert et al., 2013; Evaniew et al., 2016).

Furthermore, there have been at least two additional studies that support a lack of benefit of MP in the treatment of acute traumatic SCI. Pointillart et al. (2000) randomized 100 patients to receive nimodipine, MP (utilizing the NASCIS II protocol), both, or neither. While all groups showed improvement in their ASIA score at 1 year compared to admission, there was no significant difference between the groups and a trend towards more infectious and hemorrhagic complications in the MP group (Pointillart et al., 2000). Similarly, in another randomized trial, Matsumoto et al. (2001) reported higher rates of pneumonia and gastrointestinal hemorrhage in MP-treated patients.

Geisler et al. published two randomized controlled trials that examined the use of GM-1 ganglioside (Sygen) as a neuroprotective agent in acute traumatic SCI patients (Geisler et al., 1991, 2001). The control groups for both studies were treated with NASCIS protocol MP. Collectively, more than 800 patients received MP, a far larger cohort than treated in the NASCIS trials. The authors reported no significant difference in outcomes between use of GM-1 ganglioside and MP.

In summary, despite the purported benefit from the NASCIS II *post hoc* analysis, the overwhelming majority of the published evidence does not support the use of MP in post-SCI care. Indeed, each study has reported at least a trend towards more complications (and in some cases mortality) in the MP treatment groups. For these reasons, the use of MP in the treatment of acute SCI is not recommended in guidelines from the AANS and CNS. This level I recommendation parallels findings in traumatic brain injury, where the Corticosteroid Randomization After Significant Head injury study found higher mortality when patients were treated with corticosteroids (Edwards et al., 2005).

# COMPLEX DECISION MAKING

## Management of blunt cervical trauma-associated vascular injuries

The association of blunt cervical trauma and vascular injury was first reported in the 1950s (Suechting and French, 1955), and was increasingly recognized over time (Gurdjian et al., 1963; Willis et al., 1994; Beletsky et al., 2003). While vertebral artery injury may occur in the absence of a cervical spine fracture, it is commonly associated with fractures through the foramen transversarium, facet fracture-dislocation, or vertebral subluxation. Because of this strong association and the potentially devastating consequences of a posterior-circulation stroke, the criteria outlined in Table 15.7 (modified Denver screening criteria)

*Table 15.7*

**The Modified Denver Criteria is a protocol developed to determine which patients should be screened for blunt cerebrovascular injury**

| Denver screening criteria for blunt cerebrovascular injury |
| --- |
| Lateralizing neurologic exam unexplained by CT head |
| Infarct on CT head |
| Cervical hematoma |
| Epistaxis (massive) |
| Anisocoria/Horner's syndrome |
| GCS < 8 unexplained by CT head |
| Cervical spine fracture |
| Basilar skull fracture |
| Severe facial fracture |
| Supraclavicular seatbelt sign |
| Cervical bruit/thrill |

CT, computed tomography; GCS, Glasgow Coma Score.

are now widely used to screen for vascular injury in the trauma population (Biffl et al., 1999).

Conventional catheter angiography has historically been considered the gold standard for the diagnosis of cerebrovascular injury. Despite its high sensitivity and specificity, catheter angiography is invasive, associated with a small but measurable morbidity, and requires significant time and expertise to perform. Conversely, use of CT angiography (CTA) is noninvasive, requires less time and fewer personnel to perform, and is associated with little morbidity. Numerous studies have compared conventional catheter angiography to CTA with respect to diagnosis of cerebrovascular injury.

Biffl et al. (2006) evaluated more than 300 blunt trauma patients using the Denver screening criteria. All patients who met screening criteria were evaluated with CTA; those patients with CTA-confirmed vascular injury then underwent angiography. Conventional angiography corroborated the presence of injury in all the patients with a positive CTA. Furthermore, no patient with a normal CTA went on to develop clinically evident vascular injury. The authors concluded that CTA was an accurate and reliable method for vascular injury screening. Berne et al. (2004) published a similar experience, albeit with a much lower incidence of vascular injury. Again, no patients with a negative CTA went on to develop clinically significant vascular injury. Eastman et al. (2006) prospectively compared CTA and catheter angiography in blunt trauma patients who met the modified Denver criteria for screening. They reported 97% sensitivity and 100% specificity for CTA with respect to blunt cerebrovascular injury identification. This study, in addition to those noted above, has suggested that CTA has near 100% accuracy in this population when the modified Denver screening criteria are appropriately applied. While some recent studies suggest that CTA may have substantially better specificity than sensitivity (Roberts et al., 2013; Paulus et al., 2014), because of this class I medical evidence study, CTA is widely regarded as the new gold standard and standard of care for the diagnosis of cerebrovascular injury in patients sustaining blunt cervical trauma (Harrigan et al., 2013).

Also contentious is the treatment of a vertebral artery injury in the trauma population. Arterial injury may include endothelial disruption, pseudoaneurysm, or occlusion. Such pathology compromises cerebral blood flow and may result in embolic ischemic stroke. The natural inclination is to treat the injury with antiplatelet or anticoagulant medications in an effort to reduce the risk of stroke. However, there are no definitive longitudinal studies quantifying the risk of stroke. A significant number of patients either remain asymptomatic after injury or already experienced the ischemic insult by the time of their presentation. The potential consequences of anticoagulation may outweigh the benefits of stroke prevention in this setting, particularly if the patient has significant intracranial or systemic injury.

There have been several small, class III evidence studies evaluating the treatment of blunt cerebrovascular injury after trauma (Biffl et al., 2000; Beletsky et al., 2003; Cothren et al., 2009). There is considerable discordance among these authors both with respect to the risk of a clinically significant injury and the preferred method of prevention. While treatment with antiplatelet medications such as aspirin appears to be the safest and most widely studied option, even in the setting of concomitant intracranial hemorrhage (Callcut et al., 2012), current recommendations call for individualized treatment decisions based on the type of vascular injury, the individual patient's risk profile, and other significant systemic injuries. If no significant contraindication is present, treatment with aspirin should be considered (Harrigan et al., 2013).

It has been hypothesized that surgical intervention in addition to antiplatelet therapy or anticoagulation may have a protective role. Foreman et al. (2015) retrospectively evaluated 52 patients with traumatic vertebral artery occlusions in conjunction with cervical spinal fracture-dislocation injuries. Multivariate analysis revealed that early surgery to reduce and stabilize the cervical spine appeared to be protective against ischemic stroke. Accordingly, early surgical intervention should be considered in patients with unstable cervical fractures and a concomitant vertebral artery injury. This represents class III medical evidence.

## Deep venous thrombosis prophylaxis

Patients with acute traumatic SCI are at high risk for developing deep venous thrombosis (DVT) and pulmonary embolism (PE), particularly in the first few months following the injury (Geerts et al., 1994). Because DVT and PE are associated with substantial morbidity, their prevention and early detection are of paramount importance (DeVivo et al., 1989; Geerts et al., 1994). There are several DVT/PE prophylactic measures that have been studied in considerable detail, including the use of anticoagulation, pneumatic compression devices, and vena cava filters. While the majority of existing research consists of class III evidence, there have been several class I and II studies on this topic that have demonstrated a decrease in DVT/PE rates in patients receiving various prophylactic measures (Hachen, 1974b; Becker et al., 1987; Green et al., 1988; Merli et al., 1992; Powell et al., 1999; Aito et al., 2002).

As early as 1974, Hachen conducted a retrospective cohort study of low-dose unfractionated heparin (UFH) vs. oral anticoagulation (warfarin) in 120 acute SCI patients (Hachen, 1974b). Patients who received low-dose subcutaneous UFH had fewer thromboembolic complications than those who received oral anticoagulation. This class II study helped form the basis for the modern practice of using subcutaneous anticoagulation for DVT prophylaxis in traumatic SCI patients.

Becker et al. (1987) conducted a small (15 patients) randomized trial suggesting that use of rotating beds in the first 10 days following acute SCI may reduce the incidence of DVT.

Green et al. (1988) published the results of a prospective, randomized trial comparing the use of low-dose and adjusted-dose UFH for DVT prophylaxis in acute SCI patients. The adjusted-dose group was titrated to an activated partial thromboplastin time of 1.5 times normal. They reported that patients who received adjusted-dose UFH had fewer thromboembolic complications than patients who received the standard low-dose protocol (7% vs. 31%). However, it was also reported that these patients had a higher incidence of bleeding complications (7 of 29 patients treated with adjusted-dose protocol).

Merli et al. (1988, 1992) evaluated the use of multimodality prophylaxis in the form of UFH plus electric stimulation and pneumatic stockings, respectively. In each of their studies they reported that low-dose UFH alone was no better than placebo and that multimodality therapy was superior to UFH alone.

Over the past two decades, many clinicians and institutions have switched from UFH to low-molecular-weight heparin (LMWH). A multicenter randomized controlled trial of 107 patients compared 5000 units UFH every 8 hours in combination with intermittent pneumatic compressions with 30 mg every 12 hours of enoxaparin. There was no difference in the incidence of DVT, but significantly fewer patients in the enoxaparin group developed PE (Spinal Cord Injury Thromboprophylaxis Investigators, 2003a). Unfortunately, many patients were lost to follow-up. However, a prospective multicenter cohort study during the rehabilitation phase of patients with SCI further supported these findings (Spinal Cord Injury Thromboprophylaxis Investigators, 2003b). Many clinicians also prefer to use LMWH due to ease of use (daily dosing compared to two or three times a day) (Green et al., 2005). Clinical trials comparing different LMWH regiments have not demonstrated efficacy of one agent over another (Chiou-Tan et al., 2003; Slavik et al. 2007).

Timing of prophylaxis remains a controversial topic. Despite the lack of high-quality studies, several longitudinal studies have demonstrated that patients with acute traumatic SCI are significantly more prone to DVT development in the first 6 months after the injury compared to age-matched controls (DeVivo et al., 1989). In addition, long-term follow-up has demonstrated that

the rate of formation decreases over time (McKinley et al., 1999). As such, DVT/PE prophylaxis should be initiated within 72 hours of injury (if no systemic contraindication) and continued for at least 8–12 weeks, but may be discontinued soon in patients with useful lower-extremity motor function (Dhall et al., 2013).

Patients with acute traumatic SCI often have significant concomitant injuries, which may act as a contraindication to systemic anticoagulation. As such, several authors have described the use of inferior vena cava (IVC) filters as an alternate method for preventing PE (Wilson et al., 1994). At present there is no class I or II evidence. Existing class III evidence supports the notion that IVC filters do not prevent formation of DVT, may be ineffective at prevention of PE after several months, and may themselves carry significant morbidity (Gorman et al., 2009). As such, the routine use of IVC filters is not recommended in patients with acute traumatic SCI. However, IVC filters may be effective with established venous thromboembolic disease in patients who fail and/or have contraindications to systemic anticoagulation (Dhall et al., 2013).

At present, there is evidence to support a level I recommendation for prophylaxis against DVT/PE in acute traumatic SCI patients, preferably with LMWH. Treatment should be implemented as early as possible and should be continued for at least 3 months in patients with significant lower-extremity motor deficits (level II recommendation) (Dhall et al., 2013).

## CLINICAL TRIALS AND GUIDELINES

In some instances, it is impossible to ethically evaluate neurosurgical pathology in a randomized and controlled manner. Still other pathologies are too rare to feasibly study in a randomized fashion.

The AANS, in conjunction with the CNS, has created guidelines for the management of acute cervical spine and SCIs. Initially published in 2002, the newest guidelines from March 2013 offer more than 100 recommendations on various subjects surrounding the care of SCI patients (Hadley et al., 2002; Hadley and Walters, 2013). Based on a thorough review of the existing literature, they offer 19 level I and 16 additional level II recommendations. Those pertaining to the topics discussed in this chapter are outlined in Table 15.8.

## OUTCOME ASSESSMENT

The definitive clinical assessment of patients who sustain acute traumatic SCI involves more than the ASIA scale and AIS grade assessments described earlier in the chapter.

*Table 15.8*

**Level I and II recommendations for care of spinal cord injury (SCI) patients**

| Recommendation | Class of recommendation | Substantiating studies |
|---|---|---|
| **Triage and prehospital management** | | |
| Spinal immobilization is recommended for all trauma patients with known or suspected SCI. | II | Del Rossi et al. (2004) |
| Triage of trauma patients at the scene by EMS personnel is recommended | II | Burton et al. (2006) |
| Immobilization of awake patients who pass screening criteria is not recommended | II | Stroh and Braude (2001) |
| **Clinical assessment of SCI** | | |
| The American Spinal Injury Association standard is recommended for neurologic assessment | II | Kirshblum et al. (2002) Savic et al. (2007) |
| The Spinal Cord Independence Measure II is the preferred functional outcome assessment measure | I | Bluvshtein et al. (2011) Rudhe and van Hedel (2009) Catz et al. (2007) Itzkovich et al. (2007) |
| The International Spinal Cord Injury Basic Pain Data Set is the preferred measure to assess pain | I | Jensen et al. (2010) Bryce et al. (2007) Cardenas et al. (2002) |
| **Radiographic assessment** | | |
| 1. Awake, asymptomatic patients without neck pain, neurologic deficit, intoxication, or distracting injury do not require cervical imaging or immobilization | I | Anderson et al. (2010) Stiell et al. (2001, 2003) Hoffman et al. (2000) |
| 2. Awake, symptomatic patients should be initially evaluated with high-quality CT or three-view cervical X-rays if CT is not available | I | Bailitz et al. (2009) Mathen et al. (2007) Daffner et al. (2006) Berne et al. (2004) |
| 3. Obtunded or unevaluable patients should be initially evaluated with high-quality CT or three-view cervical X-rays if CT is not available | I | Hennessy et al. (2010) Mathen et al. (2007) Brohi et al. (2005) Diaz et al. (2003) |
| **Pharmacologic therapy** | | |
| The use of methylprednisolone for treatment of SCI is not recommended | I | Ito et al. (2009) Qian et al. (2005) Matsumoto et al. (2001) Pointillart et al. (2000) Bracken et al. (1984, 1985, 1990, 1992, 1997, 1998) |
| The use of GM-1 gangliosides for treatment of SCI is not recommended | I | Geisler et al. (1991, 2001) |
| **Management of cerebrovascular injury** | | |
| The use of CTA for vascular injury screening is recommended | I | Eastman et al. (2006) |

EMS, emergency medical services; CT, computed tomography; CTA, computed tomography angiography.

The functional severity of SCI is based on a variety of factors, such as age, mechanism of injury, time from injury to arrival at a definitive treatment center, level of injury, and presence of significant systemic injuries. The initial clinical presentation (functional ability on arrival) is important in outcome prediction (Hadley et al., 2013). An accurate and consistent description of a patient's neurologic status utilizing a simple and reproducible assessment scale facilitates interprovider communication and prognostication.

A comprehensive description of the neurologic status of a SCI patient includes a detailed neurologic exam, a functional assessment, and pain evaluation. If used properly, these scales provide a historic comparison for the SCI, allow for determination of clinically significant functional changes over time, and help predict their future recovery potential.

Functional outcome scales describe the level of human function *vis-à-vis* activities of daily living following injury. While several scales were previously used, the Spinal Cord Independence Measure (SCIM) has become the most widely embraced.

This scale was originally described in 1997 by Catz et al. in a cohort of 30 patients. It had a relatively high interrater reliability (kappa = 0.66) and has a higher sensitivity for detecting functional changes compared to the historic Functional Independence Measure (FIM) (Dodds et al., 1993). The initial SCIM scale included three subscales relating to self-care, sphincter management/respiration, and mobility. The authors updated the subscales in 2001 and included new scales for activities of daily living functionality (for example, bathing, dressing, and bowel care) (Catz et al., 2001). Itzkovich et al. (2007) described a third iteration of SCIM scale in a multinational study evaluating 425 SCI patients. Compared to the FIM scale, the SCIM III was more sensitive and responsive to changes in functional ability of SCI patients over time. Bluvshtein et al. (2011) corroborated this claim in another international study involving more than 260 patients. These two studies represent class I evidence supporting a level I recommendation for the use of the SCIM III scale as the most valid and reliable functional outcome measure for use in adult SCI patients.

Pain following acute traumatic SCI may result from structural damage to the bony canal or compression of the neural elements. Chronic pain following acute SCI may be classified as neuropathic or nociceptive, and is present in 25–80% of patients (Cardenas et al., 2002; Hadley et al., 2013). Patients with severe pain have worse outcome scores and often exhibit functional impairment out of proportion to their physical and neurologic injuries (Hadley et al., 2013).

While many authors have reported a varying degree of success with more than a dozen pain scales and assessment tools, the Spinal Cord Injury Basic Pain Data Set has been identified as the most valid and reliable scale for SCI patients.

# REFERENCES

Aito S, Pieri A, D'Andrea M et al. (2002). Primary prevention of deep venous thrombosis and pulmonary embolism in acute spinal cord injured patients. Spinal Cord 40: 300–303.

American College of Surgeons (2012). Advanced Trauma Live Support (ATLS) Student Manual. American College of Surgeons, Chicago, IL.

Anderson PA, Muchow RD, Munoz A et al. (2010). Clearance of the asymptomatic cervical spine: a meta-analysis. J Orthop Trauma 24: 100–106.

ASIA/IMSOP, 2000. International Standards for Neurological and Functional Classification of Spinal Cord Injury-Revised 2000. American Spinal Injury Association, Richmond, VA.

Babu R, Owens TR, Thomas S et al. (2013). Timing of tracheostomy after anterior cervical spine fixation. J Trauma Acute Care Surg 74: 961–966.

Bailitz J, Starr F, Beecroft M et al. (2009). CT should replace three-view radiographs as the initial screening test in patients at high, moderate, and low risk for blunt cervical spine injury: a prospective comparison. J Trauma 66: 1605–1609.

Bartholdy K, Biering-Sørensen T, Malmqvist L et al. (2014). Cardiac arrhythmias the first month after acute traumatic spinal cord injury. J Spinal Cord Med 37: 162–170.

Bauer D, Kowalski R (1988). Effect of spinal immobilization devices on pulmonary function in the healthy, nonsmoking man. Ann Emerg Med 17: 915–918.

Becker DM, Gonzalez M, Gentili A et al. (1987). Prevention of deep venous thrombosis in patients with acute spinal cord injuries: use of rotating treatment tables. Neurosurgery 20: 675–677.

Beletsky V, Nadareishvili Z, Lynch J et al. (2003). Cervical arterial dissection: time for a therapeutic trial? Stroke J Cereb Circ 34: 2856–2860.

Berne JD, Norwood SH, McAuley CE et al. (2004). Helical computed tomographic angiography: an excellent screening test for blunt cerebrovascular injury. J Trauma 57: 11–17. discussion 17–19.

Berney SC, Gordon IR, Opdam HI et al. (2011). A classification and regression tree to assist clinical decision making in airway management for patients with cervical spinal cord injury. Spinal Cord 49: 244–250.

Biffl WL, Moore EE, Offner PJ et al. (1999). Optimizing screening for blunt cerebrovascular injuries. Am J Surg 178: 517–522.

Biffl WL, Moore EE, Elliott JP et al. (2000). The devastating potential of blunt vertebral arterial injuries. Ann Surg 231: 672–681.

Biffl WL, Egglin T, Benedetto B et al. (2006). Sixteen-slice computed tomographic angiography is a reliable noninvasive screening test for clinically significant blunt cerebrovascular injuries. J Trauma 60: 745–751. discussion 751–752.

Black CA, Buderer NM, Blaylock B et al. (1998). Comparative study of risk factors for skin breakdown with cervical orthotic devices: Philadelphia and Aspen. J Trauma Nurs Off J Soc Trauma Nurses 5: 62–66.

Blaylock B (1996). Solving the problem of pressure ulcers resulting from cervical collars. Ostomy Wound Manage 42: 26–28. 30, 32–33.

Bluvshtein V, Front L, Itzkovich M et al. (2011). SCIM III is reliable and valid in a separate analysis for traumatic spinal cord lesions. Spinal Cord 49: 292–296.

Boyd CR, Corse KM, Campbell RC (1989). Emergency interhospital transport of the major trauma patient: air versus ground. J Trauma 29: 789–793. discussion 793–794.

Bracken MB, Collins WF, Freeman DF et al. (1984). Efficacy of methylprednisolone in acute spinal cord injury. JAMA 251: 45–52.

Bracken MB, Shepard MJ, Hellenbrand KG et al. (1985). Methylprednisolone and neurological function 1 year after spinal cord injury. Results of the National Acute Spinal Cord Injury Study. J Neurosurg 63: 704–713.

Bracken MB, Shepard MJ, Collins WF et al. (1990). A randomized, controlled trial of methylprednisolone or naloxone in the treatment of acute spinal-cord injury. Results of the Second National Acute Spinal Cord Injury Study. N Engl J Med 322: 1405–1411.

Bracken MB, Shepard MJ, Collins WF et al. (1992). Methylprednisolone or naloxone treatment after acute spinal cord injury: 1-year follow-up data. Results of the second National Acute Spinal Cord Injury Study. J Neurosurg 76: 23–31.

Bracken MB, Shepard MJ, Holford TR et al. (1998). Methylprednisolone or tirilazad mesylate administration after acute spinal cord injury: 1-year follow up. Results of the third National Acute Spinal Cord Injury randomized controlled trial. J Neurosurg 89: 699–706.

Brohi K, Healy M, Fotheringham T et al. (2005). Helical computed tomographic scanning for the evaluation of the cervical spine in the unconscious, intubated trauma patient. J Trauma 58: 897–901.

Brown LH, Gough JE, Simonds WB (1998). Can EMS providers adequately assess trauma patients for cervical spinal injury? Prehospital Emerg Care Off J Natl Assoc EMS Physicians Natl Assoc State EMS Dir 2: 33–36.

Brunette DD, Rockswold GL (1987). Neurologic recovery following rapid spinal realignment for complete cervical spinal cord injury. J Trauma 27: 445–447.

Bryce TN, Budh CN, Cardenas DD et al. (2007). Pain after spinal cord injury: an evidence-based review for clinical practice and research. Report of the National Institute on Disability and Rehabilitation Research Spinal Cord Injury Measures meeting. J Spinal Cord Med 30: 421–440.

Burke DC, Berryman D (1971). The place of closed manipulation in the management of flexion-rotation dislocations of the cervical spine. J Bone Joint Surg Br 53: 165–182.

Burney RE, Waggoner R, Maynard FM (1989). Stabilization of spinal injury for early transfer. J Trauma 29: 1497–1499.

Burns AS, Lee BS, Ditunno JF et al. (2003). Patient selection for clinical trials: the reliability of the early spinal cord injury examination. J Neurotrauma 20: 477–482.

Burton JH, Dunn MG, Harmon NR et al. (2006). A statewide, prehospital emergency medical service selective patient spine immobilization protocol. J Trauma 61: 161–167.

Callcut RA, Hanseman DJ, Solan PD et al. (2012). Early treatment of blunt cerebrovascular injury with concomitant hemorrhagic neurologic injury is safe and effective. J Trauma Acute Care Surg 72: 338–345. discussion 345–346.

Cardenas DD, Turner JA, Warms CA et al. (2002). Classification of chronic pain associated with spinal cord injuries. Arch Phys Med Rehabil 83: 1708–1714.

Casha S, Christie S (2011). A systematic review of intensive cardiopulmonary management after spinal cord injury. J Neurotrauma 28: 1479–1495.

Catz A, Itzkovich M, Agranov E et al. (1997). SCIM–spinal cord independence measure: a new disability scale for patients with spinal cord lesions. Spinal Cord 35: 850–856.

Catz A, Itzkovich M, Agranov E et al. (2001). The spinal cord independence measure (SCIM): sensitivity to functional changes in subgroups of spinal cord lesion patients. Spinal Cord 39: 97–100.

Catz A, Itzkovich M, Tesio L et al. (2007). A multicenter international study on the Spinal Cord Independence Measure, version III: Rasch psychometric validation. Spinal Cord 45: 275–291.

Chiou-Tan FY, Garza H, Chan KT et al. (2003). Comparison of dalteparin and enoxaparin for deep venous thrombosis prophylaxis in patients with spinal cord injury. Am J Phys Med Rehabil 82: 678–685.

Cline JR, Scheidel E, Bigsby EF (1985). A comparison of methods of cervical immobilization used in patient extrication and transport. J Trauma 25: 649–653.

Como JJ, Diaz JJ, Dunham CM et al. (2009). Practice management guidelines for identification of cervical spine injuries following trauma: update from the eastern association for the surgery of trauma practice management guidelines committee. J Trauma 67: 651–659.

Cordell WH, Hollingsworth JC, Olinger ML et al. (1995). Pain and tissue-interface pressures during spine-board immobilization. Ann Emerg Med 26: 31–36.

Cothren CC, Biffl WL, Moore EE et al. (2009). Treatment for blunt cerebrovascular injuries: equivalence of anticoagulation and antiplatelet agents. Arch Surg Chic Ill 1960 (144): 685–690.

Cowan JA, McGillicuddy JE (2008). Images in clinical medicine. Reversal of traumatic quadriplegia after closed reduction. N Engl J Med 359: 2154.

Crutchfield WG (1954). Skeletal traction in treatment of injuries to the cervical spine. J Am Med Assoc 155: 29–32.

Daffner RH, Sciulli RL, Rodriguez A et al. (2006). Imaging for evaluation of suspected cervical spine trauma: a 2-year analysis. Injury 37: 652–658.

Davies G, Deakin C, Wilson A (1996). The effect of a rigid collar on intracranial pressure. Injury 27: 647–649.

Davis JW, Kaups KL, Cunningham MA et al. (2001). Routine evaluation of the cervical spine in head-injured patients with dynamic fluoroscopy: a reappraisal. J Trauma 50: 1044–1047.

De Lorenzo RA (1996). A review of spinal immobilization techniques. J Emerg Med 14: 603–613.

Del Rossi G, Heffernan TP, Horodyski M et al. (2004). The effectiveness of extrication collars tested during the execution of spine-board transfer techniques. Spine J Off J North Am Spine Soc 4: 619–623.

DeVivo MJ, Kartus PL, Stover SL et al. (1989). Cause of death for patients with spinal cord injuries. Arch Intern Med 149: 1761–1766.

DeVivo MJ, Go BK, Jackson AB (2002). Overview of the national spinal cord injury statistical center database. J Spinal Cord Med 25: 335–338.

Dhall SS, Hadley MN, Aarabi B et al. (2013). Deep venous thrombosis and thromboembolism in patients with cervical spinal cord injuries. Neurosurgery 72 (Suppl 2): 244–254.

Diaz JJ, Gillman C, Morris JA et al. (2003). Are five-view plain films of the cervical spine unreliable? A prospective evaluation in blunt trauma patients with altered mental status. J Trauma 55: 658–663. discussion 663–664.

Dodds TA, Martin DP, Stolov WC et al. (1993). A validation of the functional independence measurement and its performance among rehabilitation inpatients. Arch Phys Med Rehabil 74: 531–536.

Doran SE, Papadopoulos SM, Ducker TB et al. (1993). Magnetic resonance imaging documentation of coexistent traumatic locked facets of the cervical spine and disc herniation. J Neurosurg 79: 341–345.

Duane TM, Cross J, Scarcella N et al. (2010). Flexion-extension cervical spine plain films compared with MRI in the diagnosis of ligamentous injury. Am Surg 76: 595–598.

Eastman AL, Chason DP, Perez CL et al. (2006). Computed tomographic angiography for the diagnosis of blunt cervical vascular injury: is it ready for primetime? J Trauma 60: 925–929. discussion 929.

Edwards P, Arango M, Balica L et al. (2005). Final results of MRC CRASH, a randomised placebo-controlled trial of intravenous corticosteroid in adults with head injury-outcomes at 6 months. Lancet Lond Engl 365: 1957–1959.

Evaniew N, Belley-Côté EP, Fallah N et al. (2016). Methylprednisolone for the treatment of patients with acute spinal cord injuries: a systematic review and meta-analysis. J Neurotrauma 33: 468–481.

Evans D (1961). Reduction of cervical dislocations. J Bone Jt Surg Br 43 (B): 552–555.

Farrington JD (1968). Extrication of victims – surgical principles. J Trauma 8: 493–512.

Foreman PM, Griessenauer CJ, Chua M et al. (2015). Corrective spinal surgery may be protective against stroke in patients with blunt traumatic vertebral artery occlusion. J Neurosurg Spine: 1–6.

Geerts WH, Code KI, Jay RM et al. (1994). A prospective study of venous thromboembolism after major trauma. N Engl J Med 331: 1601–1606.

Geisler WO, Wynne-Jones M, Jousse AT (1966). Early management of the patient with trauma to the spinal cord. Med Serv J Can 22: 512–523.

Geisler FH, Dorsey FC, Coleman WP (1991). Recovery of motor function after spinal-cord injury – a randomized, placebo-controlled trial with GM-1 ganglioside. N Engl J Med 324: 1829–1838.

Geisler FH, Coleman WP, Grieco G et al. (2001). The Sygen multicenter acute spinal cord injury study. Spine 26: S87–S98.

Gelb DE, Hadley MN, Aarabi B et al. (2013). Initial closed reduction of cervical spinal fracture-dislocation injuries. Neurosurgery 72 (Suppl 2): 73–83.

Gorman PH, Qadri SFA, Rao-Patel A (2009). Prophylactic inferior vena cava (IVC) filter placement may increase the relative risk of deep venous thrombosis after acute spinal cord injury. J Trauma 66: 707–712.

Grande CM, Barton CR, Stene JK (1988). Appropriate techniques for airway management of emergency patients with suspected spinal cord injury. Anesth Analg 67: 714–715.

Grant GA, Mirza SK, Chapman JR et al. (1999). Risk of early closed reduction in cervical spine subluxation injuries. J Neurosurg 90: 13–18.

Green BA, Eismont FJ, O'Heir JT (1987). Spinal cord injury – a systems approach: prevention, emergency medical services, and emergency room management. Crit Care Clin 3: 471–493.

Green D, Lee MY, Ito VY et al. (1988). Fixed- vs adjusted-dose heparin in the prophylaxis of thromboembolism in spinal cord injury. JAMA 260: 1255–1258.

Green D, Sullivan S, Simpson J et al. (2005). Evolving risk for thromboembolism in spinal cord injury (SPIRATE Study). Am J Phys Med Rehabil Assoc Acad Physiatr 84: 420–422.

Greg Anderson D, Voets C, Ropiak R et al. (2004). Analysis of patient variables affecting neurologic outcome after traumatic cervical facet dislocation. Spine J Off J North Am Spine Soc 4: 506–512.

Grossman RG, Frankowski RF, Burau KD et al. (2012). Incidence and severity of acute complications after spinal cord injury. J Neurosurg Spine 17: 119–128.

Gunby I (1981). New focus on spinal cord injury. JAMA 245: 1201–1206.

Gurdjian ES, Hardy WG, Lindner DW et al. (1963). Closed cervical cranial trauma associated with involvement of carotid and vertebral arteries. J Neurosurg 20: 418–427.

Hachen HJ (1974a). Emergency transportation in the event of acute spinal cord lesion. Paraplegia 12 (1): 33–37.

Hachen HJ (1974b). Anticoagulant therapy in patients with spinal cord injury. Paraplegia 12: 176–187.

Hachen HJ (1977). Idealized care of the acutely injured spinal cord in Switzerland. J Trauma 17: 931–936.

Hadley MN, Walters BC (2013). Guidelines for the management of acute cervical spine and spinal cord injuries. Neurosurgery 72: 1–259.

Hadley MN, Fitzpatrick BC, Sonntag VK et al. (1992). Facet fracture-dislocation injuries of the cervical spine. Neurosurgery 30: 661–666.

Hadley MN, Walters BC, Grabb PA (2002). Guidelines for the management of acute cervical spine and spinal cord injuries. Neurosurgery 50: S2–S199.

Hadley MN, Walters BC, Aarabi B et al. (2013). Clinical assessment following acute cervical spinal cord injury. Neurosurgery 72 (Suppl 2): 40–53.

Harrigan MR, Hadley MN, Dhall SS et al. (2013). Management of vertebral artery injuries following non-penetrating cervical trauma. Neurosurgery 72 (Suppl 2): 234–243.

Harrop JS, Sharan AD, Scheid EH et al. (2004). Tracheostomy placement in patients with complete cervical spinal cord injuries: American Spinal Injury Association Grade A. J Neurosurg 100: 20–23.

Hassid VJ, Schinco MA, Tepas JJ et al. (2008). Definitive establishment of airway control is critical for optimal outcome in lower cervical spinal cord injury. J Trauma 65: 1328–1332.

Haut ER, Kalish BT, Efron DT et al. (2010). Spine immobilization in penetrating trauma: more harm than good? J. Trauma 68: 115–120. discussion 120–121.

Hawryluk G, Whetstone W, Saigal R et al. (2015). Mean arterial blood pressure correlates with neurological recovery after human spinal cord injury: analysis of high frequency physiologic data. J Neurotrauma 32: 1958–1967.

Hector SM, Biering-Sørensen T, Krassioukov A et al. (2013). Cardiac arrhythmias associated with spinal cord injury. J Spinal Cord Med 36: 591–599.

Hennessy D, Widder S, Zygun D et al. (2010). Cervical spine clearance in obtunded blunt trauma patients: a prospective study. J Trauma 68: 576–582.

Hewitt S (1994). Skin necrosis caused by a semi-rigid cervical collar in a ventilated patient with multiple injuries. Injury 25: 323–324.

Hindman BJ, From RP, Fontes RB et al. (2015). Intubation biomechanics: laryngoscope force and cervical spine motion during intubation in cadavers-cadavers versus patients, the effect of repeated intubations, and the effect of type II odontoid fracture on C1-C2 motion. Anesthesiology 123: 1042–1058.

Hindman BJ, Fontes RB, From RP et al. (2016). Intubation biomechanics: laryngoscope force and cervical spine motion during intubation in cadavers-effect of severe distractive-flexion injury on C3-4 motion. J Neurosurg Spine: 1–11.

Hoffman JR, Mower WR, Wolfson AB et al. (2000). Validity of a set of clinical criteria to rule out injury to the cervical spine in patients with blunt trauma. National Emergency X-Radiography Utilization Study Group. N Engl J Med 343: 94–99.

Horn EM, Lekovic GP, Feiz-Erfan I et al. (2004). Cervical magnetic resonance imaging abnormalities not predictive of cervical spine instability in traumatically injured patients. Invited submission from the Joint Section Meeting on Disorders of the Spine and Peripheral Nerves, March 2004. J Neurosurg Spine 1: 39–42.

Hurlbert RJ, Hadley MN, Walters BC et al. (2013). Pharmacological therapy for acute spinal cord injury. Neurosurgery 72 (Suppl 2): 93–105.

Inoue T, Manley GT, Patel N et al. (2014). Medical and surgical management after spinal cord injury: vasopressor usage, early surgerys, and complications. J Neurotrauma 31: 284–291.

Insko EK, Gracias VH, Gupta R et al. (2002). Utility of flexion and extension radiographs of the cervical spine in the acute evaluation of blunt trauma. J Trauma 53: 426–429.

Ito Y, Sugimoto Y, Tomioka M et al. (2009). Does high dose methylprednisolone sodium succinate really improve neurological status in patient with acute cervical cord injury? A prospective study about neurological recovery and early complications. Spine 34: 2121–2124.

Itzkovich M, Gelernter I, Biering-Sorensen F et al. (2007). The Spinal Cord Independence Measure (SCIM) version III: reliability and validity in a multi-center international study. Disabil Rehabil 29: 1926–1933.

Jensen MP, Widerström-Noga E, Richards JS et al. (2010). Reliability and validity of the International Spinal Cord Injury Basic Pain Data Set items as self-report measures. Spinal Cord 48: 230–238.

Key A (1975). Cervical spine dislocations with unilateral facet interlocking. Paraplegia 13: 208–215.

Kirshblum SC, Memmo P, Kim N et al. (2002). Comparison of the revised 2000 American Spinal Injury Association classification standards with the 1996 guidelines. Am J Phys Med Rehabil Assoc Acad Physiatr 81: 502–505.

Kleyn PJ (1984). Dislocations of the cervical spine: closed reduction under anaesthesia. Paraplegia 22: 271–281.

Kolb JC, Summers RL, Galli RL (1999). Cervical collar-induced changes in intracranial pressure. Am J Emerg Med 17: 135–137.

Kossuth LC (1965). The removal of injured personnel from wrecked vehicles. J Trauma 5: 703–708.

Ledsome JR, Sharp JM (1981). Pulmonary function in acute cervical cord injury. Am Rev Respir Dis 124: 41–44.

Lee AS, MacLean JC, Newton DA (1994). Rapid traction for reduction of cervical spine dislocations. J Bone Joint Surg Br 76: 352–356.

Leelapattana P, Fleming JC, Gurr KR et al. (2012). Predicting the need for tracheostomy in patients with cervical spinal cord injury. J Trauma Acute Care Surg 73: 880–884.

Lehmann KG, Lane JG, Piepmeier JM et al. (1987). Cardiovascular abnormalities accompanying acute spinal cord injury in humans: incidence, time course and severity. J Am Coll Cardiol 10: 46–52.

Levi L, Wolf A, Belzberg H (1993). Hemodynamic parameters in patients with acute cervical cord trauma: description, intervention, and prediction of outcome. Neurosurgery 33: 1007–1016. discussion 1016–1017.

Levi AD, Tator CH, Bunge RP (1996). Clinical syndromes associated with disproportionate weakness of the upper versus the lower extremities after cervical spinal cord injury. Neurosurgery 38: 179–183. discussion 183–185.

Liew SC, Hill DA (1994). Complication of hard cervical collars in multi-trauma patients. Aust N Z J Surg 64: 139–140.

Linares HA, Mawson AR, Suarez E et al. (1987). Association between pressure sores and immobilization in the immediate post-injury period. Orthopedics 10: 571–573.

Maiman DJ, Barolat G, Larson SJ (1986). Management of bilateral locked facets of the cervical spine. Neurosurgery 18: 542–547.

Mathen R, Inaba K, Munera F et al. (2007). Prospective evaluation of multislice computed tomography versus plain radiographic cervical spine clearance in trauma patients. J Trauma 62: 1427–1431.

Matsumoto T, Tamaki T, Kawakami M et al. (2001). Early complications of high-dose methylprednisolone sodium succinate treatment in the follow-up of acute cervical spinal cord injury. Spine 26: 426–430.

Mawson AR, Biundo JJ, Neville P et al. (1988). Risk factors for early occurring pressure ulcers following spinal cord injury. Am J Phys Med Rehabil Assoc Acad Physiatr 67: 123–127.

McCabe JB, Nolan DJ (1986). Comparison of the effectiveness of different cervical immobilization collars. Ann Emerg Med 15: 50–53.

McKinley WO, Jackson AB, Cardenas DD et al. (1999). Long-term medical complications after traumatic spinal cord injury: a regional model systems analysis. Arch Phys Med Rehabil 80: 1402–1410.

McMichan JC, Michel L, Westbrook PR (1980). Pulmonary dysfunction following traumatic quadriplegia. Recognition, prevention, and treatment. JAMA 243: 528–531.

Merli GJ, Herbison GJ, Ditunno JF et al. (1988). Deep vein thrombosis: prophylaxis in acute spinal cord injured patients. Arch Phys Med Rehabil 69: 661–664.

Merli GJ, Crabbe S, Doyle L et al. (1992). Mechanical plus pharmacological prophylaxis for deep vein thrombosis in acute spinal cord injury. Paraplegia 30: 558–562.

Moerman JR, Christie BD, Sykes LN et al. (2011). Early cardiac pacemaker placement for life-threatening bradycardia in traumatic spinal cord injury. J Trauma 70: 1485–1488.

Moylan JA (1985). Trauma injuries. Triage and stabilization for safe transfer. Postgrad Med 78: 166–171. 174–175, 177.

Muchow RD, Resnick DK, Abdel MP et al. (2008). Magnetic resonance imaging (MRI) in the clearance of the cervical spine in blunt trauma: a meta-analysis. J Trauma 64: 179–189.

O'Conner P, McCormack O, Noel J et al. (2003). Anterior displacement correlates with neurological impairment in cervical facet dislocations. Int Orthop 27: 190–193.

O'Keeffe T, Goldman RK, Mayberry JC et al. (2004). Tracheostomy after anterior cervical spine fixation. J Trauma 57: 855–860.

Padayachee L, Cooper DJ, Irons S et al. (2006). Cervical spine clearance in unconscious traumatic brain injury patients: dynamic flexion-extension fluoroscopy versus computed tomography with three-dimensional reconstruction. J Trauma 60: 341–345.

Patel MB, Humble SS, Cullinane DC et al. (2015). Cervical spine collar clearance in the obtunded adult blunt trauma patient: a systematic review and practice management guideline from the Eastern Association for the Surgery of Trauma. J Trauma Acute Care Surg 78: 430–441.

Paulus EM, Fabian TC, Savage SA et al. (2014). Blunt cerebrovascular injury screening with 64-channel multidetector computed tomography: more slices finally cut it. J Trauma 76: 279–283.

Piepmeier JM, Lehmann KB, Lane JG (1985). Cardiovascular instability following acute cervical spinal cord trauma. Cent Nerv Syst Trauma J Am Paralys Assoc 2: 153–160.

Podolsky SM, Hoffman JR, Pietrafesa CA (1983). Neurologic complications following immobilization of cervical spine fracture in a patient with ankylosing spondylitis. Ann Emerg Med 12: 578–580.

Pointillart V, Petitjean ME, Wiart L et al. (2000). Pharmacological therapy of spinal cord injury during the acute phase. Spinal Cord 38: 71–76.

Pollack CV, Hendey GW, Martin DR et al. (2001). Use of flexion-extension radiographs of the cervical spine in blunt trauma. Ann Emerg Med 38: 8–11.

Powell M, Kirshblum S, O'Connor KC (1999). Duplex ultrasound screening for deep vein thrombosis in spinal cord injured patients at rehabilitation admission. Arch Phys Med Rehabil 80: 1044–1046.

Prasad VS, Schwartz A, Bhutani R et al. (1999). Characteristics of injuries to the cervical spine and spinal cord in polytrauma patient population: experience from a regional trauma unit. Spinal Cord 37: 560–568.

Qian T, Guo X, Levi AD et al. (2005). High-dose methylprednisolone may cause myopathy in acute spinal cord injury patients. Spinal Cord 43: 199–203.

Ready WJ, Whetstone WD, Ferguson AR et al. (2015). Complications and outcomes of vasopressor usage in acute traumatic central cord syndrome. J Neurosurg Spine 31: 1–7.

Rimel RW, Jane JA, Edlich RF (1981). An educational training program for the care at the site of injury of trauma to the central nervous system. Resuscitation 9: 23–28.

Rizzolo SJ, Vaccaro AR, Cotler JM (1994). Cervical spine trauma. Spine 19: 2288–2298.

Roberts DJ, Chaubey VP, Zygun DA et al. (2013). Diagnostic accuracy of computed tomography angiography for blunt cerebrovascular injury detection in trauma patients: a systematic review and meta-analysis. Ann Surg 257: 621–632.

Romero J, Vari A, Gambarrutta C et al. (2009). Tracheostomy timing in traumatic spinal cord injury. Eur Spine J Off Publ Eur Spine Soc Eur Spinal Deform Soc Eur Sect Cerv Spine Res Soc 18: 1452–1457.

Rosen PB, McSwain NE, Arata M et al. (1992). Comparison of two new immobilization collars. Ann Emerg Med 21: 1189–1195.

Rudhe C, van Hedel HJA (2009). Upper extremity function in persons with tetraplegia: relationships between strength, capacity, and the spinal cord independence measure. Neurorehabil Neural Repair 23: 413–421.

Ryken TC, Hadley MN, Walters BC et al. (2013a). Radiographic assessment. Neurosurgery 72 (Suppl 2): 54–72.

Ryken TC, Hurlbert RJ, Hadley MN et al. (2013b). The acute cardiopulmonary management of patients with cervical spinal cord injuries. Neurosurgery 72 (Suppl 2): 84–92.

San Mateo County, C., 1991. EMS System Policy Memorandum #f-3A.

Savic G, Bergström EMK, Frankel HL et al. (2007). Inter-rater reliability of motor and sensory examinations performed according to American Spinal Injury Association standards. Spinal Cord 45: 444–451.

Schafermeyer RW, Ribbeck BM, Gaskins J et al. (1991). Respiratory effects of spinal immobilization in children. Ann Emerg Med 20: 1017–1019.

Schoenfeld AJ, Bono CM, McGuire KJ et al. (2010). Computed tomography alone versus computed tomography and magnetic resonance imaging in the identification of occult injuries to the cervical spine: a meta-analysis. J Trauma 68: 109–113. discussion 113–114.

Schoenwaelder M, Maclaurin W, Varma D (2009). Assessing potential spinal injury in the intubated multi-trauma patient: does MRI add value? Emerg Radiol 16: 129–132.

Schuster R, Waxman K, Sanchez B et al. (2005). Magnetic resonance imaging is not needed to clear cervical spines in blunt trauma patients with normal computed tomographic results and no motor deficits. Arch Surg Chic Ill 1960 (140): 762–766.

Shapiro SA (1993). Management of unilateral locked facet of the cervical spine. Neurosurgery 33: 832–837. discussion 837.

Shatney CH, Brunner RD, Nguyen TQ (1995). The safety of orotracheal intubation in patients with unstable cervical spine fracture or high spinal cord injury. Am J Surg 170: 676–679. discussion 679–680.

Shrosbree RD (1979). Neurological sequelae of reduction of fracture dislocations of the cervical spine. Paraplegia 17: 212–221.

Slavik RS, Chan E, Gorman SK et al. (2007). Dalteparin versus enoxaparin for venous thromboembolism prophylaxis in acute spinal cord injury and major orthopedic trauma patients: 'DETECT' trial. J Trauma 62: 1075–1081.

Sonntag VK (1981). Management of bilateral locked facets of the cervical spine. Neurosurgery 8: 150–152.

Spinal Cord Injury Thromboprophylaxis Investigators (2003a). Prevention of venous thromboembolism in the acute treatment phase after spinal cord injury: a randomized, multicenter trial comparing low-dose heparin plus intermittent pneumatic compression with enoxaparin. J Trauma 54: 1116–1124.

Spinal Cord Injury Thromboprophylaxis Investigators (2003b). Prevention of venous thromboembolism in the rehabilitation phase after spinal cord injury: prophylaxis with low-dose heparin or enoxaparin. J Trauma 54: 1111–1115.

Star AM, Jones AA, Cotler JM et al. (1990). Immediate closed reduction of cervical spine dislocations using traction. Spine 15: 1068–1072.

Stiell IG, Wells GA, Vandemheen KL et al. (2001). The Canadian C-spine rule for radiography in alert and stable trauma patients. JAMA 286: 1841–1848.

Stiell IG, Clement CM, McKnight RD et al. (2003). The Canadian C-spine rule versus the NEXUS low-risk criteria in patients with trauma. N Engl J Med 349: 2510–2518.

Stroh G, Braude D (2001). Can an out-of-hospital cervical spine clearance protocol identify all patients with injuries? An argument for selective immobilization. Ann Emerg Med 37: 609–615.

Suechting RL, French LA (1955). Posterior inferior cerebellar artery syndrome; following a fracture of the cervical vertebra. J Neurosurg 12: 187–189.

Tator CH, Rowed DW, Schwartz ML et al. (1984). Management of acute spinal cord injuries. Can J Surg J Can Chir 27 (289–293): 296.

Tator CH, Duncan EG, Edmonds VE et al. (1993). Changes in epidemiology of acute spinal cord injury from 1947 to 1981. Surg Neurol 40: 207–215.

Theodore N, Aarabi B, Dhall SS et al. (2013a). Transportation of patients with acute traumatic cervical spine injuries. Neurosurgery 72 (Suppl 2): 35–39.

Theodore N, Hadley MN, Aarabi B et al. (2013b). Prehospital cervical spinal immobilization after trauma. Neurosurgery 72 (Suppl 2): 22–34.

Thompson SR, Zlololow DA (2012). Handbook of Splinting and Casting. Elsevier, pp. 291–295.

Thumbikat P, Hariharan RP, Ravichandran G et al. (2007). Spinal cord injury in patients with ankylosing spondylitis: a 10-year review. Spine 32: 2989–2995.

Tomycz ND, Chew BG, Chang Y-F et al. (2008). MRI is unnecessary to clear the cervical spine in obtunded/comatose trauma patients: the four-year experience of a level I trauma center. J Trauma 64: 1258–1263.

Toscano J (1988). Prevention of neurological deterioration before admission to a spinal cord injury unit. Paraplegia 26: 143–150.

Totten VY, Sugarman DB (1999). Respiratory effects of spinal immobilization. Prehospital Emerg Care Off J Natl Assoc EMS Physicians Natl Assoc State EMS Dir 3: 347–352.

Vaccaro AR, An HS, Lin S et al. (1992). Noncontiguous injuries of the spine. J Spinal Disord 5: 320–329.

Vale FL, Burns J, Jackson AB et al. (1997). Combined medical and surgical treatment after acute spinal cord injury: results of a prospective pilot study to assess the merits of aggressive medical resuscitation and blood pressure management. J Neurosurg 87: 239–246.

Vollmer D, Eichler M, Jenkins III A (2011). Spinal trauma: assessment of the cervical spine after trauma, in: Youmans Neurological Surgery. Elsevier, Amsterdam, The Netherlands, pp. 3166–3180.

Walton G (1893). A new method of reducing dislocation of cervical vertebrae. J Nerv Ment Dis 20: 609.

Williams KD (2013). Campbell's Operative Orthopaedics. Elsevier, pp. 1559–1627.

Willis BK, Greiner F, Orrison WW et al. (1994). The incidence of vertebral artery injury after midcervical spine fracture or subluxation. Neurosurgery 34: 435–441. discussion 441–442.

Wilson JT, Rogers FB, Wald SL et al. (1994). Prophylactic vena cava filter insertion in patients with traumatic spinal cord injury: preliminary results. Neurosurgery 35: 234–239. discussion 239.

Wolf A, Levi L, Mirvis S et al. (1991). Operative management of bilateral facet dislocation. J Neurosurg 75: 883–890.

Zäch GA, Seiler W, Dollfus P (1976). Treatment results of spinal cord injuries in the Swiss Paraplegic Centre of Basle. Paraplegia 14: 58–65.

*Handbook of Clinical Neurology, Vol. 140 (3rd series)*
*Critical Care Neurology, Part I*
E.F.M. Wijdicks and A.H. Kramer, Editors
http://dx.doi.org/10.1016/B978-0-444-63600-3.00016-7

Chapter 16

# Decompressive craniectomy in acute brain injury

D.A. BROWN[1] AND E.F.M. WIJDICKS[2]*

[1]*Department of Neurological Surgery, Mayo Clinic, Rochester, MN, USA*

[2]*Division of Critical Care Neurology, Mayo Clinic and Neurosciences Intensive Care Unit, Mayo Clinic Campus, Saint Marys Hospital, Rochester, MN, USA*

## Abstract

Decompressive surgery to reduce pressure under the skull varies from a burrhole, bone flap to removal of a large skull segment. Decompressive craniectomy is the removal of a large enough segment of skull to reduce refractory intracranial pressure and to maintain cerebral compliance for the purpose of preventing neurologic deterioration. Decompressive hemicraniectomy and bifrontal craniectomy are the most commonly performed procedures. Bifrontal craniectomy is most often utilized with generalized cerebral edema in the absence of a focal mass lesion and when there are bilateral frontal contusions. Decompressive hemicraniectomy is most commonly considered for malignant middle cerebral artery infarcts. The ethical predicament of deciding to go ahead with a major neurosurgical procedure with the purpose of avoiding brain death from displacement, but resulting in prolonged severe disability in many, are addressed.

This chapter describes indications, surgical techniques, and complications. It reviews results of recent clinical trials and provides a reasonable assessment for practice.

## INTRODUCTION

Removal of parts of the skull (bone flap) has a long history dating back to the Neolithic period, with archaeologic evidence of the practice from several cultures from Africa, Asia, and the Americas (Kshettry et al., 2007). Hippocrates published the first systematic description of trephination replete with a discussion of the injuries for which the intervention was appropriate (Panourias et al., 2005). Theodor Kocher published the first modern description of decompressive craniectomy (DC) with the following historic "preamble" to the now revered Monro–Kellie doctrine: "if there is no cerebrospinal fluid (CSF) pressure, but brain pressure exists, then pressure relief must be achieved by opening the skull" (Kolias et al., 2013). Employing the technique previously published by Kocher, Harvey Cushing (1908) reported use of DC for relief of "cerebral hernia" associated with brain

tumors. In the same collection of papers, he reported the first case series on the use of DC in the setting of traumatic brain injury in which he performed subtemporal craniectomy on patients following traumatic brain injury. In his small series of only 15 patients, only 2 succumbed to their injury, which represents, both then and now, a remarkable improvement in prognosis over the expected natural course. Over the subsequent century, DC has been applied to a number of clinical scenarios in which structural and functional brain anatomy is threatened by a mass lesion, as shown in Table 16.1. Whether DC improves functional outcome for patients remains a contentious issue. In this chapter, we will discuss DC with primary focus on use of the technique in traumatic brain injury and malignant middle cerebral artery (MCA) infarction, the two indications for which there has been a considerable amount of interest and research.

---

*Correspondence to: Eelco F.M. Wijdicks, MD, PhD, Department of Neurology, Mayo Clinic, 200 First Street SW, Rochester MN 55905, USA. E-mail: wijde@mayo.edu

*Table 16.1*

**Perceived indications for decompressive craniectomy***

| Year | Case description | Reference |
|------|-----------------|-----------|
| **1908** | Subtemporal craniectomy for traumatic brain injury | Cushing (1908) |
| **1976** | Reye's syndrome encephalopathy | Ausman et al. (1976) |
| **1980** | Cerebral venous and superior sagittal sinus thrombosis | Ohya and Sato (1980), Stefini et al. (1999) |
| **1981** | Hemicraniectomy for acute massive cerebral infarction | Rengachary et al. (1981) |
| **1984** | Multiple cerebrovascular occlusive disease associated with neurofibromatosis | Sasaki et al. (1984) |
| **1990** | Syringomyelia associated with Arnold–Chiari malformation | Keyaki et al. (1990) |
| **1992** | Cerebellar infarction | Chen et al. (1992) |
| **1994** | Worsening coma in acute subarachnoid hemorrhage | Fisher and Ojemann (1994) |
| **1994** | Tuberculous hypertrophic pachymeningitis involving the posterior fossa and high cervical region | Yamashita et al. (1994) |
| **1997** | Lhermitte–Duclos disease | Tuli et al. (1997) |
| **1999** | Posttraumatic pituitary apoplexy | Uchiyama et al. (1999) |
| **2000** | Mucopolysaccharidoses with compression | Kachur and Del Maestro (2000) |
| **2002** | Acute subdural empyema or bacterial meningoencephalitis | Ong et al. (2002), Raffelsieper et al. (2002) |
| **2002** | Hajdu–Cheney syndrome | Faure et al. (2002) |
| **2003** | Herpetic encephalitis | Mellado et al. (2003) |
| **2005** | Cerebral toxoplasmosis | Agrawal and Hussain (2005) |
| **2006** | Paget's disease with symptomatic basilar impression | Gabrovski et al. (2006) |
| **2008** | Pneumococcal meningitis | Perin et al. (2008) |
| **2008** | Malignant monophasic multiple sclerosis (Marburg's disease type) | Gonzalez Sanchez et al. (2010) |
| **2009** | Tumefactive demyelinating disease | Nilsson et al. (2009) |
| **2010** | Acute disseminated encephalomyelitis (ADEM) | Ahmed et al. (2010) |
| **2012** | Butane intoxication | Peyravi et al. (2012) |
| **2012** | Giant frontal mucocele | Visocchi et al. (2012) |
| **2012** | Epstein–Barr virus encephalitis | Hayton et al. (2012) |
| **2013** | Pseudotumoral acute hemicerebellitis in a child | Morais et al. (2013) |

*A PubMed search was performed using the term "decompressive craniectomy" with a Case Reports filter. The first unique mention of decompressive craniectomy for a given indication was included in the table.

## PATHOPHYSIOLOGY

The underlying rationale for DC is the Monroe–Kellie doctrine which states that any increase in intracranial volume must be offset by a concomitant decrease in another intracranial component in order to maintain intracranial pressure (ICP) (Mokri, 2001). The underlying assumption is that increasing the size of the intracranial compartment (opening the box through DC) reduces ICP and increases compliance (Quinn et al., 2011). There is good evidence that indeed decompression reduces ICP (Bor-Seng-Shu et al., 2012) although, as will be subsequently reviewed, the clinical impact of that reduction on actual patient outcomes remains controversial.

Several studies in mammalian models have been performed with the ultimate aim of understanding the physiologic impact of DC as both justification for the technique and to understand some of the reported complications (see review of complications, below). Schaller et al. (2003) used a positron emission tomography (PET)-computed tomography (CT) method to evaluate the impact of left hemicraniectomy performed on normal cats. They demonstrated reduction in cerebral blood flow and increase in the oxygen extraction fraction in the region of the craniectomy. The cerebral metabolic rate of oxygen and glucose decreased in regions with severe reduction in cerebral blood flow. These changes remained at least 24 hours, regardless of whether corrective cranioplasty was performed. Nonetheless, several animal models of DC for acute cerebral infarction have demonstrated early reperfusion, reduction in edema and infarct size following decompression (Forsting et al., 1995; Doerfler et al., 1996; Engelhorn et al., 1999, 2003). Similarly, animal models of DC for traumatic brain injury have demonstrated reduction in secondary edema and, ultimately, neuroprotection (Zweckberger et al., 2006; Tian et al., 2015), though the intervention may compromise CSF flow dynamics which, again, has implications for posthemicraniectomy complications (Karacalioglu et al., 2011).

# What (technically) is decompressive craniectomy?

DC is the removal of a large enough segment of skull to facilitate reduction of ICPs and the maintenance of cerebral compliance for the purpose of preventing neurologic deterioration. There are two technical points that are of paramount importance in DC. The first of these is that the bony decompression must be sufficiently large to prevent herniation through the craniectomy window with resultant compression of bridging veins leading to a venous infarct and a paradoxically worse outcome (Wagner et al., 2001; Whitfield et al., 2001; Jiang et al., 2005; Li et al., 2012; Tagliaferri et al., 2012; Kolias et al., 2013). To facilitate adequate bony removal and prevent associated complications, several authors recommend a minimum bone flap diameter of 11–12 cm (Wagner et al., 2001; Li et al., 2012; Tagliaferri et al., 2012). Secondly, bony decompression without wide durotomy does not provide sufficient room for brain expansion and a wide durotomy is thus an important and indeed required step in the performance of an adequate DC (Polin et al., 1997; Whitfield et al., 2001; Timofeev and Hutchinson, 2006; Timofeev et al., 2006; Guresir et al., 2011; Quinn et al., 2011; Kolias et al., 2013).

Three main techniques for DC are typically employed: subtemporal, bifrontal, and frontotemporoparietal (classically considered decompressive hemicraniectomy). The latter can be performed unilaterally or bilaterally as clinically indicated. To date, there is a paucity of studies with direct comparison of the efficacy of the various techniques. One randomized trial comparing unilateral hemicraniectomy to a temporoparietal craniectomy showed that the former provided greater reductions in ICP, mortality, and overall neurologic outcomes at the cost of an increased incidence of delayed intracranial hematomas and subdural effusions (Qiu et al., 2009). These results provide information important for further large and multicenter clinical trials on the effects of DC in patients with acute posttraumatic brain swelling.

As decompressive hemicraniectomy and bifrontal craniectomy are the most commonly performed, we will limit our discussion to these two techniques. The discussion presented herein is meant for a broad audience to foster basic understanding of the techniques, thus only a cursory technical overview will be presented. The reader is encouraged to explore the neurosurgical literature for a more thorough handling of specific neurosurgical techniques and their rationale.

## BIFRONTAL CRANIECTOMY

The bifrontal craniectomy is most often utilized in cases of generalized cerebral edema in the absence of a focal mass lesion and when there are bilateral frontal contusions (Polin et al., 1997; Quinn et al., 2011). The incision extends from the zygomatic arch immediately anterior to the tragus and courses 2–3 cm posterior to the coronal suture and then toward the contralateral zygomatic arch. Soft-tissue dissection is carried down to the level of the bone and the myocutaneous flap is brought anteriorly to the orbital rim with care taken to preserve the supraorbital nerves. Burrholes are then made in the keyholes and squamous temporal bone as well as across the midline, where they straddle the superior sagittal sinus and coronal suture. Blunt dissection is used to free the sinus from the overlying bone prior to completion of the craniectomy with a cutting drill bit equipped with a foot plate. A central tenet of this technique is dural opening and division of the anterior superior sagittal sinus and falx, without which the brain cannot fully expand anteriorly and has a significant risk of herniation against the dural edge (Polin et al., 1997; Quinn et al., 2011).

## FRONTOTEMPOROPARIETAL HEMICRANIECTOMY

This technique is the archetype of decompressive hemicraniectomy and is the most common technique employed (Quinn et al., 2011). Its utility spans traumatic brain injury, hemispheric infarction, and a plethora of other etiologies, ultimately resulting in brain compression and/or herniation. It is of particular utility when there is a mass lesion such as a compressive hematoma on the side of the decompression. The patient is positioned supine with the ipsilateral shoulder elevated and the head turned away from the craniectomy side. If the procedure is being performed in the context of a traumatic brain injury, the head is generally placed on a donut as there can be devastating injuries from unrecognized skull fractures. This is particularly true for fractures in the axial plane, which are easily missed on preoperative CT scans. It is of paramount importance to be cognizant of surface landmarks – particularly the midline – as transgression of the superior sagittal sinus can often have dire consequences in the setting of trauma, where patients are often coagulopathic and where there may be trauma to draining cortical veins. The typical incision is a reverse question mark that begins anterior to the ipsilateral tragus at the zygomatic arch and then courses posterosuperiorly over the pinna toward the external occipital protuberance, where it then curves cranially toward the vertex and ends at the anterior hairline just off the midline. It is important to preserve vascular supply to the flap, which is often severed as the incision is carried posteriorly.

An alternate incision is the "tulip" or "T-bar" incision, popularized by military neurosurgeons treating wartime injuries (Ragel et al., 2010). This incision extends from the anterior hairline toward the inion just off the midline,

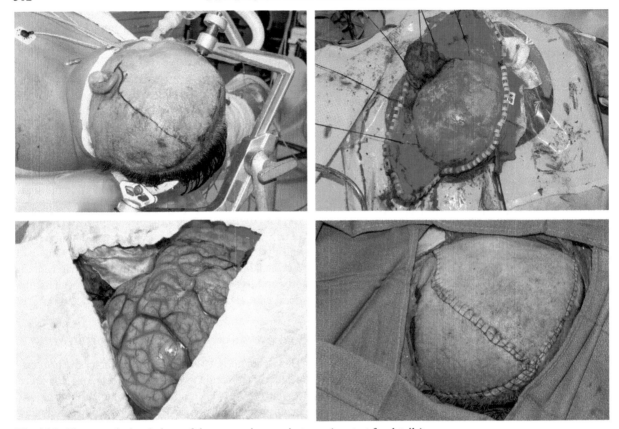

**Fig. 16.1.** Neurosurgical technique of decompressive craniectomy (see text for details).

with a separate incision beginning anterior to the ipsilateral tragus at the zygomatic arch and extending medially toward the midline sagittal incision as shown in Figure 16.1. The advantage of this is efficiency, preservation of vascular supply to the flap, and a wide opening that allows for maximizing the craniectomy. The pitfall is the risk of necrosis at the point where the incisions meet and subsequent wound complications. Once meticulous hemostasis is attained, burrholes are made at the keyhole, the squamous temporal bone, the parietal bone, and as many as necessary along the medial extent of the intended craniectomy to facilitate stripping the underlying dura without damage to the superior sagittal sinus. These latter burrholes are placed approximately 2 cm lateral to the midline to avoid inadvertent transgression of the sinus. A cutting drill with foot plate is then used to connect the burrholes, with the medial burrholes connected last to facilitate expeditious removal if there is injury to the superior sagittal sinus. The bone flap can then safely be removed to expose the frontal, temporal, parietal, and occipital lobes, as shown in Figure 16.1C.

## DECOMPRESSIVE CRANIECTOMY FOR TRAUMA

Following Cushing's report of subtemporal decompression for trauma, there was very little published literature until the 1960s and 1970s, when interest in the technique was reignited. Since that time, there have been a number of case series and retrospective analyses of the efficacy of DC to improve the outcome of patients with traumatic brain injury and refractory high ICP. Some neurosurgeons felt decompressive surgery was the only option to treat increased ICP not responding to medical interventions; others felt the procedure was basically futile. The Decompressive Craniectomy in Diffuse Traumatic Brain Injury (DECRA) study was the first randomized study to address this issue and the Randomized Evaluation of Surgery with Craniectomy for Uncontrollable Elevation of Intra-Cranial Pressure (RESCUEicp) study has recently been published.

### DECRA trial

The DECRA study was a randomized, multi-institution, multinational clinical trial aimed at determining whether DC improves functional outcome in patients with intracranial hypertension refractory to maximal medical therapy (Cooper et al., 2011). The study recruited patients between 2002 and 2010 from 15 tertiary care hospitals in Australia, New Zealand, and Saudi Arabia. Patients were between the ages of 15 and 59 admitted to an intensive care unit (ICU) with severe, nonpenetrating traumatic brain injury. "Severe" was defined as Glasgow

Coma Scale 3–8 or Marshall class III on head CT. Exclusion criteria included being "too sick to treat," dilated and unreactive pupils, mass lesions, concomitant spinal cord injury, or cardiac arrest at the scene of injury.

Maximal therapy followed currently accepted guidelines for the management of traumatic brain injury (Bratton et al., 2007a–o), with specific interventions standardized for the study (Cooper et al., 2008). A "refractory" elevation in ICP was defined as an increase $\geq 20$ mmHg for $\geq 15$ minutes (continuously or intermittently) within any 1-hour period despite maximal, first-tier interventions, including optimization of sedation, normalization of arterial carbon dioxide, hyperosmolar therapy with mannitol, hypertonic saline, neuromuscular blockade, and external ventricular drain.

Patients were randomized to surgery combined with standard medical treatment or standard treatment only within 72 hours postinjury. Stratification of patients was by center and mode of ICP determination (external ventricular drain versus ICP monitor). At all sites, surgery was performed using a standardized approach involving a large bifrontotemporoparietal craniectomy, bilateral dural opening without sectioning of the falx cerebri, or disturbance of the superior sagittal sinus (Polin et al., 1997). In patients with refractory ICP, acceptable second-tier interventions included mild hypothermia to 35°C and/or barbiturate use. Patients in the medical management arm who continued to fail therapy were allowed by protocol to cross over to DC after 72 hours had elapsed since the time of admission.

Initially, the primary outcome of the study was the proportion of patients with an unfavorable outcome – a composite of death, persistent vegetative state, or severe disability (defined as a score of 1–4 on the Extended Glasgow Outcome Scale: EGOS). However, this was revised after interim analysis to functional outcome at 6 months postinjury based on proportional odds analysis of the EGOS. The secondary outcomes were hourly ICP measurements pre- and postrandomization, intracranial hypertension index, the proportion of survivors with EGOS of 2–4 (indicating severe disability and the need for assistance with activities of daily living), the number of ICU days, in-hospital and 6-month mortality. Outcomes were assessed by blinded reviewers.

The authors screened 3478 patients, ultimately enrolling 155, 88% of whom were treated in Australia or New Zealand. There were 73 and 82 patients in the surgery versus medical management arms, respectively. Patients were similar except for a statistically significant larger proportion of patients with unreactive pupils in the surgical arm. Median age was 23.7 and 24.6 years for the surgical and standard-care arms, respectively. Among patients in the standard-care arm, 15 (18%) patients crossed over and underwent DC. In 4 (5%) of these cases, craniectomy occurred within 72 hours of admission,

contrary to the dictates of the protocol. Patients undergoing DC had reduction in ICP with fewer medical interventions for control. Surgically treated patients also had reductions in intracranial hypertension index and reduction in cerebral hypoperfusion index which were statistically significant. Furthermore, surgically treated patients spent less time on mechanical ventilation and fewer days in the ICU, although there was no statistically significant difference in the overall length of hospital stay. Despite the clear reduction in ICP, ICU days, and medical interventions for refractory ICP, this did not translate to better primary or secondary outcomes. Treatment-related complications were higher in patients who underwent DC (37% vs. 17%). Notable among these complications was the higher proportion of patients developing hydrocephalus after surgical decompression (10% vs. 1%). In fact, decompressive hemicraniectomy was associated with a higher risk of an unfavorable outcome (70% vs. 51%; $p = 0.02$).

Assessment of functional outcome at 6 months (the primary outcome) revealed a higher proportion of unfavorable outcomes in patients treated surgically with EGOS 3 versus 4 (odds ratio (OR) 1.84; 95% confidence interval (CI) 1.05–3.24; $p = 0.03$). Overall unfavorable outcomes occurred in 70% of patients undergoing craniectomy versus 51% of patients managed with standard medical care (OR 2.21; 95% CI 1.14–4.26; $p = 0.02$). Statistical significance was lost following adjustments for baseline pupil reactivity. There was no statistically significant difference in mortality between patients treated with decompressive hemicraniectomy versus those managed with standard medical care.

The authors concluded that decompressive hemicraniectomy in the setting of severe diffuse traumatic brain injury refractory to first-tier medical therapy reliably decreased ICP, ICU stay, and ventilatory support but was associated with significantly worse outcome at 6 months. They argued that the findings were potentially due at least in part to increased survival of surgical patients who were in a persistent vegetative state. Pathophysiologically, they postulated that axonal stretch in the setting of the free-brain expansion afforded by the decompression resulted in neural injury (Cooper et al., 1979; Chung et al., 2005; Stiver, 2009; Staal et al., 2010; Tang-Schomer et al., 2010). Alternatively, they speculated about the role of alterations in cerebral blood flow and metabolism on cerebral function and ultimate outcome (Timofeev et al., 2008; Soustiel et al., 2010).

## CRITIQUE OF DECRA

The unexpected negative results of the DECRA trial have spurred pre-existing controversy among neurosurgeons and neurointensivists, creating a global chasm between experts who vehemently disagree about the implications of the trial. The generalizability of the results has been called into question based on the fact that fewer than 5% of patients screened were ultimately randomized (Timmons et al., 2011). Several authors have critiqued the inadequacy of randomization as there was a significant difference in pupillary reactivity among patients treated surgically versus medically (Honeybul et al., 2011a; Timmons et al., 2011; Sahuquillo et al., 2013). In fact, Sahuquillo et al. (2013) argued that calculations using the CRASH (Olivecrona and Olivecrona, 2013) and IMPACT (Steyerberg et al., 2008) calculators resulted in a 10% difference in the risk of unfavorable outcomes based on pupillary reactivity alone. The substantial rate of crossover from medical to surgical management has been criticized, although the implications regarding the direction of the resulting bias are unclear (Honeybul et al., 2011a; Marion, 2011; Timmons et al., 2011; Cooper et al., 2012; Sahuquillo et al., 2013). Several experts have argued that the deviation from the surgical method described by Polin et al. (1997) is a major flaw in study design, as sectioning of the falx was considered a key component of the surgery, as it allowed enhancement of the anterior vector of expansion (Sahuquillo et al., 2013). Perhaps the most contentious issue has been the choice of ICP $\geq 20$ mmHg for $\geq 15$ minutes within 1 hour as the criterion for ICP intervention. Some authors contend that most practitioners would not intervene in practice even if the study ICP parameters were met, as 20 mmHg was too low and 15 minutes too short to justify any risk associated with treatment (Honeybul et al., 2011a; Servadei, 2011; Timmons et al., 2011; Sahuquillo et al., 2013). While this was a well-needed and adequately conducted study, it has caused legitimate controversy and further studies on the efficacy of decompressive hemicraniectomy are still needed. However, one justifiable question that had been raised is whether the results of the trial are convincing enough to raise ethical concerns regarding continuation of the RESCUEicp and RESCUE-ASDH trials aimed at parsing the role of surgical decompression (Bohman and Schuster, 2013).

## RESCUEicp trial

The RESCUEicp trial included 408 patients with ages 10 to 65 years and recruited over a long 10-year period spanning 2004 to 2014. The primary outcome was the extended Glasgow Outcome Scale at 6 months analyzed as an ordinal variable ranging from death to "upper good recovery" defines as no injury-related problems (Hutchinson et al., 2016). In stark contrast to the results of the DECRA trial, surgical intervention was associated with a significant increase in survival with death occurring in 26.9% of surgically managed patients versus

48.9% in patients managed medically. However, as was the case in the DECRA trial, surgical intervention resulted in an increase in the proportion of survivors that are vegetative (8.5% versus 2.1%) or severely disabled (21.9% versus 14.4%). There was no statistically significant difference in the proportion of patients in each arm with moderate disability or good recovery. Outcomes at 12 months followed a similar trend. The authors concluded that surgery conferred a survival advantage resulting in both dependent and independent living and implied that clinicians should discuss this with families of often young patients. A list of clinical trials of DC performed in the context of traumatic brain injury is shown in Table 16.2.

## DECOMPRESSIVE HEMICRANIECTOMY FOR HEMISPHERIC STROKE

The term "malignant" MCA infarction was coined to describe the sequelae of neurologic deterioration that occurs as a consequence of space-occupying cerebral edema in the context of large MCA ischemic infarctions (Rieke et al., 1995; Hacke et al., 1996; Juttler et al., 2011) although the syndrome had long been described (Schwab et al., 1997; Schwarz et al., 1998). The clinical course is rather uniform, with deterioration occurring within the first 2–3 days following the initial stroke. The incidence is approximately 10–20 per 100 000 per year and patients are approximately a full decade younger ($56 \pm 9.4$ years) than the average age of patients presenting with ischemic strokes in general (Hacke et al., 1996). Malignant MCA infarctions are associated with a mortality rate between 41 and 79% (Rieke et al., 1995; Hacke et al., 1996; Berrouschot et al., 1998; Juttler et al., 2011; Rahme et al., 2012) although both mortality and severe disability have decreased in the current era of DC (Wartenberg, 2012).

The outcome following large hemispheric ischemic infarcts is universally poor. Hacke et al. (1996) prospectively evaluated 55 patients with complete MCA territory infarction. Patients were between the ages of 18 and 70 experiencing a first ischemic stroke with documented MCA territory involvement on CT without hemorrhagic transformation. Forty-nine patients required ventilator assistance, with intubation occurring between 3 hours and 5 days. Need for intubation was a poor prognostic sign, as 43 of the 49 intubated patients died despite maximal therapy consisting of hyperventilation, hyperosmolar therapy, and barbiturate coma. ICP values greater than 30 mmHg were also associated with mortality in 24 of 26 patients. Overall mortality rate was 78% (43/55). The main cause of death in this and several prior studies was postischemic edema with concomitant raised ICP, herniation, coma, and death (Moulin et al., 1985; Hacke et al., 1996; Schwab et al., 1997; Schwarz

*Table 16.2*

**Trials of decompressive craniectomy in trauma***

| Year | Author | Conclusions |
|------|--------|-------------|
| **2001** | Taylor et al. | DHC reduces ICP, functional outcome and quality of life in children |
| **2005** | Ucar et al. | DHC reduces unfavorable outcome in patients with GCS 6–8 |
| **2005** | Meier et al. | DHC of utility within 48 hours for age < 50 without polytrauma or < 30 with polytrauma |
| **2006** | Josan and Sgouros | DHC in the first few hours postinjury may prevent secondary deterioration in children |
| **2008** | Meier et al. | Outcome post-DHC dependent on GCS, midline shift, pupillary reactivity, hydrocephalus, hyperglycemia, and acidosis |
| **2008** | Figaji et al. | DC improves ICP and cerebral oxygenation in children without increasing the proportion of disabled survivors |
| **2008** | Morgalla et al. | Long-term results justify use of DC with good outcome in ~40% |
| **2009** | Qiu et al. | DHC is superior to temporoparietal craniectomy in regard to reductions in ICP, mortality rate, and neurologic outcomes with increased risk of intracranial hematomas and subdural effusions |
| **2010** | Lemcke et al. | Prognosis after DC for TBI is unfavorable. Age, midline shift, and status of the basal cisterns on head CT were associated with the long-term outcome |
| **2011** | Cooper et al. | Bifrontotemporoparietal DC decreased ICP and ICU length of stay but was associated with worse outcomes relative to medical management |
| **2011b** | Honeybul et al. | Improved outcome at 18-month follow-up for patients with traumatic cerebral edema treated with DC. CRASH prediction model provided excellent prediction |
| **2011** | Schulz and Mauer | No significant differences in short-term outcome after limited craniotomy versus decompressive craniectomy for acute traumatic subdural hematomas in patients over 65 years of age |
| **2016** | Hutchinson et al. | Significantly improved survival and functional outcome in patients after decompressive craniectomy but also increased disability and vegetative state |

*A PubMed search was conducted using "decompressive craniectomy AND trauma" or "decompressive craniotomy AND trauma" with results narrowed to "clinical trials" only.

DHC, decompressive hemicraniectomy; ICP, intracranial pressure; GCS, Glasgow Coma Scale; DC, decompressive craniectomy; TBI, traumatic brain injury; CT, computed tomography; ICU, intensive care unit.

et al., 1998; Hofmeijer et al., 2003a, b; Vahedi et al., 2007a). Given the role of secondary edema in the ultimate demise of patients with massive MCA infarctions, there continues to be considerable interest in DC as a strategy to prevent secondary decline.

Rengachary et al. first advocated decompressive surgery for the specific indication of massive cerebral infarction in 1981 in a publication in which they described outcome of only 3 patients, all of whom had favorable outcomes. Kondziolka et al. (1988) subsequently reported their small series of 5 patients with supratentorial cerebral infarction and uncal herniation on whom they performed frontotemporal craniectomy after failure of maximal medical therapy. All 5 patients survived and were ambulatory, and 2 returned to work. Over the next decade, decompressive hemicraniectomy for malignant MCA infarctions gained traction and led to a series of studies to evaluate its efficacy.

Rieke et al. (1995) published their open, prospective trial of 32 patients (age 37–68 years; mean 48.8 years) who received DC and duraplasty compared to 21 patients (age 37–69 years; mean 58.4 years) who had nonsurgical management. Surgery was associated with a significant survival advantage, with 21 of 32 surgical patients surviving compared to only 5 survivors in the control group. Surgically treated patients were less likely to be disabled: 5 surgical patients were disabled but independent, 15 were severely disabled but not totally dependent, and 1 was asymptomatic at ICU discharge. In comparison, there were only 4 survivors in the control group, 4 of whom had global aphasia. There was no statistically significant difference in the ages of survivors versus nonsurvivors, nor was there a difference in the timing of clinical deterioration and outcome. The authors published an update to this open study in which they evaluated outcome following late versus early hemicraniectomy on mortality rate, length of time in the neurocritical care unit, and the mean Barthel index score (Schwab et al., 1998). Mortality rate was 16% when performed early, 34.4% when performed late, and 78% for nonsurgical controls. ICU stay was 13.3, 7.4, and 12.6 days for late hemicraniectomy, early hemicraniectomy, and natural history controls, respectively. Mean Barthel index was 62.6, 68.8, and 60 for late hemicraniectomy, early hemicraniectomy, and natural history controls, respectively.

The notion that there is a prognostic benefit to earlier craniectomy was explored further by Cho et al. in their 2003 study on ultra-early DC for malignant MCA infarction. The study evaluated 52 patients aged 45–80 years old who received ultra-early (<6 hours), early (>6 hours), or conservative therapy. Survival was 91.3%, 63.3%, and 20% in the ultra-early, early, and conservative groups, respectively. Furthermore, the ability to follow commands at 7 days postonset was 91.3%, 55%, and 0% for the ultra-early, early and conservative groups, respectively. The study was not powered to detect subtle differences in outcome within the treatment groups based on age. The results provided further support for a role of craniectomy for malignant infarcts and suggested that the timing of surgery is a critical factor in procuring both survival and good functional outcome. That is, the sooner, the better!

Several additional observational studies suggested efficacy of decompressive hemicraniectomy for malignant strokes (Moulin et al., 1985; Rieke et al., 1995; Hacke et al., 1996; Wagner et al., 2001; Whitfield et al., 2001; Cho et al., 2003; Hofmeijer et al., 2003a, b; Ziai et al., 2003; Malm et al., 2006; Bratton et al., 2007h, i, j, k; Chen et al., 2007; Pillai et al., 2007; Vahedi et al., 2007a; Steyerberg et al., 2008; Timofeev et al., 2008; Soustiel et al., 2010; Honeybul et al., 2011a; Juttler et al., 2011; Marion, 2011; Timmons et al., 2011; Cooper et al., 2012; Li et al., 2012; Rahme et al., 2012; Tagliaferri et al., 2012; Wartenberg, 2012; Olivecrona and Olivecrona, 2013; Sahuquillo et al., 2013; Kolias et al., 2016). A systematic review of 138 cases published by Gupta et al. (2004) suggested that the benefits of decompressive hemicraniectomy for malignant MCA infarctions were nonuniform, with younger patients (<50 years of age) less likely to be dead or severely disabled at 4 months following the procedure (80% vs. 32%). This finding was reproduced in a study from our institution, in which older age was the sole factor predictive of poor functional outcome in the aftermath of DC for malignant stroke (Rabinstein et al., 2006). Meanwhile, several key traditional techniques for conservative management, including osmolar therapy, hypothermia, and barbiturate coma, were proving to be less efficacious (Schwab et al., 1997; Schwarz et al., 1998; Schwab et al., 1999; Hofmeijer et al., 2003a; Milhaud et al., 2005). This combination of a lack of positive evidence regarding decompressive hemicraniectomy and doubts regarding conservative management led to wide variations in practice and underscored the need for high-quality randomized controlled trials to study the effects of decompressive surgery. Furthermore, the findings suggested that trials should be designed to both determine overall efficacy but also specifically, the population most likely to benefit from the Herculean effort of neurosurgical intervention.

## Randomized controlled trials of decompressive craniectomy for malignant middle cerebral artery infarction

Several randomized controlled trials were undertaken to address the aforementioned gaps in knowledge and to standardize management of patients with hemispheric infarctions. The Hemicraniectomy and Durotomy Upon Deterioration From Infarction-Related Swelling Trial (HeADDFIRST) trial was the first randomized controlled trial aimed at providing parameters for the development of robust trials to delineate the role of DC on functional outcome and survival. Three European randomized trials were undertaken in the early 2000s: Early Decompressive Craniectomy in Malignant Cerebral Artery Infarction (DECIMAL: France), Decompressive Surgery for the Treatment of Malignant Infarction of the Middle Cerebral Artery (DESTINY: Germany), and Hemicraniectomy After Middle Cerebral Artery infarction with Life-threatening Edema Trial (HAMLET: Netherlands). The Hemicraniectomy for Malignant Middle Cerebral Artery Infarction (HeMMI) was a single-center, randomized controlled clinical trial launched in the Philippines. HeMMI was launched in January 2002 and terminated in December 2009 secondary to poor recruitment. It will not be discussed further. An uncomprehensive list of studies aimed at exploring the role of decompressive hemicraniectomy for malignant cerebral infarctions is shown in Table 16.3.

### HeADDFIRST

HeADDFIRST was actually the first randomized controlled trial aimed at addressing the role of DC for malignant infarction, although the results were not published until 2014 (Frank et al., 2014). HeADDFIRST was designed as a pilot clinical trial to provide parameters for the appropriate design of phase III clinical trials aimed at assessing the benefit of DC in malignant supratentorial cerebral hemispheric infarction. The study enrolled patients from 20 North American centers (including our own) between March 2000 and September 2002. Of 4909 patients screened, 66 met all inclusion criteria, but after the consenting and randomization procedures, only 25 patients were included, one of whom subsequently withdrew.

The initial inclusion criteria included patients 18–75 years of age presenting with a unilateral MCA stroke with National Institutes of Health Stroke Scale (NIHSS) ≥ 18 who remained responsive to minor stimulation. Neuroimaging criteria were then applied to patients who passed this initial screen. Radiographic inclusion required hypodensity involving ≥ 50% of the MCA territory on CT obtained within 5 hours of symptom onset, or

*Table 16.3*

**Clinical studies of decompressive craniotomy for malignant middle cerebral artery infarction**

| Year | Author | Study |
|------|--------|-------|
| 2003 | Cho et al. | Ultra-early DHC improves survival and functional |
| 2006 | Els et al. | DHC with hypothermia poses no added risk and may improve functional outcome |
| 2006 | Malm et al. | DHC favorable in young patients who survive acute phase |
| 2006 | Rabinstein et al. | Older age associated with poor functional outcome after DHC |
| 2006 | Wang et al. | DHC improves survival but not improve function |
| 2007 | Chen et al. | Age ≥60 years associated with poor outcome after DHC |
| 2007 | Juttler et al. | DHC improves survival but not functional outcome |
| 2007 | Pillai et al. | 73% survival with a third functionally independent after DHC |
| 2007a | Vahedi et al. | DHC improves survival but not functional outcome |
| 2008 | Skoglund et al. | DHC at 1–6 years impaired but still satisfied with life |
| 2009 | Hofmeijer et al. | DHC reduces poor functional outcome and case fatality |
| 2011 | Juttler et al. | DESTINY II: ongoing trial |
| 2012 | Hernandez-Medrano et al. | DHC may improve functional outcome in younger patients |
| 2012 | Lucas et al. | DHC maintains benefit in low-experience centers |
| 2012 | Slezins et al. | DHC increases survival without increasing percentage of disabled survivors |
| 2012 | Zhao et al. | DHC improves survival and function in patients up to 80 years |
| 2013 | Geurts et al. | DHC improves survival but not functional outcome at 3 years |
| 2013 | Hofmeijer et al. | DHC improves survival and outcome but at a high cost |
| 2013 | Neugebauer et al. | DEPTH-SOS trial: ongoing trial |
| 2013 | Shao et al. | DHC enhances functional outcome with shorter hospital stay |
| 2014 | Rai et al. | DHC reduces mortality and functional outcome |
| 2014 | Frank et al. | Early mortality benefit of surgery at 21 days |

DHC, decompressive hemicraniectomy.

hypodensity of the entire MCA vascular distribution on CT performed within 48 hours of symptom onset. Patients were excluded from the trial if neurologic deterioration preceded admission to the participating hospital; or if there was a subdural or confluent parenchymal hematoma or subarachnoid hemorrhage; partial thromboplastin time > 40 seconds; international normalized ratio > 1.4; platelet count < 100 k/μL prior to correction with blood products; any pre-existing illness limiting life expectancy to less than 6 months; any significant pre-existing disability (modified Rankin score (mRS) > 2); any pre-existing or concurrent brain injury resulting in neurologic deficits in addition to that wrought by the stroke; and participation in another clinical trial. These inclusion and exclusion criteria were used to guide the design of subsequent randomized clinical trials, including the three previously summarized European trials.

Mortality at 21 days was reduced in the surgically treated patients relative to patients receiving maximal medical therapy (40% in the surgical groups, 90% CI 15–70% vs. 21% in the medically managed group, 90% CI 6–47%). At 6 months, mortality in the surgical group had risen to 36% without significant change in the medically managed controls. Death was attributed to complications of increased intracranial hypertension with brainstem compression, worsening cerebral infarction, brainstem compression, cardiac arrhythmia, and withdrawal of life support. No subgroup analysis was performed to ascertain the impact of age on outcome.

## DECIMAL

The DECIMAL trial was a multicenter, single-blind, sequential-design study undertaken in France with enrollment between December 2001 and November 2005 (Vahedi et al., 2007a). The study randomized patients between 18 and 55 years of age presenting within 24 hours of a malignant MCA infarction involving > 50% of the MCA territory and a diffusion-weighted imaging infarct volume >145 cm$^3$. Patients with pre-existing disability, serious illness, life expectancy <3 years, and those who were pregnant were excluded. The primary endpoint was survival with mRS ≤ 3 at 6 months, while the secondary endpoints were survival and functional outcome (mRS ≤ 3; Barthel index > 85) at 12 months. The trial was prematurely terminated by the governing data safety monitoring committee due to poor recruitment and a high mortality differential between the patients undergoing surgery and the medically managed controls.

At termination, 38 patients had been enrolled, 18 of whom were assigned to standard medical therapy and the remaining 20 to decompressive hemicraniectomy performed within 6 hours of randomization, up to 30 hours from onset and with required dural opening. The absolute risk reduction in death between surgery versus the medically managed control groups was 52.8% ($p < 0.0001$). Surgical patients also enjoyed improved functional outcome, with a statistically significant increase in the proportion of patients without severe disability between the surgical and control groups (75% vs. 22.2% at 1 year; $p = 0.0029$). In the subgroup analysis, older age correlated with worsening functional outcome within the surgical group but not among medically managed controls, among whom the only predictive factor was diffusion-weighted imaging infarct volume. The authors concluded that early decompressive hemicraniectomy should be offered to young patients (<55 years of age) presenting with large MCA infarcts following a comprehensive discussion with family regarding anticipated functional outcome as none of the patients had a complete recovery without deficits.

## DESTINY

The DESTINY trial recruited patients between February 2004 and October 2005. Patients were 18–60 years of age presenting with unilateral MCA infarction with subsequent randomization to DC (removal of a bone flap of at least 12 cm, including the frontal, parietal, temporal and parts of the occipital bones with exposure of the middle fossa floor and opening of the dura and subsequent insertion of a dural patch) versus medical management. The initial outcome was 30-day mortality with a functional status at 6 months (dichotomized as mRS 0–3 and 4–6) as the primary outcome. Similar to the DECIMAL trial, the DESTINY trial was terminated after recruitment of only 32 patients as there was a clear reduction in mortality among those patients randomized to surgery (survival 88% vs. 47% in the surgical and control arms, respectively; $p = 0.02$). Surgery also improved functional outcomes at 6 months, with mRS of 0–3 occurring in 70% versus 33% of patients randomized to surgery or conservative management, respectively ($p = 0.01$). The authors concluded that early DC reduced mortality and improved functional outcome. They did not address the impact of age on outcome, except to argue that an upper limit above which decompressive surgery should not be offered would require additional randomized controlled trials. True to this goal, the authors subsequently launched the DESTINY II trial. The study is a randomized controlled trial which aims to randomize patients 61 years of age or older to DC versus medical management and will be discussed below (Juttler et al., 2011).

## HAMLET

HAMLET, the third of the European trials, recruited patients 18–60 years of age between November 2002 and October 2007 in a multicenter, open, randomized trial (Hofmeijer et al., 2009). Unlike DECIMAL and DESTINY, the focus was on overall efficacy of hemicraniectomy, with less focus on the timing of surgery. Thus, patients were randomized up to 4 days out from stroke onset to surgery versus best medical treatment. The primary outcome measure was mRS at 1 year dichotomized as good (0–3) or poor (4–6). Secondary measures included mRS of 4 versus 5, case fatality, quality of life, and symptoms of depression. Surgical decompression had no effect on the primary outcome but did significantly reduce the case fatality, with absolute risk reduction of death of 38% ($p = 0.002$). Subgroup analysis, including a meta-analysis of patients from DECIMAL, DESTINY, and HAMLET, was performed to focus on the subset of patients with aphasia, those 51–60 years of age, and the time between stroke onset and randomization. Patients randomized to surgery within 48 hours following stroke onset had lower case fatality and improved function. Interestingly, there was a trend toward greater benefit of surgery in patients 51–60 years of age relative to their younger counterparts. The authors concluded that DC reduces case fatality and poor outcomes in patients with malignant infarctions treated within 48 hours of symptom onset. With delays up to 96 hours, they report that there is no evidence of benefit. The effects of surgery on reduction of case fatality rates were sustained at 3-year follow-up (Geurts et al., 2013). Surgically treated patients were more likely to reside at home (absolute risk reduction 27%; 95% CI 4–20). Finally, patients treated with surgery reported improved quality-of-life metrics between 1 and 3 years. Like the DECIMAL and DESTINY trials, HAMLET was recommended for termination by the data monitoring committee after recruitment of 64 patients as it was deemed unlikely that a statistically significant difference could be detected for the primary outcome with the projected sample size.

## POOLED ANALYSIS OF DECIMAL, DESTINY, AND HAMLET

The effect of surgical decompression was consistent across all three of the European trials, with a significant mortality benefit in surgically treated patients without stellar improvements in functional outcome. As all three studies were terminated prematurely, none attained sufficient power to detect potentially subtle differences in functional outcome – the primary outcome of interest. Thus, Vahedi et al. (2007b) pooled patients from DECIMAL, DESTINY, and HAMLET to assess the role of early (<48 hours after symptom onset) DC on functional outcome in patients 18–60 years of age presenting with malignant cerebral artery infarction. The pooled analysis included 93 patients from the three trials. The primary endpoint was outcome at 1 year dichotomized as favorable (mRS 0–4) or unfavorable (mRS 5 or death).

Decompressive surgery resulted in a significant increase in favorable outcome with mRS ≤ 4 in 75% of surgically treated versus 24% of conservatively managed patients (absolute risk reduction 51%; 95% CI 34–69%). Similarly, 43% of surgically treated versus 21% of conservatively managed patients achieved mRS ≤ 3 (absolute risk reduction 23%; 95% CI 5–41%). Certainly, the most impressive finding was the overall survival benefit of surgical intervention, with 78% of those undergoing surgery surviving to 1 year compared to 29% of medically managed patients (absolute risk reduction 50%; 95% CI 33–67%). Based on these findings, the authors reported that only 2 patients would require surgical decompression to obtain survival with mRS ≤ 4 or survival regardless of outcome. When the functional outcome requirement was slightly more stringent (mRS ≤ 3), the number needed to treat was 4. In the subgroup analyses of age, timing of randomization, and presence of aphasia, surgical decompression retained efficacy for the primary outcome of mRS ≤ 4 ($p < 0.01$).

# Decompressive hemicraniectomy in the elderly

The previously reviewed randomized trials all limited the age of patients to ≤ 60 years based on several reports of observational studies suggesting poorer outcome and/or survival in older patients (Holtkamp et al., 2001; Leonhardt et al., 2002; Ziai et al., 2003; Gupta et al., 2004; Uhl et al., 2004; Yang et al., 2005; Yao et al., 2005; Rabinstein et al., 2006; Chen et al., 2007; Arac et al., 2009; Wang et al., 2011). However, as populations across the world age and present to clinical attention progressively older, clinicians are now forced to reconsider the definition of "elderly" in regard to decompressive hemicraniectomy for malignant MCA infarcts. This has contributed to significant controversy regarding whether decompressive surgery is indicated for patients > 60 years of age. Two randomized controlled trials have specifically addressed this question.

The first randomized controlled trial specifically addressing the role of decompressive hemicraniectomy for malignant cerebral artery infarcts was published by Zhao et al. in 2012. The authors designed the study using protocols derived from the DESTINY and HAMLET trials but included patients age 18–80 years. Recruitment began in July 2008 and the study was terminated in May 2010 after recruitment of 47 patients on the advice of the safety monitoring committee. The rationale for termination was that statistical superiority of the primary endpoint had already been determined on interim analysis. The primary endpoint was functional outcome at 6 months assessed as good (mRS 0–4) or poor (5–6). The secondary outcomes were death rates at 6 months and 1 year as well as functional outcome at 6 months and 1 year dichotomized as 0–3 versus 4–6.

The outcome among all 47 enrolled patients mirrored that obtained in the European trials and will not be described here. In the subgroup analysis of patients > 60 years of age, 16 were randomized to surgery and 13 to medical therapy. Among this group, decompressive surgery conferred a clear mortality benefit at 6 months, with 12.5% mortality among the surgical group versus 61.5% among those elderly patients randomized to medical management (absolute risk reduction 49.0%; 95% CI 18.0–80.1%; number needed to treat = 2; $P = 0.016$). The survival benefit remained at 1 year, with 18.8% mortality among surgically treated patients versus 69.2% among medically treated patients (absolute risk reduction 50.5%; 95% CI 18.9–92.0; number needed to treat = 2; $p = 0.010$). Similarly, decompressive surgery conferred a benefit on functional outcome among elderly patients. At 6 months, 33.3% of surgically treated patients versus 82.6% of conservatively managed patients had mRS > 4 (absolute risk reduction 49.3%; 95% CI 24.9–73.7%; number needed to treat = 2; $p = 0.001$). The benefit on functional outcome was maintained at 1 year. When the authors analyzed the secondary outcome of mRS > 3 at 6 months and 1 year, there was a trend toward improved functional outcome among surgically treated patients, but this did not reach statistical significance. They attributed this to the fact that the study was stopped when the primary endpoint was attained and that, with additional recruitment, the secondary functional outcome would likely prove significant. In the absence of clairvoyance, additional studies or pooled analyses (akin to that performed for the European trials) will likely be needed to assess the degree of function attainable among patients > 60 years of age undergoing decompressive surgery for malignant strokes.

## DESTINY II

Results of the DESTINY II trial which limits analysis to patients > 60 were published in 2014 (Juttler et al., 2014). The authors randomized 112 patients to hemicraniectomy versus medical management within 48 hours of symptom onset following the general protocol used in the original DESTINY trial. The primary endpoint was survival without severe disability (mRS 0–4) 6 months following randomization. The authors determined that surgical intervention statistically improved the primary outcome. Among patients who underwent decompressive surgery, 38% survived with mRS 0–4 versus 18% of medically treated controls (OR 2.91; 95%CI 1.06–7.49; $p = 0.04$). Complete recovery or recovery with only slight disability (mRS 0–2) was not attained in any patient included in the study. There was a trend toward moderate disability (mRS 3) among patients treated with surgery versus medical management (7% vs. 3%), but this did not reach statistical significance. The authors concluded that hemicraniectomy increased survival without severe disability among patients over 61 years presenting with malignant MCA infarction.

Evidence continues to amass in support of decompressive hemicraniectomy to relieve cerebral edema associated with malignant supratentorial infarctions. There is little controversy now about whether this intervention increases survival, as all major randomized trials, case series, and expert opinion have shown benefit. The question is whether the added time garnered from this procedure represents life deemed by patients and their families as life worth living. Inasmuch as previous studies have shown a significant survival benefit following decompressive surgery, the data on functional outcome remain less impressive and survival with significant functional impairment and perhaps lifelong dependence remain the likely outcome. Does survival with significant dependence warrant such Herculean efforts and the divergence of often scarce resources? Obviously, this is an important discussion and should be embarked upon artfully by the clinician.

## DECOMPRESSIVE CRANIECTOMY COMBINED WITH HYPOTHERMIA

In cases of acute brain injury from trauma or stroke, prevention of secondary injury is of paramount importance and commands high priority in acute management paradigms. The utility of hypothermia in the prevention of secondary injury has long been a proven strategy for neuroprotection since the experiments by Rosomoff in the 1950s, where experimental MCA occlusion was performed in dogs in the setting of normothermia and hypothermia (Rosomoff, 1956a, b, c, d). Neuroprotection from hypothermia has been postulated to occur via several mechanisms, including reduced metabolic rate and energy depletion, decreased excitatory neurotransmitter release and signaling, improved ion homeostasis, reduction in free radical generation, reduced vascular permeability, and blood–brain barrier compromise (Doerfler et al., 2001). Several studies have evaluated whether hypothermia can improve therapeutic efficacy when combined with other therapies. One area of interest is the combination of DC with hypothermia in both stroke and traumatic brain injury.

Doerfler et al. (2001) performed MCA occlusion in Wistar rats followed by hypothermia, craniectomy, or both. They concluded that, in that model, early DC reduced infarction size and neurologic outcome. Temporary mild hypothermia on its own delayed infarct evolution but did not reduce the ultimate size of the infarct nor was there any benefit on overall functional outcome. When combined with DC, they concluded the benefits were additive. These results have been corroborated in at least two other animal models of acute cerebral injury. Jieyong et al. (2006) performed MCA occlusion in rats treated subsequently with mild hypothermia, DC, or both. They then performed molecular assessment of ischemic brain injury using both terminal deoxynucleotidyl transferase-mediated dUTP-biotin in situ nick labeling (TUNEL) staining for the detection of DNA fragmentation and immunohistochemistry for Bcl-2 and Bax, which are markers of ischemia-induced apoptosis. Mild hypothermia alone resulted in no significant reduction infarct size but did significantly decrease both TUNEL staining and Bcl-2 expression. In contrast, animals treated with mild hypothermia and DC had a significant reduction in ischemic markers and ultimately infarct size.

Hypothermia has also shown potential benefit in animals when combined with DC for traumatic brain injury. Szczygielski et al. (2010) subjected male CD-1 mice to closed-head injury followed by DC alone or in combination with mild hypothermia with the goal of assessing whether the mild hypothermia could thwart development of posttraumatic cerebral edema. They concluded that DC increased cerebral water content after closed-head injury and that mild hypothermia as an adjunct measure is effective in curtailing posttraumatic cerebral edema. A systematic review and meta-analysis of hypothermia in animal models of acute ischemic stroke suggested that hypothermia improves outcome by about one-third under conditions that may be clinically achievable for many patients and justifies the undertaking of randomized clinical trials in humans (van der Worp et al., 2007). To date, there is no clinical evidence in humans demonstrating any benefit of combining DC with hypothermia. This deficiency will be specifically addressed by the DEcompressive surgery Plus hypoThermia for Space-Occupying Stroke (DEPTH-SOS) trial.

### DEPTH-SOS trial

As previously reviewed, early DC has proven efficacy for reducing mortality and improving functional outcome in patients 18–60 years of age with malignant

MCA infarction. Nonetheless, case fatality is still at least 20% and approximately a third of survivors are severely disabled. While there is a paucity of good evidence for the neuroprotection benefit of hypothermia in humans, there is certainly enough evidence to justify clinical trials (Bernard et al., 2002; Kollmar and Schwab, 2010; Kollmar et al., 2010; van der Worp et al., 2010). The DEPTH-SOS trial is a prospective, multicenter randomized control trial that will assess the utility of moderate therapeutic hypothermia to $33 \pm 1°C$ for at least 72 hours combined with early DC performed within 48 hours in patients presenting with malignant MCA infarction. Primary outcome will be 14-day mortality, while the secondary endpoints will include functional outcome at 14 days and at 1 year as well as complications secondary to hypothermia. The trial is currently under way and promises to provide data on both the safety and feasibility of combining moderate hypothermia with decompressive surgery in patients presenting with malignant MCA infarction. This has potential implications for changing standard of care or, at the very least, providing the paradigms around which future trials are constructed.

## COMPLICATIONS OF DECOMPRESSIVE CRANIECTOMY

DC is a life-saving procedure when performed for appropriately selected patients and, as a result, there has been a dramatic rise in the frequency with which the procedure is performed (Walcott et al., 2011). While the procedure poses few technical challenges for most neurosurgeons, it is far from benign and has been directly linked to a number of clinically significant outcomes with impact on both quality and quantity of life as well as the overall cost-effectiveness of the procedure. Kurland et al. (2015) performed a thorough systematic review of complications associated with DC as well as those of the subsequent cranioplasty and their data will be reviewed here. It is important to note that the following rates were derived from a systematic review of many studies and that actual reported rates span a wide range. Overall complication rates for the initial decompressive surgery and subsequent cranioplasty were 13.4 and 6.4% respectively. They categorized complications into three broad categories: hemorrhagic, infectious/inflammatory, and disturbances of CSF dynamics, as summarized in Table 16.4.

### Hemorrhagic complications of decompressive craniectomy

Several hemorrhagic complications are frequently reported following DC. Broadly, hemorrhagic complications include new hematomas ipsilateral to the

*Table 16.4*

**Complications of decompressive craniectomy**

| Complication | Rates and description |
|---|---|
| **Hemorrhagic** | |
| New ipsilateral hematoma | 10.2% overall; 12.9% after TBI vs. 6.5% for nontraumatic ICH |
| Remote hematoma | 8.6% overall with ~77% reoperation rate |
| Hemorrhagic progression of contusion | 12.6% of TBI patients |
| Hemorrhagic transformation of infarction | 23.7% of patients undergoing DHC for MMCAI |
| **Infectious/inflammatory** | |
| Superficial wound complications | 8.1% overall; includes wound problems (necrosis, infection), subgaleal infections, etc. |
| Abscess, epidural/ subdural empyema | 5.1% overall rate with a slightly higher incidence (5.9%) when the indication is ischemic stroke |
| Meningitis and ventriculitis | 6.1% overall incidence with most cases in the setting of TBI |
| **Abnormalities in CSF flow** | |
| Hydrocephalus | 16.4% overall; 14.8% following TBI; 25.5% and 21.1% following ischemic and hemorrhagic strokes, respectively |
| Subdural hygroma | 27.4% of TBI patients and 12.5% in MMCAI |
| CSF leak/fistula | 6.3% following TBI; 8.8% following stroke |
| Syndrome of the trephined | 10% overall |
| Paradoxical herniation | Rare but increased incidence following CSF draining procedure after craniectomy |

From (Kurland et al., 2015) with permissions from Springer Science and Business Media.
TBI, traumatic brain injury; ICH, intracerebral hemorrhage; DHC, decompressive hemicraniectomy; MMCAI, malignant middle cerebral artery infarction; CSF, cerebrospinal fluid.

decompression or at a remote (sometimes contralateral) site, progression of a contusion, and transformation of an ischemic infarction. Overall, a new ipsilateral hemorrhage was reported in approximately 10.2% of patients undergoing DC for any indication, with 12.9% occurring in the setting of DC following traumatic brain injury. A remote or contralateral hematoma is a phenomenon reported only in patients undergoing DC following brain trauma. This occurred in 8.6% of cases, with 77% requiring a secondary operative intervention to relieve mass effect and mitigate neurologic deterioration. Similarly, hemorrhagic progression of a contusion was reported only in cases of trauma and occurs in 12.6% of patients following DC. Pathophysiologically, progression of contusions is thought to be the result of changing pressure dynamics that occur in the setting of opening the cranium. Hemorrhagic transformation of an ischemic infarction was found in 23.7% of malignant stroke patients in the aftermath of DC but rates as high as 43% have been reported (Kenning et al., 2012).

## Infectious and inflammatory complications of decompressive craniectomy

Several factors increase the probability of infectious and inflammatory complications following decompressive surgery. For cases that occur in the setting of trauma there can be communication of the brain to the environment through open skull defects. Further, the long curvilinear incision often employed in cases of decompressive hemicraniectomy often disturbs blood supply to the scalp flap, leading to ischemia, wound complications, and an increased risk for infections. As the dura is often left open by necessity, there is an added infectious risk both from the underlying necrotic brain acting as a Petri dish and open communication with the environment in cases where wound breakdown does occur. Necrosis of the flap, impaired wound healing, subgaleal and skin wound infections (lumped together as "superficial complications") occur in some 8.1% of all patients undergoing DC. Issues within the cranial vault (lumped together as "deep complications") include abscesses and empyemas and occur in 5.1% of TBI and 5.9% of ischemic stroke patients undergoing DC. Meningitis and ventriculitis (considered separately) occur in 6.1% of patients, with a higher predilection in patients undergoing DC for trauma. Other wound complications (not further characterized and not included in the groups above) were reported in 13.7% and 6.4% of patients undergoing DC for stroke and traumatic brain injury, respectively.

## Complications of CSF flow and dynamics

DC may alter CSF flow through disruption of meningeal anatomy, tearing of arachnoid trabeculae, blockage of arachnoid granulations, or direct leaks through fistulae. The most common manifestation of CSF flow alteration post decompressive surgery is the development of a subdural hygroma, reported in 27.4% and 12.5% of patients undergoing DC for TBI and stroke, respectively. Although most subdural hygromas spontaneously resolve in the absence of further surgical intervention, they are associated with longer hospitalization and rehabilitation and a worse neurologic outcome. Hydrocephalus was a frequently reported complication following DC, occurring

in 16.4% and 25.5% of patients undergoing DC for traumatic brain injury and stroke, respectively. CSF leaks were reported in 6.3% of patients undergoing DC for any reason with 6.7% and 8.8% reported in patients undergoing DC for trauma and stroke, respectively.

## Syndrome of the trephined

The syndrome of the trephined or "sinking skin flap syndrome" occurs as atmospheric pressure is transduced through the skin flap to the underlying brain in the absence of a bony barrier. The result is a complex constellation of symptoms attributed to reduced cerebral perfusion and altered CSF flow. This was reported in 10% of patients undergoing DC. Left untreated, this may result in a more severe and potentially lethal condition called paradoxic herniation, wherein atmospheric pressure significantly exceeds ICP, resulting in herniation of the brain beyond the tentorial notch. Early cranioplasty has been suggested by some authors to prevent this complication (Yang et al., 2008).

## Complications of cranioplasty following decompressive craniectomy

Cranioplasty following DC is necessary to correct the cosmetic defect of decompressive surgery and to obviate or mitigate the associated complications of decompression, as previously discussed. This requires a second surgical procedure and exposes the patient to all the attendant risks, including those attributed to anesthesia. The same risk categories previously reviewed for DC are relevant following cranioplasty, although overall risk in the latter appears to be lower (6.4% vs. 13.4%). Ipsilateral hematomas following cranioplasty are reported in 3.6% of cases. Superficial and deep wound and infectious complications occurred in 9.1 and 3.8% of patients, respectively. Meningitis and ventriculitis occurred at a rate on a par with that of DC at 4.5%. Bone flap infections were reported in 5.4% of patients overall. Subdural hygromas, hydrocephalus, and CSF leaks/fistulae were all reported following cranioplasty, with reduced rates of 5.8%, 7.5%, and 6.3%, respectively when compared to the initial decompression.

Resorption of the bone flap following cranioplasty is a frequent complication necessitating subsequent reoperations. Rates of resorption are highest in pediatric patients, with reports as high as 39.2% of patients. In the adult population, bone flap resorption was reported in 16% of patients overall, with reported rates of 13.5%, 12.7%, and 6.5% in patients undergoing DC for trauma, ischemic stroke, and ICH, respectively. Autologous bone remains the material of choice for cranioplasty, with the caveat that the constellation of subsequent complications is a factor of both material and technique. A detailed review of cranioplasty techniques is outside the scope of this chapter but several such sources are readily available (Goldstein et al., 2013).

## QUALITY OF LIFE AFTER DECOMPRESSIVE CRANIECTOMY

The data reviewed in this chapter support the notion that DC is a surgical intervention based on sound pathophysiologic principles and, when applied to appropriately selected patients, improves the odds of survival and overall functional outcome. Nonetheless, a significant proportion of patients remain neurologically devastated with a life of dependence. Is this a medically acceptable outcome? Should physicians offer surgery as a "life-saving" measure to patients with severe neurologic injuries with very little probability of functional recovery? Should recent predictive scores such as CRASH and IMPACT be interwoven into the informed-consent procedure? These are obviously very difficult questions and as the patients are often, by definition, unable to participate, there is a significant burden placed on both future caregivers and patient surrogates regarding the best decisions in the acute period.

The discussions have been framed by introducing the concepts of "substantial benefit," in which one predicts that the patient would now or in the future regard the outcome as "worthwhile," versus the "risk of unacceptable badness," in which the patient would describe the outcome as intolerable (Gillett, 2001; Honeybul et al., 2013). When competent healthcare workers were presented with a number of scenarios and asked if they would provide consent, most individuals refused consent when the knowledge of a poor functional outcome was provided prior to making the decision regardless of religion and race (Gillett, 2009). In contrast, when patients with severe disability 3 years out from DC for trauma were asked, knowing what they do about their outcome, whether they would have provided consent for the procedure, almost all patients answered in the affirmative (Honeybul et al., 2013). Whether this surprising result is due to a "recalibration" of expectations and "adaptation" to their level of disability remains unclear (Honeybul et al., 2016). The more troubling possibility is that some patients are unaware of their level of disability. Unfortunately, during the acute period when a decision regarding intervention needs to be made quickly, there is insufficient time to discuss the nuances with surrogate decision makers and a recurrent theme amongst next of kin was that the greatest angst regarding providing consent was that they felt there was insufficient information regarding prognosis and eventual long-term quality of life (Honeybul et al., 2013). We do not know if more improvement can be expected over time.

## CONCLUSIONS

DC is a surgical technique that reduces intracranial hypertension effectively and improves both survival and functional outcome in cases of malignant cerebral infarction. The data on traumatic brain injury are less clear. As there are significant risks associated with the procedure, with data still being gathered on overall efficacy, an individualized approach should be taken in selecting patients in order to maximize benefit and mitigate risk. Several ethical considerations are raised, such as whether the procedure is futile, in many cases creating neurologically devastated "survivors," and thus whether this is a good use of resources. These questions will require continued investigation. DC remains an important medical, surgical, and ethical decision for the neurosurgeon and critical care neurologist.

## REFERENCES

Agrawal D, Hussain N (2005). Decompressive craniectomy in cerebral toxoplasmosis. European journal of clinical microbiology & infectious diseases : official publication of the European Society of Clinical Microbiology 24 (11): 772–773.

Ahmed AI, Eynon CA, Kinton L et al. (2010). Decompressive craniectomy for acute disseminated encephalomyelitis. Neurocrit Care 13 (3): 393–395.

Arac A, Blanchard V, Lee M et al. (2009). Assessment of outcome following decompressive craniectomy for malignant middle cerebral artery infarction in patients older than 60 years of age. Neurosurg Focus 26 (6): E3.

Ausman JI, Rogers C, Sharp HL (1976). Decompressive craniectomy for the encephalopathy of Reye's syndrome. Surg Neurol 6 (2): 97–99.

Bernard SA, Gray TW, Buist MD et al. (2002). Treatment of comatose survivors of out-of-hospital cardiac arrest with induced hypothermia. N Engl J Med 346 (8): 557–563.

Berrouschot J, Sterker M, Bettin S et al. (1998). Mortality of space-occupying ('malignant') middle cerebral artery infarction under conservative intensive care. Intensive Care Med 24 (6): 620–623.

Bohman LE, Schuster JM (2013). Decompressive craniectomy for management of traumatic brain injury: an update. Curr Neurol Neurosci Rep 13 (11): 392.

Bor-Seng-Shu E, Figueiredo EG, Amorim RL et al. (2012). Decompressive craniectomy: a meta-analysis of influences on intracranial pressure and cerebral perfusion pressure in the treatment of traumatic brain injury. J Neurosurg 117 (3): 589–596.

Bratton SL, Chestnut RM, Ghajar J et al. (2007a). Guidelines for the management of severe traumatic brain injury. XV. Steroids. J Neurotrauma 24 (Suppl 1): S91–S95.

Bratton SL, Chestnut RM, Ghajar J et al. (2007b). Guidelines for the management of severe traumatic brain injury. XIV. Hyperventilation. J Neurotrauma 24 (Suppl 1): S87–S90.

Bratton SL, Chestnut RM, Ghajar J et al. (2007c). Guidelines for the management of severe traumatic brain injury. XIII.

Antiseizure prophylaxis. J Neurotrauma 24 (Suppl 1): S83–S86.

Bratton SL, Chestnut RM, Ghajar J et al. (2007d). Guidelines for the management of severe traumatic brain injury. XII. Nutrition. J Neurotrauma 24 (Suppl 1): S77–S82.

Bratton SL, Chestnut RM, Ghajar J et al. (2007e). Guidelines for the management of severe traumatic brain injury. XI. Anesthetics, analgesics, and sedatives. J Neurotrauma 24 (Suppl 1): S71–S76.

Bratton SL, Chestnut RM, Ghajar J et al. (2007f). Guidelines for the management of severe traumatic brain injury. I. Blood pressure and oxygenation. J Neurotrauma 24 (Suppl 1): S7–S13.

Bratton SL, Chestnut RM, Ghajar J et al. (2007g). Guidelines for the management of severe traumatic brain injury. X. Brain oxygen monitoring and thresholds. J Neurotrauma 24 (Suppl 1): S65–S70.

Bratton SL, Chestnut RM, Ghajar J et al. (2007h). Guidelines for the management of severe traumatic brain injury. IX. Cerebral perfusion thresholds. J Neurotrauma 24 (Suppl 1): S59–S64.

Bratton SL, Chestnut RM, Ghajar J et al. (2007i). Guidelines for the management of severe traumatic brain injury. VIII. Intracranial pressure thresholds. J Neurotrauma 24 (Suppl 1): S55–S58.

Bratton SL, Chestnut RM, Ghajar J et al. (2007j). Guidelines for the management of severe traumatic brain injury. VII. Intracranial pressure monitoring technology. J Neurotrauma 24 (Suppl 1): S45–S54.

Bratton SL, Chestnut RM, Ghajar J et al. (2007k). Guidelines for the management of severe traumatic brain injury. VI. Indications for intracranial pressure monitoring. J Neurotrauma 24 (Suppl 1): S37–S44.

Bratton SL, Chestnut RM, Ghajar J et al. (2007l). Guidelines for the management of severe traumatic brain injury. V. Deep vein thrombosis prophylaxis. J Neurotrauma 24 (Suppl 1): S32–S36.

Bratton SL, Chestnut RM, Ghajar J et al. (2007m). Guidelines for the management of severe traumatic brain injury. IV. Infection prophylaxis. J Neurotrauma 24 (Suppl 1): S26–S31.

Bratton SL, Chestnut RM, Ghajar J et al. (2007n). Guidelines for the management of severe traumatic brain injury. III. Prophylactic hypothermia. J Neurotrauma 24 (Suppl 1): S21–S25.

Bratton SL, Chestnut RM, Ghajar J et al. (2007o). Guidelines for the management of severe traumatic brain injury. II. Hyperosmolar therapy. J Neurotrauma 24 (Suppl 1): S14–S20.

Chen HJ, Lee TC, Wei CP (1992). Treatment of cerebellar infarction by decompressive suboccipital craniectomy. Stroke 23 (7): 957–961.

Chen CC, Cho DY, Tsai SC (2007). Outcome of and prognostic factors for decompressive hemicraniectomy in malignant middle cerebral artery infarction. J Clin Neurosci 14 (4): 317–321.

Cho DY, Chen TC, Lee HC (2003). Ultra-early decompressive craniectomy for malignant middle cerebral artery infarction. Surg Neurol 60 (3): 227–232. discussion 232–223.

Chung RS, Staal JA, McCormack GH et al. (2005). Mild axonal stretch injury in vitro induces a progressive series of neurofilament alterations ultimately leading to delayed axotomy. J Neurotrauma 22 (10): 1081–1091.

Cooper PR, Hagler H, Clark WK et al. (1979). Enhancement of experimental cerebral edema after decompressive craniectomy: implications for the management of severe head injuries. Neurosurgery 4 (4): 296–300.

Cooper DJ, Rosenfeld JV, Murray L et al. (2008). Early decompressive craniectomy for patients with severe traumatic brain injury and refractory intracranial hypertension – a pilot randomized trial. J Crit Care 23 (3): 387–393.

Cooper DJ, Rosenfeld JV, Murray L et al. (2011). Decompressive craniectomy in diffuse traumatic brain injury. N Engl J Med 364 (16): 1493–1502.

Cooper DJ, Rosenfeld JV, Wolfe R (2012). DECRA investigators' response to "The future of decompressive craniectomy for diffuse traumatic brain injury" by Honeybul et al. J Neurotrauma 29 (16): 2595–2596.

Cushing HI (1908). Subtemporal decompressive operations for the intracranial complications associated with bursting fractures of the skull. Ann Surg 47 (5): 641–644.

Doerfler A, Forsting M, Reith W et al. (1996). Decompressive craniectomy in a rat model of "malignant" cerebral hemispheric stroke: experimental support for an aggressive therapeutic approach. J Neurosurg 85 (5): 853–859.

Doerfler A, Schwab S, Hoffmann TT et al. (2001). Combination of decompressive craniectomy and mild hypothermia ameliorates infarction volume after permanent focal ischemia in rats. Stroke 32 (11): 2675–2681.

Els T, Oehm E, Voigt S et al. (2006). Safety and therapeutical benefit of hemicraniectomy combined with mild hypothermia in comparison with hemicraniectomy alone in patients with malignant ischemic stroke. Cerebrovasc Dis 21 (1-2): 79–85.

Engelhorn T, Doerfler A, Kastrup A et al. (1999). Decompressive craniectomy, reperfusion, or a combination for early treatment of acute "malignant" cerebral hemispheric stroke in rats? Potential mechanisms studied by MRI. Stroke 30 (7): 1456–1463.

Engelhorn T, Doerfler A, de Crespigny A et al. (2003). Multilocal magnetic resonance perfusion mapping comparing the cerebral hemodynamic effects of decompressive craniectomy versus reperfusion in experimental acute hemispheric stroke in rats. Neurosci Lett 344 (2): 127–131.

Faure A, David A, Moussally F et al. (2002). Hajdu-Cheney syndrome and syringomyelia. Case report. J Neurosurg 97 (6): 1441–1446.

Figaji AA, Fieggen AG, Argent AC et al. (2008). Intracranial pressure and cerebral oxygenation changes after decompressive craniectomy in children with severe traumatic brain injury. Acta Neurochir Suppl 102: 77–80.

Fisher CM, Ojemann RG (1994). Bilateral decompressive craniectomy for worsening coma in acute subarachnoid hemorrhage. Observations in support of the procedure. Surg Neurol 41 (1): 65–74.

Forsting M, Reith W, Schabitz WR et al. (1995). Decompressive craniectomy for cerebral infarction. An experimental study in rats. Stroke 26 (2): 259–264.

Frank JI, Schumm LP, Wroblewski K et al. (2014). Hemicraniectomy and durotomy upon deterioration from infarction-related swelling trial: randomized pilot clinical trial. Stroke 45 (3): 781–787.

Gabrovski N, Uzunov K, Gabrovski S et al. (2006). Paget's disease as a cause for symptomatic basilar impression – a case report and review of the literature. Khirurgiia 1: 47–50.

Geurts M, van der Worp HB, Kappelle LJ et al. (2013). Surgical decompression for space-occupying cerebral infarction: outcomes at 3 years in the randomized HAMLET trial. Stroke 44 (9): 2506–2508.

Gillett G (2001). The RUB. Risk of unacceptable badness. N Z Med J 114 (1130): 188–189.

Gillett G (2009). Whose best interests? Advance directives and clinical discretion. J Law Med 16 (5): 751–758.

Goldstein JA, Paliga JT, Bartlett SP (2013). Cranioplasty: indications and advances. Curr Opin Otolaryngol Head Neck Surg 21 (4): 400–409.

Gonzalez Sanchez JJ, Nora JE, de Notaris M et al. (2010). A case of malignant monophasic multiple sclerosis (Marburg's disease type) successfully treated with decompressive hemicraniectomy. J Neurol Neurosurg Psychiatry 81 (9): 1056–1057.

Gupta R, Connolly ES, Mayer S et al. (2004). Hemicraniectomy for massive middle cerebral artery territory infarction: a systematic review. Stroke 35 (2): 539–543.

Guresir E, Vatter H, Schuss P et al. (2011). Rapid closure technique in decompressive craniectomy. J Neurosurg 114 (4): 954–960.

Hacke W, Schwab S, Horn M et al. (1996). 'Malignant' middle cerebral artery territory infarction: clinical course and prognostic signs. Arch Neurol 53 (4): 309–315.

Hayton E, Wakerley B, Bowler IC et al. (2012). Successful outcome of Epstein-Barr virus encephalitis managed with bilateral craniectomy, corticosteroids and aciclovir. Pract Neurol 12 (4): 234–237.

Hernandez-Medrano I, Matute MC, Abreu F et al. (2012). Decompressive craniectomy in malignant middle cerebral artery infarction. Experience after the implementation of a response protocol. Rev Neurol 54 (10): 593–600.

Hofmeijer J, van der Worp HB, Kappelle LJ (2003a). Treatment of space-occupying cerebral infarction. Crit Care Med 31 (2): 617–625.

Hofmeijer J, van der Worp HB, Amelink GJ et al. (2003b). Surgical decompression in space-occupying cerebral infarct; notification of a randomized trial. Ned Tijdschr Geneeskd 147 (52): 2594–2596.

Hofmeijer J, Kappelle LJ, Algra A et al. (2009). Surgical decompression for space-occupying cerebral infarction (the Hemicraniectomy After Middle Cerebral Artery infarction with Life-threatening Edema Trial [HAMLET]): a multicentre, open, randomised trial. Lancet Neurol 8 (4): 326–333.

Hofmeijer J, van der Worp HB, Kappelle LJ et al. (2013). Cost-effectiveness of surgical decompression for space-occupying hemispheric infarction. Stroke 44 (10): 2923–2925.

Holtkamp M, Buchheim K, Unterberg A et al. (2001). Hemicraniectomy in elderly patients with space occupying media infarction: improved survival but poor functional outcome. J Neurol Neurosurg Psychiatry 70 (2): 226–228.

Honeybul S, Ho KM, Lind CR et al. (2011a). The future of decompressive craniectomy for diffuse traumatic brain injury. J Neurotrauma 28 (10): 2199–2200.

Honeybul S, Ho KM, Lind CR et al. (2011b). Decompressive craniectomy for diffuse cerebral swelling after trauma: long-term outcome and ethical considerations. J Trauma 71 (1): 128–132.

Honeybul S, Janzen C, Kruger K et al. (2013). Decompressive craniectomy for severe traumatic brain injury: is life worth living? J Neurosurg 119 (6): 1566–1575.

Honeybul S, Gillett GR, Ho KM (2016). Uncertainty, conflict and consent: revisiting the futility debate in neurotrauma. Acta Neurochir (Wien) 158 (7): 1251–1257.

Hutchinson PJ, Kolias AG, Timofeev IS et al. (2016). Trial of decompressive craniectomy for traumatic intracranial hypertension. N Engl J Med 375 (12): 1119–1130.

Jiang JY, Xu W, Li WP et al. (2005). Efficacy of standard trauma craniectomy for refractory intracranial hypertension with severe traumatic brain injury: a multicenter, prospective, randomized controlled study. J Neurotrauma 22 (6): 623–628.

Jieyong B, Zhong W, Shiming Z et al. (2006). Decompressive craniectomy and mild hypothermia reduces infarction size and counterregulates Bax and Bcl-2 expression after permanent focal ischemia in rats. Neurosurg Rev 29 (2): 168–172.

Josan VA, Sgouros S (2006). Early decompressive craniectomy may be effective in the treatment of refractory intracranial hypertension after traumatic brain injury. Childs Nerv Syst 22 (10): 1268–1274.

Juttler E, Schwab S, Schmiedek P et al. (2007). Decompressive Surgery for the Treatment of Malignant Infarction of the Middle Cerebral Artery (DESTINY): a randomized, controlled trial. Stroke 38 (9): 2518–2525.

Juttler E, Bosel J, Amiri H et al. (2011). DESTINY II: DEcompressive Surgery for the Treatment of malignant INfarction of the middle cerebral arterY II. Int J Stroke 6 (1): 79–86.

Juttler E, Unterberg A, Woitzik J et al. (2014). Hemicraniectomy in older patients with extensive middle-cerebral-artery stroke. N Engl J Med 370 (12): 1091–1100.

Kachur E, Del Maestro R (2000). Mucopolysaccharidoses and spinal cord compression: case report and review of the literature with implications of bone marrow transplantation. Neurosurgery 47 (1): 223–228. discussion 228–229.

Karacalioglu AO, Erdogan E, Duz B et al. (2011). The effect of about one third craniectomy on the cerebrospinal fluid flow rate as estimated by radionuclide cisternography in normal rabbits. Hell J Nucl Med 14 (1): 34–37.

Kenning TJ, Gooch MR, Gandhi RH et al. (2012). Cranial decompression for the treatment of malignant intracranial hypertension after ischemic cerebral infarction: decompressive craniectomy and hinge craniotomy. J Neurosurg 116 (6): 1289–1298.

Keyaki A, Makita Y, Nabeshima S et al. (1990). [Surgical management of syringomyelia associated with Arnold-Chiari malformation, primary IgA deficiency and chromosomal abnormality – a case report.]. Nihon geka hokan Archiv fur japanische Chirurgie 59 (2): 161–167.

Kolias AG, Kirkpatrick PJ, Hutchinson PJ (2013). Decompressive craniectomy: past, present and future. Nat Rev Neurol 9 (7): 405–415.

Kolias AG, Adams H, Timofeev I et al. (2016). Decompressive craniectomy following traumatic brain injury: developing the evidence base. Br J Neurosurg 30 (2): 246–250.

Kollmar R, Schwab S (2010). Therapeutic hypothermia in neurological critical care. Dtsch Med Wochenschr 135 (47): 2361–2365.

Kollmar R, Staykov D, Dorfler A et al. (2010). Hypothermia reduces perihemorrhagic edema after intracerebral hemorrhage. Stroke 41 (8): 1684–1689.

Kondziolka D, Bernstein M, Resch L et al. (1988). Brain tumours presenting with tics and strokes. Can Fam Physician 34: 283–286.

Kshettry VR, Mindea SA, Batjer HH (2007). The management of cranial injuries in antiquity and beyond. Neurosurg Focus 23 (1): E8.

Kurland DB, Khaladj-Ghom A, Stokum JA et al. (2015). Complications associated with decompressive craniectomy: a systematic review. Neurocrit Care 23 (2): 292–304.

Lemcke J, Ahmadi S, Meier U (2010). Outcome of patients with severe head injury after decompressive craniectomy. Acta Neurochir Suppl 106: 231–233.

Leonhardt G, Wilhelm H, Doerfler A et al. (2002). Clinical outcome and neuropsychological deficits after right decompressive hemicraniectomy in MCA infarction. J Neurol 249 (10): 1433–1440.

Li LM, Kolias AG, Guilfoyle MR et al. (2012). Outcome following evacuation of acute subdural haematomas: a comparison of craniotomy with decompressive craniectomy. Acta Neurochir (Wien) 154 (9): 1555–1561.

Lucas C, Thines L, Dumont F et al. (2012). Decompressive surgery for malignant middle cerebral artery infarcts: the results of randomized trials can be reproduced in daily practice. Eur Neurol 68 (3): 145–149.

Malm J, Bergenheim AT, Enblad P et al. (2006). The Swedish Malignant Middle cerebral artery Infarction Study: long-term results from a prospective study of hemicraniectomy combined with standardized neurointensive care. Acta Neurol Scand 113 (1): 25–30.

Marion DW (2011). Decompressive craniectomy in diffuse traumatic brain injury. Lancet Neurol 10 (6): 497–498.

Meier U, Grawe A, Konig A (2005). The importance of major extracranial injuries by the decompressive craniectomy in severe head injuries. Acta Neurochir Suppl 95: 55–57.

Meier U, Ahmadi S, Killeen T et al. (2008). Long-term outcomes following decompressive craniectomy for severe head injury. Acta Neurochir Suppl 102: 29–31.

Mellado P, Castillo L, Andresen M et al. (2003). Decompressive craniectomy in a patient with herpetic encephalitis associated to refractory intracranial hypertension. Rev Med Chil 131 (12): 1434–1438.

Milhaud D, Thouvenot E, Heroum C et al. (2005). Prolonged moderate hypothermia in massive hemispheric infarction: clinical experience. J Neurosurg Anesthesiol 17 (1): 49–53.

Mokri B (2001). The Monro-Kellie hypothesis: applications in CSF volume depletion. Neurology 56 (12): 1746–1748.

Morais RB, Sousa I, Leiria MJ et al. (2013). Pseudotumoral acute hemicerebellitis in a child. Eur J Paediatr Neurol 17 (2): 204–207.

Morgalla MH, Will BE, Roser F et al. (2008). Do long-term results justify decompressive craniectomy after severe traumatic brain injury? J Neurosurg 109 (4): 685–690.

Moulin DE, Lo R, Chiang J et al. (1985). Prognosis in middle cerebral artery occlusion. Stroke 16 (2): 282–284.

Neugebauer H, Kollmar R, Niesen WD et al. (2013). DEcompressive surgery Plus hypoTHermia for Space-Occupying Stroke (DEPTH-SOS): a protocol of a multicenter randomized controlled clinical trial and a literature review. Int J Stroke 8 (5): 383–387.

Nilsson P, Larsson EM, Kahlon B et al. (2009). Tumefactive demyelinating disease treated with decompressive craniectomy. Eur J Neurol 16 (5): 639–642.

Ohya M, Sato O (1980). A case of cerebral venous and superior sagital sinus thrombosis, treated with decompressive craniectomy (author's transl). No Shinkei Geka 8 (9): 803–810.

Olivecrona M, Olivecrona Z (2013). Use of the CRASH study prognosis calculator in patients with severe traumatic brain injury treated with an intracranial pressure-targeted therapy. J Clin Neurosci 20 (7): 996–1001.

Ong YK, Goh KY, Chan C (2002). Bifrontal decompressive craniectomy for acute subdural empyema. Childs Nerv Syst 18 (6–7): 340–343. discussion 344.

Panourias IG, Skiadas PK, Sakas DE et al. (2005). Hippocrates: a pioneer in the treatment of head injuries. Neurosurgery 57 (1): 181–189. discussion 181–189.

Perin A, Nascimben E, Longatti P (2008). Decompressive craniectomy in a case of intractable intracranial hypertension due to pneumococcal meningitis. Acta Neurochir (Wien) 150 (8): 837–842. discussion 842.

Peyravi M, Mirzayan MJ, Krauss JK (2012). Fatal outcome despite bilateral decompressive craniectomy for refractory intracranial pressure increase in butane intoxication. Clin Neurol Neurosurg 114 (4): 392–393.

Pillai A, Menon SK, Kumar S et al. (2007). Decompressive hemicraniectomy in malignant middle cerebral artery infarction: an analysis of long-term outcome and factors in patient selection. J Neurosurg 106 (1): 59–65.

Polin RS, Shaffrey ME, Bogaev CA et al. (1997). Decompressive bifrontal craniectomy in the treatment of severe refractory posttraumatic cerebral edema. Neurosurgery 41 (1): 84–92. discussion 92–84.

Qiu W, Guo C, Shen H et al. (2009). Effects of unilateral decompressive craniectomy on patients with unilateral acute post-traumatic brain swelling after severe traumatic brain injury. Crit Care 13 (6): R185.

Quinn TM, Taylor JJ, Magarik JA et al. (2011). Decompressive craniectomy: technical note. Acta Neurol Scand 123 (4): 239–244.

Rabinstein AA, Mueller-Kronast N, Maramattom BV et al. (2006). Factors predicting prognosis after decompressive hemicraniectomy for hemispheric infarction. Neurology 67 (5): 891–893.

Raffelsieper B, Merten C, Mennel HD et al. (2002). Decompressive craniectomy for severe intracranial hypertension due to cerebral infarction or meningoencephalitis. Anasthesiol Intensivmed Notfallmed Schmerzther 37 (3): 157–162.

Ragel BT, Klimo Jr P, Martin JE et al. (2010). Wartime decompressive craniectomy: technique and lessons learned. Neurosurg Focus 28 (5): E2.

Rahme R, Curry R, Kleindorfer D et al. (2012). How often are patients with ischemic stroke eligible for decompressive hemicraniectomy? Stroke 43 (2): 550–552.

Rai VK, Bhatia R, Prasad K et al. (2014). Long-term outcome of decompressive hemicraniectomy in patients with malignant middle cerebral artery infarction: a prospective observational study. Neurol India 62 (1): 26–31.

Rengachary SS, Batnitzky S, Morantz RA et al. (1981). Hemicraniectomy for acute massive cerebral infarction. Neurosurgery 8 (3): 321–328.

Rieke K, Schwab S, Krieger D et al. (1995). Decompressive surgery in space-occupying hemispheric infarction: results of an open, prospective trial. Crit Care Med 23 (9): 1576–1587.

Rosomoff HL (1956a). The effects of hypothermia on the physiology of the nervous system. Surgery 40 (2): 328–336.

Rosomoff HL (1956b). Hypothermia and cerebral vascular lesions. I. Experimental interruption of the middle cerebral artery during hypothermia. J Neurosurg 13 (4): 244–255.

Rosomoff HL (1956c). Some effects of hypothermia on the normal and abnormal physiology of the nervous system. Proc R Soc Med 49 (6): 358–364.

Rosomoff HL (1956d). Interruption of the middle cerebral artery during hypothermia. Trans Am Neurol Assoc 64–65. 81st Meeting.

Sahuquillo J, Martinez-Ricarte F, Poca MA (2013). Decompressive craniectomy in traumatic brain injury after the DECRA trial. Where do we stand? Curr Opin Crit Care 19 (2): 101–106.

Sasaki O, Ishii R, Koike T et al. (1984). Multiple cerebrovascular occlusive disease associated with neurofibromatosis. No to shinkei = Brain and nerve 36 (2): 159–166.

Schaller B, Graf R, Sanada Y et al. (2003). Hemodynamic and metabolic effects of decompressive hemicraniectomy in normal brain. An experimental PET-study in cats. Brain Res 982 (1): 31–37.

Schulz C, Mauer UM (2011). Postoperative course after acute traumatic subdural hematoma in the elderly. Does the extent of craniotomy influence outcome? Z Gerontol Geriatr 44 (3): 177–180.

Schwab S, Spranger M, Schwarz S et al. (1997). Barbiturate coma in severe hemispheric stroke: useful or obsolete? Neurology 48 (6): 1608–1613.

Schwab S, Steiner T, Aschoff A et al. (1998). Early hemicraniectomy in patients with complete middle cerebral artery infarction. Stroke 29 (9): 1888–1893.

Schwab S, Schwarz S, Bertram M et al. (1999). Moderate hypothermia for the treatment of malignant middle cerebral artery infarct. Nervenarzt 70 (6): 539–546.

Schwarz S, Schwab S, Bertram M et al. (1998). Effects of hypertonic saline hydroxyethyl starch solution and mannitol in patients with increased intracranial pressure after stroke. Stroke 29 (8): 1550–1555.

Servadei F (2011). Clinical value of decompressive craniectomy. N Engl J Med 364: 1558–1559.

Shao A, Guo S, Chen S et al. (2013). Comparison between routine and improved decompressive craniectomy on patients with malignant cerebral artery infarction without traumatic brain injury. J Craniofac Surg 24 (6): 2085–2088.

Skoglund TS, Eriksson-Ritzen C, Sorbo A et al. (2008). Health status and life satisfaction after decompressive craniectomy for malignant middle cerebral artery infarction. Acta Neurol Scand 117 (5): 305–310.

Slezins J, Keris V, Bricis R et al. (2012). Preliminary results of randomized controlled study on decompressive craniectomy in treatment of malignant middle cerebral artery stroke. Medicina (Kaunas) 48 (10): 521–524.

Soustiel JF, Sviri GE, Mahamid E et al. (2010). Cerebral blood flow and metabolism following decompressive craniectomy for control of increased intracranial pressure. Neurosurgery 67 (1): 65–72. discussion 72.

Staal JA, Dickson TC, Gasperini R et al. (2010). Initial calcium release from intracellular stores followed by calcium dysregulation is linked to secondary axotomy following transient axonal stretch injury. J Neurochem 112 (5): 1147–1155.

Stefini R, Latronico N, Cornali C et al. (1999). Emergent decompressive craniectomy in patients with fixed dilated pupils due to cerebral venous and dural sinus thrombosis: report of three cases. Neurosurgery 45 (3): 626–629. discussion. 629–630.

Steyerberg EW, Mushkudiani N, Perel P et al. (2008). Predicting outcome after traumatic brain injury: development and international validation of prognostic scores based on admission characteristics. PLoS Med 5 (8): e165. discussion e165.

Stiver SI (2009). Complications of decompressive craniectomy for traumatic brain injury. Neurosurg Focus 26 (6): E7.

Szczygielski J, Mautes AE, Schwerdtfeger K et al. (2010). The effects of selective brain hypothermia and decompressive craniectomy on brain edema after closed head injury in mice. Acta Neurochir Suppl 106: 225–229.

Tagliaferri F, Zani G, Iaccarino C et al. (2012). Decompressive craniectomies, facts and fiction: a retrospective analysis of 526 cases. Acta Neurochir (Wien) 154 (5): 919–926.

Tang-Schomer MD, Patel AR, Baas PW et al. (2010). Mechanical breaking of microtubules in axons during dynamic stretch injury underlies delayed elasticity, microtubule disassembly, and axon degeneration. Faseb J 24 (5): 1401–1410.

Taylor A, Butt W, Rosenfeld J et al. (2001). A randomized trial of very early decompressive craniectomy in children with traumatic brain injury and sustained intracranial hypertension. Childs Nerv Syst 17 (3): 154–162.

Tian R, Han L, Hou Z et al. (2015). Neuroprotective efficacy of decompressive craniectomy after controlled cortical impact injury in rats: an MRI study. Brain Res 1622: 339–349.

Timmons SD, Ullman JS, Eisenberg HM (2011). Craniectomy in diffuse traumatic brain injury. N Engl J Med 365 (4): 373. author reply 376.

Timofeev I, Hutchinson PJ (2006). Outcome after surgical decompression of severe traumatic brain injury. Injury 37 (12): 1125–1132.

Timofeev I, Kirkpatrick PJ, Corteen E et al. (2006). Decompressive craniectomy in traumatic brain injury: outcome following protocol-driven therapy. Acta Neurochir Suppl 96: 11–16.

Timofeev I, Czosnyka M, Nortje J et al. (2008). Effect of decompressive craniectomy on intracranial pressure and cerebrospinal compensation following traumatic brain injury. J Neurosurg 108 (1): 66–73.

Tuli S, Provias JP, Bernstein M (1997). Lhermitte-Duclos disease: literature review and novel treatment strategy. Can J Neurol Sci 24 (2): 155–160.

Ucar T, Akyuz M, Kazan S et al. (2005). Role of decompressive surgery in the management of severe head injuries: prognostic factors and patient selection. J Neurotrauma 22 (11): 1311–1318.

Uchiyama H, Nishizawa S, Satoh A et al. (1999). Posttraumatic pituitary apoplexy – two case reports. Neurol Med Chir 39 (1): 36–39.

Uhl E, Kreth FW, Elias B et al. (2004). Outcome and prognostic factors of hemicraniectomy for space occupying cerebral infarction. J Neurol Neurosurg Psychiatry 75 (2): 270–274.

Vahedi K, Vicaut E, Mateo J et al. (2007a). Sequential-design, multicenter, randomized, controlled trial of early decompressive craniectomy in malignant middle cerebral artery infarction (DECIMAL Trial). Stroke 38 (9): 2506–2517.

Vahedi K, Hofmeijer J, Juettler E et al. (2007b). Early decompressive surgery in malignant infarction of the middle cerebral artery: a pooled analysis of three randomised controlled trials. Lancet Neurol 6 (3): 215–222.

van der Worp HB, Sena ES, Donnan GA et al. (2007). Hypothermia in animal models of acute ischaemic stroke: a systematic review and meta-analysis. Brain 130 (Pt 12): 3063–3074.

van der Worp HB, Macleod MR, Kollmar R et al. (2010). Therapeutic hypothermia for acute ischemic stroke: ready to start large randomized trials? J Cereb Blood Flow Metab 30 (6): 1079–1093.

Visocchi M, Esposito G, Della Pepa GM et al. (2012). Giant frontal mucocele complicated by subdural empyema:

treatment of a rare association. Acta Neurol Belg 112 (1): 85–90.

Wagner S, Schnippering H, Aschoff A et al. (2001). Suboptimum hemicraniectomy as a cause of additional cerebral lesions in patients with malignant infarction of the middle cerebral artery. J Neurosurg 94 (5): 693–696.

Walcott BP, Kuklina EV, Nahed BV et al. (2011). Craniectomy for malignant cerebral infarction: prevalence and outcomes in US hospitals. PLoS One 6 (12): e29193.

Wang KW, Chang WN, Ho JT et al. (2006). Factors predictive of fatality in massive middle cerebral artery territory infarction and clinical experience of decompressive hemicraniectomy. Eur J Neurol 13 (7): 765–771.

Wang DZ, Nair DS, Talkad AV (2011). Acute decompressive hemicraniectomy to control high intracranial pressure in patients with malignant MCA ischemic strokes. Curr Treat Options Cardiovasc Med 13 (3): 225–232.

Wartenberg KE (2012). Malignant middle cerebral artery infarction. Curr Opin Crit Care 18 (2): 152–163.

Whitfield PC, Patel H, Hutchinson PJ et al. (2001). Bifrontal decompressive craniectomy in the management of posttraumatic intracranial hypertension. Br J Neurosurg 15 (6): 500–507.

Yamashita K, Suzuki Y, Yoshizumi H et al. (1994). Tuberculous hypertrophic pachymeningitis involving the posterior fossa and high cervical region – case report. Neurol Med Chir 34 (2): 100–103.

Yang XF, Yao Y, Hu WW et al. (2005). Is decompressive craniectomy for malignant middle cerebral artery infarction of any worth? J Zhejiang Univ Sci B 6 (7): 644–649.

Yang XF, Wen L, Shen F et al. (2008). Surgical complications secondary to decompressive craniectomy in patients with a head injury: a series of 108 consecutive cases. Acta Neurochir (Wien) 150 (12): 1241–1247. discussion 1248.

Yao Y, Liu W, Yang X et al. (2005). Is decompressive craniectomy for malignant middle cerebral artery territory infarction of any benefit for elderly patients? Surg Neurol 64 (2): 165–169. discussion 169.

Zhao J, Su YY, Zhang Y et al. (2012). Decompressive hemicraniectomy in malignant middle cerebral artery infarct: a randomized controlled trial enrolling patients up to 80 years old. Neurocrit Care 17 (2): 161–171.

Ziai WC, Port JD, Cowan JA et al. (2003). Decompressive craniectomy for intractable cerebral edema: experience of a single center. J Neurosurg Anesthesiol 15 (1): 25–32.

Zweckberger K, Eros C, Zimmermann R et al. (2006). Effect of early and delayed decompressive craniectomy on secondary brain damage after controlled cortical impact in mice. J Neurotrauma 23 (7): 1083–1093.

*Handbook of Clinical Neurology, Vol. 140 (3rd series)*
*Critical Care Neurology, Part I*
E.F.M. Wijdicks and A.H. Kramer, Editors
http://dx.doi.org/10.1016/B978-0-444-63600-3.00017-9

Chapter 17

# Diagnosis and management of spinal cord emergencies

E.P. FLANAGAN[1]* AND S.J. PITTOCK[1,2]

[1]*Department of Neurology, Mayo Clinic, Rochester, MN, USA*

[2]*Department of Laboratory Medicine and Pathology, Mayo Clinic, Rochester, MN, USA*

## Abstract

Most spinal cord injury is seen with trauma. Nontraumatic spinal cord emergencies are discussed in this chapter. These myelopathies are rare but potentially devastating neurologic disorders. In some situations prior comorbidity (e.g., advanced cancer) provides a clue, but in others (e.g., autoimmune myelopathies) it may come with little warning. Neurologic examination helps distinguish spinal cord emergencies from peripheral nervous system emergencies (e.g., Guillain–Barré), although some features overlap. Neurologic deficits are often severe and may quickly become irreversible, highlighting the importance of early diagnosis and treatment. Emergent magnetic resonance imaging (MRI) of the entire spine is the imaging modality of choice for nontraumatic spinal cord emergencies and helps differentiate extramedullary compressive causes (e.g., epidural abscess, metastatic compression, epidural hematoma) from intramedullary etiologies (e.g., transverse myelitis, infectious myelitis, or spinal cord infarct). The MRI characteristics may give a clue to the diagnosis (e.g., flow voids dorsal to the cord in dural arteriovenous fistula). However, additional investigations (e.g., aquaporin-4-IgG) are often necessary to diagnose intramedullary etiologies and guide treatment. Emergency decompressive surgery is necessary for many extramedullary compressive causes, either alone or in combination with other treatments (e.g., radiation) and preoperative neurologic deficit is the best predictor of outcome.

## INTRODUCTION

Myelopathies are rare but potentially devastating neurologic disorders. In some situations prior comorbidity (e.g., advanced cancer) provides a clue but in others (e.g., autoimmune myelopathies) it may come with little warning. Most acute spinal cord injuries in the neurosciences unit are traumatic and are discussed in Chapter 15 of this volume.

In this chapter we will discuss the rare acute myelopathies which will need immediate medical or neurosurgical management. Many patients present with puzzling symptomatology and may quickly worsen in the intensive care unit, even requiring mechanical ventilation when cervical segments get involved.

## EPIDEMIOLOGY

Spinal cord emergencies are rare but devastating neurologic disorders with a variety of causes. Age, sex, and race

are important factors to take into account when considering the likely cause of the spinal cord emergency. Spinal epidural abscesses have an incidence of 0.88/100 000, are commonest in those aged 50–70 and males predominate (Ptaszynski et al., 2007; Pradilla et al., 2009). Autopsy studies report approximately 5% of cancer patients have epidural spinal cord compression (Barron et al., 1959). Dural arteriovenous fistula (AVF) (in which males also predominate) and spinal cord infarcts both peak from age 50 to 70 years. In young and middle-aged adults multiple sclerosis (MS) and neuromyelitis optica spectrum disorders (NMOSDs) are more frequent, while in children and younger adults acute disseminated encephalomyelitis (ADEM), intramedullary arteriovenous malformations (AVMs), and cavernous hemangiomas are most prevalent. Caucasians living furthest from the equator are more predisposed to MS, while those of African descent are more predisposed to NMOSD (Flanagan et al., 2016b) and spinal cord sarcoidosis.

*Correspondence to: Dr. Eoin Flanagan, Mayo Clinic, Department of Neurology, 200 First St SW, Rochester MN 55905, USA. Tel: +1-507-538-1038, Fax: +1-507-538-6012, E-mail: flanagan.eoin@mayo.edu

# NEUROPATHOLOGY

Knowledge of the etiologies of extrinsic compression of the spinal cord requires an understanding of spinal anatomy. The spinal cord is encased within the thecal sac, bordered anteriorly by the vertebral body and intervertebral discs (nucleus pulposus and annulus fibrosis), posteriorly by the posterior spinal processes, and laterally by the pedicles and lamina. Between the bony thecal sac and outer layer of the cord (the dura) lies the epidural space, which contains fat and venous plexuses. The epidural space is widest and contains most fat in the thoracolumbar region and thus this is the most common site of epidural abscess. The subdural space is a potential space between dura and arachnoid. Between the arachnoid and pia is the subarachnoid space in which cerebrospinal fluid (CSF) is contained.

## Metastatic epidural spinal cord compression

The most common region affected is the thoracic spine due to higher volume of bony tissue. The most common causes are lung, breast, and prostate carcinoma due to their high prevalence in the population. Certain other cancers are overrepresented, including non-Hodgkin's lymphoma, multiple myeloma, and renal cell carcinoma (Cole and Patchell, 2008). In children Ewing's sarcoma and neuroblastomas predominate. Arterial seeding of the vertebral body is the first step, followed by growth posteriorly into the thecal sac. Initially the epidural venous plexus is compressed, resulting in edema (which can be reversed with steroids). Further compression results in vascular injury with ischemia followed by secondary infarction of the cord. In such cases, the paraparesis progresses in a subacute to chronic fashion. Malignant vertebral collapse and bony fragments extending into the thecal sac may cause acute paraplegia. With lymphoma, paravertebral masses may extend through the intervertebral foramen and compress the cord, rather than extending from the vertebral body metastases.

## Spinal epidural abscess

The abscess may arise from direct hematogenous inoculation of the epidural space from systemic infection, infections at distant sites, or from contiguous spread to the epidural space from an intervertebral pyogenic infectious discitis and vertebral osteomyelitis. Direct inoculation may also occur during spinal surgery or with epidural catheters (more common with prolonged catheters (e.g., for pain control) rather than short-lived catheters for obstetric indications). The abscess typically extends three to five vertebral segments and is usually posterior to the cord. Neurologic deficits are usually from direct compression, but thrombophlebitis may contribute. The abscess may contain frank pus, but after a few weeks surgical excision may only reveal granulation tissue, leading to difficulty isolating an organism; preceding empiric antibiotics may also decrease the yield. The pathogen is usually bacterial, with *Staphylococcus aureus* accounting for two-thirds of cases, 40% of which may be methicillin-resistant (MRSA). *Streptococcus* and *Escherichia coli* are other common pathogens. Polymicrobial abscess may occur and explain worsening when treating a single isolated pathogen. Tuberculosis is a common cause in endemic regions. *Pseudomonas* is a recognized cause in intravenous drug users.

## Epidural spinal hematoma

This is most frequently encountered after spine surgery and may be asymptomatic. Spontaneous spinal epidural hematoma is rare and potentially venous in origin as the epidural venous system is valveless and unprotected from changes in abdominal pressure.

## Spinal cord infarct

The cervicothoracic cord is supplied by a single anterior spinal artery and two posterior spinal arteries that arise predominantly from the vertebral arteries. Cervical, thoracic intercostal, and lumbar arteries, known as radiculomedullary arteries, all contribute to spinal cord perfusion and include the artery of the lumbar enlargement (artery of Adamkiewicz) that arises from T9–T12. Sulcocommissural and pial branches supply the interior of the cord. The anterior horn cells are most vulnerable to ischemia and selective injury in watershed spinal cord infarction may result in predominantly lower motor neuron findings on examination (Flanagan and McKeon, 2014). Spinal artery infarction occurs most often as a complication of aortic surgery (although epidural hematoma needs to be excluded) but atherosclerotic disease, thromboembolism (e.g., from atrial fibrillation), systemic hypotension, hypoperfusion from vertebral dissection/thrombosis, vasculitis (medium- or large-vessel), and decompression sickness are recognized causes. With fibrocartilaginous embolism an increased axial load combined with simultaneous Valsalva or minor trauma is thought to result in retrograde embolization of the nucleus pulposus into a spinal artery. In aortic dissection, secondary obstruction of lumbar and intercostal arteries or the artery of Adamkiewicz results in cord ischemia (Gaul et al., 2008).

## Vascular malformations

These usually occur in the thoracic cord. Dural AVFs account for 70% of spinal vascular malformations, and arise in the dural sleeve of the nerve root from acquired abnormal communication between a radicular artery and radiculomedullary vein. Venous congestion ensues and occasionally progresses to venous infarction.

Intramedullary AVMs and cavernous malformations typically manifest with an acute myelopathy from an accompanying bleed.

## Autoimmune, demyelinating, and other inflammatory myelopathies

NMOSDs are the best understood of the inflammatory myelopathies due to the discovery in 2004 of its highly specific serum biomarker, aquaporin-4 (AQP-4)-IgG. AQP-4 is the most abundant water channel in the central nervous system (CNS) and is located on astrocytic end-feet. The binding of the pathogenic AQP4-IgG (secreted by plasmablasts under the influence of interleukin-6) results in activation of complement, breakdown of the blood–brain barrier, damage to the astrocyte, and secondary demyelination (Lucchinetti et al., 2002; Hinson et al., 2009, 2012; Chihara et al., 2011; Flanagan and Weinshenker, 2014).

Advances in our knowledge of NMOSD pathogenesis have led to early studies of more targeted maintenance immunotherapies showing promise, including inhibitors of the complement pathway (eculizumab) and interleukin-6 antagonists (tocilizumab) (Pittock et al., 2013; Araki et al., 2014). MS is a CNS inflammatory immune-mediated disease which results in inflammation, demyelination (often followed by remyelination), and axonal injury. ADEM is a CNS inflammatory demyelinating disease that is an autoimmune disorder triggered by an environmental stimulus (infection or vaccination) in a patient who is genetically predisposed. The syndrome of ADEM may be caused by AQP-4-IgG or myelin oligodendrocyte glycoprotein-IgG (MOG-IgG) (McKeon et al., 2008; Misu et al., 2015). Sarcoidosis is a multisystem granulomatous disease that usually involves the lung and is associated with noncaseating granulomas; spinal cord sarcoidosis frequently presents in an acute or subacute manner (Flanagan et al., 2016a).

## CLINICAL PRESENTATION

It is essential that one consider the setting when evaluating spinal cord emergencies, as there will often be clues to guide the clinician to the correct diagnosis. For example, a patient with widely metastatic lung cancer presenting with acute paraplegia is likely to have epidural metastatic spinal cord compression; an anticoagulated patient with rapidly progressive paraplegia may have an epidural hematoma; fever, back pain, and neurologic deficits raise the possibility of spinal epidural abscess. A summary of the causes of spinal cord emergencies and clinical clues to their diagnosis are outlined in Table 17.1. There are a wide array of infectious causes of intramedullary myelitis that vary by region and thus these are summarized separately in Table 17.2.

Pain is common in spinal cord emergencies. With metastatic epidural compression pain is worse when supine (e.g., at night) due to lengthening of the spine and distension of the venous plexuses. Localized pain in the thoracic region (uncommon with musculoskeletal spine disease) should warrant particular attention. Pain worse with movement may indicate spine instability from a pathologic fracture. Thoracic spine pain radiating to the back accompanied by lower-extremity weakness should raise the possibility of aortic dissection. Severe radicular pain (often asymmetric) often accompanies cauda equina syndrome, while perineal pain may occur in conus medullaris syndrome.

Weakness in epidural compression (from abscess or metastases) is common by the time of diagnosis and quickly becomes irreversible, highlighting the importance of early diagnosis and treatment. Weakness is more prominent and more asymmetric with cauda equina syndrome than conus medullaris syndrome. In spinal cord infarction weakness may occur hyperacutely but, unlike with cerebral infarction, it is not uncommon for weakness to progress over minutes to hours. Although rare, recurrent episodes of spinal cord ischemia have been described (initially by Dejerine in 1911) with aortic disease and steal syndromes.

Sensory changes are common and discussed below. Bowel and bladder impairment is a late finding in metastatic epidural spinal cord compression from metastases or abscesses and it is very rare to encounter this in isolation, unless the conus region is involved. With cauda equina syndrome, urinary retention or urine incontinence (from loss of urethral sphincter tone) may occur. Coexisting or prior optic neuritis suggests NMOSD, MS, or ADEM. Concomitant or prior episodes of intractable nausea and vomiting (with or without hiccups) suggests the characteristic area postrema involvement in NMOSD. Myelitis in the setting of connective tissue disorders (lupus, Sjögren's syndrome, antiphospholipid syndrome) is often due to AQP-4-IgG-seropositive NMOSD coexisting rather than a neurologic manifestation of the systemic autoimmune disease (Pittock et al., 2008; Wingerchuk and Weinshenker, 2012). AQP-4-IgG-seropositive NMOSD myelitis also appears to be more frequent than expected in those with a history of neurologic autoimmunity (myasthenia gravis and $N$-methyl-$D$-aspartate-receptor encephalitis) (McKeon et al., 2009; Titulaer et al., 2014). Longitudinally, extensive myelitis has been reported with posterior reversible encephalopathy syndrome and in this setting may be a manifestation of AQP-4-IgG-seropositive NMOSD (Magana et al., 2009; de Havenon et al., 2014). NMOSD may also rarely occur in a paraneoplastic context (Pittock and Lennon, 2008). Spinal cord sarcoidosis may present acutely or subacutely and a majority are accompanied by a longitudinally extensive lesion mimicking NMOSD (Flanagan et al., 2016a). In a recent comparative study of myelitis in NMOSD and spinal cord sarcoidosis the presence of tonic spasms, female sex, coexisting

*Table 17.1*

Etiologies and clinical pearls in the diagnosis of nontraumatic spinal cord emergencies

| Etiology of acute myelopathy | Clinical pearls |
| --- | --- |
| **Neoplastic** | |
| Metastatic epidural spinal cord compression | Known cancer/myeloma history, risk factors for cancer (e.g., smoker); this is the initial cancer presentation in 20% |
| Extramedullary myeloid tumors | Known hematologic malignancy |
| Intramedullary metastasis | Known cancer/myeloma history, risk factors for cancer (e.g., smoker) |
| Primary spinal cord tumors | Lymphoma may present subacutely; others usually chronic |
| **Infectious** | Immunocompromised, spinal procedures |
| Epidural abscess | Fevers/chills/night sweats; intravenous drug user |
| Intramedullary infectious myelitis (Table 17.2) | |
| **Vascular** | |
| Hematoma | |
|     Epidural, subdural, subarachnoid | Post spinal procedure, coagulopathy, preceding trauma, small-vessel vasculitis, prior radiation |
|     Intramedullary "hematomyelia" | AVM, cavernous malformation, hemorrhagic metastasis, bleeding diathesis, Osler–Weber–Rendu, prior radiation |
| Spinal cord infarct | Post aortic surgery, hypotensive injury, aortic (or vertebral) dissection, multiple vascular risk factors, other causes (endocarditis, intravascular lymphoma, thrombophilia) |
| Fibrocartilaginous embolism | Young women, preceding trauma/Valsalva |
| Vascular malformation | |
|     Dural arteriovenous fistula | Older men, stepwise deterioration precipitated by exercise/Valsalva |
|     AVM/cavernous malformation | Older children/young adults; usually manifest due to hemorrhage |
| Venous congestive | Venous anomalies of inferior vena cava |
| **Structural** | |
| Osteoporotic vertebral collapse | Known osteoporosis, steroid use |
| Herniated disc | Known degenerative disc disease/prior spine surgery |
| Atlantoaxial subluxation | Down syndrome, rheumatoid arthritis |
| Spondylotic | Prior history of spine surgery |
| Epidural lipomatosis | Obese, corticosteroid use |
| Surfer's myelopathy | Novice surfers |
| **Inflammatory/demyelinating/ autoimmune** | |
| Neuromyelitis optica spectrum disorder | Females; African descent; history of lupus, Sjögren's or myasthenia gravis; accompanying optic neuritis or nausea/vomiting; tonic spasms/Lhermitte's |
| Multiple sclerosis | Young Caucasian women, Lhermitte's, sensory useless hand from proprioceptive deficit |
| ADEM | Children, recent infection/vaccination |
| Spinal cord sarcoidosis | African-American, systemic/pulmonary symptoms |
| MOG-IgG myelitis | Conus involvement; ADEM |
| Connective tissue disease-associated* | Synovitis, oral/genital ulcers (Behçet's) |
| Paraneoplastic (sometimes necrotizing) | Known cancer, cancer risk factors (e.g., smoking) |
| Idiopathic transverse myelitis | |
| **Toxic/metabolic** | |
| Vitamin $B_{12}$ deficiency | Usually chronic but can present acutely in setting of nitrous oxide use |
| Lathrysm | Africa, Asia from grasspea ingestion |
| Konzo | Cassava bean ingestion in tropics |
| Heroin | May cause an acute or subacute combined degeneration-like presentation |
| **Iatrogenic** | |
| Radiation | History of spinal irradiation |
| Medications | Cytarabine and methotrexate well-recognized cause of subacute combined degeneration; cisplatin and pyridoxine excess cause sensory ataxia |
| Positioning | Worsening of spinal cord disorder in those undergoing MRI under anesthesia |

*Table 17.1*

**Continued**

| Etiology of acute myelopathy | Clinical pearls |
|---|---|
| **Miscellaneous** | |
| Electrocution myelopathy | Recent electrocution |
| Decompression sickness | Scuba divers |
| Functional paraplegia | Recent psychologic stressor, inconsistencies on examination |

*Aquaporin-4-IgG should be tested in cases of long myelitis accompanying connective tissue disorders; this often represents coexisting neuromyelitis optica spectrum disorder rather than a neurologic manifestation of an autoimmune disease.

AVM, arteriovenous malformation; ADEM, acute disseminated encephalomyelitis; MOG, myelin oligodendrocyte glycoprotein; IgG, immunoglobulin G; MRI, magnetic resonance imaging.

*Table 17.2*

**Summary of selected well-recognized causes of intramedullary infectious myelopathies including their geographic predominance, clinical clues, and diagnosis**

| Infection | Predominant geographic region(s) if applicable | Preferred diagnostic test | Clinical clues |
|---|---|---|---|
| **Bacterial** | | | |
| Intramedullary pyogenic abscess | | Surgical drainage and isolation of organism | Known systemic infection |
| *Borrelia burgdorferi* | North-east USA, Central Europe | Serum and CSF serology | Tick bite, erythema migrans rash, polyarthritis |
| *Treponema pallidum* | | Serum rapid plasma reagin; CSF VDRL | Sensory ataxia, infarct (meningovascular) |
| Mycobacterium tuberculosis | Developing countries | CSF ZN stain, culture and TB PCR | HIV; meningomyelitis |
| **Viruses** | | | |
| HSV 1, 2 | | CSF PCR | May be necrotizing; genital/oral herpes |
| VZV | | CSF PCR, IgM | Zoster rash; may cause vasculopathy |
| CMV | | CMV PCR | Polyradiculomyelitis in HIV; may be necrotizing |
| EBV | | EBV PCR | Postviral immune-mediated myelitis |
| West Nile virus | Africa, Middle East, Russia, USA | CSF IgM | Acute flaccid paralysis |
| Enterovirus (D68, 70, 71; Cocksackie A, B) | May occur in outbreaks (e.g., D68 Colorado 2014) | CSF PCR | Acute flaccid paralysis |
| Poliovirus | Africa, India | CSF PCR | Acute flaccid paralysis |
| HIV | | HIV serology | Acute infection at time of initial presentation; chronic myelopathy more common |
| Rabies | Developing countries (dog bites); USA (bats) | PCR from skin biopsy in Neck beneath hair line | Bat/dog bites (developing countries); hydrophobia |
| **Parasites** | | | |
| Schistosomiasis | Central/South America; sub-Saharan Africa | Serum and CSF serology; demonstration of eggs in urine/stool | Swimming in fresh water; eosinophilia (serum/CSF) |

CSF, cerebrospinal fluid; VDRL, Venereal Disease Research Laboratory; ZN, Ziehl–Neelsen; TB, tuberculosis; PCR, polymerase chain reaction; HIV, human immunodeficiency virus; HSV, herpes simplex virus; VZV, varicella-zoster virus; CMV, cytomegalovirus; EBV, Epstein–Barr virus; IgM, immunoglobulin M.

autoimmunity, and shorter time to nadir favored NMOSD, while constitutional symptoms favored spinal cord sarcoidosis (Flanagan et al., 2016a). Dural AVF typically causes a chronic progressive myelopathy but 5% present with an acute myelopathy and episodes of superimposed stepwise worsening occur in up to 25% (Fugate et al., 2012). Worsening with exertion (neurogenic claudication) and mixed upper and lower motor neuron involvement are also described (Fugate et al., 2012).

## Spinal shock

Spinal shock is used to describe flaccid areflexic para- or quadriplegia with mute plantar responses from acute spinal cord injury. In this situation it may mimic peripheral nervous system emergencies (e.g., cauda equina syndrome or Guillain–Barré syndrome).

## Neurogenic shock

This phenomenon, well recognized in traumatic spinal cord injury, may also be seen with nontraumatic spinal cord emergencies. Hypotension results from pooling of blood in vessels that lack sympathetic tone in the extremities below the level of the lesion. Unopposed vagal activity may result in accompanying bradycardia.

## Examination patterns

Upper motor neuron pattern weakness is typical, involving lower-extremity flexors and upper-extremity extensors. Hyperreflexia and increased tone help differentiate spinal cord disorders from peripheral nervous system (e.g., Guillain–Barré syndrome or cauda equina syndrome), neuromuscular junction disorder (e.g., myasthenia), or myopathic (e.g., rhabdomyolysis) emergencies. Rectal tone is reduced in cauda equina syndrome. Absent reflexes, fasciculations, and atrophy suggest either exclusive or combined lower motor neuron involvement. An inverted brachioradialis or inverted biceps jerk causes an absent reflex with spread resulting in paradoxic finger flexion and arm extension respectively. It results from C5–6 root injury at the site of compression and upper motor neuron involvement below that level. Superficial abdominal reflexes above the umbilicus (T8–10) and below the umbilicus (T10–T12) are assessed by gently scratching the skin from each quadrant towards the umbilicus and assessing for abdominal contraction. They are absent in thoracic cord lesions, but may also be difficult to elicit in obese or elderly patients.

A sensory level suggests a thoracic or lower cervical lesion. Loss of pain and temperature with preserved dorsal column function (vibration, joint position, light touch) are typical of anterior spinal artery infarction. Acute dorsal column dysfunction may occur with nitrous

oxide-associated vitamin $B_{12}$ deficiency (after surgical/dental procedures or due to misuse by dentists). Saddle anesthesia suggests cauda equina syndrome. Sacral sparing may occur with central cord lesion, as sacral fibers are laminated laterally within spinothalamic tracts.

Assessing for blood pressure or pulse differences between both arms may give a clue to aortic dissection-associated paraparesis. Detection of lymphadenopathy may give a clue to an underlying malignancy. It is important to assess for features that may suggest a functional neurologic disorder (inconsistencies in the examination, psychologic stressors). As functional overlay may occur with organic neurologic injury, unless the diagnosis is unequivocal further investigations may be necessary.

# NEURODIAGNOSTICS AND IMAGING

## Neuroimaging

### EXTRAMEDULLARY LESIONS

Magnetic resonance imaging (MRI) of the entire spine is the imaging modality of choice for acute nontraumatic spinal cord emergencies. Its excellent visualization of soft tissues and the intramedullary spinal cord and its safety in those with a coagulopathy make it preferable to computed tomography (CT) myelogram, which also risks introduction of infection to the subarachnoid space in lumbosacral spinal epidural abscess. Imaging of the entire spine is important as patients with metastatic or abscess-related compression may compress the cord at multiple sites and the clinical localization may not always fit with the location of the pathology (e.g., dural AVF) (Rabinstein, 2015). Metastatic spinal cord compression may reveal vertebral bony metastases or a paraspinal mass (Fig. 17.1B2) extending into the thecal sac and compressing the cord. The epidural abscess is noted by a T1 hypointense and T2 hyperintense lesion with a rim of enhancing granulation tissue epidurally which indents the thecal sac, resulting in cord compression (Fig. 17.1A1). A similar appearance without gadolinium enhancement suggests spinal epidural hematoma (Fig. 17.2C); heterogeneity of signal may occur in anticoagulation-associated epidural hematoma. Vertebral osteomyelitis with T1 hypointensity and loss of cortical bone margins and increased T2 signal in the disc indicates discitis and frequently accompanies spinal epidural abscess (Fig. 17.1B). CT or CT myelogram may be useful in patients in whom MRI is contraindicated (e.g., pacemakers incompatible with MRI). Plain radiographs are not useful in the diagnosis of epidural abscess or metastatic compression given their limited sensitivity and specificity. Intramedullary T2 signal hyperintensity may accompany severe compression. Intramedullary gadolinium enhancement may occur in spondylotic

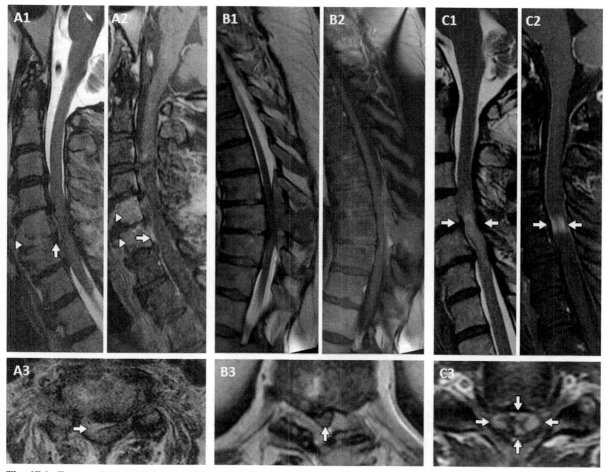

**Fig. 17.1.** Extramedullary etiologies of spinal cord compression. Sagittal T2-weighted magnetic resonance imaging (MRI) of the cervical spine reveals a ventral spinal epidural abscess (**A1**, arrow), with accompanying infectious discitis also evident (**A1**, arrowhead). The T1-weighted images postgadolinium reveal enhancement within the ventral epidural space consistent with epidural abscess on sagittal (**A2**, arrow) and axial images (**A3**, arrow); concomitant vertebral osteomyelitis is also evident (**A2**, arrowheads). Thoracic spine MRI reveals spinal cord compression from a paraspinal mass dorsal to the thoracic cord which extends into the thecal sac and is evident on sagittal T2- (**B1**), axial T2- (**B3**, arrow) and sagittal T1-weighted images after gadolinium administration (**B2**). A biopsy revealed lymphoma as the cause of the mass. Cervical spine MRI reveals spondylotic changes (**C1**, arrows) along with intramedullary T2 signal extending over multiple vertebral segments (**C1**) with a transverse band of gadolinium enhancement on sagittal T1-weighted postgadolinium images (**C2**, arrows) that forms a circumferential pattern on axial images sparing the gray matter (**C3**, arrows). This pattern of enhancement was consistent with a diagnosis of spondylotic compressive myelopathy with enhancement. (**C**, Adapted with permission from Flanagan, 2016).

myelopathy and is frequently mistaken for tumor or inflammation. This may lead to iatrogenic injury from spinal cord biopsy or unnecessary immunosuppression (Flanagan et al., 2014b). A specific "pancake-like" flat transverse band of enhancement (Fig. 17.1C) has three major characteristics (Flanagan et al., 2014b):

1. Width is greater than or equal to its height (Fig. 17.1C2).
2. It is located at the center of a spindle-shaped T2 hyperintensity (Fig. 17.1C1).
3. Axial circumferential enhancement spares gray matter (Fig. 17.1C3).

## INTRAMEDULLARY LESIONS

In spinal cord infarction emergency MRI is recommended unless there is a suspicion for aortic dissection, in which case its confirmation and treatment are prioritized. The MRI may be normal, particularly in the first few hours. T2 signal change within cord parenchyma is nonspecific but may be "pencil-like" on sagittal images and have an "owl- or snake-eye" appearance on axial images (Fig. 17.2A), the latter reflecting preferential gray-matter injury which is most vulnerable to ischemia (Flanagan and McKeon, 2014). Restricted diffusion helps suggest infarct but in the cord diffusion-weighted

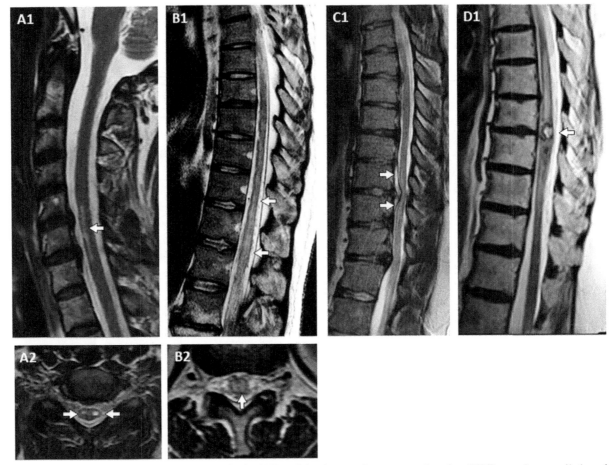

**Fig. 17.2.** Vascular myelopathy emergencies. Sagittal T2-weighted magnetic resonance imaging (MRI) reveals a pencil-shaped T2 hyperintensity in the anterior spinal cord (**A1**) that has an owl/snake-eye pattern on axial images (**A2**) consistent with a spinal cord infarct; the significance of the associated spondylotic changes at the level of the T2 lesion was uncertain in this case, but could suggest fibrocartilaginous embolism as the underlying cause. A longitudinally extensive T2 hyperintensity in the distal thoracic cord extending to the conus is shown with dorsal flow voids (**B1**, arrows) and central T2 hyperintensity on axial images (**B2**, arrow) suggested dural arteriovenous fistula. An L1 dural arteriovenous fistula was later confirmed on formal spinal angiography (not shown). Thoracic spine MRI reveals a ventral epidural lesion compressing the cord that occurred after trauma in the setting of amphetamine use; the signal characteristics were most consistent with a ventral epidural hematoma. (**C1**, arrows) A "popcorn"-like lesion with central T2 hyperintensity and surrounding T2 hypointensity and accompanying longitudinally extensive signal hyperintensity extending above and below the lesion is shown (**D1**). These characteristics were most consistent with a cavernous malformation.

imaging is limited by artifact. Concomitant vertebral body infarct is a useful confirmatory feature but rarely present. Intervertebral disc disease at the site of infarction may suggest fibrocartilaginous embolism. "Owl-eye or snake-eye" patterns were also noted in a recent infectious/postinfectious acute flaccid paralysis outbreak in children and young adults with enterovirus D68 outbreak in Colorado (Messacar et al., 2015); West Nile virus myelitis shows similar MRI abnormalities.

The vast majority of dural AVFs are in the lower thoracic or upper lumbar regions, but clinical examination is not reliable at localizing the fistula and thus entire neuroaxis MRI is necessary. Classically, it causes a thoracic

longitudinally extensive swollen T2 hyperintensity (secondary to venous congestion) with extension to the conus and flow voids dorsal to the cord from enlarged veins (Fig. 17.2B). Enlarged gadolinium enhancing veins dorsal to the cord and intramedullary gadolinium enhancement may occur. MR angiography (MRA) may help with further localization of the fistula, but formal spinal angiogram is the gold standard and essential in dural AVF diagnosis. Intramedullary AVMs show clusters of flow voids within the spinal cord parenchyma, while cavernous malformations have a characteristic "popcorn" appearance with heterogeneous signal abnormality (Fig. 17.2D).

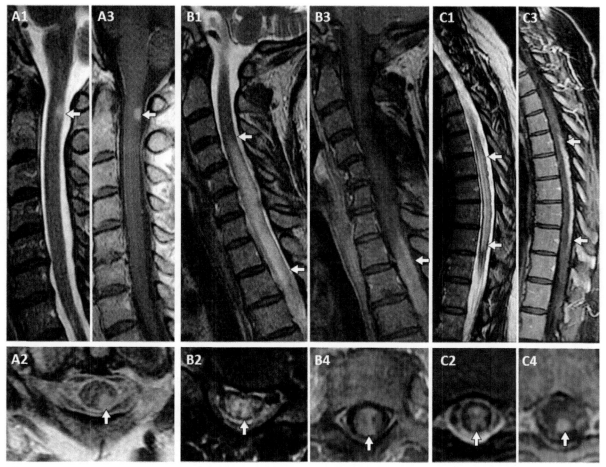

**Fig. 17.3.** Typical magnetic resonance imaging of spinal cord lesions of multiple sclerosis, aquaporin-4-IgG-seropositive neuro-myelitis optica spectrum disorder (NMOSD), and spinal cord sarcoidosis. A typical short multiple sclerosis myelitis lesion is shown with T2 hyperintensity in the dorsal cord extending approximately one vertebral level on sagittal images (**A1**) and located in the left dorsal columns on axial images (**A2**). The lesion is noted to enhance on sagittal T1-weighted images postgadolinium (**A3**). A characteristic aquaporin-4-IgG-seropositive NMOSD myelitis lesion with a longitudinally extensive T2 hyperintensity extending greater than three vertebral segments (**B1**, arrows) and involving the central cord on axial images (**B2**, arrow) with patchy gadolinium enhancement (**B3** and **B4**, arrows). A typical spinal cord sarcoidosis lesion is shown with a longitudinally extensive T2-hyperintense lesion (**C1**) involving the central cord (**C2**) (that would be indistinguishable from an NMOSD lesion based on T2-weighted images alone) and a gadolinium enhancement pattern that is suspicious for sarcoid showing intense long linear sub-pial enhancement extending in from the dorsal cord (**C3** and **C4**). (Adapted from Flanagan, 2014b with permission.)

MS spinal cord lesions are typically short, spanning fewer than three vertebral segments, located in the periphery of the cord on axial images (dorsal or lateral columns), and may have accompanying swelling and gadolinium enhancement (Fig. 17.3A). In contrast, NMOSDs are most often accompanied by a longitudi-nally extensive T2 hyperintensity extending three or more vertebral segments, centrally located on axial images and frequently associated with spinal cord swell-ing (Fig. 17.3B1 and B2). However, in approximately 14% NMOSD lesions are short (Flanagan et al., 2015). Bright spotty lesions suggest NMOSD and appear as focal syrinx-like hyperintensities within the T2 lesion (Hyun et al., 2015). Most spinal cord sarcoidosis cases

do not have a history of prior systemic sarcoid and are accompanied by a longitudinally extensive T2 lesion, thus mimicking NMOSD (Flanagan et al., 2016a). In a recent study comparing NMOSD and spinal cord sar-coidosis, linear dorsal subpial enhancement extending over multiple vertebral segments (Fig. 17.3C3 and C4) and persistent enhancement (>2 months) favored sar-coidosis, while ring enhancement (although present in only one-third) favored NMOSD; however, indistinct patchy rostrocaudal enhancement is most often seen with NMOSD lesions (Fig. 17.3B3 and 17.3B4) (Flanagan et al., 2016a).

Lesions involving the conus are described in MOG-IgG-associated long myelitis (Kitley et al., 2014). The

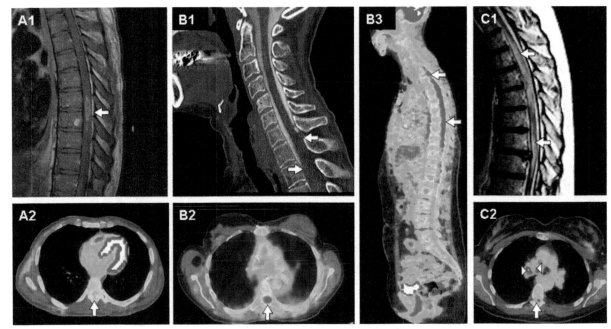

**Fig. 17.4.** Fluorodeoxyglucose positron emission tomography (FDG-PET) hypermetabolism in neoplastic spinal cord lesions and spinal cord sarcoidosis. (**A**) Intramedullary spinal cord lung metastasis demonstrating gadolinium enhancement in a "rim and flame" pattern on sagittal T1-weighted magnetic resonance imaging (MRI) (**A1**, white arrow) with corresponding moderate hypermetabolism (yellow/red color) on FDG-PET (**A2**, white arrow; maximum standardized uptake value (SUV$_{max}$), 2.8). (**B**) Grade III astrocytoma demonstrating spinal block on computed tomography myelogram in the upper thoracic spine (**B1**, white arrow) with corresponding intense hypermetabolism (red color) on axial and sagittal FDG-PET (**B2** and **B3**, white arrows; SUV$_{max}$, 5.1). (**C**) Spinal cord neurosarcoidosis showing thoracic cord longitudinally extensive T2 signal hyperintensity on MRI (**C1**, white arrows) and corresponding FDG-PET hypermetabolism (red color) (**C2**, regular white arrows; SUV$_{max}$, 6.3) and additional FDG-PET hypermetabolism of perihilar lymph nodes (**C2**, block arrows). (Reproduced from Flanagan et al., 2013, with permission.)

spinal cord characteristics of ADEM lesions are less well defined, but long and short lesions occur. Paraneoplastic myelopathies may show tract-specific signal abnormalities with enhancement or have severe necrosis (Urai et al., 2009; Flanagan et al., 2011b). A rim of enhancement surrounding a region of less avid enhancement with a flame pattern at its superior or inferior border suggests intramedullary metastasis (Fig. 17.4A1) (Rykken et al., 2013). A summary of a selection of gadolinium enhancement patterns that are associated with intramedullary acute and subacute myelopathies is shown in Figure 17.5.

## MRI HEAD

An MRI of the head is helpful when evaluating those with CNS inflammatory demyelinating diseases. At NMOSD onset, the MRI will often be normal. However, the presence of abnormalities within surrounding the third and fourth ventricle is characteristic of NMOSD and area postrema lesions accompanying nausea and vomiting episodes are especially informative (Pittock et al., 2006). In patients with a short transverse myelitis episode and the presence of two or more typical brain lesions (juxtacortical, periventricular, or infratentorial),

85% will go on to develop MS within 15 years while 15% without this finding develop MS (Brex et al., 2002). Typical lesions are ovoid or form Dawson's fingers on sagittal FLAIR images. With ADEM, multifocal lesions frequently involving the deep gray matter are described. The presence of basilar meningitis may suggest spinal cord sarcoidosis.

## MRI LUMBAR SPINE

This is required emergently when assessing cauda equina syndrome, which generally shows a central disc extrusion.

## POSITRON EMISSION TOMOGRAPHY

[18]F-fluorodeoxyglucose positron emission tomography (PET) is often used to assess for an underlying malignancy or to stage a known cancer. In such cases, the spinal cord glucose metabolism should also be assessed, as intramedullary hypermetabolic lesions are more common with neoplastic (Fig. 17.4A1 and B2–3) than nonsarcoid inflammatory causes (Flanagan et al., 2013); spinal cord sarcoid is frequently hypermetabolic within

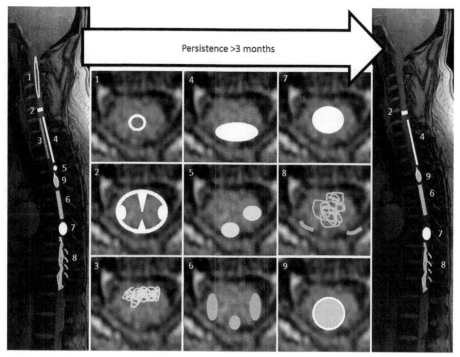

**Fig. 17.5.** Summary of intramedullary gadolinium enhancement patterns by etiology and their evolution in acute and subacute myelitis. Sagittal (left, images at initial presentation shown, and right panel, persistently enhancing lesions on follow-up images shown) and axial (middle panels) patterns of gadolinium enhancement. Brighter regions represent higher intensity of enhancement. **1**, neuromyelitis optica spectrum (elongated ring appearance in approximately one-third – the remainder usually patchy); **2**, cervical spondylotic myelopathy ("pancake-like" or "transverse band" on sagittal images – width of enhancement greater than or equal height – at middle of T2 hyperintensity and associated with moderate or severe stenosis and demonstrating circumferential white-matter enhancement sparing gray matter on axial images; enhancement only present in 7% of spondylotic myelopathies, but when present often mimics tumor or inflammation); **3**, anterior spinal artery infarct (patchy in anterior spinal cord; owl eyes or snake eyes may be seen particularly on follow-up MRI); **4**, spinal cord sarcoidosis (dorsal subpial linear enhancement extending over multiple segments); **5**, multiple sclerosis (dorsal cord or lateral cord; may be nonenhancing; often asymmetric); **6**, paraneoplastic symmetric tract-specific enhancement; **7**, primary intramedullary spinal cord lymphoma (bright homogeneous enhancement; may be multiple); **8**, dural arteriovenous fistula (patchy enhancement; enhancing veins dorsal to spinal cord may be seen; may or may not be associated with gadolinium enhancement); **9**, intramedullary spinal cord metastases (thin rim of more intense enhancement surrounding enhancing lesion with a flame-like appearance superiorly – can also be inferior to lesion). (Adapted with permission from Flanagan, 2016).

the cord and lungs (Fig. 17.4C2), although use of corticosteroids prior to imaging can reduce the metabolic activity.

## CEREBROSPINAL FLUID

CSF cytology or flow cytometry may be diagnostic in intramedullary spinal cord lymphoma and repeated studies may increase the yield, but spinal cord biopsy may be needed (Flanagan et al., 2011c). CSF studies help exclude infectious causes of myelitis (Table 17.2), but its basic characteristics may also help narrow the differential diagnosis. In MS excess oligoclonal bands or an increased IgG index occur in approximately 85%. The cell count is usually <50/μL and the protein is often <100 mg/dL; higher values are a red flag for other disorders such as NMOSD, spinal cord sarcoidosis,

infectious myelitis, or lymphoma. With NMOSD a lymphocytic pleocytosis occurs in about two-thirds and may rarely be eosinophilic. With spinal cord sarcoidosis a CSF pleocytosis is noted in over 90% and CSF hypoglycorrhachia, although uncommon, favors this diagnosis over other inflammatory myelopathies (Flanagan et al., 2016a). An elevated white cell count with a neutrophilic predominance should raise suspicion for an infectious etiology (bacterial, fungal, or mycobacterial), but may be encountered in the acute setting with inflammatory myelopathies. CSF infectious evaluation should include serology, Gram stain, bacterial, mycobacterial, and fungal cultures and polymerase chain reaction testing for viruses (Table 17.2). Albuminocytologic dissociation with markedly elevated protein but normal cell count may suggest Guillain–Barré syndrome or arise in the setting of a spinal block (Fig. 17.4B1).

## NEURAL AUTOANTIBODIES

Serum AQP-4-IgG is the gold standard for NMO/ NMOSD diagnosis and is sensitive ($\approx 80\%$) and highly specific (99–100%); newer-generation cell-based assays are most accurate (Jiao et al., 2013). With older-generation enzyme-linked immunosorbent assay (ELISA), the risk of false positives is fivefold higher (Pittock et al., 2014). False negatives may occur when CSF is only tested (as it is less sensitive than serum) or when testing is performed after immunosuppression treatment. The most frequently detected neural antibodies accompanying a paraneoplastic myelopathy are amphiphysin and collapsin response mediator protein-5 (CRMP5) IgG. AQP4-IgG may also rarely occur in a paraneoplastic context (Pittock and Lennon, 2008). The absence of a paraneoplastic autoantibody does not exclude a paraneoplastic myelopathy and in those with a high suspicion, CT body or PET imaging should be obtained (McKeon et al., 2010; Flanagan et al., 2011a). Serum MOG-IgG assays are also useful when evaluating acute myelitis but this test is not yet widely available.

## SPINAL CORD BIOPSY

Spinal cord biopsy is necessary in some spinal cord emergencies and at tertiary referral centers may be performed safely with a low risk of complications (Cohen-Gadol et al., 2003). However, given its eloquent location and potential for severe morbidity, extensive investigations to try to achieve the diagnosis by other methods and a careful assessment of the risk–benefit ratio are needed prior to pursuing this. Cord biopsy may useful in diagnosing spinal cord sarcoidosis (in patients in whom CT chest or PET-CT is unrevealing) or primary spinal cord tumors (e.g., primary intramedullary spinal cord lymphoma) (Flanagan et al., 2011c). It is generally not recommended in patients with known active systemic malignancy who present with intramedullary metastases, as in this situation the diagnosis can be made with the clinical setting and a compatible radiologic lesion and pathologic confirmation of spinal cord involvement is generally not necessary (Flanagan et al., 2012).

## Other investigations

A chest X-ray in the acute setting showing a widened mediastinum suggests aortic dissection and transesophageal echocardiogram or chest CT is confirmatory. Vascular imaging (MRA, CT angiography) of neck vessels is recommended to exclude vertebral dissection as the cause in cervical cord infarcts; other traditional stroke workup should be undertaken, including transesophageal echocardiogram, electrocardiogram, and Holter monitor as well as fasting lipids and glucose. In spinal

epidural abscess, elevations in erythrocyte sedimentation rate, C-reactive protein, and peripheral white blood cell count are frequently found, although not universal. Blood cultures should be obtained and fine-needle abscess aspiration may be considered. With vascular myelopathies (infarct, hematoma) thrombophilia screen or coagulation screen for bleeding diathesis (e.g., international normalized ratio, platelets) may be undertaken. Other blood tests for evaluating myelopathy include antinuclear antibody, SSA/SSB antibodies, double-stranded DNA antibodies, vitamin $B_{12}$ and methylmalonic acid, copper, angiotensin-converting enzyme, toxicology screen (including urine testing), and infectious serologies. Blood testing to assess for malignancy may include serum lactate dehydrogenase, peripheral smear, serum protein electrophoresis with immunofixation, and prostate-specific antigen. Body imaging with CT or PET and sex-specific tests (mammogram, testicular ultrasound) should also be considered if a neoplastic or paraneoplastic etiology is suspected (McKeon et al., 2010). Nerve conduction studies and electromyogram may be useful when the neurologic localization is uncertain (e.g., suspicion for Guillain–Barré).

# HOSPITAL COURSE AND MANAGEMENT

## Respiratory failure and spinal shock

In cases of quadriparesis assessing and protecting the airway are the first steps. While respiratory failure is a rare complication of spinal cord injury, initial assessment of the need for intubation and mechanical ventilation should not be overlooked, particularly in high cervical myelopathies.

Indications for intubation are pooling secretions, periods of deoxygenation, and need for a facemask to correct hypoxemia. In some patients hypercarbia emerges quickly and can only be recognized with a new arterial blood gas. Treatment of spinal shock, if present, is supportive with fluids, inotropes, or vasopressors either alone or in combination. Atropine or temporary pacing may be necessary for severe bradycardia. If untreated, multiorgan failure and death may ensue.

## Metastatic epidural spinal cord compression

Corticosteroids are established as the initial treatment modality of choice for acute metastatic epidural spinal cord compression. Steroids decrease spinal cord edema and may have a tumoricidal effect with certain neoplasms (e.g., lymphoma). A single randomized controlled trial showed the benefit of 96 mg of intravenous dexamethasone followed by 96 mg/day orally for 3 days and then a 10-day taper in combination with spinal irradiation compared to those with spinal irradiation alone showing improved ambulation rates at 3 months (81% vs. 63%) and 6 months (59% vs. 33%) (Sorensen et al., 1994). The optimal dose remains uncertain, as further comparative studies have suggested lower doses (10 mg dexamethasone load, followed by 16 mg daily and a taper) may be equivalent (and associated with fewer steroid-related side effects), although these were somewhat underpowered (Cole and Patchell, 2008). Radiation treatment is the standard of care in these patients, but evidence for this is limited to retrospective case series and those with radiosensitive tumors do better (Cole and Patchell, 2008). In general the approach is to treat those with a poor prognosis with a short course and those with a better prognosis (good performance status, oligometastatic disease, controlled primary tumor) with a more prolonged course. Decompressive surgical tumor resection and spine stabilization have also been shown to be beneficial, particularly in those with an unstable spine or radioresistant tumors (Cole and Patchell, 2008). The role of chemotherapy is uncertain. However, the exact treatment utilized should be individualized depending on the scenario and is discussed further in Chapter 39.

### Spinal epidural abscess

A team approach is best and typically involves neurologists, infectious disease physicians, and neuro- or orthopedic surgeons. Surgical decompression and abscess drainage in conjunction with systemic antibiotics is the treatment of choice for the vast majority of patients with spinal cord emergencies from epidural abscesses (Darouiche, 2006). Surgery may be deferred rarely in patients who refuse surgery or have very high perioperative risk and in whom the organism has been isolated from blood cultures or aspiration (Pradilla et al., 2009). Complete surgical removal of any infected spinal instrumentation (e.g., spinal cord stimulator) is necessary if applicable. While awaiting culture results, empiric systemic antibiotic coverage of staphylococcus (and streptococcus) with vancomycin (to cover MRSA), Gram-negative bacilli with a third- or fourth-generation cephalosporin is recommended; anaerobic coverage with metronidazole may also be considered. Antibiotics are then tailored to the organism identified and its sensitivities. Systemic antibiotics are required for 6–8 weeks. Worsening or recurrence despite treatment of the isolated organism may suggest a polymicrobial infection and should also prompt a search for an alternative source such as esophageal tear (cervical region) or spinal-intestinal fistula (thoracolumbar) (Darouiche, 2006).

### Spinal epidural hematoma

Stopping anticoagulation and/or antiplatelet medications and reversal of anticoagulation is the first step, if applicable. For warfarin-associated epidural hematoma, 10 mg of intravenous vitamin K may be given by slow infusion (1 mg/min or slower to reduce the risk of anaphylaxis); faster-acting agents are also indicated, such as prothrombin-complex concentrate complex or fresh frozen plasma. For heparin-associated epidural hematoma protamine is used. For newer anticoagulants prothrombin complex concentrate and antifibrinolytics (e.g., tranexamic acid) are given. Platelet infusions are recommended when marked thrombocytopenia is present. Surgical removal of hemorrhage may follow reversal of coagulopathy. Early surgical decompression with laminectomy is generally the treatment of choice in those with myelopathy and spontaneous epidural hematoma. In those with pain but without other neurologic deficits close monitoring may be considered.

### Spinal cord infarction

In spinal cord infarction secondary to aortic surgery increasing perfusion of the cord through collaterals with blood pressure augmentation (with volume and vasopressors) and lumbar drainage (at 8–12 mm Hg) has been reported to be helpful, although it has not yet been formally assessed in a clinical trial (Cheung et al., 2005). Its utility in other causes of spinal cord infarct is uncertain. The potential use of thrombolysis for spinal cord infarct is hampered by the typical diagnostic uncertainty, delay to diagnosis, need for MRI confirmation, and the most frequent cause (aortic surgery) being an absolute contraindication; however, rare case reports of its use exist (Restrepo and Guttin, 2006). In cases where diagnostic uncertainty remains, a trial of intravenous corticosteroids may be considered if inflammatory causes are a competing diagnostic possibility. Treatment of the underlying cause is important when identified (e.g., cardiogenic embolism). Antiplatelet treatment may be recommended in cryptogenic cases for secondary stroke prevention, particularly in those with vascular risk factors.

### Spinal cord infarct due to aortic dissection

Surgical treatment of the dissection may result in improvement of neurologic function and is usually necessary emergently. Lumbar drainage should be considered if a delay to surgical correction occurs and may be beneficial as removal of CSF lowers the increased intraspinal pressure and improves spinal cord perfusion (Blacker et al., 2003).

### Vascular malformations

For dural AVF surgical treatment with disconnection of the draining arterialized vein is the standard treatment with excellent success and low morbidity (Rabinstein, 2015). Endovascular treatment by embolizing the proximal arterialized vein during spinal angiography is an emerging alternative treatment, but rates of recurrence are higher than with surgical treatment (Rabinstein, 2015). Treatment is always recommended, even in patients who have prolonged paraplegia, as improvements may still occur (Rabinstein, 2015). Intramedullary AVMs are best treated with staged endovascular occlusion, but some of the feeding arteries can also supply the cord and thus occlusion of these vessels may result in clinical worsening. For cavernous malformations treatment is complete surgical resection with the goal of preventing further bleeding episodes.

## Spondylotic compressive myelopathies

In the setting of spinal cord emergency from cervical stenosis decompressive surgery (anterior or posterior approach) is usually recommended. In cases with associated gadolinium enhancement, persistent enhancement for months to years after successful surgery is typical and may lead to diagnostic confusion but, in the absence of clinical worsening, should not dissuade one from this diagnosis (Flanagan et al., 2014).

## Inflammatory demyelinating myelitis

The initial acute treatment of CNS inflammatory demyelinating spinal cord emergencies (NMOSD, MS, ADEM, MOG IgG-associated) is 1 gram of intravenous methylprednisolone once daily for 5 days. In cases with residual severe disability a course of plasma exchange (1.5 plasma volume every other day for five to seven treatments) is often recommended. Plasma exchange has been shown to improve outcomes in a randomized sham-controlled study in patients with attacks from CNS inflammatory demyelinating disease refractory to steroids (Weinshenker et al., 1999). A recent retrospective review of acute treatments in NMOSD reported better outcomes in those who receive plasma exchange, suggesting one should have a very low threshold for escalation to plasma exchange in cases of NMOSD myelopathy and leading some to advocate its use in all cases of NMOSD myelopathy (Kleiter et al., 2016; Weinshenker, 2016). For spinal cord sarcoidosis prolonged oral corticosteroids for 3–6 months followed by a slow taper is the treatment of choice; it may be preceded by 1 gram of intravenous methylprednisolone once daily for 5 days, but short-term steroids often result in early relapse. Tumor necrosis-alpha inhibitors (e.g., infliximab) or other steroid-sparing immunosuppressants may be helpful in refractory cases (Flanagan et al., 2016a). Maintenance immunosuppressant or immunomodulatory treatment is also imperative in NMOSD

(Flanagan and Weinshenker, 2014) and in most MS patients, but a discussion of this is beyond the scope of this chapter.

With ADEM, a slow oral steroid taper may be initiated for the first 3 months, as that is when the risk of relapse is highest, although most cases are monophasic. For paraneoplastic myelopathies detection and treatment of the underlying cancer are the first step and immunotherapy is also often used, but response to treatment is poor and most become wheelchair-dependent (Flanagan et al., 2011b). Tonic spasms are involuntary painful contractions of extremities that last 30 seconds to 3 minutes. They may be triggered by hyperventilation or movement and are due to ephaptic transmission within the spinal cord. They occur more often with NMOSD than MS (Kim et al., 2012) and respond well to low-dose carbamazepine (e.g., 100 mg bid).

## Infectious myelopathies

Treatment of infectious myelitis will depend on the organism isolated, although with many viral myelitis etiologies (e.g., West Nile-virus associated myelitis) treatment is supportive. Further discussion of the treatment of infectious myelopathies is beyond the scope of this chapter.

## Autonomic dysreflexia

This is an underrecognized complication of spinal cord injury above the T6 level. It is due to an exaggerated sympathetic response to a noxious stimulus below the level of the lesion. The pathophysiology relates to autonomic innervation. A strong sensory input is transmitted to the spinal cord and ascends to thoracolumbar sympathetics. This results in a spinal reflex that evokes a strong sympathetic response (possibly from an associated hyperresponsiveness of alpha-adrenergic receptors). This causes severe vasoconstriction in the splanchnic vessels and peripheral arterial hypertension ensues. In response, the intact baroreceptors detecting high blood pressure send inhibitory impulses from the brainstem to the thoracolumbar sympathetic nerves but cannot reach them due to spinal cord injury. The nucleus ambiguous also sends parasympathetic input to the heart, resulting in bradycardia, but it is insufficient to offset the strong sympathetic surge and hypertension continues.

In addition to bradycardia, prominent parasympathetic activity above the level of injury causes pupil constriction, flushing, sweating, and nasal stuffiness. Below the level of injury the sympathetic tone predominates, resulting in pale, cool skin and piloerection. The majority of triggers (85%) are bladder or bowel in origin (bladder distension, urinary tract infections, bowel/bladder procedures, fecal impaction, or constipation). Skin issues (pressure sores, tight clothing), sexual activity, pregnancy, or other injury (e.g., fracture) are other potential triggers. The clinical features include headache, sweating, flushing, piloerection, and increased blood pressure. Management includes sitting the patient upright, removal of tight clothing, searching for and removing the noxious stimulus, and blood pressure management (rapidly acting agents are preferred, e.g., nitrates, hydralazine, nifedipine).

## OUTCOME PREDICTION

The best predictor of neurologic outcome for cord compression from epidural compression is the neurologic status at the time of diagnosis (further emphasizing the importance of early diagnosis). The prognosis for metastatic epidural spinal cord compression is poor, with a median survival of between 3 and 6 months. The risk of mortality with spinal epidural abscess ranges from 6 to 32%, while with spinal cord infarct it is 10–25%. Despite the severity of initial disability with spinal cord infarct meaningful recovery may occur and 41% of survivors were ambulatory at final follow-up in one study (Robertson et al., 2012). Neuropathic pain is a frequent long-term complication. Patients with NMOSD tend to have more severe episodes with less recovery than patients with MS (Jiao et al., 2014). Therefore, these patients tend to accumulate disability with each attack, making maintenance immunosuppression critical in this group of patients. Most disability with MS results from the secondary progressive course that occurs in the majority of MS patients but rarely, if ever, occurs with NMOSD (Wingerchuk et al., 2007). Increased CSF glial fibrillary acidic protein (an astrocyte biomarker) is associated with poorer outcome in NMOSD and it is more elevated than myelin basic protein, emphasizing astrocytic damage is greater than demyelination in NMOSD (Takano et al., 2010). With paraneoplastic myelopathy the prognosis is poor and most become wheelchair-dependent (Flanagan et al., 2011b).

## NEUROREHABILITATION

Early involvement of physical and occupational therapy is important for patients with spinal cord disorders to help manage complications of neurogenic bowel and bladder, gait impairment, and spasticity. Many of these patients require antispasticity drugs (e.g., baclofen) and prolonged inpatient rehabilitation may be helpful for recovery in many such patients.

## DISCLOSURES

Dr. Flanagan has no disclosures to report.

Dr. Pittock is a named inventor on patents (#12/678,350 filed 2010 and #12/573,942 filed 2008) that relate to functional AQP4/NMO-IgG assays and NMO-IgG as a cancer marker, and receives research support from Alexion Pharmaceuticals, the Guthy-Jackson Charitable Foundation, and the National Institutes of Health (NS065829). Dr. Pittock has provided consultation to Alexion Pharmaceuticals, MedImmune, and Chugai Pharma, but has received no personal fees or personal compensation for these consulting activities. All compensation for consulting activities is paid directly to Mayo Clinic.

## REFERENCES

Araki M, Matsuoka T, Miyamoto K et al. (2014). Efficacy of the anti-IL-6 receptor antibody tocilizumab in neuromyelitis optica: a pilot study. Neurology 82: 1302–1306.

Barron KD, Hirano A, Araki S et al. (1959). Experiences with metastatic neoplasms involving the spinal cord. Neurology 9: 91–106.

Blacker DJ, Wijdicks EF, Ramakrishna G (2003). Resolution of severe paraplegia due to aortic dissection after CSF drainage. Neurology 61: 142–143.

Brex PA, Ciccarelli O, O'Riordan JI et al. (2002). A longitudinal study of abnormalities on MRI and disability from multiple sclerosis. N Engl J Med 346: 158–164.

Cheung AT, Pochettino A, McGarvey ML et al. (2005). Strategies to manage paraplegia risk after endovascular stent repair of descending thoracic aortic aneurysms. Ann Thorac Surg 80: 1280–1288. discussion 1288–1289.

Chihara N, Aranami T, Sato W et al. (2011). Interleukin 6 signaling promotes anti-aquaporin 4 autoantibody production from plasmablasts in neuromyelitis optica. Proc Natl Acad Sci U S A 108: 3701–3706.

Cohen-Gadol AA, Zikel OM, Miller GM et al. (2003). Spinal cord biopsy: a review of 38 cases. Neurosurgery 52: 806–815. discussion 815–806.

Cole JS, Patchell RA (2008). Metastatic epidural spinal cord compression. The Lancet Neurology 7: 459–466.

Darouiche RO (2006). Spinal epidural abscess. N Engl J Med 355: 2012–2020.

de Havenon A, Joos Z, Longenecker L et al. (2014). Posterior reversible encephalopathy syndrome with spinal cord involvement. Neurology 83: 2002–2006.

Flanagan EP, Weinshenker BG (2014). Neuromyelitis optica spectrum disorders. Curr Neurol Neurosci Rep 14: 483.

Flanagan EP, Lennon VA, Pittock SJ (2011a). Autoimmune myelopathies. Continuum 17: 776–799.

Flanagan EP, McKeon A, Lennon VA et al. (2011b). Paraneoplastic isolated myelopathy: clinical course and neuroimaging clues. Neurology 76: 2089–2095.

Flanagan EP, O'Neill BP, Porter AB et al. (2011c). Primary intramedullary spinal cord lymphoma. Neurology 77: 784–791.

Flanagan EP, O'Neill BP, Habermann TM et al. (2012). Secondary intramedullary spinal cord non-Hodgkin's lymphoma. J Neurooncol 107: 575–580.

Flanagan EP, Hunt CH, Lowe V et al. (2013). [(18)F]-fluorodeoxyglucose-positron emission tomography in patients with active myelopathy. Mayo Clin Proc 88: 1204–1212.

Flanagan EP, McKeon A, Weinshenker BG (2014a). Anterior spinal artery infarction causing man-in-the-barrel syndrome. Neurology Clinical Practice 4: 268–269.

Flanagan EP, Krecke KN, Marsh RW et al. (2014b). Specific pattern of gadolinium enhancement in spondylotic myelopathy. Ann Neurol 76: 54–65.

Flanagan EP, Weinshenker BG, Krecke KN et al. (2015). Short myelitis lesions in aquaporin-4-IgG-positive neuromyelitis optica spectrum disorders. JAMA Neurol 72: 81–87.

Flanagan EP (2016). Autoimmune myelopathies. Handb Clin Neurol 133: 327–351. http://dx.doi.org/10.1016/B978-0-444-63432-0.00019-0. PubMed PMID: 27112686.

Flanagan EP, Kaufmann TJ, Krecke KN et al. (2016a). Discriminating long myelitis of neuromyelitis optica from sarcoidosis. Ann Neurol 79: 437–447.

Flanagan EP, Cabre P, Weinshenker BG et al. (2016b). Epidemiology of aquaporin-4 autoimmunity and neuromyelitis optica spectrum. Ann Neurol 79: 775–783.

Fugate JE, Lanzino G, Rabinstein AA (2012). Clinical presentation and prognostic factors of spinal dural arteriovenous fistulas: an overview. Neurosurg Focus 32. E17.

Gaul C, Dietrich W, Erbguth FJ (2008). Neurological symptoms in aortic dissection: a challenge for neurologists. Cerebrovasc Dis 26: 1–8.

Hinson SR, McKeon A, Fryer JP et al. (2009). Prediction of neuromyelitis optica attack severity by quantitation of complement-mediated injury to aquaporin-4-expressing cells. Arch Neurol 66: 1164–1167.

Hinson SR, Romero MF, Popescu BF et al. (2012). Molecular outcomes of neuromyelitis optica (NMO)-IgG binding to aquaporin-4 in astrocytes. Proc Natl Acad Sci U S A 109: 1245–1250.

Hyun JW, Kim SH, Jeong IH et al. (2015). Bright spotty lesions on the spinal cord: an additional MRI indicator of neuromyelitis optica spectrum disorder? J Neurol Neurosurg Psychiatry 86: 1280–1282.

Jiao Y, Fryer JP, Lennon VA et al. (2013). Updated estimate of AQP4-IgG serostatus and disability outcome in neuromyelitis optica. Neurology 81: 1197–1204.

Jiao Y, Fryer JP, Lennon VA et al. (2014). Aquaporin 4 IgG serostatus and outcome in recurrent longitudinally extensive transverse myelitis. JAMA Neurol 71: 48–54.

Kim SM, Go MJ, Sung JJ et al. (2012). Painful tonic spasm in neuromyelitis optica: incidence, diagnostic utility, and clinical characteristics. Arch Neurol 69: 1026–1031.

Kitley J, Waters P, Woodhall M et al. (2014). Neuromyelitis optica spectrum disorders with aquaporin-4 and myelin-oligodendrocyte glycoprotein antibodies: a comparative study. JAMA Neurol 71: 276–283.

Kleiter I, Gahlen A, Borisow N et al. (2016). Neuromyelitis optica: evaluation of 871 attacks and 1,153 treatment courses. Ann Neurol 79: 206–216.

Lucchinetti CF, Mandler RN, McGavern D et al. (2002). A role for humoral mechanisms in the pathogenesis of Devic's neuromyelitis optica. Brain : a journal of neurology 125: 1450–1461.

Magana SM, Matiello M, Pittock SJ et al. (2009). Posterior reversible encephalopathy syndrome in neuromyelitis optica spectrum disorders. Neurology 72: 712–717.

McKeon A, Lennon VA, Lotze T et al. (2008). CNS aquaporin-4 autoimmunity in children. Neurology 71: 93–100.

McKeon A, Lennon VA, Jacob A et al. (2009). Coexistence of myasthenia gravis and serological markers of neurological autoimmunity in neuromyelitis optica. Muscle Nerve 39: 87–90.

McKeon A, Apiwattanakul M, Lachance DH et al. (2010). Positron emission tomography-computed tomography in paraneoplastic neurologic disorders: systematic analysis and review. Arch Neurol 67: 322–329.

Messacar K, Schreiner TL, Maloney JA et al. (2015). A cluster of acute flaccid paralysis and cranial nerve dysfunction temporally associated with an outbreak of enterovirus D68 in children in Colorado, USA. Lancet 385: 1662–1671.

Misu T, Sato DK, Nakashima I et al. (2015). MOG-IgG serological status matters in paediatric ADEM. J Neurol Neurosurg Psychiatry 86: 242.

Pittock SJ, Lennon VA (2008). Aquaporin-4 autoantibodies in a paraneoplastic context. Arch Neurol 65: 629–632.

Pittock SJ, Lennon VA, Krecke K et al. (2006). Brain abnormalities in neuromyelitis optica. Arch Neurol 63: 390–396.

Pittock SJ, Lennon VA, de Seze J et al. (2008). Neuromyelitis optica and non organ-specific autoimmunity. Arch Neurol 65: 78–83.

Pittock SJ, Lennon VA, McKeon A et al. (2013). Eculizumab in AQP4-IgG-positive relapsing neuromyelitis optica spectrum disorders: an open-label pilot study. The Lancet Neurology 12: 554–562.

Pittock SJ, Lennon VA, Bakshi N et al. (2014). Seroprevalence of aquaporin-4-IgG in a northern California population representative cohort of multiple sclerosis. JAMA Neurol 71: 1433–1436.

Pradilla G, Ardila GP, Hsu W et al. (2009). Epidural abscesses of the CNS. The Lancet Neurology 8: 292–300.

Ptaszynski AE, Hooten WM, Huntoon MA (2007). The incidence of spontaneous epidural abscess in Olmsted County from 1990 through 2000: a rare cause of spinal pain. Pain Med 8: 338–343.

Rabinstein AA (2015). Vascular myelopathies. Continuum 21: 67–83.

Restrepo L, Guttin JF (2006). Acute spinal cord ischemia during aortography treated with intravenous thrombolytic therapy. Texas Heart Institute journal / from the Texas Heart Institute of St. Luke's Episcopal Hospital, Texas Children's Hospital 33: 74–77.

Robertson CE, Brown Jr RD, Wijdicks EF et al. (2012). Recovery after spinal cord infarcts: long-term outcome in 115 patients. Neurology 78: 114–121.

Rykken JB, Diehn FE, Hunt CH et al. (2013). Rim and flame signs: postgadolinium MRI findings specific for non-CNS intramedullary spinal cord metastases. AJNR Am J Neuroradiol 34: 908–915.

Sorensen S, Helweg-Larsen S, Mouridsen H et al. (1994). Effect of high-dose dexamethasone in carcinomatous metastatic spinal cord compression treated with radiotherapy: a randomised trial. Eur J Cancer 30A: 22–27.

Takano R, Misu T, Takahashi T et al. (2010). Astrocytic damage is far more severe than demyelination in NMO: a clinical CSF biomarker study. Neurology 75: 208–216.

Titulaer MJ, Hoftberger R, Iizuka T et al. (2014). Overlapping demyelinating syndromes and anti-N-methyl-D-aspartate receptor encephalitis. Ann Neurol 75: 411–428.

Urai Y, Matsumoto K, Shimamura M et al. (2009). Paraneoplastic necrotizing myelopathy in a patient with advanced esophageal cancer: an autopsied case report. J Neurol Sci 280: 113–117.

Weinshenker BG (2016). What is the optimal sequence of rescue treatments for attacks of neuromyelitis optica spectrum disorder? Ann Neurol 79: 204–205.

Weinshenker BG, O'Brien PC, Petterson TM et al. (1999). A randomized trial of plasma exchange in acute central nervous system inflammatory demyelinating disease. Ann Neurol 46: 878–886.

Wingerchuk DM, Weinshenker BG (2012). The emerging relationship between neuromyelitis optica and systemic rheumatologic autoimmune disease. Mult Scler 18: 5–10.

Wingerchuk DM, Pittock SJ, Lucchinetti CF et al. (2007). A secondary progressive clinical course is uncommon in neuromyelitis optica. Neurology 68: 603–605.

*Handbook of Clinical Neurology*, Vol. 140 (3rd series)
*Critical Care Neurology, Part I*
E.F.M. Wijdicks and A.H. Kramer, Editors
http://dx.doi.org/10.1016/B978-0-444-63600-3.00018-0

Chapter 18

# Diagnosis and management of acute encephalitis

J.J. HALPERIN*

*Overlook Medical Center, Summit, NJ, and Sidney Kimmel Medical College of Thomas Jefferson University, Philadelphia, PA, USA*

## Abstract

Encephalitis is typically viral (approximately half of diagnosed cases) or autoimmune (about a quarter) with the remainder remaining undiagnosable at this time. All require general supportive care but only a minority requires intensive care admission – in these intubation, to protect the airway or to treat status epilepticus with anesthetic drugs, may be needed. In some dysautonomia with wide blood pressure fluctuations is the principal concern. Remarkably, in addition to supportive care, specific treatment options are available for the majority – immune-modulating therapy for those with autoimmune disorders, antiviral therapy for herpes simplex 1 and 2, and varicella-zoster encephalitis. Flavivirus infections (West Nile, Japanese encephalitis, tick-borne encephalitis) remain the most common other identified cause of encephalitis but no specific intervention is available. Overall long-term outcomes are favorable in the majority of patients with encephalitis, a proportion that hopefully will improve with further advances in diagnostic technology and therapeutic interventions.

## INTRODUCTION

Encephalitis, by definition "inflammation of the brain parenchyma associated with neurologic dysfunction" (Tunkel et al., 2008), occurs as the result of either a central nervous system (CNS) infection or an immune-mediated attack on the brain. Fortunately, both are rare. Both groups of disorders range from acute medical emergencies to more indolent and often difficult-to-diagnose disorders. In some patients an etiologic diagnosis is readily ascertainable; in many no pathogen or underlying pathophysiologic mechanism can be identified. Some aspects of patient management are common to all, regardless of etiology, while some disorders require specific treatment that can dramatically alter outcome. The clinical imperative is to initiate those aspects of care that are essential regardless of etiology while simultaneously implementing a strategy to address those disorders that require specific therapeutic interventions.

CNS infections present an interesting paradox. Due in large part to the brain's structural protection in the bony skull, and its cellular protection by the blood–brain

(BBB) and blood–cerebrospinal fluid (CSF) barriers, these infections are extremely rare. On the other hand, the organisms that cause most cases of meningitis and encephalitis are quite prevalent – as just one example, one-third of the world's population has symptomatic herpes simplex infection (Widener and Whitley, 2014). The reason one individual infected with these pathogens develops a CNS infection and thousands of others do not presumably relates to a combination of host genetics and immune responses, co-occurring environmental factors and random effects, but the relative roles of these elements are largely unknown.

CNS infections can be divided into those primarily involving the subarachnoid space – by definition, meningitis – and those involving brain (encephalitis) and/or spinal cord (encephalomyelitis) parenchyma (Table 18.1). Most CNS infections are due to viral infections. Meningitis most commonly is viral (particularly enteroviruses, but many others as well), is not life-threatening and typically has full recovery. Bacterial meningitis, on the other hand, most commonly caused by *Streptococcus pneumoniae*,

*Correspondence to: J.J. Halperin, MD, Overlook Medical Center, 99 Beauvoir Avenue, Summit NJ 07078, USA. Tel: +1-908-522-3501, E-mail: john.halperin@atlantichealth.org

*Table 18.1*

Diagnostic criteria for encephalitis, as proposed by the International Encephalitis Consortium

---

**Major criterion (required)**
Patients presenting to medical attention with altered mental status (defined as decreased or altered level of consciousness, lethargy or personality change) lasting $\geq 24$ hours with no alternative cause identified
**Minor criteria (two required for possible encephalitis; $\geq 3$ required for probable or confirmed encephalitis)**
Documented fever $\geq 38°C$ (100.4°F) within the 72 hours before or after presentation
Generalized or partial seizures not fully attributable to a pre-existing seizure disorder
New onset of focal neurologic findings
Cerebrospinal fluid white blood cell count $\geq 5/mm^3$
Abnormality of brain parenchyma on neuroimaging suggestive of encephalitis that is either new from prior studies or appears acute in onset
Abnormality on electroencephalography that is consistent with encephalitis and not attributable to another cause

---

Reproduced from Venkatesan et al. (2013), with permission from Oxford University Press.

---

*Neisseria meningitidis*, group B streptococcus, and *Listeria monocytogenes*, is often a life-threatening illness. Mortality is generally not a consequence of the infection within the subarachnoid space as such but rather of either secondary involvement of brain parenchyma – often related to inflammatory involvement of the large brain arteries and veins that pass through the subarachnoid space – or the more serious systemic effects of bacteremia and sepsis leading to shock. Important in the consideration of treatment options in encephalitis, while corticosteroids have been shown to lessen neurologic sequelae in meningitis due to *S. pneumoniae* (Brouwer et al., 2015) if given shortly before or concurrent with antibiotics, the potential role of corticosteroids in nonbacterial brain infections is far more complex and controversial.

Since it is impossible to consider treatment of encephalitis without understanding its pathogenesis, this chapter will focus on both diagnosis and management. Although it is commonly stated that an etiology is determined in about 50% of encephalitis cases (Mailles et al., 2012; Venkatesan et al., 2013), a recent review of the Mayo Clinic experience was more optimistic (Singh et al., 2015) – although the referral nature of the Mayo Clinic's patient population may have skewed this somewhat. That notwithstanding, an etiology was identified in 70% of 198 patients: viral in 95 (48%), autoimmune in 44 (22%) (similar to the proportion identified in a recent British population-based study (Granerod et al., 2013)), and indeterminate in the remainder. Herpes simplex was the etiologic agent in 37 of 95, varicella-zoster (VZV) in 22, West Nile virus (WNV) in 18, Epstein–Barr in 6, and human immunodeficiency virus (HIV) in 3. Since specific treatment is available for autoimmune disorders, herpesviruses, and HIV, it is critically important to appreciate that treatment beyond supportive care is available for >50% of patients with encephalitis. The other important insight from the Mayo Clinic experience was that, of their 198 patients, only 76 required admission to an intensive care

unit, of whom only 50 required mechanical ventilation. Only 5 had global cerebral edema – all important considerations in clinical management.

## EPIDEMIOLOGY

Disorders that present initially as meningitis – bacterial, mycobacterial, or fungal – are dealt with in Chapter 19 of this volume. Infections of the brain parenchyma that are more indolent in presentation, such as the spirochetoses, are unlikely to present in a critical care setting and so will not be addressed further. Similarly others, such as amebic meningoencephalitis (Booth et al., 2015), can ultimately require critical care but are so rare that they will similarly not be considered further. Rather the focus here will be on viral pathogens. These infections can be divided into three broad categories based on their mechanisms of transmission. The first consists of organisms that only infect humans – primarily various herpesviruses (herpes simplex 1 and 2 (HSV1 and HSV2), VZV, human herpesvirus 6 (HHV6)), but also JC virus and several others as well. The common characteristic of all is that these are near-ubiquitous human infections in which humans act as the reservoir host, vector, and victim. Only rarely, for reasons that are often inapparent, do these infections transform from their baseline indolent state – in which they are either carried asymptomatically or at worst cause painful cutaneous eruptions – to cause a devastating brain infection. Because large segments of the human population carry these infections, these forms of encephalitis are often referred to as endemic. Encephalitis occurs completely sporadically, with no seasonal, geographic, or environmental pattern.

In contrast to this are epidemic forms of encephalitis – disorders in which other species serve as reservoir hosts and human infection is ecologically incidental and self-limited – i.e., person-to-person spread plays a minimal, if any, role in disease dissemination. This group includes the arthropod-borne viruses – WNV – now arguably the most common form of encephalitis in the USA, Japanese encephalitis virus (JEV), the most common cause worldwide, and tick-borne encephalitis virus (TBE), a quite prevalent cause of encephalomyelitis in Europe and Russia.

Arboviruses, a microbiologically unfortunate grouping that includes many classes of viruses that happen to share the property of being transmitted by ticks (TBE, Powassan) or mosquitoes (all others), generally require the interaction of at least two nonhuman species for humans to become infected. A reservoir host maintains the virus in the environment. As well exemplified by the outbreak of WNV in the USA, when first introduced into the ecosystem this virus may be highly lethal in susceptible hosts. However, with time the most lethal strains and most susceptible hosts are selected out and a surviving population of hosts remains in the ecosystem. Since transmission from one animal to another requires a vector (mosquito, tick), and since in the most heavily populated regions of the world there is a marked seasonality to proliferation of and feeding by these poikilothermic arthropods, these infections have a marked seasonality. Moreover, since the animal hosts do not maintain an active viremia indefinitely, the number of viremic hosts is low in spring, but may gradually increase during warm-weather months, as both feeding arthropods and infected viremic reservoir hosts multiply with repeated feedings. In areas where this builds to a critical mass, outbreaks of arthropod-borne encephalitis occur in late summer and early autumn – until cold weather ends arthropod feeding. If in a given area in a given season the number of infected reservoir hosts never exceeds the necessary threshold, human infections remain rare. Presumably these mechanisms account for not only the seasonality of WNV encephalitis but also the spread of it across the continental USA, initially occurring in the northeast, where it killed most susceptible avian hosts, then each year moving further west until it established its current habitat in the central USA from the Midwest to the Rocky Mountain states.

Rabies, in contrast, can infect many mammalian species but is spread by direct animal-to-animal contact, without an intervening vector. As this infection is virtually invariably lethal, the nature of the reservoir host is conceptually different. Since any individual animal (including humans) is infectious for only a limited period of time, persistence of infection in the ecosystem requires a large population of susceptible hosts. No individual animal can serve as a reservoir or vector for any appreciable period of time but the population as a whole – be it a populous bat colony, innumerable feral dogs in India, or large numbers of infected raccoons – can maintain the infection in the environment. Infected humans typically receive postexposure vaccination,

and never develop transmissible infection, or are isolated once symptomatic, so person-to-person transmission is exceedingly rare. This requirement for a population of reservoir hosts provides an important opportunity, such as the mass vaccination of dogs, which nearly eliminated this infection in Western Europe and North America.

These epidemiologic considerations can be quite helpful in diagnosing individual patients. Arthropod-borne virus-mediated encephalitis occurs in areas where the virus is known to be present in reservoir hosts (geographic selection) at times of year that arthropods are active (>55°F, 13°C) (seasonal variation). Rabies occurs in patients who have had potential exposure to rabid animals (India and other areas of the developing and underdeveloped world; North American areas with bat infestation or infected raccoons), i.e., geographic selection. Encephalitis due to the various herpesviruses occurs with neither geographic nor temporal clustering.

## CLINICAL PRESENTATION

One of the many challenges in the management of patients with encephalitis is that, while early antiviral treatment is essential to maximize the likelihood of a good recovery, early recognition and diagnosis of these brain infections can be difficult. Altered mental status, or encephalopathy, is considered a virtually invariant element of encephalitis (Venkatesan et al., 2013) (Table 18.2), but encephalopathy is so common among patients presenting with acute illnesses as to have very little specificity or predictive value for a CNS infection. Fever is considered a "minor criterion" (Venkatesan et al., 2013) for the diagnosis, but again the number of febrile encephalopathic patients presenting to the average emergency department far exceeds the number of patients likely to have encephalitis. The key to early

*Table 18.2*

**Most common agents of meningitis and encephalitis, and their relative annual frequency in the USA**

| Organism | Cases/year in USA |
| --- | --- |
| **Bacterial meningitis** | |
| *Streptococcus pneumoniae* | 3000–6000 (CDC, 2015e) |
| *Neisseria meningitidis* | 500–700 (CDC, 2015d) |
| Group B streptococcus (GBS) | Approximately 500 (Schuchat, 1998; CDC, 2015b) |
| *Listeria monocytogenes* | Approximately 250 (CDC) |
| **Viral encephalitis** | |
| West Nile | 1000–2500 |
| Herpes simplex | 1250 |
| Varicella-zoster | Approximately 800 |
| Autoimmune encephalitis | Approximately 500–600 |

diagnosis often rests on obtaining an accurate history and appropriate neurologic examination. Since brain infection is typically focal, at least early on, patients often experience focal symptoms or manifest focal signs, with behavioral concomitants of temporal-lobe involvement in HSV1 encephalitis, brainstem, and extrapyramidal findings in those with WNV and other flavivirus and occasionally other encephalitides (including rare HSV1 cases). Recognizing these focal abnormalities in the context of a more global encephalopathy and promptly initiating treatment can be life-saving.

The International Encephalitis Consortium (Venkatesan et al., 2013) has proposed that the diagnosis of encephalitis (Table 18.2) requires altered mental status for at least 24 hours, with no other identifiable cause, combined with two or more (two for possible encephalitis, three for probable or definite) of the following: fever within 72 hours before or after presentation; seizures not attributable to a pre-existing seizure disorder; new onset of focal neurologic findings; CSF pleocytosis; new abnormalities on brain imaging and/or characteristic EEG abnormalities.

Against this background, the first step in diagnosis is obviously in suspecting that the patient has a CNS infection, rather than just a toxic-metabolic encephalopathy. In arbovirus-mediated encephalitis there is often a viral prodrome. WNV may produce a febrile illness with gastrointestinal symptoms; other viruses may be more nonspecific. Encephalitis is typically only considered in patients with an altered level of consciousness (Venkatesan et al., 2013).

In many of these disorders the pathogen begins multiplying in the CNS days before symptoms are evident. Once symptoms begin, it is important to differentiate between the fluctuations in consciousness and cognition that are typical of toxic/metabolic encephalopathies in patients who are very ill, and focal abnormalities suggestive of encephalitis. Seizures or alterations in language or memory (déjà vu) or primary sensory modalities (olfactory hallucinations) are highly suggestive of HSV1 involvement of the medial temporal lobes. Areflexia or brainstem abnormalities suggest WNV or other flaviviruses. A history of craniofacial shingles raises the possibility of VZV.

## NEURODIAGNOSTICS AND NEUROIMAGING

With any signs or symptoms that suggest structural brain abnormalities, brain imaging can be highly informative – magnetic resonance imaging (MRI) being much more sensitive than computed tomography (CT) in most instances. In looking for early evidence of infection it is helpful to remember that cellular edema in infectious processes can result in increased signal on diffusion-weighted imaging, and this may be evident substantially

earlier than changes on T2 or other sequences. Although it is often stated (correctly) that CSF may be normal early in encephalitis, this probably occurs in fewer than 5% of patients (Widener and Whitley, 2014). Similarly, it is commonplace to be concerned about doing lumbar punctures in patients with raised intracranial pressure (Solomon et al., 2012). However, if the increase is not due to strongly asymmetric structural changes applying pressure across one of the unyielding intracranial connective tissue structures (tentorium, falx, foramen magnum), the risk of not identifying and treating the correct causative organism probably outweighs that of herniation.

Cerebrospinal diagnostic testing generally should include nonspecific markers of inflammation (white and red cell count, protein and glucose concentrations) and more specific ones. Viral culture often takes days; for most infections polymerase chain reaction (PCR) is now highly sensitive and specific. CSF PCR for HSV1, HSV2, VZV, and enteroviruses will identify 90% of cases due to known viral pathogens (Solomon et al., 2012). Immunologic markers (IgG, IgM antibodies) may be useful but this typically depends on the rapidity of the particular infection. Since it takes several weeks for specific antibody levels to be measurable, this is not overly helpful in diagnosis of fulminant encephalitis or infections in which the majority of the population can be expected to carry antibodies (HSV). On the other hand, antibody markers may be helpful in flavivirus infections where clinical sensitivity of PCR may be lower and brain infection develops somewhat more slowly. PCR may also be helpful in following treatment response, at least in HSV encephalitis. Although it is true that PCR cannot differentiate between the DNA of viable organisms and the detritus of dead ones, the empiric observation is that PCR positivity declines with successive weeks of treated HSV encephalitis, suggesting that, at least in this infection, this may provide a useful marker of treatment response.

Electroencephalography (EEG) has a time-honored role in the diagnosis of HSV encephalitis, with fairly characteristic periodic discharges. Generally, though, findings are nonspecific. Although EEG can be helpful in problematic cases, with current imaging and PCR technology, this is rarely required diagnostically. On the other hand, since patients with encephalitis may develop nonconvulsive status epilepticus, it can still provide clinically valuable information in the appropriate setting. In addition EEG remains important to detect seizures in patients with autoimmune encephalitis.

## HOSPITAL COURSE IN SPECIFIC DISORDERS

### Herpes encephalitis

Herpes simplex is often referred to as the commonest form of viral encephalitis, with an annual incidence of

2–4/million (Solomon et al., 2012). Most cases are due to HSV1; in about 10%, primarily in neonates or the immunocompromised, HSV2 is responsible. HSV2 typically involves the brain as part of a disseminated infection. Brain involvement is similarly quite disseminated. HSV1, in contrast, typically initially involves the medial temporal and orbital-frontal cortex, an anatomic predilection explained in two different ways – either the virus spreads from the oronasopharynx along the olfactory nerves, or reactivated virus travels along the intracranial portions of the trigeminal nerves, with innervation of the middle temporal fossa arising from the same trigeminal division as that to the oral mucosa. It is thought that about one-third of HSV1 encephalitis cases are attributable to primary infection; the remaining two-thirds are due to reactivation of latent infection (Widener and Whitley, 2014). In either event it appears that virus multiplies locally in the brain for a few days before initial symptoms occur, with symptoms perhaps related as much to the inflammatory response as to virus-induced cell death. The interaction of HSV with the neuronal cellular machinery and the host immune response seems tailor-made to enable the virus' lifelong symbiotic existence in sensory neurons. One viral protein blocks the process by which degraded viral proteins are transported to the cell surface for major histocompatibility class class 1 presentation to the immune system. Others block programmed cell death. Others interfere with intracellular protein synthesis. It is easy to see how these various processes, normally functioning to permit viral persistence in viable neurons, could, if out of control, facilitate extreme viral multiplication, severe neuronal injury, necrosis, and widespread brain damage.

Limbic involvement, with appropriate clinical phenomenology and imaging changes, is highly characteristic but probably not sufficiently sensitive and specific to allow definitive diagnosis. Patients typically present with headache, fever, and confusion. CSF examination generally confirms an inflammatory process. Early in the disease, there can be a polymorphonuclear leukocyte predominance, a moderately hemorrhagic component, and even mild hypoglycorrhachia. With time CSF protein climbs and lymphocytes come to predominate.

PCR has become the diagnostic procedure of choice. Although sensitivity and specificity are typically said to approach 100%, very early in infection PCR may be negative (Lakeman and Whitley, 1995; Venkatesan et al., 2013). If the index of suspicion is high, CSF should be re-examined 3–7 days after presentation. PCR typically remains positive during the first week of treatment; by week 2 half of tested patients are negative. Positivity declines further with time: it has been proposed that PCR positivity at the end of treatment should trigger prolonging antiviral therapy (Widener and Whitley, 2014).

Absent antiviral therapy, HSV1 encephalitis carries an approximately 70% mortality, with major neurologic morbidity in most survivors. Standard treatment is intravenous acyclovir 30 mg/kg/day for 21 days (typically given in three divided doses, adjusted appropriately for impaired renal function). Treatment should begin immediately but may be discontinued if PCR on a sample obtained after more than a few days of symptoms is negative. This necrotizing encephalitis is highly epileptogenic; patients with HSV encephalitis should be maintained on anticonvulsants.

Herpes zoster has long been known to cause a CNS vasculitis; more recent studies show this virus to be responsible for a substantial proportion of cases of viral encephalitis as well (Singh et al., 2015). This infection lacks the limbic localization of HSV encephalitis but should be suspected in individuals with craniofacial shingles, acute VZV infection, or who are immunocompromised and have a disorder that follows a potentially vascular distribution (Langan et al., 2014; Nagel et al., 2015). As with HSV1, PCR provides a potent diagnostic tool. Treatment is with the same daily dose of acyclovir as HSV1 – 30 mg/kg/day, in three divided doses. The usual recommendation is for 14 days of therapy. <LIZ>

HHV6 is similarly nonlocalizing. Like HSV1, it is more likely to cause seizures, particularly in children. This most commonly occurs as part of roseola in children or as an encephalitis in immunocompromised adults. Treatment is with foscarnet 60 mg/kg every 8 hours. Optimal duration of therapy is not clearly defined.

The greatest area of controversy relates to the role of corticosteroids in treatment of HSV encephalitis (Solomon et al., 2012). Despite a general reluctance to use steroids in infections, their positive effect in pneumococcus meningitis, and the presence of significant cerebral edema in HSV encephalitis has led to efforts to clarify their potential impact. This has been tempered by the knowledge that CD8+ T cells normally reside in the trigeminal ganglion, help prevent HSV activation, and are suppressed by corticosteroids (Ramos-Estebanez et al., 2014). Unfortunately the proposed trial to assess this question (Martinez-Torres et al., 2008) was eventually closed because of a failure to enroll sufficient numbers of patients.

A recent systematic review (Ramos-Estebanez et al., 2014) summarized animal studies as showing a beneficial effect when corticosteroids were given some time after viral inoculation; if given before or concurrent with inoculation, outcomes were worse. A number of case reports suggest a potential beneficial role of adjunctive steroids. Very few case series have addressed this question (Nakano et al., 2003; Kamei et al., 2005). In one, 3 patients treated with corticosteroids within 5 days of symptom onset seemed to do well, while there was no evident benefit in the 2 treated weeks after onset. In the other (Kamei et al., 2005), larger retrospective review of 45 patients treated for HSV encephalitis, those who received corticosteroids seemed to have better outcomes. Although the question remains unresolved, there are sufficient data that, pending more compelling studies, it is probably worth considering steroids in severely ill patients with significant cerebral edema.

## Flavivirus encephalitides

The arboviruses most often responsible for human encephalitis are flaviviruses (Asnis and Cruppi, 2007) – a group that includes WNV, JEV, and the tick-borne encephalitis complex viruses, including Powassan. Infections due to these single-stranded RNA viruses share several important clinical properties. All cause far more asymptomatic than symptomatic infections. The majority of symptomatic patients develop a nonspecific febrile illness, with only a small minority developing clinically evident brain involvement.

## WEST NILE VIRUS

WNV has been the most common cause of arboviral encephalitis in the USA since its first appearance in 1999. With between 500 and 3000 cases of neuroinvasive disease in the USA annually (CDC, 2015f), it has an overall incidence of 2–6/million, in some years rivaling, if not exceeding, that of HSV1. Unlike HSV1, though, WNV has a distinct geographic pattern (Fig. 18.1) (CDC, 2015a). Mosquitoes transmit the infection among the birds that serve as its primary reservoir host. Humans are infected incidentally. Other vertebrate species (e.g., horses) may develop viremia but generally not for a sufficiently prolonged period of time or with a sufficiently high viral load to play a meaningful role in disease transmission.

In the approximately 20–25% of WNV-infected patients who become symptomatic (Mostashari et al., 2001; Zou et al., 2010), fever, chills, maculopapular rash,

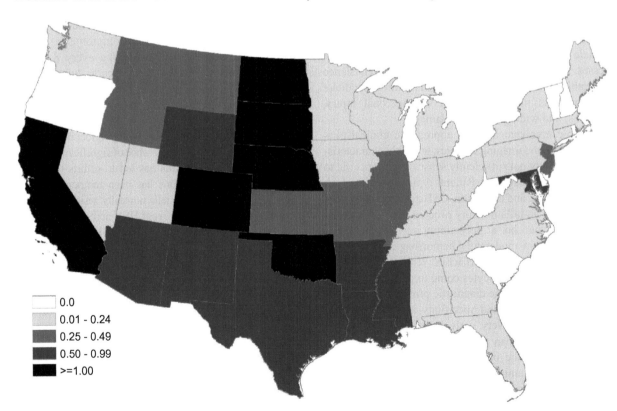

West Nile virus neuroinvasive disease incidence reported to ArboNET, by state, United States, 2015

| | |
|---|---|
| | 0.0 |
| | 0.01 - 0.24 |
| | 0.25 - 0.49 |
| | 0.50 - 0.99 |
| | >=1.00 |

Source: ArboNET, Arboviral Diseases Branch, Centers for Disease Control and Prevention

**Fig. 18.1.** Average annual incidence of West Nile virus neuroinvasive disease reported to the Centers for Disease Control and Prevention by state, 1999–2014. (Reproduced from CDC, 2015a.)

generalized weakness, headache, joint, muscle, and eye pain are the most common symptoms. Overall, 1 patient in 140 infected individuals develops meningoencephalitis, with a prominent age effect – namely, this occurs in 1/300 individuals under the age of 65 but 1/50 age 65 or older. Fatal disease appears to occur only in those over 50 or in the immunocompromised.

Involvement tends to involve gray matter preferentially. A subset of patients (about 10% of those hospitalized) develops a polio-like acute lower motor neuron syndrome clinically resembling Guillain–Barré syndrome (Ahmed et al., 2000) with rapidly progressive flaccid paralysis. A predilection for the basal ganglia in others results in a range of movement disorders (as do JEV and Eastern equine encephalitis). Seizures are quite uncommon.

Diagnostically a CSF pleocytosis is typical; neutrophils may predominate early on (Asnis and Cruppi, 2007). Because infection incubates for days to weeks presymptomatically, serology may be informative at the time of presentation. On the other hand seroprevalence is quite high, so demonstration of IgM in CSF or serum is particularly helpful, as is demonstration of seroconversion. Symptomatic patients are often viremic, so PCR of blood as well as CSF can be helpful. There is significant cross-reactivity – both in PCR and serologic assays – among the different flaviviruses, so laboratories often have to perform additional testing to differentiate among the different infections. Brain imaging studies are nonspecific, although involvement of the basal ganglia should raise the possibility of an arboviral encephalitis.

Treatment of West Nile encephalitis is largely supportive. There has been longstanding interest in using intravenous immunoglobulin (IVIg) – either conventional or from donors with high-titer anti-WNV antibodies. Despite a substantial body of anecdotal evidence (Shimoni et al., 2012; Yango et al., 2014) there remain few systematic data that definitively address this possible therapeutic approach.

### JAPANESE ENCEPHALITIS VIRUS

JEV, the most common agent of arboviral encephalitis worldwide, is prevalent in China and nearby areas of Nepal, India, and Southeast Asia. Like WNV, involvement of the deep gray nuclei, including the brainstem and basal ganglia, leads to frequent parkinsonian features as well as eye movement abnormalities. Coma is more common than in WNV, but asymptomatic infection and nonencephalitic febrile illnesses similarly account for the majority of infections. As in WNV, flaccid paralysis is not uncommon (Solomon et al., 2012).

MRI can demonstrate changes in the basal ganglia –in combination with inflammatory CSF and appropriate epidemiologic exposure, this should raise the possibility of this infection.

### TICK-BORNE ENCEPHALITIS

TEV is the most common cause of encephalitis in Russia and central Europe, with about 10 000 cases reported annually (Granger et al., 2010). Like other flaviviruses, two-thirds of infections are asymptomatic (Granger et al., 2010). Similar to Powassan and deer tick encephalitis viruses (El Khoury et al., 2013) and not unlike WNV and JEV infection, these viruses have a predilection for gray matter – particularly the anterior horn of the spinal cord, where they can cause a segmental polio-like disorder. Patients may develop altered mental status and movement disorders, with tremors and parkinsonian features; seizures may occur as well. Although there is no specific treatment, there are widely available vaccines that have been highly effective at reducing incidence in those countries where their use has been encouraged.

## Rabies

Rabies, well described for millennia (Halperin, 2007), is highly unusual among zoonoses in that it is spread among mammalian hosts without intervening vectors. Once rabies becomes symptomatic and transmissible, the host generally rapidly becomes incapacitated and dies. Consequently it is only by sustaining transmission in a fairly large population of competent hosts that infection can persist. Worldwide, the most common hosts/vectors are dogs. In underdeveloped parts of the world the population of rabid dogs is so great that there are over 50 000 cases of human rabies annually worldwide. Widespread vaccination of domestic canines virtually eliminated human rabies from Western Europe and the USA; 34 cases were reported in the USA between 2003 and 2015. At least 11 of these were probably contracted in other countries and 4 were the result of organ transplantation from an individual who died with undiagnosed rabies. Despite this impressively low risk, concerns about contact with other potentially rabid species lead to up to 60 000 postexposure vaccinations annually in the USA (Fig. 18.2) (CDC, 2015c).

Rabies virus cannot penetrate intact skin but can enter through abrasions or mucosal surfaces. A surface glycoprotein (G protein) extends through the virion's lipid coat and specifically binds the muscle acetylcholine receptor molecules. Virus then multiplies asymptomatically, in muscle or elsewhere. Once sufficiently numerous, virions are picked up in sensory and motor nerve terminals, and transported back to the CNS.

Clinically rabies takes one of two forms – both rapidly lethal. The majority of patients develop "furious" rabies,

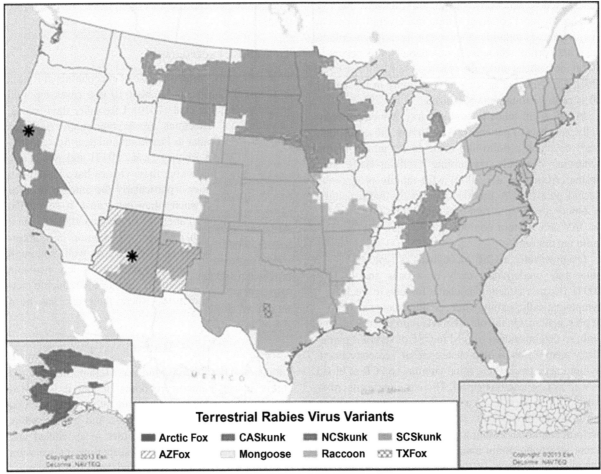

**Fig. 18.2.** Distribution of major rabies virus variants among vector species in the USA and Puerto Rico, 2009 through 2013. (Reproduced from CDC, 2015c.)

initially developing behavioral changes due to brain involvement; survival is generally a week or less. About one-third develop "dumb" rabies, in which rapidly progressive flaccid paralysis precedes the development of cerebral involvement; survival from initial symptom is up to 2 weeks. Dysautonomia is prominent in many and can be the direct precipitant of the fatal outcome. A very small number of individuals who became symptomatic despite receiving postexposure prophylaxis has survived. One 15-year-old who did not receive vaccine, treated with induced coma, ketamine, midazolam, ribavirin, and amantadine, survived symptomatic rabies, albeit with neurologic sequelae (Willoughby et al., 2005). Despite some enthusiasm for what has come to be known as "the Milwaukee protocol," with several additional possible survivors reported (Caicedo et al., 2015; Lu et al., 2015), the general sense has been that this approach is ineffective (Jackson, 2013; Appolinario and Jackson, 2015), leaving no therapeutic interventions other than postexposure prophylactic vaccination and palliative care measures in those who become symptomatic.

## Immune-mediated encephalitis

Once thought to be an extremely rare concomitant of neoplastic disease, autoimmune encephalitis is being recognized with increasing frequency in patients with no evidence of neoplasia. As typified in the Mayo Clinic series (Singh et al., 2015) and British population data (Granerod et al., 2013), this is most often associated with antibodies directed against the $N$-methyl-D-aspartate (NMDA) receptor (NMDAR)or voltage-gated potassium channels (VGKC), occasionally with antibodies to thyroid peroxidase, collapsin response mediator protein 5 (CRMP5), glutamate decarboxylase (GAD65), or Purkinje cells. In this disorder symptoms are typically more subacute. In addition to behavioral changes, patients may develop orofacial dyskinesias, choreoathetosis, and faciobrachial dystonia. Intractable seizures, including status epilepticus, are not uncommon (Solomon et al., 2012). Patients with demonstrable NMDAR or VGKC antibodies should be screened for malignancies, including ovarian teratomas, screening that should include vaginal ultrasound, although teratomas are now found in a distinct minority of these patients.

One important recent variant of this disorder occurs following HSV encephalitis (Armangue et al., 2015). It has long been recognized that a minority of HSV encephalitis patients develop recrudescent symptoms following completion of apparently successful antiviral treatment, including some with negative CSF HSV PCR at the end of therapy. Adult patients with this "relapse" typically develop worsening neurobehavioral symptoms or seizures after the acute illness seems to be under control. In children choreoathetosis seems quite common. Typically suspected to be a recrudescence of the suppressed infection, there is now quite good evidence that this is commonly mediated by a postviral autoimmune process, with the majority of patients having anti-NMDAR antibodies. These patients may therefore benefit from immunotherapies.

There are no high-level studies of different treatment approaches in autoimmune encephalitis, although it is clear that immunosuppression is helpful. British guidelines recommend prolonged corticosteroid courses (0.5 mg/kg/day, prednisolone), with IVIg or plasmapheresis for acute symptoms (Solomon et al., 2012). In the Mayo series outcomes were comparably favorable in patients receiving IVIg and those receiving 5-day courses of high-dose corticosteroids, while all those receiving plasmapheresis had good outcomes (Singh et al., 2015) ($p = 0.002$), suggesting that this might be the preferred approach in highly symptomatic individuals.

## HOSPITAL MANAGEMENT

Patients with encephalitis are acutely ill and require supportive medical management. In any such patient initial assessment must address the basics – airway protection, adequate respiration, and circulation. Medical considerations peculiar to encephalitis include not infrequent autonomic instability and hyponatremia, both of which require careful fluid and electrolyte management.

Although increased intracranial pressure is always a concern in patients with an inflammatory intracranial process, this seems to be a relatively infrequent issue in patients with encephalitis, a fortunate circumstance given the conflicting evidence on use of corticosteroids. Beyond this special consideration, management of patients with raised intracranial pressure is described in detail in Chapter 5 of this volume. Among patients with encephalitis, elevated intracranial pressure arises most commonly in patients with HSV, where animal studies and clinical series suggest that, if corticosteroids are given following initiation of antiviral agents, outcomes are improved – but importantly, no worse than if steroids are not used.

Mass effect in the temporal lobe may become clinically relevant, requiring neurosurgical decompression.

Seizures are common in HSV and autoimmune encephalitis, less so with other etiologies, where infection, though typically more prominent in gray than white matter, tends to involve deep structures (thalamus, basal ganglia) and brainstem. When seizures and status epilepticus occur, appropriate treatment is necessary and further detailed in Chapter 9.

As described above, therapeutic interventions specific to encephalitis are both tailored to the mechanism in the individual patient, and potentially quite effective. In the absence of definitive evidence of an alternative etiology, in any patient with an acute encephalitic presentation acyclovir is typically initiated for possible HSV immediately after a lumbar puncture. If a lumbar puncture cannot be accomplished within hours of presentation, acyclovir should be initiated first, as PCR usually remains positive in the first days to a week of treatment. If PCR is negative on the initial CSF sample (and if necessary on a follow-up sample obtained 3–7 days after presentation), this medication can be stopped. Antiviral treatment is typically continued for 3 weeks. Although it has generally been suggested that CSF may be rechecked for HSV PCR at the end of this time, recent evidence indicates that recrudescent symptoms following such treatment are likely autoimmune, not infectious. In light of this, should symptoms recur following 3 weeks of treatment, it would seem prudent to repeat the lumbar puncture, looking for both HSV by PCR and anti-NMDAR antibodies, then treat based on the results.

If the initial presentation is typical for HSV encephalitis and there is significantly raised intracranial pressure, corticosteroids may be initiated following the administration of acyclovir. Seizures are so frequent in HSV encephalitis that antiseizure medications should be initiated routinely, as they should be in any encephalitis patient who develops seizures. In patients with disseminated HSV (1 or 2) acyclovir should similarly be administered rapidly.

In patients with VZV encephalitis acyclovir is similarly effective. Notably, a subset of such patients present with primarily cerebellar involvement. This is thought to be more a parainfectious than infectious process and is commonly treated with corticosteroids, typically in combination with acyclovir (Solomon et al., 2012). Finally, HHV6 is treated with foscarnet.

## NEUROREHABILITATION

Protracted recovery is expected in many patients. In HSV encephalitis older age, worsening to coma, and restricted diffusion on brain MRI, but also delay in the administration of intravenous acyclovir predicted a poor outcome in herpes simplex encephalitis. Presence of seizures, focal neurologic deficits, EEG abnormalities, and location or extension of fluid-attenuated inversion recovery/T2 abnormalities did not influence functional outcome (Singh et al., 2016).

## CONCLUSIONS

With advances in both our understanding of its pathogenesis and the development of effective antiviral agents, the majority of patients with encephalitis can be successfully treated. Both acute and long-term outcomes can be remarkably favorable in those in whom an etiology is identified and appropriate treatment instituted rapidly (Mailles et al., 2012). Diagnostic tools, including PCR for likely pathogens, and the identification of relevant antibodies in autoimmune encephalitis, have greatly improved the outcome for many of these patients.

### REFERENCES

Ahmed S, Libman R, Wesson K et al. (2000). Guillain-Barre syndrome: an unusual presentation of West Nile virus infection. Neurology 55: 144–146.

Appolinario CM, Jackson AC (2015). Antiviral therapy for human rabies. Antivir Ther 20: 1–10.

Armangue T, Moris G, Cantarin-Extremera V et al. (2015). Autoimmune post-herpes simplex encephalitis of adults and teenagers. Neurology 85: 1736–1743.

Asnis DS, Cruppi RS (2007). West Nile virus. In: J Halperin (Ed.), Encephalitis: Diagnosis and Treatment. Informa Healthcare, New York, NY.

Booth PJ, Bodager D, Slade TA et al. (2015). Primary amebic meningoencephalitis associated with hot spring exposure during international travel - Seminole County, Florida, July 2014. MMWR Morb Mortal Wkly Rep 64: 1226.

Brouwer MC, McIntyre P, Prasad K et al. (2015). Corticosteroids for acute bacterial meningitis. Cochrane Database Syst Rev 9, CD004405.

Caicedo Y, Paez A, Kuzmin I et al. (2015). Virology, immunology and pathology of human rabies during treatment. Pediatr Infect Dis J 34: 520–528.

CDC. Listeria (listeriosis) [online]. CDC. Available: http://www.cdc.gov/listeria/statistics.html [accessed October 25, 2015].

CDC (2015a). Average annual incidence of West Nile virus neuroinvasive disease reported to CDC by state, 1999–2014 [online]. CDC. Available: http://www.cdc.gov/westnile/resources/pdfs/data/6-wnv-neuro-incidence-by-state-map_1999-2014_06042015.pdf. [accessed November 15, 2015].

CDC (2015b). Group B strep *GBS) [online]. CDC. Available: http://www.cdc.gov/groupbstrep/clinicians/clinical-overview.html. [accessed October 25, 2015].

CDC (2015c). Human rabies [online]. Available: http://www.cdc.gov/rabies/location/usa/surveillance/human_rabies.html. [accessed November 28, 2015].

CDC (2015d). Meningococcal disease: technical & clinical information [online]. CDC. Available: http://www.cdc.gov/meningococcal/clinical-info.html. [accessed October 25, 2015].

CDC (2015e). Pneumococcal disease [online]. Available: http://www.cdc.gov/pneumococcal/clinicians/clinical-features.html. [accessed October 25, 2015].

CDC (2015f). West Nile virus neuroinvasive disease cases reported to CDC by state of residence, 1999–2014 [online]. CDC. Available: http://www.cdc.gov/westnile/resources/pdfs/data/3-west-nile-virus-cases-reported-to-cdc-by-state_1999-2014_06082015.pdf. [accessed November 15, 2015].

El Khoury MY, Hull RC, Bryant PW et al. (2013). Diagnosis of acute deer tick virus encephalitis. Clin Infect Dis 56: e40–e47.

Granerod J, Cousens S, Davies NW et al. (2013). New estimates of incidence of encephalitis in England. Emerg Infect Dis 19.

Granger D, Lopansri B, Butcher D et al. (2010). Tick-borne encephalitis among U.S. travelers to Europe and Asia – 2000–2009. MMWR Morb Mortal Wkly Rep 59: 335–338.

Halperin J (2007). Rabies. In: J Halperin (Ed.), Encephalitis: diagnosis and treatment. Informa Healthcare, New York, NY.

Jackson AC (2013). Current and future approaches to the therapy of human rabies. Antiviral Res 99: 61–67.

Kamei S, Sekizawa T, Shiota H et al. (2005). Evaluation of combination therapy using aciclovir and corticosteroid in adult patients with herpes simplex virus encephalitis. J Neurol Neurosurg Psychiatry 76: 1544–1549.

Lakeman FD, Whitley RJ (1995). Diagnosis of herpes simplex encephalitis: application of polymerase chain reaction to cerebrospinal fluid from brain-biopsied patients and correlation with disease. National Institute of Allergy and Infectious Diseases Collaborative Antiviral Study Group. J Infect Dis 171: 857–863.

Langan SM, Minassian C, Smeeth L et al. (2014). Risk of stroke following herpes zoster: a self-controlled case-series study. Clin Infect Dis 58: 1497–1503.

Lu A, Shah P, Shen P et al. (2015). Temporal evolution on MRI of successful treatment of rabies. Clin Imaging 39: 893–896.

Mailles A, De Broucker T, Costanzo P et al. (2012). Long-term outcome of patients presenting with acute infectious encephalitis of various causes in France. Clin Infect Dis 54: 1455–1464.

Martinez-Torres F, Menon S, Pritsch M et al. (2008). Protocol for German trial of acyclovir and corticosteroids in herpes-simplex-virus-encephalitis (GACHE): a multicenter, multinational, randomized, double-blind, placebo-controlled German, Austrian and Dutch trial [ISRCTN45122933]. BMC Neurol 8: 40.

Mostashari F, Bunning ML, Kitsutani PT et al. (2001). Epidemic West Nile encephalitis, New York, 1999: results of a household-based seroepidemiological survey. Lancet 358: 261–264.

Nagel MA, White T, Khmeleva N et al. (2015). Analysis of varicella-zoster virus in temporal arteries biopsy positive and negative for giant cell arteritis. JAMA Neurol 72: 1281–1287.

Nakano A, Yamasaki R, Miyazaki S et al. (2003). Beneficial effect of steroid pulse therapy on acute viral encephalitis. Eur Neurol 50: 225–229.

Ramos-Estebanez C, Lizarraga KJ, Merenda A (2014). A systematic review on the role of adjunctive corticosteroids in herpes simplex virus encephalitis: is timing critical for safety and efficacy? Antivir Ther 19: 133–139.

Schuchat A (1998). Epidemiology of group B streptococcal disease in the United States: shifting paradigms. Clin Microbiol Rev 11: 497–513.

Shimoni Z, Bin H, Bulvik S et al. (2012). The clinical response of West Nile virus neuroinvasive disease to intravenous immunoglobulin therapy. Clin Pract 2. e18.

Singh TD, Fugate JE, Rabinstein AA (2015). The spectrum of acute encephalitis: causes, management, and predictors of outcome. Neurology 84: 359–366.

Singh TD, Fugate JE, Hocker S et al. (2016). Predictors of outcome in HSV encephalitis. J Neurol 263: 277–289.

Solomon T, Michael BD, Smith PE et al. (2012). Management of suspected viral encephalitis in adults – Association of British Neurologists and British Infection Association National Guidelines. J Infect 64: 347–373.

Tunkel AR, Glaser CA, Bloch KC et al. (2008). The management of encephalitis: clinical practice guidelines by the Infectious Diseases Society of America. Clin Infect Dis 47: 303–327.

Venkatesan A, Tunkel AR, Bloch KC et al. (2013). Case definitions, diagnostic algorithms, and priorities in encephalitis: consensus statement of the international encephalitis consortium. Clin Infect Dis 57: 1114–1128.

Widener RW, Whitley RJ (2014). Herpes simplex virus. Handb Clin Neurol 123: 251–263.

Willoughby JR RE, Tieves KS, Hoffman GM et al. (2005). Survival after treatment of rabies with induction of coma. N Engl J Med 352: 2508–2514.

Yango AF, Fischbach BV, Levy M et al. (2014). West Nile virus infection in kidney and pancreas transplant recipients in the Dallas-Fort Worth Metroplex during the 2012 Texas epidemic. Transplantation 97: 953–957.

Zou S, Foster, Gregory A et al. (2010). West Nile fever characteristics among viremic persons identified through blood donor screening. J Infect Dis 202: 1354–1361.

*Handbook of Clinical Neurology, Vol. 140 (3rd series)*
*Critical Care Neurology, Part I*
E.F.M. Wijdicks and A.H. Kramer, Editors
http://dx.doi.org/10.1016/B978-0-444-63600-3.00019-2

Chapter 19

# Management of bacterial central nervous system infections

M.C. BROUWER AND D. VAN DE BEEK*

*Department of Neurology, Center for Infection and Immunity, Academic Medical Center, University of Amsterdam, Amsterdam, The Netherlands*

## Abstract

Bacterial infections of the central nervous system present as a medical emergency, thus requiring rapid diagnosis and immediate treatment. The most prevalent bacterial infections seen in the intensive care unit can be summarized as acute bacterial meningitis, subdural empyema, intracerebral abscess, and ventriculitis, which all commonly involve the brain parenchyma. The infections can either be community-acquired or hospital-acquired, e.g., after neurosurgical intervention, as a complication of severe neurotrauma or related to indwelling cerebrospinal fluid drains. Community-acquired bacterial meningitis is most commonly caused by the pneumococcus (*Streptococcus pneumoniae*) and meningococcus (*Neisseria meningitidis*), and is often complicated by hearing loss, cerebrovascular complications, and seizures. Brain abscesses are frequently associated with contiguous or metastatic foci of infection such as otitis, sinusitis, pneumonia, or endocarditis which need to be detected and treated early during disease course. Despite optimal treatment, many patients are at risk for both major systemic and neurologic complications, leading to a substantial mortality and risk of major disability in survivors. Empiric treatment depends on regional antibiotic resistance patterns of common pathogens. For subdural empyema and brain abscesses, neurosurgical drainage of the infection is required alongside prolonged antibiotic treatment.

## INTRODUCTION

Bacterial infections of the central nervous system (CNS) require rapid diagnosis and immediate treatment. Despite optimal treatment, many patients develop severe disease and are at risk for both systemic and neurologic complications, leading to a substantial mortality and risk of sequelae in survivors. The most commonly encountered patients in the emergency department or neurosciences intensive care unit are those with meningitis, subdural empyema, intracerebral abscess, and ventriculitis, which all commonly involve the brain parenchyma, resulting in encephalitis. The infections can be community-acquired or hospital-acquired (e.g., after neurosurgical intervention, as a complication of severe neurotrauma, or related to ventriculostomies). A substantial proportion of patients with community-acquired bacterial CNS infections have a focus of infection outside the CNS,

such as mastoiditis, pneumonia, and endocarditis, which should be actively sought for and treated. Empiric treatment depends on local epidemiology and regional antibiotic resistance patterns of common pathogens. This chapter provides an overview of these challenging infections. A multidisciplinary approach involving the infectious disease consultant and otorhinolaryngologist early is essential.

## EPIDEMIOLOGY

### Community-acquired bacterial meningitis

The incidence of acute community-acquired bacterial meningitis is 0.9–2.6/100 000 persons per year in high-income countries, resulting in an estimated 4000 cases in the USA annually (Thigpen et al., 2011; Bijlsma et al., 2016). The incidence has substantially decreased

*Correspondence to: Diederik van de Beek, Department of Neurology, Center of Infection and Immunity Amsterdam (CINIMA), Academic Medical Center, University of Amsterdam, P.O. Box 22660, 1100DD Amsterdam, The Netherlands. Tel: +31-205663842, Fax: +31-205669374, E-mail: D.vandeBeek@amc.uva.nl

in the past 25 years, which is mostly due to implementation of vaccination strategies against the most common pathogens in pediatric bacterial meningitis: *Haemophilus influenzae* type b (Hib), *Streptococcus pneumoniae,* and *Neisseria meningitidis* (McIntyre et al., 2012). Routine vaccination of children against Hib has resulted in a 99% reduction of *H. influenzae* meningitis in the developed world, and is currently also available in most developing countries (Brouwer et al., 2010b; McIntyre et al., 2012). Following the introduction of Hib vaccination, *S. pneumoniae* has become the most common pathogen beyond the neonatal period and bacterial meningitis has become a disease predominantly of adults (Brouwer et al., 2010b). Currently, *S. pneumoniae* is identified in approximately 70% of bacterial meningitis cases. The introduction of conjugate vaccines against seven serotypes of *S. pneumoniae* (PCV7) has reduced the rate of invasive pneumococcal infections in young children and in older persons (McIntyre et al., 2012). These serotypes were selected based on their prevalence among children aged 6 months to 2 years, and a reduced susceptibility to antibiotics. However, following the introduction serotype replacement occurred, leading to the introduction of the 10- and 13-valent pneumococcal conjugate vaccines (McIntyre et al., 2012). Recent data showed this has impacted pneumococcal meningitis incidence, with a specific decrease among vaccine serotypes, and no evidence of increase in nonvaccine serotypes (Bijlsma et al., 2016).

*N. meningitidis* most commonly causes bacterial meningitis in young adults and can occur as sporadic cases and epidemics (Stephens et al., 2007; Bijlsma et al., 2014a). The meningococcus is identified in 10–15% of cases nowadays and its incidence shows a peak in winter and early spring. Small outbreaks typically occur in young adults living in close quarters, such as dormitories of military camps or schools. The incidence of meningococcal meningitis and causative serogroups varies greatly around the world. Major epidemics of meningococcal disease of serogroup A, C, and W135 have occurred periodically in sub-Saharan Africa (referred to as the "meningitis belt"), Europe, Asia, and South America. During these epidemics, attack rates can reach several hundred per 100 000, with devastating consequences. Following an epidemic outbreak of serogroup C disease in the late 1990s in several European countries the conjugated group C vaccine (MenC) was introduced. This has resulted in a sharp decrease of group C meningococcal disease, which in part was attributed to herd immunity (Bijlsma et al., 2014b). Currently, most cases of meningococcal meningitis in the USA and Europe are caused by serogroup B (Thigpen et al., 2011; Bijlsma et al., 2014a), for which a multicomponent meningococcal B protein vaccine (4CMenB) has been developed (Read et al., 2014). Clinical trials showed this vaccine to be immunogenic in

infants and adults, and resulted in decreased carriage (Read et al., 2014). However, as the incidence has spontaneously declined over the past decade, this vaccine has not been widely introduced (Bijlsma et al., 2014a). A major achievement in reduction of meningococcal disease has been achieved in several African countries following introduction of the serogroup A vaccine, which led to over 99% reduction in cases.

A less frequent cause of community-acquired meningitis is *Listeria monocytogenes,* which causes meningitis preferentially in neonates, immunosuppressed individuals, the elderly, and cancer patients (Koopmans et al., 2013). Small outbreaks of *L. monocytogenes* infections have been associated with contaminated food products. Other less common causes of community-acquired bacterial meningitis currently are *Haemophilus influenzae, Staphylococcus aureus,* and *Streptococcus pyogenes,* which are all associated with specific predisposing conditions (otitis, sinusitis, or endocarditis).

## Hospital-acquired bacterial meningitis

Bacterial meningitis also occurs in hospitalized patients ("physician-associated meningitis" or "nosocomial meningitis"). In a large city hospital, almost 40% of cases were reported to be nosocomial (Durand et al., 1993). Most cases occur in patients undergoing neurosurgical procedures, including implanting of neurosurgical devices, and in patients with severe neurotrauma (van de Beek et al., 2010). The organisms causing nosocomial meningitis differ markedly from those causing community-acquired meningitis and include Gram-negative rods (*Escherichia coli, Klebsiella* spp., *Pseudomonas aeruginosa, Acinetobacter* spp., *Enterobacter* spp., and others), staphylococci and streptococci other than *S. pneumoniae.*

## Brain abscess

The incidence of brain abscesses has been estimated at 0.4–0.9 per 100 000, but in specific risk groups incidence can be substantially higher, for instance in human immunodeficiency virus (HIV)/acquired immunodeficiency syndrome (AIDS)-infected patients (Nicolosi et al., 1991). Brain abscesses are predominantly found in men (70%), with a mean age of 34 years (Brouwer et al., 2014a). In a meta-analysis of 9699 patients, the most common causative micro-organisms were found to be *Streptococcus* and *Staphylococcus* species, causing 34% and 18% of cases respectively. Gram-negative enteric bacteria (*Klebsiella* spp., *Proteus* spp., *Escherichia coli* and Enterobacteriacae) constitute the third large group, being responsible for 15% of cases (Brouwer et al., 2014a). One-fourth of patients with brain abscesses are found to have a polymicrobial infection. Most reported cases were community-acquired and associated with contiguous or metastatic foci of infection (Brouwer et al., 2014a). Posttraumatic and postneurosurgical brain abscesses constituted 14% and 9% of cases respectively (Brouwer et al., 2014a).

## Subdural empyema

In studies reporting on focal bacterial infections of the CNS, 15–20% of cases consist of subdural empyema. More specific data on the incidence of subdural empyema are lacking. A large retrospective cohort study of 699 patients showed 62% of patients were male and the mean age was 15 years (range 1 month to 72 years). Most patients (75%) with subdural empyema have sinusitis or mastoiditis, while 10% of empyemas develop as a complication of bacterial meningitis (Nathoo et al., 1999). When complicating bacterial meningitis, subdural empyema is most often caused by *Streptococcus pneumoniae* (Jim et al., 2012), whereas other *Streptococcus* and *Staphylococcus* species are more common in patients with otitis, sinusitis, and trauma. In 20% of patients with positive cultures, multiple bacterial strains are identified (polymicrobial infection).

## NEUROPATHOLOGY

### Bacterial meningitis

During bacterial meningitis there is diffuse inflammation of the pia mater and arachnoid, with migration of neutrophil leukocytes into the cerebrospinal fluid (CSF) (Nau et al., 1999). This leads to pus accumulation over the surface of the brain, specifically around its base, the cranial nerves, and the spinal cord. The meningeal vessels become dilated and congested and may show endothelial inflammation, leading to microhemorrhages and infarction (Vergouwen et al., 2010). Leukocyte infiltration and inflammation of the ventricle result in ventriculitis, with concomitant loss of the ependymal lining and gliosis of subependymal cell layers. Accumulation of pus and swelling of brain structures due to inflammation may block CSF circulation, causing obstructive hydrocephalus or spinal block. Thickening due to high protein and leukocyte content of CSF results in decreased CSF uptake and subsequent resorption hydrocephalus and increased intracranial pressure (ICP). In many cases death may be attributable to related septicemia and especially patients with meningococcal septicemia may develop acute pulmonary edema.

### Brain abscess

Histopathologic features in patients with brain abscess can be described in several stages, of which the first stage is early cerebritis, which occurs after initial hematogenous seeding of bacteria or infection *per continuitatem*

from paranasal sinuses, mastoiditis, or through traumatic or postoperative skull defects (Brouwer et al., 2014b). This stage may progress to a perivascular inflammatory response surrounding a necrotic center with increased edema in the surrounding white matter. Subsequently, the necrotic center reaches its maximum size and capsule formation starts with fibroblasts and neovascularization. The capsule thickens with abundance of reactive collagen. Inflammation, necrosis, and edema extend beyond the capsule.

## CLINICAL PRESENTATION

### Community-acquired bacterial meningitis

Early recognition is important in bacterial meningitis patients to initiate treatment and thereby improve prognosis (Brouwer et al., 2012). However, initial signs and symptoms are often nonspecific and have poor test characteristics to differentiate between bacterial meningitis, other infections, and other neurologic diseases. A study in children and adolescents with meningococcal disease, of which meningitis was diagnosed in one-third of patients, analyzed symptoms and signs prior to hospital admission retrospectively (Thompson et al., 2006). This study showed the first symptoms consisted of headache, fever, and irritability, while typical meningitis symptoms such as neck stiffness, altered mental status, and rash developed late during disease.

The clinical presentation of bacterial meningitis differs per age group and causative pathogen. Infants often present with nonspecific signs and symptoms of poor feeding, fever, and irritability, while older children are more likely to present with signs of meningeal irritation and brain inflammation (Brouwer et al., 2010b). In adults the classic triad of fever, neck stiffness, and altered mental status was found in 41–44% of episodes, whereas 95% had at least two out of four symptoms of headache, fever, neck stiffness, and altered mental status (van de Beek et al., 2004; Bijlsma et al., 2016). A petechial rash was identified in 8–26% of patients, and is indicative of meningococcal infection in 70–90% of patients with a rash. Several studies assessed the diagnostic accuracy of neck stiffness, Kernig's sign, and Brudzinski's sign for detecting bacterial meningitis (Brouwer et al., 2012). These clinical findings have low diagnostic accuracy for prediction of meningitis, defined as increased CSF white blood cell count (combined sensitivity neck stiffness 31%, Brudzinski 9%, Kernig 11%). Therefore, the absence of these findings cannot exclude bacterial meningitis. Focal neurologic deficits, such as aphasia or hemiparesis, are identified in 20–25% of patients, and cranial nerve palsies are found upon presentation in 10% (Bijlsma et al., 2016). Focal deficits may indicate cerebral infarctions, which occur in up to 25% of patients during disease course, but can also indicate a concomitant brain abscess (2%), empyema (3%), or cerebral hemorrhage (3%). Cranial nerve palsies are though to originate from increased ICP or inflammation of the nerve upon its exit through the meninges. Most commonly affected cranial nerves are the oculomotor, abducens, facial, and vestibulocochlear nerves. Seizures are reported in 15–20% of bacterial meningitis episodes, of which 5% occur prehospital and the remainder occur during hospitalization (Zoons et al., 2008). Seizures occur more frequently in patients with cerebrovascular complications early during bacterial meningitis and may also indicate empyema or brain abscess.

Foci of infection outside the nervous system may suggest the bacterial etiology. Otitis and sinusitis are commonly identified in bacterial meningitis and are most frequently found in pneumococcal meningitis and meningitis due to *H. influenzae*. Half of the patients with pneumococcal meningitis have otitis or sinusitis and therefore early consultation of an ear, nose, and throat (ENT) physician is warranted to evaluate whether operative treatment of the infective focus is indicated. Pneumonia is present in 9% of meningitis cases and also most frequently found in pneumococcal meningitis (Bijlsma et al., 2016). Patients with meningococcal meningitis have a petechial rash in 60–70% of cases. A rash may also be seen in bacterial meningitis patients with concomitant endocarditis, which is found in 2% of cases. In these patients, *Staphylococcus aureus* is a common pathogen besides the pneumococcus (Lucas et al., 2013). Sepsis may co-occur in bacterial meningitis due to any pathogen and is associated with poor prognosis. *Listeria moncytogenes* meningitis is associated with a prolonged duration of disease prior to presentation.

## Hospital-acquired bacterial meningitis

The diagnosis of hospital-acquired bacterial meningitis is usually troublesome (van de Beek et al., 2010). Fever and a decreased level of consciousness are the most commonly reported symptoms in hospital-acquired meningitis, but these are nonspecific (Baltas et al., 1994). Patients developing bacterial meningitis following neurotrauma or neurosurgery often already have an altered mental status due to the nature of the injury, sedation, or postoperative brain edema. Fever can occur after surgery without infection or the patient may have another focus of infection, for instance, a urinary tract infection or hospital-acquired pneumonia. Patients with a CSF drain-related meningitis may only have a low-grade fever and general malaise (Vinchon and Dhellemmes, 2006). Neck stiffness is observed in less than 50% of patients (van de Beek et al., 2010).

## Brain abscess

Patients with brain abscesses can present with a multitude of symptoms and signs, including seizures, fever, focal neurologic deficits, and symptoms of increased ICP such as headache, papilledema, and loss of vision (Brouwer et al., 2014b). The most common symptom is headache, which occurs in 69% of cases. Nausea and/or vomiting is seen in half of the patients and 53% have fever upon presentation (Brouwer et al., 2014a). An altered mental status is observed in 43% of patients and neurologic deficits occur in 48% of cases. Neck stiffness is present in 32% of patients and most often found in patients with concomitant meningitis. Up to 25% present with seizures, which can be focal or generalized. The classic triad of fever, headache, and focal neurologic deficits is present in only 20% of patients and therefore not very useful (Brouwer et al., 2014a). Time from onset of symptoms to diagnosis is on average 8 days.

## Subdural empyema

Few studies systematically analyzed the clinical characteristics of subdural empyema. The largest available cohort study performed in South Africa including 699 patients showed that 77% of patients have fever as presenting symptom (Nathoo et al., 1999). Neck stiffness was present in 74% of patients and only 32% were reported to have headache upon presentation. Seizures upon admission occurred in 39% of cases, of which 29% consisted of a focal seizure and 10% were generalized. As the majority of patients have sinusitis, otitis, meningitis, or a dental focus of infection, consultation of an ENT physician and a dentist is indicated.

## NEURODIAGNOSTICS AND IMAGING

### Community-acquired bacterial meningitis

Bacterial meningitis can only be confirmed by examination of CSF. Therefore, there is an urgent need to perform a lumbar puncture. In a small proportion of patients a lumbar puncture is hazardous as brain shift may worsen due to the removal of CSF at the lumbar level, which may ultimately result in compression of the brainstem and eventually death. To prevent this rare event, cranial imaging can be performed to rule out space-occupying lesions such as brain abscesses, brain infarctions, generalized edema, or subdural empyema (Brouwer et al., 2012). Cranial imaging, however, is known to delay the time to antibiotic treatment, and was found to negatively influence outcome (Aronin et al., 1998). Studies showed that the majority of patients receive cranial imaging before lumbar puncture, even when there is no clear indication to do this (van de Beek et al., 2004). In a prospective study in 301 patients with suspected bacterial meningitis, 235 (78%) received cranial imaging before the lumbar puncture (Hasbun et al., 2001). Abnormalities were shown in 24% of patients and 5% had mass lesions causing brain shift. Clinical predictors of space-occupying lesions in this study were new-onset seizures, an immunocompromised state (e.g., HIV, patients on immunosuppressive therapy), papilledema, focal neurologic deficits, and a moderate to severe impairment of consciousness. These items were included in major review articles as directive for when to perform or withhold cranial computed tomography (CT) (van de Beek et al., 2006; Brouwer et al., 2012). In patients in whom cranial imaging is indicated before lumbar puncture, empiric treatment for bacterial meningitis with antibiotics and dexamethasone is advised prior to the scan. Other contraindications for immediate lumbar puncture are coagulation disorders, such as diffuse intravascular coagulation or use of anticoagulants. Furthermore, if a patient presents with septic shock, lumbar puncture should be postponed until the patient has been stabilized. In all patients in whom a lumbar puncture is not performed before initiation of antibiotic treatment, blood cultures should be drawn before the antibiotics are given. This increases the chance of detecting the causative pathogen, which is essential for antibiotic susceptibility testing and rationalizing antibiotic treatment.

Besides detection of intracranial lesions contraindicating a lumbar puncture, cranial imaging is often performed to identify mastoiditis or sinusitis as a cause of bacterial meningitis. These infections need to be detected early on during the disease course to determine whether surgical treatment of these foci of infection is needed. Furthermore, in patients with a suspected CSF, leak thin-slice CT of the sinuses and mastoid, and often also magnetic resonance imaging (MRI) with three-dimensional constructive interference in steady state images are indicated to detect the leak and facilitate the workup towards repair surgery. These investigations can be done after the diagnosis has been confirmed by CSF examination.

During bacterial meningitis ICP is increased, which is reflected by an elevated opening pressure found at the lumbar puncture. Over half of the patients have an opening pressure over 400 mm$^3$ water (upper limit of normal is 200 mm$^3$) (Bijlsma et al., 2016). Characteristic findings in CSF or bacterial meningitis are a (strongly) elevated leukocyte count, high total protein contact, low glucose concentration, and low ratio of CSF to blood glucose. A study in 422 patients with bacterial of viral meningitis showed CSF glucose concentration <1.9 mmol/L, CSF to blood glucose ratio <0.23, CSF protein concentration >2.2 g/L, CSF leukocyte count >2000/μL, and CSF neutrophil count >1180/μL were

strong individual predictors of bacterial meningitis (Spanos et al., 1989). In two large cohort studies, it was shown that 88–96% patients have one of these predictors (van de Beek et al., 2004; Bijlsma et al., 2016). A substantial proportion of patients (~10%) have < 100 leukocytes/mL, which may lead to a misinterpretation of CSF results and a diagnosis of viral meningitis. Especially patients with *L. monocytogenes* meningitis, stem cell transplantation recipients, patients with active cancer, and those using immunosuppressive drugs often have a low CSF white cell count. Therefore in these patient groups extra caution should be kept for bacterial meningitis, even though CSF abnormalities are not typical (Koopmans et al., 2013).

The gold standard for diagnosing bacterial meningitis is CSF culture, which is positive in 80–90% of patients with community-acquired bacterial meningitis, when the lumbar puncture is performed prior to antibiotic treatment (Brouwer et al., 2010b). If CSF is collected after initiation of treatment, the yield of culture decreases by 10–20%. Gram staining is a simple and inexpensive method to confirm the diagnosis and identify the pathogen. The reported yield of CSF Gram stain differs per pathogen: in pneumococcal meningitis the reported range of positivity is 70–90% and for meningococcal meningitis this is 30–90%. In the past decade polymerase chain reaction (PCR) on CSF has been increasingly used for the diagnosis of bacterial meningitis. The reported sensitivity was 79–100% for *Streptococcus pneumoniae* meningitis and 91–100% for *N. meningitidis* (Brouwer et al., 2010b). The specificity was generally high – between 95 and 100% for all micro-organisms. PCR was shown to have incremental value compared to CSF culture and Gram stain (Corless et al., 2001; Tzanakaki et al., 2005).

A study from Burkina Faso in 409 bacterial meningitis patients showed 33% of patients could not be diagnosed with conventional methods and were diagnosed with PCR only (Parent et al., 2005). In several countries PCR has become the standard method for confirmation of meningococcal disease. The UK meningococcal reference unit showed 1099 of 1925 (57%) invasive meningococcal disease episodes were diagnosed by PCR only (Heinsbroek et al., 2013). A Spanish study in children with meningococcal disease showed similar results: 46 of 188 cases were confirmed only by PCR (Munoz-Almagro et al., 2009). PCR was negative in 5% of culture-positive cases in this study. PCR is especially useful in patients who received intravenous antibiotic treatment prior to the lumbar puncture, as CSF and blood cultures in these patients are often negative. A disadvantage of PCR compared to CSF culture is the lack of antimicrobial susceptibility data. Studies analyzing the test characteristics of *L. monocytogenes* PCR in meningitis showed culture-positive CSF samples were positive with PCR as well (Le Monnier et al., 2011). The incremental value of PCR in *Listeria* meningitis next to culture is currently unclear.

Other diagnostic methods for rapid diagnosis in bacterial meningitis are latex agglutination and immunochromatography antigen testing. The reported sensitivity of latex agglutination testing in CSF differs per causative micro-organism: for *S. pneumoniae* between 59% and 100%, and for *N. meningitidis* between 22 and 93% (Brouwer et al., 2010b). In clinical conditions latex agglutination testing has not shown to provide additional value over other tests. In a study of 176 children treated with antibiotic before the lumbar puncture in whom CSF culture remained negative, no latex agglutination test was positive (Nigrovic et al., 2004). Another study showed the sensitivity of latex agglutination tests decreased from 60% to 9% in patients in whom treatment was started before the lumbar puncture was performed. Because of the limited value of latex agglutination these tests are not advised in the diagnosis of bacterial meningitis when other methods are available, such as Gram staining (Brouwer et al., 2010b). Immunochromatographic antigen testing to detect *S. pneumoniae* in CSF was studied in 450 children with suspected acute bacterial meningitis (Saha et al., 2005). The test was 100% sensitive and specific for diagnosing pneumococcal meningitis. Another study including 1179 CSF samples from children in Bangladesh with suspected bacterial meningitis also revealed high sensitivity (98.6%) and specificity (99.3%) (Moisi et al., 2009). False-positive results have been reported in patients with meningitis due to other streptococcal species. Further studies assessing its usefulness in clinical practice are awaited.

Serum inflammatory markers may contribute to the diagnosis when differentiating between viral and bacterial meningitis. Studies have suggested serum concentrations of C-reactive protein and procalcitonin to be discriminatory between bacterial and viral meningitis in children (Dubos et al., 2008). A study in 507 children reported a C-reactive protein level >40 mg/L to have a 93% sensitivity and 100% specificity (Sormunen et al., 1999). A study in 105 adults also showed good sensitivity and specificity of procalcitonin when differentiating between bacterial meningitis, viral meningitis, or no meningitis (Ray et al., 2007). However, other bacterial infections such as sepsis and pneumonia are often included in the differential diagnosis of bacterial meningitis, and in these situations C-reactive protein and procalcitonin may be of little value for the diagnosis of bacterial meningitis.

Blood cultures are valuable for detection of the causative organism and establish susceptibility patterns if CSF cultures are negative or if a lumbar puncture cannot be performed, for instance, in patients with coagulopathy (Brouwer et al., 2010b). Blood cultures are positive in 75% of pneumococcal meningitis patients and 40–60% of patients with meningococcal meningitis. The yield of blood cultures was shown to decrease by 20% if patients are treated with antibiotic prior to the blood culture (Nigrovic et al., 2008).

## Hospital-acquired bacterial meningitis

The diagnosis of hospital-acquired bacterial meningitis is based on CSF cultures, and in all patients with suspected meningitis following trauma, neurosurgery, or with an external CSF drain, both anaerobic and aerobic cultures should be taken (van de Beek et al., 2010). Prolonged incubation is required before CSF culture can be confirmed to be negative. More rapid diagnostic methods such as CSF Gram stain were shown to have excellent specificity but poor sensitivity. CSF leukocyte count may also be useful but cannot be used to rule out hospital-acquired bacterial meningitis. A prospective study in patients with an external CSF drain showed 22% of patients with a culture-proven bacterial meningitis had normal CSF leukocyte count. An elevated CSF leukocyte, which is usually diagnostic for CNS infections, may be due to hemorrhage or inflammation following surgery. Several alternative diagnostic markers have been studied, such as CSF lactate and serum procalcitonin. Serum procalcitonin showed poor predictive value of postoperative meningitis, while studies reported both good and poor test characteristics of CSF lactate (Choi and Choi, 2013; Munoz-Gomez et al., 2015).

## Brain abscess

Brain abscesses are diagnosed with CT, which provides a rapid method of detecting the size, number, perifocal edema, and location of abscesses (Brouwer et al., 2014b). However, CT does not differentiate well between cerebral abscesses, metastases, and sometimes primary brain tumors. MRI with diffusion-weighed imaging is therefore indicated in patients with suspected brain abscesses for differentiation from primary necrotic or cystic tumors (Brouwer et al., 2014b). A study of 115 patients with a total of 147 lesions in the brain included 97 patients with brain abscess and showed that diffusion-weighted imaging had a sensitivity and specificity for the differentiation of brain abscesses from primary or metastatic cancers of 96% (Fig. 19.1) (Reddy et al., 2006). Blood parameters of infection, such as leukocyte count or C-reactive protein, were normal in a substantial proportion of patients (Brouwer et al., 2014a). Blood cultures show the causative pathogen in 28% of cases while CSF cultures were positive in 24% of patients (Brouwer et al., 2014a). Clinical deterioration attributed

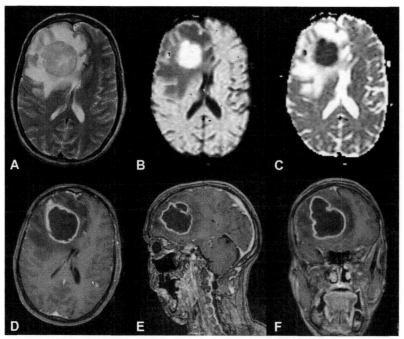

**Fig. 19.1.** Magnetic resonance imaging of patient with a brain abscess showing a large brain abscess in the frontal lobe with perifocal edema on T2-weighted imaging (**A**), with hyperintense signal on diffusion-weighted imaging (DWI: **B**) and hyperintense signal on apparent diffusion coefficient imaging (ADC: **C**), typical for brain abscess. (**D–F**) Axial, sagittal, and coronal T1 images with contrast enhancement of the abscess wall.

to a lumbar puncture was however reported in 7% of cases in whom it was performed. Therefore, lumbar punctures must only be performed when cranial imaging shows no brain shift due to the abscess and there is a suspected concomitant meningitis (Brouwer et al., 2014b). Aspiration of the abscess for confirming the diagnosis and the pathogen is often indicated and simultaneously reduces the abscess' size. Using stereotactic neurosurgery, almost all brain abscesses over 1 cm can be targeted for stereotactic aspiration, regardless of location (Brouwer et al., 2014b). Microbiologic evaluation of CSF, blood, or aspirate from the abscess should include a Gram stain, aerobic, and anaerobic cultures. When tuberculosis, fungi, yeasts, or *Nocardia* is included in the differential diagnosis, the appropriate microbiologic investigations for these pathogens should be performed as well. PCR-based 16S ribosomal DNA sequencing may provide a definitive etiologic diagnosis. In a study of 71 patients, of whom 30 had positive cultures, ribosomal DNA sequencing identified bacteria in 59 patients (Al Masalma et al., 2012).

### Subdural empyema

Subdural empyema is diagnosed by cranial imaging (CT or MRI), which shows fluid collection between the cerebral convexity and the skull, adjacent to the falx cerebri or the tentorium. Diffusion-weighted imaging is advocated to enable differentiation between subdural effusion and subdural empyema, in which empyema shows high signal intensity on diffusion-weighted imaging and low signal on apparent diffusion coefficient imaging (Fig. 19.2) (Wong et al., 2004). However, in patients with suspected empyema, for instance, as a complication of bacterial meningitis, mastoiditis, or post neurosurgery, any subdural fluid collection should be considered infectious and treated with a prolonged course of antibiotics. Often neurosurgical evacuation of the empyema is warranted to reduce mass effect and bacterial load. Simultaneously, pus can be acquired for identification of the causative micro-organism by Gram stain and culture. A lumbar puncture is contraindicated because of the risk of brain shift and cerebral herniation. In a cohort of 280 patients with subdural empyema in whom a lumbar puncture was performed, clinical deterioration attributed to the lumbar puncture occurred in 33 patients (12%) (Nathoo et al., 1999).

## HOSPITAL COURSE AND MANAGEMENT

### Community-acquired bacterial meningitis

Patients with suspected bacterial meningitis benefit from rapid initiation of treatment and therefore empiric treatment with antibiotics and dexamethasone should be started directly after the lumbar puncture is performed or before the patient goes to the radiology department,

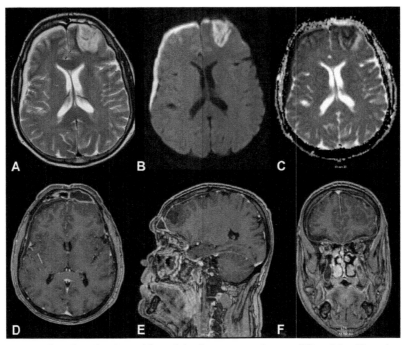

**Fig. 19.2.** Magnetic resonance imaging of patient with a subdural empyema edema on T2-weighted imaging most extensive on the right convexity with extension into a frontal sulcus of the left frontal lobe (**A**), with hyperintense signal on diffusion-weighted imaging (DWI: **B**) and hypointense signal on apparent diffusion coefficient imaging (ADC: **C**). (**D–F**) Axial, sagittal, and coronal T1 images with contrast enhancement of the frontal sinus and empyema in the right convexity subdural space, which extends to the anterior cranial fossa (**F**).

when cranial imaging is indicated prior to the lumbar puncture. The choice of antibiotics depends on local epidemiology and antibiotic-susceptibility patterns (Table 19.1) (Brouwer et al., 2010b). This usually results in a combined regimen of vancomycin plus a third-generation cephalosporin (ceftriaxone or cefotaxime) (Brouwer et al., 2010b; van de Beek et al., 2012). Only in regions where the rate of ceftriaxone resistance to *S. pneumoniae* is low (<1%), monotherapy with a third-generation cephalosporin usually suffices (van de Beek et al., 2012). When *L. monocytogenes* is suspected based on predisposing conditions (immunocompromised state or age >50 years), amoxicillin or ampicillin should be added.

After identification of the pathogen, antibiotic treatment can be modified according to the results of susceptibility testing (Table 19.2). The prevalence of reduced susceptibility of *S. pneumoniae* to penicillin and third-generation cephalosporins has increased over the past decades. Treatment consists of penicillin or amoxicillin/ampicillin if the strain is fully susceptible to penicillin, ceftriaxone or cefotaxime if the strain has reduced susceptibility to penicillin but is fully susceptible to ceftriaxone or cefotaxime, and vancomycin plus ceftriaxone or cefotaxime if there is reduced susceptibility to ceftriaxone or cefotaxime (Brouwer et al., 2010b; van de Beek et al., 2012). When meningococcus is cultured,

susceptible strains are to be treated with penicillin and strains with reduced susceptibility with ceftriaxone of cefotaxime. *Listeria* is treated with amoxicillin for a duration of 3 weeks. Some experts advise to add an aminoglycoside to amoxicillin in the treatment of *Listeria* meningitis because of increased bacterial killing *in vitro*. Retrospective studies provide conflicting data on the effectiveness of aminoglycosides in *Listeria* meningitis (Mylonakis et al., 1998; Mitja et al., 2009).

Outcome of bacterial meningitis has been related to the severity of the inflammatory response in the CNS. Experimental studies showed that adjuvant treatment with corticosteroids reduced the inflammation and thereby could improve outcome. Subsequent trials in children with *H. influenzae* meningitis showed adjunctive dexamethasone reduced hearing loss in the 1980s. In total, 25 randomized controlled trials have been performed so far and showed conflicting results (Brouwer et al., 2015). A large trial of European adults with bacterial meningitis showed dexamethasone reduced mortality and unfavorable outcome, while randomized controlled trials in children in South America and Malawi, and in adults in Viet Nam and Malawi showed no benefit (de Gans and van de Beek, 2002; Molyneux et al., 2002; Nguyen et al., 2007; Scarborough et al., 2007; Brouwer et al., 2015) A Cochrane meta-analysis showed corticosteroids were associated with a nonsignificant reduction in mortality

*Table 19.1*

**Recommendations for initial antibiotic therapy in patients with suspected or proven bacterial central nervous system infection**

| Predisposing factor | Common bacterial pathogens | Initial management |
|---|---|---|
| **Community-acquired bacterial meningitis** | | |
| Age <1 month | *Streptococcus agalactiae, Escherichia coli, Listeria monocytogenes, Klebsiella* species | Ampicillin plus cefotaxime or ampicillin plus an aminoglycoside |
| 2–60 years | *Neisseria meningitidis, Streptococcus pneumoniae* | Vancomycin plus cefotaxime/ ceftriaxone |
| >60 years | *N. meningitidis, S. pneumoniae, L. monocytogenes,* aerobic Gram-negative bacilli | Vancomycin plus cefotaxime/ ceftriaxone plus ampicillin* |
| With risk factor present[†] | *S. pneumoniae, L. monocytogenes, Haemophilus influenzae* | Vancomycin plus cefotaxime/ ceftriaxone plus ampicillin* |
| **Hospital-acquired bacterial meningitis** | | |
| Postneurosurgical infection | Gram-negative bacilli, *Staphylococcus aureus,* coagulase-negative staphylococci | Vancomycin plus cefepime, ceftazidime, or meropenem |
| Ventricular or lumbar cererbrospinal fluid drain | Coagulase-negative staphylococci, *S. aureus,* Gram-negative bacilli, *Propionibacterium acnes* | Vancomycin plus cefepime, ceftazidime, or meropenem |
| Penetrating trauma | *S. aureus,* coagulase-negative staphylococci, Gram-negative bacilli | Vancomycin plus cefepime, ceftazidime, or meropenem |
| Basilar skull fracture | *Streptococcus pneumoniae, Haemophilus influenzae,* group A β-hemolytic streptococci | Vancomycin plus a third-generation cephalosporin |
| **Other** | | |
| Brain abscess | *Streptococcus* and *Staphylococcus* species | Cefotaxime or ceftriaxone plus metronidazole |
| Subdural empyema | *Streptococcus* and *Staphylococcus* species | Cefotaxime or ceftriaxone plus metronidazole |

Modified from Brouwer et al. (2010b, 2014b); van de Beek et al. (2010, 2012).

*In areas with very low penicillin resistance and cephalosporin resistance rates, combination therapy of amoxicillin and third-generation cephalosporin may be considered.

[†]Alcoholism, altered immune status due to use of immunosuppressive drugs, cancer, HIV, and diabetes mellitus.

(17.8% vs. 19.9%). Corticosteroids were associated with lower rates of severe hearing loss and neurologic sequelae. A subgroup analysis showed that corticosteroids reduced mortality in pneumococcal meningitis, but not in meningococcal or *H. influenzae* meningitis. In high-income countries, corticosteroids reduced severe hearing loss, any hearing loss, and short-term neurologic sequelae. There was no beneficial effect of corticosteroid therapy in low-income countries (Brouwer et al., 2015). Following incorporation of adjunctive dexamethasone in treatment guidelines, it has been implemented as routine therapy in a dose of 10 mg QID for 4 days started before or with the first dose of antibiotics (Brouwer et al., 2010a).

Phase IV studies in the Netherlands and USA suggested a decrease in mortality following the introduction of adjunctive dexamethasone (Castelblanco et al., 2014; Bijlsma et al., 2016). Currently, 80–90% of patients are treated with adjunctive dexamethasone. The study in the Netherlands showed there was also a treatment benefit in patients with nonpneumococcal meningitis, implying it can safely be given to all patients with suspected bacterial meningitis, irrespective of causative bacteria. Several

other adjunctive treatments have been tested in randomized controlled trials in the past 25 years, including acetaminophen, glycerol, and therapeutic hypothermia (Ajdukiewicz et al., 2011; Pelkonen et al., 2011; Kasanmoentalib et al., 2013; Mourvillier et al., 2013). None of these treatments showed a beneficial effect on outcome.

Patients with bacterial meningitis are prone to develop neurologic or systemic complications (Bijlsma et al., 2016). Neurologic complications can consist of stroke, including cerebral infarctions (25%), hemorrhage (3%), and sinus thrombosis (1%) (Schut et al., 2012b). Seizures during admission occur in 10–15% of patients and may indicate development of subdural empyema (Zoons et al., 2008). Other neurologic complications are hearing loss, which, depending on the pathogen, occurs in 5–25% of patients (Heckenberg et al., 2012). Furthermore, hydrocephalus may develop and is usually associated with a poor prognosis despite ventriculostomy placement (Kasanmoentalib et al., 2010). Patients with new neurologic deficits during clinical course or a new decrease in consciousness should receive prompt cranial imaging to detect treatable complications. An

*Table 19.2*

**Antimicrobial therapy in community-acquired bacterial meningitis based on cerebrospinal fluid culture results and susceptibility testing**

| Micro-organism, susceptibility | Standard therapy | Alternative therapies |
|---|---|---|
| **Streptococcus pneumoniae** | | |
| ***Penicillin MIC*** | | |
| <0.1 mg/L | Penicillin G or ampicillin | Cefotaxime or ceftriaxone, chloramphenicol |
| 0.1–1.0 mg/L | Cefotaxime or ceftriaxone | Cefepime, meropenem |
| >2.0 mg/L | Vancomycin plus cefotaxime or ceftriaxone | Fluoroquinolone |
| ***Cefotaxime or ceftriaxone MIC*** | | |
| >1.0 mg/L | Vancomycin plus cefotaxime or ceftriaxone | Fluoroquinolone |
| **Neisseria meningitidis** | | |
| ***Penicillin MIC*** | | |
| <0.1 mg/L | Penicillin G or ampicillin | Cefotaxime or ceftriaxone, chloramphenicol |
| 0.1–1.0 mg/L | Cefotaxime or ceftriaxone | Chloramphenicol, fluoroquinolone, meropenem |
| *Listeria monocytogenes* | Penicillin G or ampicillin | Trimethoprim–sulfamethoxazole, meropenem |
| Group B streptococcus | Penicillin G or ampicillin | Cefotaxime or ceftriaxone |
| *Escherichia coli* and other Enterobacteriaceae | Cefotaxime or ceftriaxone | Aztreonam, fluoroquinolone, meropenem, trimethoprim–sulfamethoxazole, ampicillin |
| *Pseudomonas aeruginosa* | Ceftazidime or cefepime | Aztreonam, ciprofloxacin, meropenem |
| **Haemophilus influenzae** | | |
| β-Lactamase-negative | Ampicillin | Cefotaxime or ceftriaxone, cefepime, chloramphenicol, fluoroquinolone |
| β-Lactamase-positive | Cefotaxime or ceftriaxone | Cefepime, chloramphenicol, fluoroquinolone |

MIC, minimum inhibitory concentration.

electroencephalogram may be indicated if there is decreased consciousness without apparent cause on cranial imaging to exclude nonconvulsive status epilepticus. Systemic complications consist of septic shock and respiratory failure which may be due to systemic infection or pneumonia (van de Beek et al., 2004). Hyponatremia is a common, but usually self-limiting, complication of bacterial meningitis that is particularly common in *Listeria* meningitis (Koopmans et al., 2013). Arthritis (and possibly need for debridement) is not a rare complication.

## Hospital-acquired bacterial meningitis

Treatment of hospital-acquired bacterial meningitis consists of high-dose antibiotics covering a broad spectrum of potential pathogens. The advised treatment for patients with postneurosurgical meningitis, a ventricular or lumbar CSF drain, or penetrating trauma, is vancomycin plus cefepime, ceftazidime, or meropenem. For patients with meningitis following a skull-base fracture, treatment consists of vancomycin plus a third-generation cephalosporin (van de Beek et al., 2010). The initiation of treatment is based on the clinical suspicion, but in a substantial proportion of patients microbiologic examination (Gram stain and cultures) remains negative and the question remains

whether meningitis actually occurred. The British Society for Antimicrobial Chemotherapy advices treatment for all patients with suspected postoperative meningitis, but discontinuation after 72 hours if cultures remain negative (Infection in Neurosurgery Working Party of the British Society for Antimicrobial Chemotherapy, 2000). This approach has been prospectively evaluated in 75 patients with suspected postoperative meningitis and showed that stopping antibiotics after 3 days in culture-negative patients is safe and effective (Zarrouk et al., 2007). However, this needs to be assessed separately for each patient, because prior antibiotic treatment may render cultures negative despite bacterial infections.

## Brain abscess

Empiric antibiotic treatment for brain abscesses consists of ceftriaxone and metronidazole to cover both aerobic and anaerobic pathogens (Brouwer et al., 2014b). This can be adjusted according to the culture results. If a pathogen is cultured from blood, the risk of polymicrobial brain abscess must be taken into account before narrowing down the spectrum of antibiotic treatment. In patients with large abscesses, antibiotic treatment alone may fail and reduction of the abscess size through aspiration is needed to enhance recovery. In a review of the literature it was shown that an 88% majority of patients was operated for brain abscess, while the remainder were treated with antibiotics alone (Brouwer et al., 2014a). Excision of the abscess can be considered in superficial abscesses, although with the advent of minimally invasive neurosurgical techniques using stereotactic aspiration, this is becoming less common. A feared complication of brain abscesses is rupture of the abscess into the ventricles, which results in acute hydrocephalus and ventriculitis, and is associated with a high mortality (Brouwer et al., 2014b). Hydrocephalus is also common in patients with a posterior fossa abscess. Epilepsy is a common complication and needs to be treated with antiepileptic drugs. Prophylactic use of antiepileptic drugs has not been studied in brain abscess patients, but was not shown to be effective in other types of space-occupying lesions in the brain (brain tumors). Neurologic deficits may increase during clinical course due to growth of the abscess or an increase in perifocal edema. Corticosteroids are used in 55% of patients with brain abscesses reported in the literature to reduce surrounding edema, although no trials have been performed to determine whether this is beneficial (Brouwer et al., 2014a). As corticosteroids reduce the passage of antibiotics into the nervous system and thereby into the brain abscess, it is only advised in patients in whom edema is likely to result in cerebral herniation (Brouwer et al., 2014b).

## Subdural empyema

Treatment for subdural empyema consists of antibiotic treatment combined with removal of the empyema, usually through burrhole drainage or craniotomy (Nathoo et al., 1999). Simultaneously, the focus of infection can be treated if it is adjacent to the empyema, for instance, mastoiditis or otitis (Fig. 19.2). Antibiotic treatment is similar to that of brain abscesses and consists of cefotaxime or ceftriaxone combined with metronidazole. Seizures are a frequent complication and focal neurologic deficits may increase if the empyema progresses.

## CLINICAL TRIALS AND GUIDELINES

### Community-acquired bacterial meningitis

In recent years several randomized clinical trials have been published on adjunctive treatment of community-acquired bacterial meningitis. An intensive care unit-based study on moderate hypothermia in patients with severe pneumococcal meningitis showed hypothermia was associated with worse outcome, in contrast to previous case series and animal experiments (Mourvillier et al., 2013). Several studies were performed on the effect of glycerol in bacterial meningitis. Glycerol reduces ICP and was first reported to reduce hearing loss in children in South America (Peltola et al., 2007). However, other trials in Africa showed no beneficial effect in children and potential harm of glycerol in adults (Blaser et al., 2010; Molyneux et al., 2014). The effect of acetaminophen was studied in randomized controlled trials in Malawi and Angola, but showed no significant improvement in outcome (Pelkonen et al., 2011; Molyneux et al., 2014). Currently ongoing clinical trials include a Spanish study on prophylactic phenytoin in bacterial meningitis patients to prevent seizures (NCT01478035) and a follow-up trial on acetaminophen in Angola (NCT01540838) (Brouwer et al., 2016).

Guidelines for diagnosis and treatment of community-acquired bacterial meningitis have been published by the Infectious Disease Society of America (IDSA) in 2004, by the European Federation of Neurological Sciences (EFNS) in 2008, and, most recently, by the European Society for Clinical Microbiology and Infectious Diseases (ESCMID) in 2016 (Brouwer and van de Beek, 2015; van de Beek et al., 2016). Antibiotic treatment advice between guidelines is roughly similar, as is the advice on when to perform cranial imaging before lumbar puncture. Differences in the guidelines include the advice to start adjunctive dexamethasone only in patients with suspected *S. pneumoniae* or *H. influenzae* meningitis in the IDSA and EFNS guidelines, whereas the ESCMID guideline recommends including dexamethasone in all patients with suspected or proven bacterial meningitis and consider discontinuing dexamethasone only if other pathogens are identified (Brouwer and van de Beek, 2015). The latter is in line with a recent observational study suggesting dexamethasone was similarly effective in nonpneumococcal meningitis cases (Bijlsma et al., 2016).

### Hospital-acquired bacterial meningitis

Few randomized controlled trials have been performed in hospital-acquired bacterial meningitis. These include a trial on exchange of external ventricular CSF drains 5 days after insertion, which did not result in a reduction of the number of drain-related infections (Wong et al., 2002). Furthermore, a trial comparing intravenous to intraventricular treatment with vancomycin in patients with staphylococcal ventriculitis was performed in 10 patients. This showed higher vancomycin concentration in CSF, but the trial was too small to determine whether intraventricular was superior to intravenous treatment (Pfausler et al., 2003). Currently, no active trials on hospital-acquired bacterial meningitis have been identified in the clinical trials registry (www.clinicaltrials.gov).

## COMPLEX CLINICAL DECISIONS

### Community-acquired bacterial meningitis

Patients with bacterial meningitis may present in a deplorable state and in these patients death may seem imminent. However, the decision on when to discontinue treatment should not be taken too early. A study on patients presenting with a minimal score on the Glasgow Coma Scale, i.e., those who do not have a verbal, motor, or eye-opening response to voice or pain, showed that, out of 30 such patients, 7 had a good clinical outcome (22%) and 12 (40%) survived (Lucas et al., 2014). The decision to discontinue treatment and timing to do so of course depend on multiple factors such as patient's age and comorbid conditions.

Controversy exists on whether to treat the elevated ICP in bacterial meningitis patients, which can occur due to brain swelling or hydrocephalus. Several multistep treatment strategies, including hyperventilation, osmotic agents, CSF drainage and, in exceptional cases, hemicraniectomy, have been described to reduce the ICP in retrospective observational studies, and have been suggested to improve outcome (Edberg et al., 2011; Abulhasan et al., 2013; Glimaker et al., 2014). No randomized controlled trial have been performed and results varied considerably between observational studies. Furthermore, the control groups which were used to compare the intervention groups, did not come from the same population (Glimaker et al., 2014). As the described interventions may also cause substantial harm, further studies are needed before these treatment strategies can be advised for routine use in patients with bacterial meningitis. As the majority of patients have elevated ICP at the initial lumbar puncture and many of them have good outcome, treatment based on ICP alone is not known TO MODIFY OUTCOME (Bijlsma et al., 2016). In a recent large series of patients with ICP monitoring ventriculostomy was used far more often than parenchymal monitors and guided control of ICP, but with only a few successful outcomes with ICP >20 mmHg (Edberg et al., 2011). In animal experiments hypertonic saline (3%) bolus doses are remarkably more successful in control of ICP when compared with mannitol, but there are no comparative studies in humans (Liu et al., 2011). Hypertonic saline may control the commonly observed hyponatremia and maintain a more adequate volume status.

### Brain abscess and subdural empyema

Data on timing of antibiotic treatment for bacterial brain abscesses or subdural empyema are not available. In general 6–8 weeks of intravenous treatment is advised (Tunkel, 2010; Brouwer et al., 2014b), with potential extension if the patient has not shown sufficient clinical improvement or radiologic resolution of the abscess. The Infection in Neurosurgery Working Party of the British Society for Antimicrobial Chemotherapy recommended only 1–2 weeks of intravenous therapy for bacterial brain abscess patients. After such treatment, and depending on the clinical response, a change to an oral regimen is advised (de Louvois et al., 2000). In selected patients this approach has been described to be successful, but it is not considered to be standard therapy. Criteria for evaluating treatment are the neurologic condition of the patient and abscess size on cranial imaging. For both brain abscesses and subdural empyema cranial imaging should be performed immediately if there is clinical deterioration, after 1–2 weeks if there is no improvement, and on a biweekly basis for up to 3 months until clinical recovery is evident (Brouwer et al., 2014b). Further neurosurgery is indicated if there is clinical deterioration with an increase in abscess or empyema size on imaging, despite the use of antimicrobial therapy. If subdural empyema resolves within the 6 weeks of standard treatment, a shorter duration of antibiotic treatment can be considered.

## OUTCOME PREDICTION

Identifying patients at high risk of an unfavorable outcome may be important for counseling patients and their families, as well as deciding upon optimal patient management such as level of care. In community-acquired bacterial meningitis, many risk scores have been developed but only a few have been externally validated in separate datasets. Three validated risk scores have been developed to predict outcome of bacterial meningitis or pneumococcal meningitis (Table 19.3). Predicted outcomes in the studies on all bacterial meningitis patients were a combination of death or neurologic deficits at discharge (Aronin et al., 1998), and unfavorable outcome, defined as a score of 1–4 on the Glasgow Outcome Scale (Aronin et al., 1998; Weisfelt et al., 2008). One risk score has been developed for pneumococcal meningitis with death as predicted outcome (Hoen et al., 1993). Characteristics associated with poor outcome in the risk scores by Aronin et al. (1998) were blood pressure, altered mental status, and baseline seizures. For the score by Weisfelt et al., age, heart rate, score on the Glasgow Coma Scale (GCS), cranial nerve palsy, CSF leukocytes < 1000/mL, and the results of CSF Gram staining were identified as prognostic factors (Hoen et al., 1993). External validation of this Dutch study showed the risk score could not be extrapolated to bacterial meningitis patients from cohorts in Vietnam and Malawi (Schut et al., 2012a). Finally, the risk score by Hoen et al. (1993) for pneumococcal meningitis was based on the following prognostic factors: GCS score ≥7, age > 45 years, CSF

*Table 19.3*

**Calculation of identified risk scores and suggested cut-off values for high risk**

| Population | Study | Score calculation* | Output |
|---|---|---|---|
| Bacterial meningitis | Aronin et al. (1998) | (systolic BP $\leq$ 90 mmHg or a $>$ 40 mmHg decrease) + (altered mental status) + (baseline seizures) | High risk if $\geq$ 2 risk factors present |
| Bacterial meningitis | Weisfelt et al. (2008) | 1/[1 + exp(−lp)], where lp = −1.83 + 0.02*(age in years) + 1.09*(pulse >120/min) −0.13*(GCS) + 0.91*(cranial nerve palsy) + 1.37*(CSF leukocytes < 1000/μL) + 0*(Gram-negative cocci) + 1.29*(Gram-positive cocci) + 0.19*(no bacteria) + 0.24*(other Gram result) | Risk calculated by use of nomogram (Weisfelt et al., 2008) |
| Pneumococcal meningitis | Hoen et al. (1993) | 1/[1 + exp(−lp)], where lp = −2.36*(GCS score $\geq$ 7) + 1.90*(age > 45 years) −1.89*(CSF glucose $\geq$ 0.6 mmol/l) + 1.30*(concomitant pneumonia) −0.24 | High risk > 0.7 |

BP, blood pressure; GCS, Glasgow Coma Score; CSF, cerebrospinal fluid.

glucose $\geq$ 0.6 mmol/L, and concomitant pneumonia (Hoen et al., 1993). Whether these risk scores are applied in clinical practice is unclear.

## NEUROREHABILITATION

Neurorehabilitation may be indicated for patients with focal neurologic sequelae due to bacterial meningitis, cerebral abscess, or subdural empyema. Approximately one-third of patients surviving bacterial meningitis will have sequelae or persisting complaints. A systematic review analyzed sequelae of bacterial meningitis in children and showed hearing loss occurred in 34% of survivors, seizures in 13%, motor deficits in 12%, cognitive defects in 9%, hydrocephalus in 7%, and visual loss in 6% (Edmond et al., 2012). One in five children had multiple sequelae. Common sequelae in adults are neurologic deficits due to cerebral infarctions, hearing loss, and cognitive slowness (Hoogman et al., 2007; Heckenberg et al., 2012; Schut et al., 2012b). To improve successful return to school for children and to society for adults, recognition of these sequelae is essential. When returning home, neuropsychologic sequelae may come to light that hinder functioning in work and at home. Patients, family members, and caregivers should be informed about the potential sequelae and when to contact their physician. Neuropsychologic sequelae in children often consist of failure to learn in school and poor development of cognitive abilities for their age. Learning problems were found in 10–20% of children and 12–33% of children had to repeat school years or required referral to a special-needs school after pneumococcal meningitis in one Dutch follow-up study (Koomen et al., 2004). In a Dutch study including 155 adult survivors of bacterial meningitis and 72 healthy controls, neuropsychologic examination revealed that 32% had cognitive defects compared to 6% in the control group. The most apparent

defect was cognitive slowness (Hoogman et al., 2007). A follow-up study in the same population 9 years after bacterial meningitis found that psychologic functioning and quality of life had returned to normal on a group level, but some cognitive slowness persisted on an individual level (Schmand et al., 2010). Cognitive neurorehabilitation is indicated when neuropsychologic examination shows the above-mentioned abnormalities.

Hearing loss is a common complication of bacterial meningitis and may require treatment a couple of weeks after meningitis occurred (Worsoe et al., 2010). Especially in young children hearing loss may go undetected for a period of time, which negatively influences speech development. Cochlear implants may be indicated to improve hearing, and should be placed in a timely fashion, as cochlear fibrosis and calcification may occur within a couple of weeks after meningitis, and limit the function of the implant. Therefore, it is necessary to identify hearing loss quickly in both children and adults with bacterial meningitis, and hearing evaluation should be performed during admission. In patients with over 30 dB hearing loss or progressive hearing loss over time, contrast-enhanced MRI, repeated hearing evaluation, and consultation with a cochlear implantation specialist are indicated.

## REFERENCES

Abulhasan YB, Al-Jehani H, Valiquette MA et al. (2013). Lumbar drainage for the treatment of severe bacterial meningitis. Neurocrit Care 19: 199–205.

Ajdukiewicz KM, Cartwright KE, Scarborough M et al. (2011). Glycerol adjuvant therapy in adults with bacterial meningitis in a high HIV seroprevalence setting in Malawi: a double-blind, randomised controlled trial. Lancet Infect Dis 11: 293–300.

Al Masalma M, Lonjon M, Richet H et al. (2012). Metagenomic analysis of brain abscesses identifies specific bacterial associations. Clin Infect Dis 54: 202–210.

Aronin SI, Peduzzi P, Quagliarello VJ (1998). Community-acquired bacterial meningitis: risk stratification for adverse clinical outcome and effect of antibiotic timing. Ann Intern Med 129: 862–869.

Baltas I, Tsoulfa S, Sakellariou P et al. (1994). Posttraumatic meningitis: bacteriology, hydrocephalus, and outcome. Neurosurgery 35: 422–426.

Bijlsma MW, Bekker V, Brouwer MC et al. (2014a). Epidemiology of invasive meningococcal disease in the Netherlands, 1960–2012: an analysis of national surveillance data. Lancet Infect Dis 14: 805–812.

Bijlsma MW, Brouwer MC, Spanjaard L et al. (2014b). A decade of herd protection after introduction of meningococcal serogroup C conjugate vaccination. Clin Infect Dis 59: 1216–1221.

Bijlsma MW, Brouwer MC, Kasanmoentalib ES et al. (2016). Community-acquired bacterial meningitis in adults in the Netherlands, 2006–14: a prospective cohort study. Lancet Infect Dis 16: 339–347.

Blaser C, Klein M, Grandgirard D et al. (2010). Adjuvant glycerol is not beneficial in experimental pneumococcal meningitis. BMC Infect Dis 10: 84.

Brouwer MC, van de Beek D (2015). Earlier treatment and improved outcome in adult bacterial meningitis following guideline revision promoting prompt lumbar puncture. Clin Infect Dis 61: 664–665.

Brouwer MC, Heckenberg SG, de Gans J et al. (2010a). Nationwide implementation of adjunctive dexamethasone therapy for pneumococcal meningitis. Neurology 75: 1533–1539.

Brouwer MC, Tunkel AR, van de Beek D (2010b). Epidemiology, diagnosis, and antimicrobial treatment of acute bacterial meningitis. Clin Microbiol Rev 23: 467–492.

Brouwer MC, Thwaites GE, Tunkel AR et al. (2012). Dilemmas in the diagnosis of acute community-acquired bacterial meningitis. Lancet 380: 1684–1692.

Brouwer MC, Coutinho JM, van de Beek D (2014a). Clinical characteristics and outcome of brain abscess: systematic review and meta-analysis. Neurology 82: 806–813.

Brouwer MC, Tunkel AR, McKhann 2nd GM et al. (2014b). Brain abscess. N Engl J Med 371: 447–456.

Brouwer MC, McIntyre P, Prasad K et al. (2015). Corticosteroids for acute bacterial meningitis. Cochrane Database Syst Rev 9. CD004405.

Brouwer MC, Wijdicks EF, van de Beek D (2016). What's new in bacterial meningitis. Intensive Care Med 42: 415–417.

Castelblanco RL, Lee M, Hasbun R (2014). Epidemiology of bacterial meningitis in the USA from 1997 to 2010: a population-based observational study. Lancet Infect Dis 14: 813–819.

Choi SH, Choi SH (2013). Predictive performance of serum procalcitonin for the diagnosis of bacterial meningitis after neurosurgery. Infect Chemother 45: 308–314.

Corless CE, Guiver M, Borrow R et al. (2001). Simultaneous detection of *Neisseria meningitidis, Haemophilus influenzae,* and *Streptococcus pneumoniae* in suspected cases of meningitis and septicemia using real-time PCR. J Clin Microbiol 39: 1553–1558.

de Gans J, van de Beek D (2002). Dexamethasone in adults with bacterial meningitis. N Engl J Med 347: 1549–1556.

de Louvois J, Brown EM, Bayston R et al. (2000). The rational use of antibiotics in the treatment of brain abscess. Br J Neurosurg 14: 525–530.

Dubos F, Korczowski B, Aygun DA et al. (2008). Serum procalcitonin level and other biological markers to distinguish between bacterial and aseptic meningitis in children: a European multicenter case cohort study. Arch Pediatr Adolesc Med 162: 1157–1163.

Durand ML, Calderwood SB, Weber DJ et al. (1993). Acute bacterial meningitis in adults. A review of 493 episodes. N Engl J Med 328: 21–28.

Edberg M, Furebring M, Sjolin J et al. (2011). Neurointensive care of patients with severe community-acquired meningitis. Acta Anaesthesiol Scand 55: 732–739.

Edmond K, Scott S, Korczak V et al. (2012). Long term sequelae from childhood pneumonia; systematic review and meta-analysis. PLoS One 7. e31239.

Glimaker M, Johansson B, Halldorsdottir H et al. (2014). Neuro-intensive treatment targeting intracranial hypertension improves outcome in severe bacterial meningitis: an intervention-control study. PLoS One 9. e91976.

Hasbun R, Abrahams J, Jekel J et al. (2001). Computed tomography of the head before lumbar puncture in adults with suspected meningitis. N Engl J Med 345: 1727–1733.

Heckenberg SG, Brouwer MC, van der Ende A et al. (2012). Hearing loss in adults surviving pneumococcal meningitis is associated with otitis and pneumococcal serotype. Clin Microbiol Infect 18: 849–855.

Heinsbroek E, Ladhani S, Gray S et al. (2013). Added value of PCR-testing for confirmation of invasive meningococcal disease in England. J Infect 67: 385–390.

Hoen B, Viel JF, Gerard A et al. (1993). Mortality in pneumococcal meningitis: a multivariate analysis of prognostic factors. Eur J Med 2: 28–32.

Hoogman M, van de Beek D, Weisfelt M et al. (2007). Cognitive outcome in adults after bacterial meningitis. J Neurol Neurosurg Psychiatry 78: 1092–1096.

Infection in Neurosurgery Working Party of the British Society for Antimicrobial Chemotherapy (2000). The management of neurosurgical patients with postoperative bacterial or aseptic meningitis or external ventricular drain-associated ventriculitis. Br J Neurosurg 14: 7–12.

Jim KK, Brouwer MC, van der Ende A et al. (2012). Subdural empyema in bacterial meningitis. Neurology 79: 2133–2139.

Kasanmoentalib ES, Brouwer MC, van der Ende A et al. (2010). Hydrocephalus in adults with community-acquired bacterial meningitis. Neurology 75: 918–923.

Kasanmoentalib ES, Brouwer MC, van de Beek D (2013). Update on bacterial meningitis: epidemiology, trials and genetic association studies. Curr Opin Neurol 26: 282–288.

Koomen I, Grobbee DE, Roord JJ et al. (2004). Prediction of academic and behavioural limitations in school-age survivors of bacterial meningitis. Acta Paediatr 93: 1378–1385.

Koopmans MM, Brouwer MC, Bijlsma MW et al. (2013). Listeria monocytogenes sequence type 6 and increased rate of unfavorable outcome in meningitis: epidemiologic cohort study. Clin Infect Dis 57: 247–253.

Le Monnier A, Abachin E, Beretti JL et al. (2011). Diagnosis of *Listeria monocytogenes* meningoencephalitis by real-time PCR for the hly gene. J Clin Microbiol 49: 3917–3923.

Liu S, Li L, Luo Z et al. (2011). Superior effect of hypertonic saline over mannitol to attenuate cerebral edema in a rabbit bacterial meningitis model. Crit Care Med 39: 1467–1473.

Lucas MJ, Brouwer MC, van der Ende A et al. (2013). Endocarditis in adults with bacterial meningitis. Circulation 127: 2056–2062.

Lucas MJ, Brouwer MC, van der Ende A et al. (2014). Outcome in patients with bacterial meningitis presenting with a minimal Glasgow Coma Scale score. Neurol Neuroimmunol Neuroinflamm 1: e9.

McIntyre PB, O'Brien KL, Greenwood B et al. (2012). Effect of vaccines on bacterial meningitis worldwide. Lancet 380: 1703–1711.

Mitja O, Pigrau C, Ruiz I et al. (2009). Predictors of mortality and impact of aminoglycosides on outcome in listeriosis in a retrospective cohort study. J Antimicrob Chemother 64: 416–423.

Moisi JC, Saha SK, Falade AG et al. (2009). Enhanced diagnosis of pneumococcal meningitis with use of the Binax NOW immunochromatographic test of *Streptococcus pneumoniae* antigen: a multisite study. Clin Infect Dis 48 (Suppl 2): S49–S56.

Molyneux EM, Walsh AL, Forsyth H et al. (2002). Dexamethasone treatment in childhood bacterial meningitis in Malawi: a randomised controlled trial. Lancet 360: 211–218.

Molyneux EM, Kawaza K, Phiri A et al. (2014). Glycerol and acetaminophen as adjuvant therapy did not affect the outcome of bacterial meningitis in Malawian children. Pediatr Infect Dis J 33: 214–216.

Mourvillier B, Tubach F, van de Beek D et al. (2013). Induced hypothermia in severe bacterial meningitis: a randomized clinical trial. JAMA 310: 2174–2183.

Munoz-Almagro C, Rodriguez-Plata MT, Marin S et al. (2009). Polymerase chain reaction for diagnosis and serogrouping of meningococcal disease in children. Diagn Microbiol Infect Dis 63: 148–154.

Munoz-Gomez S, Wirkowski E, Cunha BA (2015). Post craniotomy extra-ventricular drain (EVD) associated nosocomial meningitis: CSF diagnostic criteria. Heart Lung 44: 158–160.

Mylonakis E, Hohmann EL, Calderwood SB (1998). Central nervous system infection with Listeria monocytogenes. 33 years' experience at a general hospital and review of 776 episodes from the literature. Medicine (Baltimore) 77: 313–336.

Nathoo N, Nadvi SS, van Dellen JR et al. (1999). Intracranial subdural empyemas in the era of computed tomography: a review of 699 cases. Neurosurgery 44: 529–535. discussion 535–526.

Nau R, Soto A, Bruck W (1999). Apoptosis of neurons in the dentate gyrus in humans suffering from bacterial meningitis. J Neuropathol Exp Neurol 58: 265–274.

Nguyen TH, Tran TH, Thwaites G et al. (2007). Dexamethasone in Vietnamese adolescents and adults with bacterial meningitis. N Engl J Med 357: 2431–2440.

Nicolosi A, Hauser WA, Musicco M et al. (1991). Incidence and prognosis of brain abscess in a defined population: Olmsted County, Minnesota, 1935–1981. Neuroepidemiology 10: 122–131.

Nigrovic LE, Kuppermann N, McAdam AJ et al. (2004). Cerebrospinal latex agglutination fails to contribute to the microbiologic diagnosis of pretreated children with meningitis. Pediatr Infect Dis J 23: 786–788.

Nigrovic LE, Malley R, Macias CG et al. (2008). Effect of antibiotic pretreatment on cerebrospinal fluid profiles of children with bacterial meningitis. Pediatrics 122: 726–730.

Parent dC I, Traore Y, Gessner BD et al. (2005). Bacterial meningitis in Burkina Faso: surveillance using field-based polymerase chain reaction testing. Clin Infect Dis 40: 17–25.

Pelkonen T, Roine I, Cruzeiro ML et al. (2011). Slow initial beta-lactam infusion and oral paracetamol to treat childhood bacterial meningitis: a randomised, controlled trial. Lancet Infect Dis 11: 613–621.

Peltola H, Roine I, Fernandez J et al. (2007). Adjuvant glycerol and/or dexamethasone to improve the outcomes of childhood bacterial meningitis: a prospective, randomized, double-blind, placebo-controlled trial. Clin Infect Dis 45: 1277–1286.

Pfausler B, Spiss H, Beer R et al. (2003). Treatment of staphylococcal ventriculitis associated with external cerebrospinal fluid drains: a prospective randomized trial of intravenous compared with intraventricular vancomycin therapy. J Neurosurg 98: 1040–1044.

Ray P, Badarou-Acossi G, Viallon A et al. (2007). Accuracy of the cerebrospinal fluid results to differentiate bacterial from non bacterial meningitis, in case of negative gram-stained smear. Am J Emerg Med 25: 179–184.

Read RC, Baxter D, Chadwick DR et al. (2014). Effect of a quadrivalent meningococcal ACWY glycoconjugate or a serogroup B meningococcal vaccine on meningococcal carriage: an observer-blind, phase 3 randomised clinical trial. Lancet 384: 2123–2131.

Reddy JS, Mishra AM, Behari S et al. (2006). The role of diffusion-weighted imaging in the differential diagnosis of intracranial cystic mass lesions: a report of 147 lesions. Surg Neurol 66: 246–250.

Saha SK, Darmstadt GL, Yamanaka N et al. (2005). Rapid diagnosis of pneumococcal meningitis: implications for treatment and measuring disease burden. Pediatr Infect Dis J 24: 1093–1098.

Scarborough M, Gordon SB, Whitty CJ et al. (2007). Corticosteroids for bacterial meningitis in adults in sub-Saharan Africa. N Engl J Med 357: 2441–2450.

Schmand B, de Bruin E, de Gans J et al. (2010). Cognitive functioning and quality of life nine years after bacterial meningitis. J Infect 61: 330–334.

Schut ES, Brouwer MC, Scarborough M et al. (2012a). Validation of a Dutch risk score predicting poor outcome in adults with bacterial meningitis in Vietnam and Malawi. PLoS One 7: e34311.

Schut ES, Lucas MJ, Brouwer MC et al. (2012b). Cerebral infarction in adults with bacterial meningitis. Neurocrit Care 16: 421–427.

Sormunen P, Kallio MJ, Kilpi T et al. (1999). C-reactive protein is useful in distinguishing Gram stain-negative bacterial meningitis from viral meningitis in children. J Pediatr 134: 725–729.

Spanos A, Harrell Jr FE, Durack DT (1989). Differential diagnosis of acute meningitis. An analysis of the predictive value of initial observations. JAMA 262: 2700–2707.

Stephens DS, Greenwood B, Brandtzaeg P (2007). Epidemic meningitis, meningococcaemia, and *Neisseria meningitidis*. Lancet 369: 2196–2210.

Thigpen MC, Whitney CG, Messonnier NE et al. (2011). Bacterial meningitis in the United States, 1998–2007. N Engl J Med 364: 2016–2025.

Thompson MJ, Ninis N, Perera R et al. (2006). Clinical recognition of meningococcal disease in children and adolescents. Lancet 367: 397–403.

Tunkel AR (2010). Brain abscess. In: GL Mandell, JE Bennett, R Dolin (Eds.), Principles and practice of infectious diseases, 7th edn. Churchill Livingstone, Philadelphia.

Tzanakaki G, Tsopanomichalou M, Kesanopoulos K et al. (2005). Simultaneous single-tube PCR assay for the detection of *Neisseria meningitidis, Haemophilus influenzae* type b and *Streptococcus pneumoniae*. Clin Microbiol Infect 11: 386–390.

van de Beek D, de Gans J, Spanjaard L et al. (2004). Clinical features and prognostic factors in adults with bacterial meningitis. N Engl J Med 351: 1849–1859.

van de Beek D, de Gans J, Tunkel AR et al. (2006). Community-acquired bacterial meningitis in adults. N Engl J Med 354: 44–53.

van de Beek D, Drake JM, Tunkel AR (2010). Nosocomial bacterial meningitis. N Engl J Med 362: 146–154.

van de Beek D, Brouwer MC, Thwaites GE et al. (2012). Advances in treatment of bacterial meningitis. Lancet 380: 1693–1702.

van de Beek D, Cabellos C, Dzupova O et al. (2016). ESCMID guideline: diagnosis and treatment of acute bacterial meningitis. Clin Microbiol Infect 22 (suppl. 3): S37–S62.

Vergouwen MD, Schut ES, Troost D et al. (2010). Diffuse cerebral intravascular coagulation and cerebral infarction in pneumococcal meningitis. Neurocrit Care 13: 217–227.

Vinchon M, Dhellemmes P (2006). Cerebrospinal fluid shunt infection: risk factors and long-term follow-up. Childs Nerv Syst 22: 692–697.

Weisfelt M, van de Beek D, Spanjaard L et al. (2008). A risk score for unfavorable outcome in adults with bacterial meningitis. Ann Neurol 63: 90–97.

Wong GK, Poon WS, Wai S et al. (2002). Failure of regular external ventricular drain exchange to reduce cerebrospinal fluid infection: result of a randomised controlled trial. J Neurol Neurosurg Psychiatry 73: 759–761.

Wong AM, Zimmerman RA, Simon EM et al. (2004). Diffusion-weighted MR imaging of subdural empyemas in children. AJNR Am J Neuroradiol 25: 1016–1021.

Worsoe L, Caye-Thomasen P, Brandt CT et al. (2010). Factors associated with the occurrence of hearing loss after pneumococcal meningitis. Clin Infect Dis 51: 917–924.

Zarrouk V, Vassor I, Bert F et al. (2007). Evaluation of the management of postoperative aseptic meningitis. Clin Infect Dis 44: 1555–1559.

Zoons E, Weisfelt M, de Gans J et al. (2008). Seizures in adults with bacterial meningitis. Neurology 70: 2109–2115.

*Handbook of Clinical Neurology,* Vol. 140 (3rd series)
*Critical Care Neurology, Part I*
E.F.M. Wijdicks and A.H. Kramer, Editors
http://dx.doi.org/10.1016/B978-0-444-63600-3.00020-9

Chapter 20

# Management of infections associated with neurocritical care

L. RIVERA-LARA[1], W. ZIAI[2], AND P. NYQUIST[3]*

[1]*Department of Anesthesiology and Critical Care Medicine and Neurology,*
*Johns Hopkins University School of Medicine, Baltimore, MD, USA*

[2]*Departments of Anesthesiology and Critical Care Medicine, and Neurology and Neurosurgery, Johns Hopkins University*
*School of Medicine, Baltimore, MD, USA*

[3]*Departments of Anesthesiology and Critical Care Medicine, Neurology and Neurosurgery, and General Internal Medicine,*
*Johns Hopkins University School of Medicine, Baltimore, MD, USA*

**Abstract**

The reported incidence of hospital-acquired infections (HAIs) in the neurointensive care unit (NICU) ranges from 20% to 30%. HAIs in US hospitals cost between $28 and $45 billion per year in direct medical costs. These infections are associated with increased length of hospital stay and increased morbidity and mortality. Infection risk is increased in NICU patients due to medication side-effects, catheter and line placement, neurosurgical procedures, and acquired immune suppression secondary to steroid/barbiturate use and brain injury itself. Some of these infections may be preventable but many are not. Their appearance do not always constitute a failure of prevention or physician error. Neurointensivists require indepth knowledge of common nosocomial infections, their diagnosis and treatment, and an approach to evidence-based practices that improve processes of care and reduce HAIs.

## INTRODUCTION

Data from the National Nosocomial Infection Surveillance system and Centers for Disease Control and Prevention (CDC) show that hospital-acquired infections (HAIs) represent a significant proximal cause of mortality in hospitals and intensive care units (ICUs). In 2002 HAIs resulted in almost 100 000 deaths (Orsi et al., 2006; Klevens et al., 2007). The Centers for Medicare and Medicaid Services have recently mandated denial of payment to hospitals for costs associated with "preventable infection" (Calfee, 2012). Most neurointensive ICU (NICU) infections are nosocomial and related to indwelling arterial lines, urinary catheters, external ventricular drains (EVDs), and ventilators. Other nonnosocomial primary infections of the nervous system are also treated in the NICU, including encephalitis, meningitis, and ventriculitis. Susceptibility to infection is often increased in

the NICU related to acquired immune suppression from brain injury and exposure to the associated stress of intensive care (Poungvarin et al., 1987; Wolach et al., 2001; Morris et al., 2011; Hunter, 2012; Conway Morris et al., 2013). This chapter reviews the prevention, diagnosis, and management of infections associated with NICU care.

## INFECTIONS IN THE NEUROSCIENCES INTENSIVE CARE UNIT

### Pneumonia

Ventilator-associated pneumonia (VAP) is defined as pneumonia that occurs 48–72 hours after endotracheal intubation and contributes to half of all cases of hospital-acquired pneumonia (HAP) (American Thoracic Society

*Correspondence to: Paul Nyquist, MD, MPH, Department of Anesthesiology and Critical Care Medicine, Johns Hopkins University, 1800 Orleans Street/Phipps 455, Baltimore MD 21287-7840, USA. Tel: +1-410-955-2611, Fax: +1-410-614-7903, E-mail: pnyquis1@jhmi.edu

and Infectious Diseases Society of America, 2005). VAP is estimated to occur in 9–27% of all mechanically ventilated patients (Chastre and Fagon, 2002; American Thoracic Society and Infectious Diseases Society of America, 2005). Measurements of attributable mortality of VAP range from 20% to 50% in medical ICU patients (Safdar et al., 2005). Additionally, VAP is the most commonly reported nosocomial infection in mechanically ventilated patients and accounts for 50% of all antibiotics given in the ICU (Vincent et al., 1995; Hunter, 2012). VAP is associated with increased duration of mechanical ventilation, increased length of ICU stay, and increased healthcare costs (Rello et al., 2002; Koenig and Truwit, 2006; Amin, 2009).

Estimates of prevalence and incidence of VAP vary due to inconsistency in the instruments for case definition. Most diagnostic criteria incorporate core variables, including the presence of new or progressive infiltrates, signs of systemic infection (fever, white blood cell count), changes in sputum characteristics, and detection of a causative agent (American Thoracic Society and Infectious Diseases Society of America, 2005). Miner studied differences in incidences by case definition in VAP in a single cohort of surgical ICU patients and reported estimated incidences ranged from 4% to 48%, using the Johanson definition and CDC definition respectively (Minei et al., 2000) (http://www.cdc.gov/nhsn/pdfs/pscmanual/6pscvapcurrent.pdf).

In 2012 the National Healthcare Safety Network (NHSN) reported that the incidence of VAP in neurocritical care units ranged from 2.1 (neurosurgical units) to 3.0 (neurologic units) per 1000 ventilator days (Dudeck et al., 2013). Variable VAP rates are reported in the NICU, with incidence ranging from 4% to 31.3% (Josephson et al., 2010; Kuusinen et al., 2012; Kalanuria et al., 2015). In the NICU VAP diagnosis is more problematic due to the ubiquitous nature of clinical findings related to primary brain injury, such as fever, leukocytosis, and altered mental status. The clinical factors most likely to differentiate surveillance defined versus clinically treated VAP in a NICU population are change in sputum character, tachypnea, oxygen desaturation, persistent infiltrate on chest X-ray, and higher clinical pulmonary infection score (Table 20.1). Unexpectedly, a positive sputum culture is not strongly associated (Kalanuria et al., 2015). In a large prospective observational cohort study of HAIs in neurosurgical patients, length of stay was significantly longer among infected versus noninfected patients (median 54 vs. 11 days respectively, $p < 0.01$) and mortality was significantly associated with HAIs, with an increased relative risk of 2.04 (95% confidence interval (CI) 1.30–3.20; $p < 0.01$) (Orsi et al., 2006). However, other studies have shown no association between VAP and increased mortality

*Table 20.1*

**The clinical pulmonary infection score (CPIS)**

| Assessed parameter | Result | Score |
|---|---|---|
| Temperature (°C) | 36.5–38.4°C | 0 |
| | 38.5–38.9°C | 1 |
| | ≤36 or ≥39°C | 2 |
| Leukocytes in blood (cells/mm³) | 4000–11 000/mm³ | 0 |
| | <4000 or >11 000/mm³ | 1 |
| | ≥500 band cells | 2 |
| Tracheal secretions (subjective visual scale) | None | 0 |
| | Mild/nonpurulent | 1 |
| | Purulent | 2 |
| Radiographic findings (on chest radiography, excluding CHF and ARDS) | No infiltrate | 0 |
| | Diffuse/patchy infiltrate | 1 |
| | Localized infiltrate | 2 |
| Culture results (endotracheal aspirate) | No or mild growth | 0 |
| | Moderate or florid growth | 1 |
| | Moderate or florid growth and pathogen consistent with Gram stain | 2 |
| Oxygenation status (defined by $Pao_2$: $Fio_2$) | >240 or ARDS | 0 |
| | ≤240 and absence of ARDS | 2 |

Adapted from Kalanuria et al. (2014).
CHF, congestive heart failure; ARDS, acute respiratory distress syndrome.

in intubated NICU patients (Josephson et al., 2010). The presence of neurologic disease has been identified as an independent risk factor for development of VAP and for failure of VAP resolution with initial antibiotic therapy (Cook, 2000; Shorr et al., 2008). Neurologic patients are particularly vulnerable to pneumonia due to decreased consciousness, dysphagia, and impaired protective airway reflexes (Berrouane et al., 1998).

## CAUSATIVE ORGANISMS

The causative organism in VAP often depends on the duration of mechanical ventilation. Early-onset VAP, occurring within 4 days of intubation, is usually attributed to antibiotic-sensitive pathogens, such as *Haemophilus influenzae, Streptococcus pneumoniae,* and methicillin-sensitive *Staphylococcus aureus, Escherichia coli, Klebsiella pneumoniae, Enterobacter* species, *Proteus* species, and *Serratia marcescens.* Late-onset VAP occurring later than 4 days after intubation is more likely caused by multidrug-resistant (MDR) pathogens, such as *Pseudomonas aeruginosa, Acinetobacter,*

*Table 20.2*

**Pathogens that caused ventilator-associated pneumonia (VAP) with their frequency in hospital-acquired pneumonia**

| VAP pathogens | Frequency |
| --- | --- |
| *Pseudomonas* | 24.4% |
| *Staphylococcus aureus* | 20.4% |
| Enterobacteriaceae (*Klebsiella* spp., | 14.1% |
| *Escherichia coli*, *Proteus* spp., *Enterobacter* | |
| spp., *Serratia* spp., *Citrobacter* spp.) | |
| *Streptococcus* species | 12.1% |
| *Haemophilus* species | 9.8% |
| *Acinetobacter* species | 7.9% |
| *Neisseria* species | 2.6% |
| Coagulase-negative staphylococcus | 1.4% |
| Others (*Corynebacterium*, *Moraxella*, | 4.7% |
| *Enterococcus*, fungi, virus) | |

Modified from Vincent et al. (1995); Chastre and Fagon (2002); American Thoracic Society and Infectious Diseases Society of America (2005); Bhattacharya (2013).

methicillin-resistant *S. aureus* (MRSA), and extended-spectrum beta-lactamase-producing bacteria (American Thoracic Society and Infectious Diseases Society of America, 2005; Hunter, 2012) (Table 20.2). MDR bacteria are the causative organism in one-quarter to one-third of VAP cases and carry a significantly increased mortality risk (Depuydt et al., 2008). Common risk factors for MDR bacterial infection include history of hospital admission for $\geq 2$ days in the past 90 days, nursing-home residents, chemotherapy, or antibiotics in the last 30 days, exposure to more than two classes of antibiotics during hospitalization, septic shock, high frequency of antibiotic resistance in the hospital, hemodialysis at outpatient centers, and poor functional status prior to illness (American Thoracic Society and Infectious Diseases Society of America, 2005; Hunter, 2012; Martin-Loeches et al., 2014).

## DIAGNOSIS

Daily bedside evaluation in conjunction with chest radiography is suggestive, but not definitive for the presence or absence of VAP (Petersen et al., 1999). Differential diagnosis of pulmonary infiltrates includes aspiration pneumonitis, pulmonary embolism, pulmonary hemorrhage, acute respiratory distress syndrome, infiltrative tumor, lung contusion, radiation pneumonitis, and congestive heart failure. In general the correlation of chest radiography with autopsy-proven pneumonia lacks precision (Wunderink et al., 1992).

Presently, there is general consensus that VAP should be suspected when there are new or persistent infiltrates on chest radiograph with two or more of the following:

fever, leukocytosis/leukopenia, and purulent tracheobronchial secretions (Fabregas et al., 1999).

Many of the weaknesses in diagnosing VAP have been addressed by revised CDC surveillance definitions for VAP. Diagnostic criteria such as radiographic infiltrates, altered mental status, fever, and leukocytosis/leukopenia have been removed and replaced by persistent clinical findings. Newer guidelines emphasize variables such as persistent positive quantitative or semiquantitative cultures. They exclude clinically confusing or imprecise findings such as mixed respiratory or oral flora, *Candida*, coagulase-negative *Staphylococcus*, and *Enterococcus* (Luna et al., 1997). The new CDC algorithm, however, is for surveillance purposes and not for clinical use.

### ASPIRATION AND BRONCHIAL CULTURES

The American Thoracic Society (ATS) and the Infectious Diseases Society of America (IDSA) guidelines recommend obtaining lower respiratory tract samples for culture and microbiology, ideally before antibiotics are started (American Thoracic Society and Infectious Diseases Society of America, 2005). There are several methods for obtaining microbiologic samples. Invasive sampling methods requiring bronchoscopy include bronchoalveolar lavage (BAL) and protected specimen brushing (PSB). The mini-BAL and tracheobronchial aspiration are blind methods not requiring bronchoscopy. Clinical trials comparing the two strategies have failed to show an advantage to direct bronchoscopy as compared to blind methods (Chastre et al., 1995; Kirtland et al., 1997; The Canadian Critical Care Trials Group, 2006). Once specimens are obtained, the sample is sent for Gram stain, differential white cell count, culture, and sensitivity. The Gram stain can provide crucial initial clues to the type of organism(s) and identify purulence (defined as $\geq 25$ neutrophils and $\leq 10$ squamous epithelial cells per low-power field (American Thoracic Society and Infectious Diseases Society of America, 2005).

Culture analysis can be quantitative or semiquantitative. Diagnostic thresholds for tracheobronchial aspiration, BAL, and PSB are $10^6$, $10^4$, and $10^3$ colony-forming units (CFU) per milliliter, respectively (Chastre et al., 1995; American Thoracic Society and Infectious Diseases Society of America, 2005). Semiquantitative cultures are reported as heavy, moderate, light, or no growth. Heavy and moderate growth are considered indicative of VAP (American Thoracic Society and Infectious Diseases Society of America, 2005). A meta-analysis of three randomized trials comparing quantitative versus semiquantitative cultures failed to identify an impact on mortality or length of stay (Berton et al., 2012).

## Treatment

In general, antibiotics should be administered empirically for VAP for a high degree of clinical suspicion. Delayed antimicrobial therapy is associated with increased mortality (Iregui et al., 2002). VAP diagnosis can be confirmed or refuted once cultures return after 2–3 days. At that time culture results should guide continued antibiotic therapy if clinically necessary. The treatment of VAP is guided by recommendations of the ATS and the IDSA in conjunction with local institutional surveillance data on prevalence and resistance patterns and patient-specific risk factors for MDR organisms (American Thoracic Society and Infectious Diseases Society of America, 2005). Inappropriate initial antibiotic therapy independently increases the risk for mortality in VAP three- to sevenfold (Iregui et al., 2002; Jackson and Shorr, 2006).

For patients with early VAP, without risk factors for MDR bacteria, one of the following options is appropriate: second- or third-generation cephalosporin (ceftriaxone or cefuroxime), ampicillin sulbactam, fluoroquinolone (levofloxacin or moxifloxacin), or ertapenem. When institutional data suggest higher prevalence of Gram-negative resistant bacilli (*Enterobacter* spp., *Serratia* spp., *Pseudomonas* spp.), piperacillin-tazobactam, cefepime, or a carbapenem may be used as monotherapy (American Thoracic Society and Infectious Diseases Society of America, 2005).

Patients with late-onset VAP or risk of MDR bacteria can be treated with monotherapy, including antipseudomonal cephalosporin (cefepime or ceftazidime), piperacillin-tazobactam, antipseudomonal carbapenem (imipenem), or aztreonam (for patients with a penicillin allergy). Combination therapy for *Pseudomonas aeruginosa* and *Acinetobacter* is controversial and its recommendation varies institutionally due to the high rate of resistance to monotherapy (Kalanuria et al., 2014). A meta-analysis compared treatment failure of monotherapy versus combination therapy for VAP in 41 trials and found that monotherapy is not inferior to combination therapy in the empiric treatment for VAP (Aarts et al. 2008). However, this data do not permit specific recommendations regarding the additional utility of empirical coverage against methicillin-resistant *S. aureus*, as all studies evaluating linezolid or vancomycin included methicillin-resistant *S. aureus* coverage in the comparator arm.

Additional Gram-negative coverage for combination therapy includes antipseudomonal fluoroquinolone (ciprofloxacin or levofloxacin), aminoglycoside (gentamicin, tobramycin or amikacin) or colistin (if highly resistant *Pseudomonas* or *Acinetobacter* is suspected). In some ICUs, 50–70% of *Staphylococcus aureus* are MRSA. Therefore, vancomycin or linezolid should be added if a high local incidence of MRSA is documented

*Table 20.3*

**Comparison of recommended initial empiric therapy for ventilator-associated pneumonia (VAP) according to time of onset**

| Early-onset VAP | Late-onset VAP |
| --- | --- |
| Second- or third-generation cephalosporin, e.g.: | Cephalosporin |
| Ceftriaxone: 2 grams daily | e.g., Cefepime: 1–2 grams every 8 hours |
| Cefuroxime: 1.5 grams every 8 hours | Ceftazidime 2 grams every 8 hours |
| Cefotaxime: 2 grams every 8 hours | or |
| or | Carbapenem |
| Fluoroquinolones | e.g., Imipenem+cilastin: 500 mg every 6 hours or 1 gram every 8 hours |
| e.g., Levofloxacin: 750 mg daily | Meropenem: 1 gram every 8 hours |
| Moxifloxacin: 400 mg daily | or |
| or | Beta-lactam/beta-lactamase inhibitor |
| Aminopenicillin+beta-lactamase inhibitor, e.g., | e.g., Piperacillin+tazobactam: 4.5 grams every 6 hours |
| Ampicillin+sulbactam: 3 grams every 8 hours | plus |
| or | Aminoglycoside |
| Ertapenem 1 gram daily | e.g., Amikacin: 20 mg/kg/day |
| | Gentamicin: 7 mg/kg/day |
| | Tobramycin: 7 mg/kg/day |
| | or |
| | Antipseudomonal fluoroquinolone |
| | e.g., Ciprofloxacin 400 mg every 8 hours |
| | Levofloxacin 750 mg daily |
| | plus |
| | Coverage for MRSA |
| | e.g., vancomycin 15 mg/kg every 12 hours |
| | or |
| | Linezolid 600 mg every 12 hours |

Adapted from Kalanuria et al. (2014).
MRSA, methicillin-resistant *Staphylococcus aureus*.
Optimal dosage includes adjusting for hepatic and renal failure. Trough levels for vancomycin (15–20 µg/mL), amikacin (<5 µg/mL), gentamicin (<1 µg/mL), and tobramycin (<1 µg/mL) should be measured frequently to avoid untoward systemic side effects. All recommended doses are for intravenous infusion. Usual duration of therapy is 8 days unless treatment is for multidrug-resistant organisms, in which case treatment will be for 14 days.

(Jackson and Shorr, 2006) (Table 20.3). Vancomycin is administered by weight-based dosing (at 15 mg/kg every 8–12 hours) and should be adjusted by renal clearance. Trough levels should be maintained at 15–20 g/mL

(American Thoracic Society and Infectious Diseases Society of America, 2005). The duration of therapy is guided by clinical response; 8 days is the usual duration for early-onset VAP (Chastre et al., 2003). For late-onset VAP, or if MDR organisms are suspected or identified, duration of treatment with an effective agent ranges from 8 to 14 days. There is an associated increase in recurrence of nonfermenting Gram-negative bacilli infections (like *Pseudomonas* or *Acinetobacter*) (Chastre et al., 2003; Capellier et al., 2012; Dimopoulos et al., 2013).

Considering the high prevalence of VAP, prevention has assumed increasing importance in ventilator management. The following measures have reduced VAP in clinical trials: oral care with chlorhexidine (Chan et al., 2007; Labeau et al., 2011), use of probiotics (e.g., *Lactobacillus rhamnosus*) (Morrow et al., 2010), elevation of the head of the bed to more than 30° (Drakulovic et al., 1999), use of specially designed endotracheal tubes with subglottic suction to drain tracheal secretions (Lorente et al., 2007; Muscedere et al., 2011), silver-coated endotracheal tubes (Kollef et al., 2008; Fernandez et al., 2012), avoidance of reintubation (Kollef, 2004), minimization of transport out of the ICU, and the use of daily weaning trials to facilitate early extubation (Kollef, 2004). Each day a patient remains intubated increases the risk of VAP by 1–3% (Kollef, 2004).

## Bacteremia

Bacteremia is the second most common HAI in the NICU (Orsi et al., 2006). Most hospital-acquired bacteremias are associated with indwelling vascular catheters, especially central venous catheters (CVCs) (Fowler et al., 2005). The crude mortality rate resulting from bacteremia has been estimated at 27% (Wisplinghoff et al., 2004). Risk factors for bacteremia include intravascular catheter placement, and host factors such as immunosuppression, older age, malnutrition, and total parenteral nutrition. Catheter location remains a controversial risk factor; although several studies (Maki et al., 2006) found a similar risk of infectious complications among subclavian, internal jugular, and femoral vein insertion sites. A more recent meta-analysis of 10 studies (3250 subclavian, 3053 internal jugular, and 1554 femoral vein CVCs), of which one was randomized, reported fewer catheter-associated infections for the subclavian vein site (1.3 compared to 2.7 per 1000 catheter days for alternative sites) (Parienti et al., 2012).

The risk for catheter-related bacteremia (CRB) (per 1000 catheter days, with 95% confidence intervals) has been estimated at 2.7 (2.6–2.9) for noncuffed CVCs, 1.7 (1.2–2.3) for arterial catheters, 1.6 (1.5–1.7) for cuffed and tunneled CVCs, and 1.1 (0.9–1.3) for peripherally inserted central catheters (Maki et al., 2006). However, other studies have shown that the CRB risk for CVCs is the same as for peripherally inserted catheters in hospitalized patients (Nolan et al., 2016). Aseptic technique is essential for avoidance of infection and lines placed without aseptic technique in emergent conditions have a higher associated risk of infection (Maki et al., 2006). A meta-analysis of randomized controlled trials favors the use of cutaneous chlorhexidine over povidone-iodine for optimal antiseptic technique (Chaiyakunapruk et al., 2002).

### DIAGNOSIS AND MICROBIOLOGY

The most frequent pathogens associated with CRB are *Staphylococcus epidermidis* (37%), *S. aureus* (13%), *Enterococcus* (13%), *Enterobacter-Klebsiella* (11%), *Candida* spp. (8%), *Serratia* (5%), and others (*Escherichia coli, Pseudomonas* spp.). Gram-negative organisms are especially common in patients with malignancies (Ropper, 2004). According to IDSA guidelines, a blood infection occurring in the presence of a CVC without other apparent source should be suspected CRB (Mermel et al., 2009). Purulence or inflammation at the insertion site is a specific but insensitive sign (Safdar and Maki, 2002). Signs of sepsis, such as hypotension and mental status changes, may also indicate CRB. True confirmation of a catheter source requires the following: (1) the same organism is grown from peripheral blood and the catheter tip culture with growth of >15 CFUs; or (2) the central blood sample is read as positive ≥2 hours earlier than a peripheral blood sample inoculated at the same time; or (3) both catheter and peripheral cultures grow the same organisms and the colony count from the catheter-drawn blood is three to five times greater than that drawn by venepuncture (Bouza et al., 2007; Mermel et al., 2009). Complications by *S. aureus* bacteremia should be investigated. Echocardiography, preferably by transesophageal echocardiogram, the gold standard, should be performed if there is any suspicions for endocarditis. The best time to look for vegetations is on days 5–7. Other possible complications include osteomyelitis, epidural abscess, and septic arthritis.

### TREATMENT

Short- and long-term catheters should be removed from patients with CRB when associated with any of the following conditions: hemodynamic instability or sepsis, endocarditis, suppurative thrombophlebitis, or infections due to *S. aureus,* Gram-negative bacilli, enterococci, fungi, mycobacteria, and pathogens that are difficult to eradicate (e.g., *Bacillus* species, *Micrococcus* species, or propionibacteria). For patients in whom catheter salvage is attempted, additional blood cultures should be obtained; if blood cultures remain positive despite

72 hours of antimicrobial therapy, the catheter should be removed. Catheter tip culture should be performed when a catheter is removed for suspected CRB (Mermel et al., 2009). Catheter dysfunction may reflect the presence of an infected thrombus, therefore alteplase and other thrombolytic agents are not recommended as adjunctive therapy for patients with CRB.

Antimicrobial therapy is often initiated empirically. The initial choice of antibiotics depends on the severity of the patient's clinical disease, the risk factors for infection, and the likely pathogens associated with the intravascular device. Vancomycin is the empiric therapy of choice in the ICU as the most likely pathogens are methicillin-resistant coagulase-negative staphylococci. Daptomycin is appropriate if the vancomycin minimum inhibitory concentration (MIC) is $\geq 2$ $\mu$g/mL. The addition of empiric therapy against *Pseudomonas* (e.g., cefepime, piperacillin-tazobactam, meropenem) is indicated in patients who are critically ill, have sepsis or neutropenia, or who have a femoral catheter in place. Patients who are critically ill and have recent colonization or infection with an MDR Gram-negative pathogen should receive two antimicrobial agents of different classes with Gram-negative activity as initial therapy. Antibiotic therapy should be tailored according to available subsequent culture and susceptibility results. Blood cultures should be redrawn after initiation of therapy to assure clearance of bacteremia. If candidemia is suspected (CRB involving a femoral catheter, total parenteral nutrition, hematologic malignancy, transplant patient, and prolonged broad-spectrum antibiotic use), empiric treatment should be administered. Fluconazole can be used for patients without azole exposure in the previous 3 months and in healthcare settings where the risk of *Candida krusei or C. glabrata* infection is very low. Otherwise, an echinocandin (e.g., caspofungin) is the recommended choice (Mermel et al., 2009).

The recommended duration of therapy is 14 days, with day 1 defined as the first day with negative cultures. Four to six weeks of therapy is recommended when bacteremia or fungemia persists for more than 72 hours after catheter removal, in bacteremia resulting from infection with *S. aureus* in patients with diabetes, with an immunocompromised state, or with a prosthetic intravascular device; and when endocarditis, suppurative thrombophlebitis, or metastatic infectious foci are identified (Mermel et al., 2009).

Antibiotic treatment is not recommended in some situations involving positive cultures associated with an indwelling or recently removed CVC. These include a positive culture from a removed catheter tip not accompanied by clinical signs of infection, positive cultures from an indwelling CVC associated with negative associated peripheral blood cultures, and phlebitis in the absence of infection (topical antimicrobials are preferred) (Mermel et al., 2009).

## Urinary tract infections

Urinary tract infections (UTIs) are the second most common HAI in patients admitted to ICUs and the third most common in patients admitted to NICUs, accounting for 22.7–36.6% of HAIs (Vincent et al., 1995; Zolldann et al., 2005; Orsi et al., 2006; Edwards et al., 2008). Incidence and prevalence also vary widely due to inconsistencies in the definition of "significant bacteriuria." The prevalence of UTIs in ICU patients is between 8% and 21% (Eriksen et al., 2005; Laupland et al., 2005). Approximately 20% of hospital-acquired bacteremias arise from the urinary tract, and the mortality associated with this condition is 10% (Gould et al., 2010). A meta-analysis demonstrated that catheter-associated UTI is associated with significant increases in mortality and length of stay in critically ill patients (Chant et al., 2008). Eighty percent of hospital-acquired UTIs are attributable to indwelling urethral catheters (Foxman, 2002; Klevens et al., 2007). Other risk factors include diabetes mellitus, older age, female sex, severe underlying illness, and bacterial colonization of the drainage bag (Platt et al., 1986; Wald et al., 2008).

### DIAGNOSIS AND MICROBIOLOGY

Most ICU-acquired catheter-associated UTIs (CAUTI) are monomicrobial (88–95%) (Laupland et al., 2005; Bagshaw and Laupland, 2006). The predominant pathogens are: *E. coli* (39%), *P. aeruginosa* (22%), *Enterococcus* (15%), *Acinetobacter* spp. (11%), *Klebsiella* spp. (11%), and *Proteus* (11%). *Candida* spp. account for one-third of all ICU-acquired UTIs (Leone et al., 2003; Laupland et al., 2005). According to the IDSA, a CAUTI is defined as culture growth of $\geq 10^3$ CFU/mL of uropathogenic bacteria in the presence of symptoms or signs compatible with UTI with no other identified source of infection in a patient with an indwelling urethral or suprapubic catheter, or intermittent catheterization. Signs and symptoms compatible with CAUTIs include new-onset or worsening fever, rigors, altered mental status, malaise, or lethargy with no other identified cause. Other significant signs and symptoms include flank pain, costovertebral angle tenderness, acute hematuria, and pelvic discomfort. In contrast, catheter-associated asymptomatic bacteriuria is defined by culture growth of $\geq 10^5$ CFU/mL of uropathogenic bacteria in patients with an indwelling urethral or suprapubic catheter, or intermittent catheterization in a patient without clinical symptoms (Hooton et al., 2010). Less than one-quarter of hospitalized patients with catheter-associated bacteriuria develop UTI symptoms

(Kunin and McCormack, 1966; Saint, 2000; Tambyah and Maki, 2000a).

Pyuria (white blood cell count $\geq 10$ cells/$\mu$L) can be present in catheterized patients with asymptomatic bacteriuria, and has a low sensitivity for predicting growth in catheterized patients (Tambyah and Maki, 2000b). Therefore, the IDSA recommends against using the degree of pyuria to differentiate CAUTI from catheter-associated asymptomatic bacteriuria. A urine culture should be obtained prior to initiating treatment for presumed UTI because of the wide spectrum of potential infecting organisms and the increased likelihood of antimicrobial resistance. The urine culture should be obtained from the freshly placed catheter prior to the initiation of antimicrobial therapy in patients with long-term indwelling catheters. In a symptomatic patient, this should be done immediately prior to initiating antimicrobial therapy. In patients with short-term catheterization, it is recommended that specimens be obtained by sampling through the catheter port using aseptic technique or, if a port is not present, by puncturing the catheter tubing with a needle and syringe. Culture specimens should not be obtained from the drainage bag (Hooton et al., 2010).

## TREATMENT

Uncomplicated UTI (not CAUTI) diagnosed early in the ICU stay can be treated with trimethoprim/sulfamethoxazole or ciprofloxacin. For empiric treatment of CAUTI with Gram-negative rods, third-generation cephalosporins (e.g., ceftriaxone) or a fluoroquinolone (ciprofloxacin or levofloxacin) are recommended. Vancomycin is the drug of choice for empiric treatment of Gram-positive cocci (Hooton et al., 2010). Attention to bacterial susceptibility is important. Follow-up of culture results is essential. There has been increasing resistance to third-generation cephalosporins (5 and 20% for *E. coli* and *Klebsiella pneumonia*, respectively) and increasing *P. aeruginosa* resistance to imipenem (Gaynes and Edwards, 2005).

For patients without severe illness who have uncomplicated UTI, 3–7 days of antibiotic treatment is sufficient. Seven days is recommended for patients with a CAUTI who have prompt resolution of symptoms, although 5 days can be enough in patients who are not critically ill. Ten to 14 days of therapy is recommended for those with a delayed response and in septic patients (Hooton et al., 2010).

*Candida albicans* and *C. glabrata* are the most frequent uropathogens associated with CAUTI (Leone et al., 2003). Colonized patients, without evidence of infection, do not require treatment. However, the indwelling catheter should be changed or removed.

Parenteral fluconazole for 14 days is the best option for treating a candiduria due to *C. albicans*, and voriconazole is more effective against non-*C. albicans* (Edwards et al., 1997). Antimicrobial treatment should be tailored to the specific organism isolated and susceptibility data. Treatment is not necessary for asymptomatic bacteriuria and should be avoided due to concerns of increasing antimicrobial resistance. Routine screening is not recommended.

## PREVENTION

The most effective strategy to reduce the incidence of UTIs is to reduce the use of internal or external catheters. Indwelling catheters should be placed only when indicated and should be removed as soon as possible. The Centers for Medicare and Medicaid Services stopped offering additional reimbursements for patients discharged with a diagnosis of CAUTI from October 2008 (Wald and Kramer, 2007). Since then, numerous studies have examined the impact of different interventions to reduce this complication. In the NICU, Titsworth et al. (2012) reported a decrease in catheter utilization rates from 100% to 73% following implementation of an evidence-based UTI prevention bundle (avoidance of catheter insertion, maintenance of sterility, product standardization, and early catheter removal). Reduction in utilization rates correlated strongly with a decrease in the CAUTI rate from 13.3 to 4.0 infections per 1000 catheter days.

## Ventriculitis

Bacterial ventriculitis (BV) is inflammation of the ventricular drainage system due to bacterial infection of the cerebrospinal fluid (CSF) (Lewis et al., 2016). BV is associated with CSF shunts, EVD, or any other intracranial device. Hemorrhagic CSF further contributes to the increased incidence of EVD-associated infections in patients with aneurysmal subarachnoid hemorrhage (10%) and intraventricular hemorrhage (13.7%) (Sundbarg et al., 1988; Holloway et al., 1996; Lozier et al., 2002). Other risk factors for BV include type of EVD, insertion technique, management, frequency of CSF sampling, and EVD duration. Published EVD-related BV rates range from 3.8% to 23.2%, with reported mortality rates from 10% to 75% (Lozier et al., 2002; Korinek et al., 2005; Beer et al., 2008). Infection risk increases significantly after 5 days of placement and peaks at days 9–11 after placement (Holloway et al., 1996; Rebuck et al., 2000; Lyke et al., 2001; Lozier et al., 2002; Beer et al., 2008). Despite this high risk, the CDC does not specifically define device-related infection or EVDs as it does for ventilators, Foley catheters, and CVCs. There are up to

17 different definitions of ventriculostomy-related infection in the literature (Lewis et al., 2015), with variation based on a heterogeneous population in terms of laboratory and clinical findings. CSF shunt-related infection is reported in 8–40% of patients, with most infections occurring within 1 month of implantation (Armstrong et al., 2000). Ventricular infection superimposed on an already injured brain significantly increases length of stay, morbidity, and mortality (Beer et al. 2008; Williamson et al., 2014).

## MICROBIOLOGY

The most common pathogens involved in EVD and CSF shunt infections are Gram-positive organisms such as *Staphylococcus epidermidis, S. aureus, Propionibacterium acnes, Streptococcus* sp. and fungi (*Candida albicans*). Up to 25% of infections are caused by Gram-negative organisms such as *Escherichia coli, Klebsiella* species, *Acinetobacter,* and *Pseudomonas* species (Armstrong et al., 2000; Tunkel et al., 2004). In traumatic brain-injured patients and/or following brain surgery, aerobic Gram-negative bacilli, including *Pseudomonas* species, *Staphylococcus aureus,* and *S. epidermidis,* are the most common pathogens (Tunkel et al., 2004).

## DIAGNOSIS

Ventriculitis is diagnosed by the presence of clinical symptoms and a positive CSF analysis. The clinical symptoms of ventriculitis include fever and signs of meningitis (nuchal rigidity, decreased mental status, seizures, etc.). A positive CSF culture with absent symptoms should lead the clinician to suspect colonization or contamination. Contamination constitutes an isolated positive CSF culture in the absence of abnormal CSF findings. EVD catheter colonization is defined by multiple positive CSF cultures with "expected" CSF profiles and lack of clinical signs other than fever (Lozier et al., 2002). A positive CSF analysis for BV includes a positive Gram stain and culture with increased protein, decreased glucose, and CSF pleocytosis.

Presently there are no specific data on identification of causative organisms in ventriculitis. Most assumptions about accuracy are extrapolated from data on the accuracy of Gram stain in identifying the causative bacterium in community-acquired bacterial meningitis, which is only 60–90% sensitive with a specificity >97% (Tunkel, 2001). The likelihood of visualizing the bacterium on Gram stain correlates with the CSF concentration of bacteria – concentrations of $\leq 10^3$ CFU/mL are associated with a positive Gram stain result 25% of the time; $10^3$–$10^5$ CFU/mL yields a positive Gram stain result in 60% of patients, and CSF concentrations of $>10^5$ CFU/mL lead to positive microscopy results in 97% of cases (La Scolea and Dryja, 1984). The likelihood of having a positive Gram stain also depends on the specific pathogen (Gray and Fedorko, 1992): 90% of cases caused by *Streptococcus pneumoniae,* 86% of cases caused by *Haemophilus influenzae,* 75% of cases caused by *Neisseria meningitidis,* 50% of cases caused by Gram-negative bacilli, and approximately one-third of cases of meningitis caused by *Listeria monocytogenes* have positive Gram stain results (Mylonakis et al., 1998).

In patients who have already suffered a neurologic injury that causes inflammation and breakdown of the blood–brain barrier, the diagnosis of ventriculitis can be challenging, as CSF may already contain blood with increased protein, inflammatory cells, and decreased glucose depending on the underlying pathology. Especially in postoperative neurosurgery cases, determination of a high lactate concentration can assist with diagnosis. In one study of 73 patients, CSF lactate values (cutoff, 4 mmol/L), in comparison with CSF/blood glucose ratios (cutoff, 0.4), were associated with higher sensitivity (0.88 vs. 0.77), specificity (0.98 vs. 0.87), and positive (0.96 vs. 0.77) and negative (0.94 vs. 0.87) predictive values for bacterial meningitis (Leib et al., 1999). CSF lactate is not, however, useful for suspected community-acquired bacterial meningitis. Factors that may elevate CSF lactate include cerebral hypoxia/ischemia, anaerobic glycolysis, vascular compromise, and metabolism of CSF leukocytes (Leib et al., 1999). Current guidelines recommend that, in the postoperative neurosurgical patient, initiation of empiric antimicrobial therapy should be considered if CSF lactate concentrations are $\geq 4.0$ mmol/L, pending results of additional studies (Tunkel et al., 2004).

## TREATMENT

Recommended empiric therapy for BV is a combination of vancomycin and cefepime for adults with ventriculitis post neurosurgery, CSF shunt infections, head trauma, skull fractures, and penetrating trauma. Alternative agents include vancomycin plus ceftazidime or vancomycin plus meropenem (Tunkel et al., 2004). Targeted antimicrobial therapy and duration are based on presumptive pathogen identification by CSF Gram stain and culture and response to treatment. In most cases treatment is continued for 10–14 days; for aerobic Gram-negative bacilli, therapy may be continued for up to 21 days (Tunkel et al., 2004). Some experts advocate for a shorter course of 5–7 days if the EVD is exchanged (Beer et al., 2008). A fungal infection with *Candida* species should be managed with voriconazole and the polyene amphotericin B for 2 weeks since the last negative CSF culture; treatment with echinocandins such as caspofungin is still controversial due to poor central nervous system penetration with undetectable levels in CSF with systemic treatment (Beer et al., 2008).

## INTRAVENTRICULAR ADMINISTRATION OF ANTIBIOTICS

In addition to antimicrobial therapy, infected hardware should be removed, replaced, or externalized when appropriate (Ziai and Lewin, 2008). The ventricles can act as a persistent reservoir of infection and inflammation, resulting in extreme difficulty in eradicating infection and potential blockade of CSF outflow tracts (Salmon, 1972). Intraventricular (IVT) administration of antibiotics may be effective in selected cases, although indications remain controversial (Bayston et al., 1987). The first IVT administration of antibiotics was performed more than 50 years ago (Clifford and Stewart, 1961; Flint et al., 2013). The rationale for administration of antibiotics directly into the ventricles is compelling, because meningeal inflammation, which enhances the ability of antimicrobials to penetrate the blood–brain barrier, is less pronounced in ventriculitis (Pfausler et al., 1997) and the ventricles can act as persistent reservoirs of infection (Salmon, 1972). Under these conditions, penetration of systemic β-lactams and glycopeptides into the CSF is poor and results in subtherapeutic concentrations in the CSF and high failure rates (Yogev and Davis, 1980; Gump, 1981; Fan-Havard et al., 1990).

IVT antibiotics can lead to rapid CSF sterilization in postneurosurgical patients with meningitis and ventriculitis (mean time $2.9 \pm 2.7$ days, range 1–12 days) (Flint et al., 2013). The relapse rate of ventriculitis is also very low among patients treated by IVT antibiotics. Although randomized controlled trials would be helpful to clarify specific indications for intraventricular or lumbar intrathecal antibiotics, there is some agreement that intrathecal administration of antibiotics appears to be an effective and safe treatment for central nervous system infections caused by MDR organisms (Flint et al., 2013). The typical indications are: (1) failure to achieve adequate CSF antimicrobial concentrations with nontoxic drug doses, or (2) persistently positive CSF cultures despite intravenous dosing with an appropriate antibiotic, and exhaustion of all appropriate means of source control (Ziai and Lewin, 2009). The choice of intrathecal antibiotic depends on the CSF pathogen; frequently used antibiotics include gentamicin, vancomycin, colistin, meropenem, and netilmicin. Target antimicrobial concentrations in the CSF are not well established, although drug concentrations at least 10 times the MIC are recommended to achieve rapid bactericidal activity (Nau et al., 1998). Intrathecal antibiotics are administered at 24-hour intervals and for 48–72 hours after sterilization of the CSF in most cases.

## PREVENTION OF VENTRICULITIS

As with all HAIs, prevention is key to decreased morbidity and mortality. Korinek et al. (2005) demonstrated that meticulous EVD care can prolong EVD use and minimize infection rates. In this study, implementation of protocolized EVD insertion and nursing care reduced the incidence of EVD-related ventriculitis by almost half (9.9% vs. 4.6%, $p < 0.05$). A recent meta-analysis examining the impact of antibiotic- and silver-impregnated EVD on the risk of infection found that both antibiotic- and silver-impregnated EVDs were more effective than standard EVDs for the prevention of catheter-related infection. There is no conclusive evidence guiding preference of antibiotic- or silver-impregnated EVDs (Cui et al., 2015). A prospective study of 866 patients failed to find additional protection against ventriculitis with prolonged systemic antibiotic prophylaxis (1 g IV cefazolin every 8 hours until catheter removal) for patients treated with antibiotic-coated EVDs. Furthermore, prolonged systemic antibiotic therapy following placement of EVDs was associated with a higher rate of nosocomial infections and increased cost (Murphy et al., 2015). It is not recommended to exchange EVDs with the aim of preventing ventriculitis. In a retrospective study of 199 patients with 269 EVDs, second and third EVDs in previously uninfected patients were more likely to become infected than first EVDs, suggesting that EVD-associated infections are acquired by introduction of bacteria on insertion of the drain rather than by subsequent retrograde colonization (Lo et al., 2007).

## Postneurosurgical wound infections

The incidence of postneurosurgical wound infection is from <1 to 8%, with reported mortality as high as 14% (van Ek et al., 1986; Patir et al., 1992; Korinek, 1997; McClelland and Hall, 2007). A recent meta-analysis reported a significantly lower incidence of postcraniotomy infections in North America as compared to European countries (2.2 vs. 5.7%, $p = 0.001$) (McClelland and Hall, 2007). After initial inoculation approximately 100 000 bacterial organisms per gram of tissue are required to produce a postoperative wound infection, which commonly manifests as meningitis, brain abscess, subdural empyema (SDE), and/or epidural abscess (Marion, 1991; Borges, 1992).

### SUBDURAL EMPYEMA

SDE occurs after neurosurgery in 4% of cases (Hall and Truwit, 2008). Signs and symptoms of SDE usually present within 1–8 weeks (mean 2 weeks) after the neurosurgical procedure, and include headache, meningismus, fever, confusion, nausea, vomiting, seizures, and focal neurologic deficits. Staphylococci and Gram-negative bacilli are the most common pathogens. Pus can be found over the convexities, layering along the tentorium cerebelli, or in the interhemispheric fissure, where spread is dependent on gravity; with 1–10% of SDEs located in the posterior fossa (Nathoo et al., 1997). Laboratory abnormalities may include elevated white blood cell count and positive blood cultures. Lumbar puncture is not recommended due to increased risk for cerebral herniation. If performed, protein is usually elevated, and if meningitis is present, CSF white blood cell count is elevated with positive cultures. On computed tomography (CT) SDE appears as a hypodense collection with peripheral enhancement. On magnetic resonance imaging (MRI), SDE has decreased signal on T1-weighted imaging (T1WI) and increased signal on T2WI (Hall and Truwit, 2008). SDE can be differentiated from reactive subdural effusions by diffusion-weighted imaging (DWI) (SDE exhibits reduced diffusion with an apparent diffusion coefficient (ADC) lower than that of normal cortical gray matter, in contrast to reactive effusions which do not show DWI changes) (Wong et al., 2004). The recommended management for SDEs includes surgical drainage and antibiotic therapy. Surgical drainage is performed in up to 96% of cases and enables source control (Nathoo et al., 1999). Empiric treatment for patients who have undergone neurosurgical procedures consists of vancomycin plus a fourth-generation cephalosporin (i.e., cefepime). Cultures should be sent from the surgical drainage and appropriate antibiotic therapy should be tailored accordingly and continued for 3–6 weeks depending on the clinical response.

## BRAIN ABSCESS

Abscess formation is an uncommon but serious complication after neurosurgical procedures. Immunocompromised patients and head trauma patients with penetrating brain injury are at higher risk (Tenney, 1986; Calfee and Wispelwey, 2000). Patients typically present 2 weeks postsurgery complaining of headache. Low-grade fevers are present in over 50%; seizures and signs of increased intracranial pressure may be present. Over 60% of patients have a focal neurologic deficit or altered level of consciousness (Hall and Truwit, 2008). In postneurosurgical cases, the most common pathogens are skin-colonizing bacteria, such as *Staphylococcus aureus* and *S. epidermidis,* or Gram-negative bacilli (Yang et al., 2006).

The first stage of brain abscess is early cerebritis (Britt et al., 1981). This leads to a perivascular

inflammation dispersed concentrically around the necrotic center and increased edema in the surrounding white matter. Subsequently a capsule forms around the necrotic center through accumulation of fibroblasts and neovascularization. The capsule thickens with an abundance of reactive collagen. Inflammation and edema often extend beyond the capsule (Brouwer et al., 2014). Patients commonly have elevated peripheral white blood cell count. Lumbar puncture should be performed only when there is clinical suspicion of meningitis or abscess rupture into the ventricular system and with consideration of the risk of cerebral herniation. Herniation is estimated to occur in 15–20% of patients who have a lumbar puncture with cerebral abscess (Brouwer et al., 2014).

Head CT is highly sensitivity for the detection of abscess (95–99%) with relatively poor specificity. Other mass lesions, such as brain metastasis, resolving hematoma, and radiation necrosis, may appear identical. Cerebritis appears as an ill-defined hypodense area enhancing homogeneously with contrast on CT. Once encapsulation occurs, the abscess appears as a ring-enhancing lesion with contrast CT. Vasogenic edema around the abscess is hyperintense on T2WI, the center of the abscess is isointense or hyperintense, and the capsule is hypointense. The capsule enhances clearly with intravenous contrast on MRI. DWI is usually hyperintense inside the abscess with a low ADC (Hall and Truwit, 2008).

When CSF analysis fails to identify a causative pathogen, surgical aspiration should be considered to isolate the organism and to reduce the abscess diameter. With the use of modern stereotactic neurosurgical techniques, a 1-cm brain abscess is amenable to stereotactic aspiration, regardless of location (Brouwer et al., 2014). Medical therapy alone may be appropriate if the causative pathogen has been identified and the abscess measure less than 2.5 in diameter or when the abscess is located in deep or eloquent brain. Other reasons for medical management include poor surgical candidacy, and concurrent meningitis, ventriculitis, or hydrocephalus that requires CSF shunting which may become infected at the time of abscess drainage (Hall and Truwit, 2008). The established practice for neurosurgical intervention for abscesses above 2.5 cm originates from a case study of 16 patients by Mamelak et al. (1995), in which surgical drainage was performed on abscesses larger than 2.5 cm.

Empiric antibiotic therapy is defined by mechanism of infection, predisposing conditions, local antimicrobial susceptibility, and on the ability of the antimicrobial agent to penetrate the abscess (Brouwer et al., 2014). Empiric treatment following neurosurgical procedures or head trauma with skull fractures consists of vancomycin plus a fourth-generation cephalosporin (i.e., cefepime) and metronidazole for 6–8 weeks (Brouwer et al., 2014).

## CONCLUSION

HAIs occur in approximately 30% of patients in the NICU and are associated with substantial morbidity and mortality. Significant strides in reducing central line-associated blood stream infection and VAP rates are now being applied to CAUTI and EVD-associated infections. These include patient-centered, interdisciplinary urinary catheter management algorithms to reduce urinary catheter utilization and CAUTI, and strict protocols for EVD placement and maintenance using bundle approaches, which have been shown to be cost-effective and to have better outcomes than implementation of individual single practices.

## REFERENCES

Aarts MA, Hancock JN, Heyland D et al. (2008). Empiric antibiotic therapy for suspected ventilator-associated pneumonia: a systematic review and meta-analysis of randomized trials. Crit Care Med 36 (1): 108–117.

American Thoracic Society, Infectious Diseases Society of America (2005). Guidelines for the management of adults with hospital-acquired, ventilator-associated, and healthcare-associated pneumonia. Am J Respir Crit Care Med 171 (4): 388–416.

Amin A (2009). Clinical and economic consequences of ventilator-associated pneumonia. Clin Infect Dis 49 (Suppl 1): S36–S43.

Armstrong W, McGillicuddy I (2000). Infections of the central nervous system. In: H Crockard, J Hoff (Eds.), Neurosurgery: the scientific basis of clinical practice, 3rd edn. Vol. 2. Blackwell Science, Oxford, pp. 757–783.

Bagshaw SM, Laupland KB (2006). Epidemiology of intensive care unit-acquired urinary tract infections. Curr Opin Infect Dis 19 (1): 67–71.

Bayston R, Hart CA, Barnicoat M (1987). Intraventricular vancomycin in the treatment of ventriculitis associated with cerebrospinal fluid shunting and drainage. J Neurol Neurosurg Psychiatry 50 (11): 1419–1423.

Beer R, Lackner P, Pfausler B et al. (2008). Nosocomial ventriculitis and meningitis in neurocritical care patients. J Neurol 255 (11): 1617–1624.

Berrouane Y, Daudenthun I, Riegel B et al. (1998). Early onset pneumonia in neurosurgical intensive care unit patients. J Hosp Infect 40 (4): 275–280.

Berton DC, Kalil AC, Teixeira PJ (2012). Quantitative versus qualitative cultures of respiratory secretions for clinical outcomes in patients with ventilator-associated pneumonia. Cochrane Database Syst Rev 1: Cd006482.

Bhattacharya S (2013). Early diagnosis of resistant pathogens: how can it improve antimicrobial treatment? Virulence 4 (2): 172–184.

Borges LF (1992). Infections in neurologic surgery. Host defenses. Neurosurg Clin N Am 3 (2): 275–278.

Bouza E, Alvarado N, Alcala L et al. (2007). A randomized and prospective study of 3 procedures for the diagnosis of catheter-related bloodstream infection without catheter withdrawal. Clin Infect Dis 44 (6): 820–826.

Britt RH, Enzmann DR, Yeager AS (1981). Neuropathological and computerized tomographic findings in experimental brain abscess. J Neurosurg 55 (4): 590–603.

Brouwer MC, Tunkel AR, McKhann 2nd GM et al. (2014). Brain abscess. N Engl J Med 371 (5): 447–456.

Calfee DP (2012). Crisis in hospital-acquired, healthcare-associated infections. Annu Rev Med 63: 359–371.

Calfee DP, Wispelwey B (2000). Brain abscess. Semin Neurol 20 (3): 353–360.

Capellier G, Mockly H, Charpentier C et al. (2012). Early-onset ventilator-associated pneumonia in adults randomized clinical trial: comparison of 8 versus 15 days of antibiotic treatment. PLoS One 7: e41290.

Chaiyakunapruk N, Veenstra DL, Lipsky BA et al. (2002). Chlorhexidine compared with povidone-iodine solution for vascular catheter-site care: a meta-analysis. Ann Intern Med 136 (11): 792–801.

Chan EY, Ruest A, Meade MO et al. (2007). Oral decontamination for prevention of pneumonia in mechanically ventilated adults: systematic review and meta-analysis. BMJ 334 (7599): 889.

Chant C, Dos Santos CC, Saccucci P et al. (2008). Discordance between perception and treatment practices associated with intensive care unit-acquired bacteriuria and funguria: a Canadian physician survey. Crit Care Med 36 (4): 1158–1167.

Chastre J, Fagon JY (2002). Ventilator-associated pneumonia. Am J Respir Crit Care Med 165 (7): 867–903.

Chastre J, Fagon JY, Bornet-Lecso M et al. (1995). Evaluation of bronchoscopic techniques for the diagnosis of nosocomial pneumonia. Am J Respir Crit Care Med 152 (1): 231–240.

Chastre J, Wolff M, Fagon J et al. (2003). Comparison of 8 vs 15 days of antibiotic therapy for ventilator-associated pneumonia in adults: a randomized trial. JAMA 290: 2588–2598.

Clifford HE, Stewart GT (1961). Intraventricular administration of a new derivative of polymyxin B in meningitis due to *Ps. pyocyanea*. Lancet 2 (7195): 177–180.

Conway Morris A, Anderson N, Brittan M et al. (2013). Combined dysfunctions of immune cells predict nosocomial infection in critically ill patients. Br J Anaesth 111 (5): 778–787.

Cook D (2000). Ventilator associated pneumonia: perspectives on the burden of illness. Intensive Care Med 26 (Suppl 1): S31–S37.

Cui Z, Wang B, Zhong Z et al. (2015). Impact of antibiotic- and silver-impregnated external ventricular drains on the risk of infections: a systematic review and meta-analysis. Am J Infect Control 43 (7): e23–e32.

Depuydt PO, Vandijck DM, Bekaert MA et al. (2008). Determinants and impact of multidrug antibiotic resistance in pathogens causing ventilator-associated-pneumonia. Crit Care 12 (6): R142.

Dimopoulos G, Poulakou G, Pneumatikos IA et al. (2013). Short- vs long-duration antibiotic regimens for ventilator-associated pneumonia: a systematic review and meta-analysis. Chest 144 (6): 1759–1767.

Drakulovic MB, Torres A, Bauer TT et al. (1999). Supine body position as a risk factor for nosocomial pneumonia in mechanically ventilated patients: a randomised trial. Lancet 354 (9193): 1851–1858.

Dudeck MA, Weiner LM, Allen-Bridson K et al. (2013). National Healthcare Safety Network (NHSN) report, data summary for 2012, device-associated module. Am J Infect Control 41 (12): 1148–1166.

Edwards Jr JE, Bodey GP, Bowden RA et al. (1997). International conference for the development of a consensus on the management and prevention of severe candidal infections. Clin Infect Dis 25 (1): 43–59.

Edwards JR, Peterson KD, Andrus ML et al. (2008). National Healthcare Safety Network (NHSN) report, data summary for 2006 through 2007, issued November 2008. Am J Infect Control 36 (9): 609–626.

Eriksen HM, Iversen BG, Aavitsland P (2005). Prevalence of nosocomial infections in hospitals in Norway, 2002 and 2003. J Hosp Infect 60 (1): 40–45.

Fabregas N, Ewig S, Torres A et al. (1999). Clinical diagnosis of ventilator associated pneumonia revisited: comparative validation using immediate post-mortem lung biopsies. Thorax 54 (10): 867–873.

Fan-Havard P, Nahata MC, Bartkowski MH et al. (1990). Pharmacokinetics and cerebrospinal fluid (CSF) concentrations of vancomycin in pediatric patients undergoing CSF shunt placement. Chemotherapy 36 (2): 103–108.

Fernandez JF, Levine SM, Restrepo MI (2012). Technologic advances in endotracheal tubes for prevention of ventilator-associated pneumonia. Chest 142 (1): 231–238.

Flint AC, Rao VA, Renda NC et al. (2013). A simple protocol to prevent external ventricular drain infections. Neurosurgery 72 (6): 993–999. discussion 999.

Fowler Jr VG, Miro JM, Hoen B et al. (2005). *Staphylococcus aureus* endocarditis: a consequence of medical progress. JAMA 293 (24): 3012–3021.

Foxman B (2002). Epidemiology of urinary tract infections: incidence, morbidity, and economic costs. Am J Med 113 (Suppl 1A): 5s–13s.

Gaynes R, Edwards JR (2005). Overview of nosocomial infections caused by Gram-negative bacilli. Clin Infect Dis 41 (6): 848–854.

Gould CV, Umscheid CA, Agarwal RK et al. (2010). Guideline for prevention of catheter-associated urinary tract infections 2009. Infect Control Hosp Epidemiol 31 (4): 319–326.

Gray LD, Fedorko DP (1992). Laboratory diagnosis of bacterial meningitis. Clin Microbiol Rev 5 (2): 130–145.

Gump DW (1981). Vancomycin for treatment of bacterial meningitis. Rev Infect Dis 3 (suppl): S289–S292.

Hall WA, Truwit CL (2008). The surgical management of infections involving the cerebrum. Neurosurgery 62 (Suppl 2): 519–530. discussion 530–531.

Holloway KL, Barnes T, Choi S et al. (1996). Ventriculostomy infections: the effect of monitoring duration and catheter exchange in 584 patients. J Neurosurg 85 (3): 419–424.

Hooton TM, Bradley SF, Cardenas DD et al. (2010). Diagnosis, prevention, and treatment of catheter-associated urinary tract infection in adults: 2009 International Clinical Practice Guidelines from the Infectious Diseases Society of America. Clin Infect Dis 50 (5): 625–663.

Hunter JD (2012). Ventilator associated pneumonia. BMJ 344. e3325.

Iregui M, Ward S, Sherman G et al. (2002). Clinical importance of delays in the initiation of appropriate antibiotic treatment for ventilator-associated pneumonia. Chest 122 (1): 262–268.

Jackson WL, Shorr AF (2006). Update in ventilator-associated pneumonia. Curr Opin Anaesthesiol 19 (2): 117–121.

Josephson SA, Moheet AM, Gropper MA et al. (2010). Ventilator-associated pneumonia in a neurologic intensive care unit does not lead to increased mortality. Neurocrit Care 12 (2): 155–158.

Kalanuria AA, Zai W, Mirski M (2014). Ventilator-associated pneumonia in the ICU. Crit Care 18 (2): 208.

Kalanuria AA, Fellerman D, Nyquist P et al. (2015). Variability in diagnosis and treatment of ventilator-associated pneumonia in neurocritical care patients. Neurocrit Care 23 (1): 44–53.

Kirtland SH, Corley DE, Winterbauer RH et al. (1997). The diagnosis of ventilator-associated pneumonia: a comparison of histologic, microbiologic, and clinical criteria. Chest 112 (2): 445–457.

Klevens RM, Edwards JR, Richards Jr CL et al. (2007). Estimating health care-associated infections and deaths in U.S. hospitals, 2002. Public Health Rep 122 (2): 160–166.

Koenig SM, Truwit JD (2006). Ventilator-associated pneumonia: diagnosis, treatment, and prevention. Clin Microbiol Rev 19 (4): 637–657.

Kollef MH (2004). Prevention of hospital-associated pneumonia and ventilator-associated pneumonia. Crit Care Med 32 (6): 1396–1405.

Kollef MH, Afessa B, Anzueto A et al. (2008). Silver-coated endotracheal tubes and incidence of ventilator-associated pneumonia: the NASCENT randomized trial. JAMA 300 (7): 805–813.

Korinek AM (1997). Risk factors for neurosurgical site infections after craniotomy: a prospective multicenter study of 2944 patients. The French Study Group of Neurosurgical Infections, the SEHP, and the C-CLIN Paris-Nord. Service Epidemiologie Hygiene et Prevention. Neurosurgery 41 (5): 1073–1079. discussion 1079–81.

Korinek AM, Reina M, Boch AL et al. (2005). Prevention of external ventricular drain-related ventriculitis. Acta Neurochir (Wien) 147 (1): 39–45. discussion 45–46.

Kunin CM, McCormack RC (1966). Prevention of catheter-induced urinary-tract infections by sterile closed drainage. N Engl J Med 274 (21): 1155–1161.

Kuusinen P, Ala-Kokko T, Jartti A et al. (2012). The occurrence of pneumonia diagnosis among neurosurgical patients: the definition matters. Neurocrit Care 16 (1): 123–129.

La Scolea Jr LJ, Dryja D (1984). Quantitation of bacteria in cerebrospinal fluid and blood of children with meningitis and its diagnostic significance. J Clin Microbiol 19 (2): 187–190.

Labeau SO, Van de Vyver K, Brusselaers N et al. (2011). Prevention of ventilator-associated pneumonia with oral antiseptics: a systematic review and meta-analysis. Lancet Infect Dis 11 (11): 845–854.

Laupland KB, Bagshaw SM, Gregson DB et al. (2005). Intensive care unit-acquired urinary tract infections in a regional critical care system. Crit Care 9 (2): R60–R65.

Leib SL, Boscacci R, Gratzl O et al. (1999). Predictive value of cerebrospinal fluid (CSF) lactate level versus CSF/blood glucose ratio for the diagnosis of bacterial meningitis following neurosurgery. Clin Infect Dis 29 (1): 69–74.

Leone M, Albanese J, Garnier F et al. (2003). Risk factors of nosocomial catheter-associated urinary tract infection in a polyvalent intensive care unit. Intensive Care Med 29 (7): 1077–1080.

Lewis A, Wahlster S, Karinja S et al. (2015). Ventriculostomy-related infections: the performance of different definitions for diagnosing infection. Br J Neurosurg 1–8.

Lewis A, Wahlster S, Karinja S et al. (2016). Ventriculostomy-related infections: the performance of different definitions for diagnosing infection. Br J Neurosurg 30 (1): 49–56.

Lo CH, Spelman D, Bailey M et al. (2007). External ventricular drain infections are independent of drain duration: an argument against elective revision. J Neurosurg 106 (3): 378–383.

Lorente L, Lecuona M, Jimenez A et al. (2007). Influence of an endotracheal tube with polyurethane cuff and subglottic secretion drainage on pneumonia. Am J Respir Crit Care Med 176 (11): 1079–1083.

Lozier AP, Sciacca RR, Romagnoli MF et al. (2002). Ventriculostomy-related infections: a critical review of the literature. Neurosurgery 51 (1): 170–181. discussion 181–182.

Luna CM, Vujacich P, Niederman MS et al. (1997). Impact of BAL data on the therapy and outcome of ventilator-associated pneumonia. Chest 111 (3): 676–685.

Lyke KE, Obasanjo OO, Williams MA et al. (2001). Ventriculitis complicating use of intraventricular catheters in adult neurosurgical patients. Clin Infect Dis 33 (12): 2028–2033.

Maki DG, Kluger DM, Crnich CJ (2006). The risk of bloodstream infection in adults with different intravascular devices: a systematic review of 200 published prospective studies. Mayo Clin Proc 81 (9): 1159–1171.

Mamelak AN, Mampalam TJ, Obana WG et al. (1995). Improved management of multiple brain abscesses: a combined surgical and medical approach. Neurosurgery 36 (1): 76–85. discussion 85–86.

Marion DW (1991). Complications of head injury and their therapy. Neurosurg Clin N Am 2 (2): 411–424.

Martin-Loeches I, Diaz E, Valles J (2014). Risks for multidrug-resistant pathogens in the ICU. Curr Opin Crit Care 20 (5): 516–524.

McClelland 3rd S, Hall WA (2007). Postoperative central nervous system infection: incidence and associated factors in 2111 neurosurgical procedures. Clin Infect Dis 45 (1): 55–59.

Mermel LA, Allon M, Bouza E et al. (2009). Clinical practice guidelines for the diagnosis and management of intravascular catheter-related infection: 2009 Update by the Infectious Diseases Society of America. Clin Infect Dis 49 (1): 1–45.

Minei JP, Hawkins K, Moody B et al. (2000). Alternative case definitions of ventilator-associated pneumonia identify different patients in a surgical intensive care unit. Shock 14 (3): 331–336. discussion 336–337.

Morris AC, Brittan M, Wilkinson TS et al. (2011). C5a-mediated neutrophil dysfunction is RhoA-dependent and predicts infection in critically ill patients. Blood 117 (19): 5178–5188.

Morrow LE, Kollef MH, Casale TB (2010). Probiotic prophylaxis of ventilator-associated pneumonia: a blinded, randomized, controlled trial. Am J Respir Crit Care Med 182 (8): 1058–1064.

Murphy RK, Liu B, Srinath A et al. (2015). No additional protection against ventriculitis with prolonged systemic antibiotic prophylaxis for patients treated with antibiotic-coated external ventricular drains. J Neurosurg 122 (5): 1120–1126.

Muscedere J, Rewa O, McKechnie K et al. (2011). Subglottic secretion drainage for the prevention of ventilator-associated pneumonia: a systematic review and meta-analysis. Crit Care Med 39 (8): 1985–1991.

Mylonakis E, Hohmann EL, Calderwood SB (1998). Central nervous system infection with Listeria monocytogenes. 33 years' experience at a general hospital and review of 776 episodes from the literature. Medicine (Baltimore) 77 (5): 313–336.

Nathoo N, Nadvi SS, van Dellen JR (1997). Neurosurgery 41 (6): 1263–1268. discussion 1268–1269.

Nathoo N, Nadvi SS, van Dellen JR et al. (1999). Intracranial subdural empyemas in the era of computed tomography: a review of 699 cases. Neurosurgery 44 (3): 529–535. discussion 535–536.

Nau R, Sorgel F, Prange HW (1998). Pharmacokinetic optimisation of the treatment of bacterial central nervous system infections. Clin Pharmacokinet 35 (3): 223–246.

Nolan ME, Yadav H, Cawcutt KA et al. (2016). Complication rates among peripherally inserted central venous catheters and centrally inserted central catheters in the medical intensive care unit. J Crit Care 31 (1): 238–242.

Orsi GB, Scorzolini L, Franchi C et al. (2006). Hospital-acquired infection surveillance in a neurosurgical intensive care unit. J Hosp Infect 64 (1): 23–29.

Patir R, Mahapatra AK, Banerji AK (1992). Risk factors in postoperative neurosurgical infection. A prospective study. Acta Neurochir (Wien) 119 (1–4): 80–84.

Parienti JJ, du Cheyron D, Timsit JF et al. (2012). Meta-analysis of subclavian insertion and nontunneled central venous catheter-associated infection risk reduction in critically ill adults. Crit Care Med 40 (5): 1627–1634. http://dx.doi.org/10.1097/CCM.0b013e31823e99cb.

Petersen IS, Aru A, Skodt V et al. (1999). Evaluation of pneumonia diagnosis in intensive care patients. Scand J Infect Dis 31 (3): 299–303.

Pfausler B, Haring HP, Kampfl A et al. (1997). Cerebrospinal fluid (CSF) pharmacokinetics of intraventricular vancomycin in patients with staphylococcal ventriculitis associated with external CSF drainage. Clin Infect Dis 25 (3): 733–735.

Platt R, Polk BF, Murdock B et al. (1986). Risk factors for nosocomial urinary tract infection. Am J Epidemiol 124 (6): 977–985.

Poungvarin N, Bhoopat W, Viriyavejakul A et al. (1987). Effects of dexamethasone in primary supratentorial intracerebral hemorrhage. N Engl J Med 316 (20): 1229–1233.

Rebuck JA, Murry KR, Rhoney DH et al. (2000). Infection related to intracranial pressure monitors in adults: analysis of risk factors and antibiotic prophylaxis. J Neurol Neurosurg Psychiatry 69 (3): 381–384.

Rello J, Ollendorf D, Oster G et al. (2002). Epidemiology and outcomes of ventilator-associated pneumonia in a large US database. Chest 122: 2115–2121.

Ropper AH (2004). Neurological and neurosurgical intensive care. Fever and Infections in the Neurological Intensive Care Unit. Lippincott, Williams & Wilkins, Philadelphia, PA.

Safdar N, Maki DG (2002). Inflammation at the insertion site is not predictive of catheter-related bloodstream infection with short-term, noncuffed central venous catheters. Crit Care Med 30 (12): 2632–2635.

Safdar N, Dezfulian C, Collard HR et al. (2005). Clinical and economic consequences of ventilator-associated pneumonia: a systematic review. Crit Care Med 33 (10): 2184–2193.

Saint S (2000). Clinical and economic consequences of nosocomial catheter-related bacteriuria. Am J Infect Control 28 (1): 68–75.

Salmon JH (1972). Ventriculitis complicating meningitis. Am J Dis Child 124 (1): 35–40.

Shorr AF, Cook D, Jiang X et al. (2008). Correlates of clinical failure in ventilator-associated pneumonia: insights from a large, randomized trial. J Crit Care 23 (1): 64–73.

Sundbarg G, Nordstrom CH, Soderstrom S (1988). Complications due to prolonged ventricular fluid pressure recording. Br J Neurosurg 2 (4): 485–495.

Tambyah PA, Maki DG (2000a). Catheter-associated urinary tract infection is rarely symptomatic: a prospective study of 1,497 catheterized patients. Arch Intern Med 160 (5): 678–682.

Tambyah PA, Maki DG (2000b). The relationship between pyuria and infection in patients with indwelling urinary catheters: a prospective study of 761 patients. Arch Intern Med 160 (5): 673–677.

Tenney JH (1986). Bacterial infections of the central nervous system in neurosurgery. Neurol Clin 4 (1): 91–114.

The Canadian Critical Care Trials Group (2006). A randomized trial of diagnostic techniques for ventilator-associated pneumonia. N Engl J Med 355 (25): 2619–2630.

Titsworth WL, Hester J, Correia T et al. (2012). Reduction of catheter-associated urinary tract infections among patients in a neurological intensive care unit: a single institution's success. J Neurosurg 116 (4): 911–920.

Tunkel AR (2001). Bacterial meningitis. Lippincott Williams & Wilkins, Philadelphia.

Tunkel AR, Hartman BJ, Kaplan SL et al. (2004). Practice guidelines for the management of bacterial meningitis. Clin Infect Dis 39 (9): 1267–1284.

van Ek B, Bakker FP, van Dulken H et al. (1986). Infections after craniotomy: a retrospective study. J Infect 12 (2): 105–109.

Vincent JL, Bihari DJ, Suter PM et al. (1995). The prevalence of nosocomial infection in intensive care units in Europe. Results of the European Prevalence of Infection in Intensive Care (EPIC) Study. EPIC International Advisory Committee. JAMA 274 (8): 639–644.

Wald HL, Kramer AM (2007). Nonpayment for harms resulting from medical care: catheter-associated urinary tract infections. JAMA 298 (23): 2782–2784.

Wald HL, Ma A, Bratzler DW et al. (2008). Indwelling urinary catheter use in the postoperative period: analysis of the national surgical infection prevention project data. Arch Surg 143 (6): 551–557.

Williamson RA, Phillips-Bute BG, McDonagh DL et al. (2014). Predictors of extraventricular drain-associated bacterial ventriculitis. J Crit Care 29 (1): 77–82.

Wisplinghoff H, Bischoff T, Tallent SM et al. (2004). Nosocomial bloodstream infections in US hospitals: analysis of 24,179 cases from a prospective nationwide surveillance study. Clin Infect Dis 39 (3): 309–317.

Wolach B, Sazbon L, Gavrieli R et al. (2001). Early immunological defects in comatose patients after acute brain injury. J Neurosurg 94 (5): 706–711.

Wong AM, Zimmerman RA, Simon EM et al. (2004). Diffusion-weighted MR imaging of subdural empyemas in children. AJNR Am J Neuroradiol 25 (6): 1016–1021.

Wunderink RG, Woldenberg LS, Zeiss J et al. (1992). The radiologic diagnosis of autopsy-proven ventilator-associated pneumonia. Chest 101 (2): 458–463.

Yang KY, Chang WN, Ho JT et al. (2006). Postneurosurgical nosocomial bacterial brain abscess in adults. Infection 34 (5): 247–251.

Yogev R, Davis AT (1980). Neurosurgical shunt infections. A review. Childs Brain 6 (2): 74–81.

Ziai WC, Lewin 3rd JJ (2008). Update in the diagnosis and management of central nervous system infections. Neurol Clin 26 (2): 427–468. viii.

Ziai WC, Lewin 3rd JJ (2009). Improving the role of intraventricular antimicrobial agents in the management of meningitis. Curr Opin Neurol 22 (3): 277–282.

Zolldann D, Spitzer C, Hafner H et al. (2005). Surveillance of nosocomial infections in a neurologic intensive care unit. Infect Control Hosp Epidemiol 26 (8): 726–731.

*Handbook of Clinical Neurology*, Vol. 140 (3rd series)
*Critical Care Neurology, Part I*
E.F.M. Wijdicks and A.H. Kramer, Editors
http://dx.doi.org/10.1016/B978-0-444-63600-3.00021-0

Chapter 21

# Determinants of prognosis in neurocatastrophes

K. SHARMA AND R.D. STEVENS*

*Division of Neurosciences Critical Care, Johns Hopkins University School of Medicine, Baltimore, MD, USA*

## Abstract

A neurocatastrophe or severe brain injury (SBI) is a central nervous system insult associated with a high likelihood of death or severe disability. While many etiologic processes may lead to SBI, the most common and best-studied clinical paradigms are traumatic brain injury and anoxic-ischemic encephalopathy following cardiac arrest. Clinical phenotypes following SBI include acute and chronic disorders of consciousness as well as a range of cognitive and behavioral impairments. A fundamental task for medical teams working in the acute phase is to estimate SBI recovery probabilities with the highest degree of accuracy possible. Predictions made on the basis of single features or variables lack discrimination and are generally supplanted by multivariable models that combine clinical, imaging, and laboratory data into tractable scoring systems. Yet existing scores fail to classify outcomes with the accuracy that would support individual patient-level decision making. Improved prognostication will likely depend on the use of molecular and imaging data that capture unique biologic features in individual patients with SBI. The integration of these additional layers of information will require iterative computational approaches.

## DEFINITION OF SEVERE BRAIN INJURY

One of the challenges in predicting recovery from acute neurologic injury lies in the variability of phenotypic manifestations and clinical trajectories which depend on many determinants, including the preexisting clinical and neurologic state of the patient, the specific etiology and pathophysiology of brain injury, the anatomic distribution of damage, and the relative preponderance of postinjury plasticity and neurodegeneration (Cramer, 2008; Stevens and Sutter, 2013; Geurts et al., 2014; Carmichael et al., 2016). The location of injury is an immediately recognizable prognosticator. Thus a hemispheric cerebral infarction may not cause coma, whereas a much smaller stroke in the dorsal paramedian midbrain or pons might be responsible for an irreversible loss of consciousness (Parvizi and Damasio, 2003; Seet et al., 2005). Overall, while prognostic models must integrate the magnitude of clinical deficits and the anatomic distribution of

injury, these characteristics are not sufficient for accurate outcome classification.

For the purpose of this review, we define neurocatastrophe or severe brain injury (SBI) as an insult severe enough to cause an acute and persistent loss of consciousness and to entail a significant likelihood of death or of long-term functional dependence (Stevens and Sutter, 2013). Although progressive conditions like demyelinating or neurodegenerative diseases may result in an analogous phenotype, we will restrict the discussion in this chapter to acute neurologic injury only. A special emphasis will be made on traumatic brain injury (TBI) and anoxic-ischemic encephalopathy (AIE), which are the leading and best-studied clinical paradigms of SBI. The prognostic considerations discussed here arise when the inciting neural insult unfolds over a discrete period of minutes to hours. The potential for functional recovery in these circumstances informs all phases of care for these patients.

---

*Correspondence to: Robert D. Stevens, MD, Division of Neuroscience Critical Care, Johns Hopkins University School of Medicine, 600 N. Wolfe St, Phipps 455, Baltimore MD 21287, USA. Tel: +1-410-955-7481, Fax: +1-410-614-7903, E-mail: rstevens@jhmi.edu

## ETIOLOGIC CLASSIFICATION OF SEVERE BRAIN INJURY

A number of etiologic processes may result in a phenotype of SBI. However, a preponderance of published observations regarding prognosis and the potential for recovery have been realized in patients with AIE following cardiac arrest and in TBI (Geurts et al., 2014). These types of injury may particularly lend themselves to investigation of recovery prediction as they represent a temporally discrete insult, often occurring in a previously undiseased neurologic context. Research on recovery from vascular events such as ischemic stroke, intracerebral hemorrhage (ICH), and aneurysmal subarachnoid hemorrhage (SAH) can also yield valuable prognostic clues. On the other hand, the trajectory of recovery from other etiologies of SBI (e.g., autoimmune encephalitis) may be more difficult to predict in the acute setting given natural histories which remain insufficiently characterized (Titulaer et al., 2013); in these situations, it is therefore more challenging to establish predictive models on the basis of acute injury markers.

## TRAJECTORIES OF RECOVERY

The clinical trajectory following SBI may be considered in terms of three linked processes that overlap temporally and mechanistically: (1) recovery of consciousness; (2) recovery of higher neuropsychologic processing; and (3) return of functional independence.

### Recovery of consciousness

Recovery of consciousness may be viewed conceptually as a matrix of disorders of consciousness (DOC) that are distributed along the two principal axes: content/complexity of cognitive functioning (awareness) on the one hand, and the level of arousal (vigilance, wakefulness) on the other (Laureys et al., 2004). Recent evidence obtained with functional neuroimaging has suggested that a subset of patients who exhibit a clinical phenotype of unconsciousness may have patterns of neural activation that are analogous to those seen in conscious subjects (Monti et al., 2010; Cruse et al., 2011). Thus, it has been proposed that clinical characterization of DOC should refer to the more descriptive "levels of (motor) responsiveness" rather than the interpretive "levels of consciousness" (Giacino et al., 2014). Phenotypic accounts of DOC include a range of descriptive terms such as lethargy, obtundation, stupor, akinetic mutism, and apallic syndrome; since there is limited consensus on the biologic meaning of these different terms, there has been a push to adopt objective scoring systems to evaluate conscious states. The best known among these are the Glasgow Coma Scale (GCS: Teasdale and Jennett, 1974), Full Outline of UnResponsiveness (FOUR) score (Wijdicks et al., 2005), and the Coma Recovery Scale (Giacino et al., 1991, 2004).

Coma is a state of eyes-closed unarousable unresponsiveness (Posner and Plum, 2007). Coma patients lack both wakefulness and awareness. In response to stimuli, the comatose patient may grimace and exhibit stereotyped extension, flexion, or withdrawal responses in the extremities, but the patient does not make localizing or purposeful movements (Posner and Plum, 2007). The vegetative state (VS) is characterized by the return of an arousal phenotype without signs of awareness (Jennett and Plum, 1972; Multi-Society Task Force on PVS, 1994a, b). Patients in the VS have spontaneous eye opening, but do not attend to stimuli, and there is no evidence of language comprehension, verbal or gestural communication, or reproducible purposeful behavioral responses to visual, auditory, tactile, or noxious stimuli. Recently, the term "unresponsive wakefulness syndrome" was proposed to convey the phenotype of VS more accurately (Laureys et al., 2010). The minimally conscious state (MCS) identifies a condition of severely impaired arousal in which there is fragmented, but unequivocal, evidence of self or environmental awareness (Giacino et al., 2002). Patients in MCS may visually attend to and track stimuli, have purposeful motor activity, follow commands, and demonstrate contextually relevant facial expression or speech. A key feature of MCS is that these meaningful behaviors occur in an intermittent and unpredictable fashion, hence repeated examination is generally required to establish the diagnosis. VS/unresponsive wakefulness syndrome or MCS may occur as transitional states during neurologic recovery, or conversely they may persist indefinitely with minimal improvement (Katz et al., 2009; Nakase-Richardson et al., 2012). Lastly, the term "emerged from the MCS" or EMCS is used to denote those DOC patients who, in contradistinction to MCS, have recovered reliable and consistent communication or functional object use (Giacino et al., 2002).

### Recovery of higher neuropsychologic processing

The restoration of conscious awareness is associated with the emergence of higher-order mental processes, including perception, attention, directed motor planning, executive function, memory, language, and emotion. Neuropsychologic function may be assessed with the help of an array of cognitive batteries which test global or domain-specific capabilities (Fields et al., 2011). These batteries have been for the most part established and validated for the evaluation of patients with or at risk for dementia; their face and construct validity in patients recovering from SBI are less well established. Moreover, a plausible description, let alone an understanding, of the sequence or pattern governing the individual and cohesive recovery of cognitive domains following specific types of SBI is lacking. Cognition depends to a large degree on integration between widely distributed regions of the cerebral cortex; their restoration following injury, it is postulated, is reflective of either reactivation of intact cerebral networks and/or adaptive cortical reorganization (Grefkes and Fink, 2011; Carmichael et al., 2016). Notwithstanding insights which have been gained on the neural basis of recovery in patients with focal lesions (e.g., stroke) and for selected functions (e.g., motor recovery) (Granziera et al., 2012; Forkel et al., 2014), far less is known regarding the recovery of cognition, in particular when injury is diffuse or multifocal, as is the case with TBI or AIE.

## Recovery of functional independence

Alongside the restoration of cognition, arguably the most meaningful development for patients and their families is the recovery of functional independence. In its widest sense, functional independence refers to a matrix of intrinsic and learned capabilities that are necessary for physical, mental, social, and professional health and well-being. In the clinical realm, functional status is measured and classified with the help of activity/disability scoring systems or scales, of which several have been extensively validated in patients recovering from SBI. These include the Barthel index (Mahoney and Barthel, 1965) and modified Rankin scale (van Swieten et al., 1988), used primarily in patients with stroke, ICH, and SAH; the Glasgow Outcome Scale (Jennett and Bond, 1975), Extended Glasgow Outcome Scale (Jennett et al., 1981), and Disability Rating Scale (Rappaport et al., 1982), used in patients with TBI; and the Cerebral Performance Category scale, used in AIE (Brain Resuscitation Clinical Trial I Study Group, 1986).

## NEUROBIOLOGY

Conscious awareness has been linked to coupled, integrated activity between discrete neuronal populations in the thalamus and cortical association areas (Laureys et al., 2000; Llinas and Steriade, 2006; Ching et al., 2010). Electroencephalography (EEG) activity reflective of collective synaptic activity in neocortical and hippocampal neurons is thought to stem largely from this system (Llinas and Steriade, 2006). The overall level of arousal, in turn, is regulated by the ascending reticular arousal system (ARAS), a distributed multineurotransmitter neuronal system originating in the dorsal pons and midbrain (Parvizi and Damasio, 2003). The thalamic

projections of the ARAS regulate thalamocortical activity associated with sleep and wakefulness. ARAS projections to the hypothalamus and basal forebrain are relayed by secondary projections to multiple cortical sites that regulate arousal (Saper et al., 2005). Widespread activity in prefrontal and parietal cortices correlates temporally with reports of conscious awareness in experimental paradigms comparing conscious to nonconscious information processing (Dehaene and Changeux, 2011). This multisite cortical activation has been hypothesized to represent the neural underpinning of a "global workspace" of internal cognitive information needed for conscious awareness to emerge (Dehaene and Naccache, 2001).

DOC occur when there is reduced activity of neurons in the thalamocortical and/or corticocortical systems (Llinás and Steriade, 2006). Synaptic deafferentation and/or deefferentation of the thalamus, cortex, and striatum, as occurs in SBI, results in an inability to maintain patterns of multifocal brain integration needed for conscious awareness (Timofeev et al., 2000; Brown et al., 2010). The spectrum of DOC described in the previous section has been linked to damage to structures of the ARAS anywhere from the originating neurons in the brainstem to the thalamus, hypothalamus, or basal forebrain (Gosseries et al., 2014). DOC may also result from bilateral thalamic or cortical damage, or disconnection of the thalamocortical or corticocortical pathways (Posner and Plum, 2007; Giacino et al., 2014). Recovery of conscious awareness is, in turn, associated with restoration of integration within distributed cortical systems (Vanhaudenhuyse et al., 2010; Boly et al., 2011; Rosanova et al., 2012; Di Perri et al., 2016).

## PROGNOSTIC VARIABLES

### Age

Age has been reported as a significant predictor of mortality and functional outcome in SBI across etiologies (Hemphill et al., 2001; Mushkudiani et al., 2007; Rosengart et al., 2007; Dragancea et al., 2015). In TBI, many studies analyze age as an ordinal variable organized in ranges (e.g., 0–20, 20–40, 40–60, >60 years). Fewer studies have analyzed the association between outcome and age as a continuous variable; these studies indicate both an inflection point around age 30–40 years, above which outcome becomes increasingly worse, and a fairly continuous relation across all ages, which may be approximated by a linear function (Mushkudiani et al., 2007; Perel et al., 2008; Tokutomi et al., 2008).

In cardiac arrest, a weak inverse association between advanced age (>80 years) and survival to discharge has been noted in studies of out-of-hospital (Longstreth et al., 1990; Kim et al., 2000; Rea et al., 2003) and in-hospital arrest patients (Ebell et al., 2013), although in other studies no such association was seen (Wuerz et al., 1995).

Age is independently associated with mortality and functional outcome after ischemic stroke (Wahlgren et al., 2008; Cooray et al., 2016), and the same robust association has been noted in patients with ICH (Hemphill et al., 2001, 2009); Godoy et al., 2006; Rost et al., 2008 and SAH (Ogilvy and Carter, 1998; Rosengart et al., 2007).

## Neurologic presentation

The severity of neurologic injury, as assessed by clinical examination, is one of the most consistently reported predictors of outcome in many injury models. Abolition of the pupillary light reflex may indicate brainstem dysfunction or compression, and is associated with mortality in TBI independent of the GCS (Hoffmann et al., 2012; Majdan et al., 2015). The GCS (Teasdale and Jennett, 1974) has been widely adopted as a simple method to numerically express the clinically observed features of consciousness. Studies in TBI, cardiac arrest, ischemic stroke, ICH, and SAH patients have shown an association between lower score on the GCS and worse short- and longer-term survival or functional outcome (Rordorf et al., 2000; Hemphill et al., 2001; Marmarou et al., 2007; Perel et al., 2008; van Heuven et al., 2008; Schefold et al., 2009; Degos et al., 2012). The motor component of the GCS has the highest predictive value in prognostic models of TBI and AIE (Steyerberg et al., 2008; Perel et al., 2008; Dragancea et al., 2015). The predictive value of the verbal and eye opening subscores of the GCS is diminished in many SBI patients due to concurrent intubation, sedation, or lesions causing aphasia, aphonia, or in the presence of facial or ocular injury impeding eye evaluation. The GCS also does not directly assess impairment in brainstem responses, which are independently associated with poor outcomes in SBI.

The FOUR score overcomes some of the shortcomings of the GCS by including an assessment of pupillary light reflex, corneal reflex, cough reflex, and breathing pattern (Wijdicks et al., 2005). Head-to-head comparisons suggest that GCS and FOUR have equivalent predictive accuracy in discriminating outcomes of patients with TBI and AIE (Fugate et al., 2010a; McNett et al., 2014; Saika et al., 2015; Kasprowicz et al., 2016).

Among patients with AIE, early studies demonstrated that death or severe disability could be predicted on the basis of a limited number of clinical signs, including abnormal motor responses and the lack of brainstem reflexes like pupillary light reactivity, corneal and oculocephalic or oculovestibular responses (Bates et al., 1977; Levy et al., 1985). In a more contemporary cohort of 500

patients with nontraumatic coma, the pupillary and, to a lesser degree, oculocephalic responses were the clinical findings most predictive of 6-month functional outcome (Greer et al., 2012). However, current prospective evaluations in AIE patients who were treated with targeted temperature management (TTM) challenge the predictive accuracy of clinical findings, in particular the association between absent or abnormal motor responses and poor outcome, with false-positive rates of up to 24% in recent reports (Rossetti et al., 2010a; Bouwes et al., 2012; Dragancea et al., 2015). The reduced prognostic significance of clinical findings in AIE patients treated with TTM is further borne out in three recently published meta-analyses (Kamps et al., 2013; Sandroni et al., 2013; Golan et al., 2014).

## Structural neuroimaging

Cranial computed tomographic (CT) scanning is an integral part of the evaluation in the acute phase of virtually all patients with SBI owing to widespread accessibility, speed of acquisition, and sensitivity to acute hemorrhage or lesions that require immediate intervention. In survivors of cardiac arrest, early anoxic-ischemic damage is suggested by a loss of differentiation between gray and white matter (Torbey et al., 2000; Cocchi et al., 2010; Inamasu et al., 2010, 2011; Kim et al., 2013; Scheel et al., 2013; Cristia et al., 2014; Gentsch et al., 2015; Langkjaer et al., 2015; Lee et al., 2015; Hanning et al., 2016), which is believed to indicate a relative loss of gray-matter density due to neuronal cell death; however, in many cases of AIE, CT is unrevealing.

In the TBI population, several features readily identified on cranial CT scan have major prognostic significance. These include shift of midline structures, encroachment of the basal cisterns, cerebral infarction, SAH, intraventricular hemorrhage, diffuse injury, and extra-axial hematomas. Combinations of individual CT characteristics in a multivariable model like the Marshall (Marshall et al., 1992) or Rotterdam (Maas et al., 2005) CT scores provide good discrimination between patients with favorable and unfavorable outcome. Notwithstanding, cranial CT lacks the resolution to detect early stages of diffuse or multifocal traumatic axonal injury (TAI), which is the biologic hallmark of TBI across the severity spectrum, and likely one of its most important prognostic determinants (Hill et al., 2016).

While CT may be insensitive to tissue changes occurring in the hyperacute phase (3–6 hours) of ischemic stroke, subsequent indicators of parenchymal edema are predictive of the extent of tissue infarction, response to reperfusion therapy (Hill et al., 2006; Finlayson et al., 2013; Soize et al., 2013; Yaghi et al.,

2014), and may help predict risk of fatal or malignant infarction (Haring et al., 1999; Kim et al., 2010; Minnerup et al., 2011). Cranial CT is critical in the evaluation of patients with intracranial hemorrhage. In ICH, CT readily identifies hematoma location, hematoma volume and growth, perihematomal edema, and the presence of intraventricular extension, all of which are predictors of survival and functional outcome (Hemphill et al., 2001, 2009; Gebel et al., 2002; Huttner et al., 2006; Delcourt et al., 2012; Sato et al., 2014; Murthy et al., 2015; Purrucker et al., 2016). Recently, several groups have examined the significance of the focal contrast extravasation on contrast-enhanced cranial CT – the so-called "spot sign" – obtained in the acute phase of ICH. These studies consistently demonstrate a robust association between the presence, size, and number of spot signs and unfavorable post-ICH outcome (Wada et al., 2007; Delgado Almandoz et al., 2010; Demchuk et al., 2012).

Brain magnetic resonance imaging (MRI) is the method of choice to characterize brain damage in SBI. The prognostic value of MRI in the acute setting of traumatic and non-TBI is being actively investigated. In patients with traumatic coma, there is an inverse correlation between number of axial white-matter lesions detected acutely using T2-weighted or fluid-attenuated inversion recovery (FLAIR) sequences and long-term functional status (Yanagawa et al., 2000; Carpentier et al., 2006). Lesions of the corpus callosum, pons, midbrain, and basal ganglia are predictive of poor outcome, especially when they are bilateral (Weiss et al., 2008; Skandsen et al., 2011). However, conventional MR sequences lack specificity and sufficient sensitivity for detection and characterization of TAI. In rodent models of TBI, diffusion-weighted MRI (Alsop et al., 1996; Albensi et al., 2000; Immonen et al., 2009) and, in particular, diffusion tensor imaging (DTI) (MacDonald et al., 2007; Tu et al., 2016), are sensitive to TAI-associated white-matter damage and correlate with behavioral deficits. In patients with severe TBI, there is evidence that quantitative assessment and localization of white-matter damage using DTI may be equal or superior to clinical prediction of long-term functional outcome (Kraus et al., 2007; Sidaros et al., 2008; Tollard et al., 2009; Galanaud et al., 2013). Using proton MR spectroscopy, cellular changes in the form of altered neuronal energy metabolism and viability, cell membrane damage, and gliosis can all be robustly observed and quantified, even in tissues that may appear normal using conventional morphologic MRI sequences. These changes have been linked to worse long-term outcome (Garnett et al., 2000a) and may have increased prognostic accuracy when combined with DTI information (Tollard et al., 2009).

With regard to AIE, findings from brain MRI, and in particular diffusion-weighted sequences, contain valuable prognostic information (Wijman et al., 2009; Mlynash et al., 2010; Greer et al., 2011; Hirsch et al., 2016). In one cohort, mean whole-brain apparent diffusion coefficient measured 2–5 days after cardiac arrest discriminated between 6-month functional outcome categories more accurately than clinical assessment (Wijman et al., 2009). In other studies, reduced regional values in the putamen and in occipital, parietal, and temporal cortices and in the putamen correlated with poor outcomes (Wu et al., 2009; Choi et al., 2010). Recently it was reported that white-matter damage as detected by quantitative DTI is widespread after cardiac arrest and classified 1-year functional outcome with a reasonable degree of accuracy (Luyt et al., 2012). MR spectroscopy may provide complementary information by identifying metabolic abnormalities associated with neuronal and glial damage, and increase the sensitivity for predicting unfavorable outcome (Khong et al., 2004; Wartenberg et al., 2004).

## Functional and metabolic neuroimaging

By mapping the functional MRI (fMRI) signal, regional activation of the brain may be inferred at rest, during passive stimulus presentation, or in response to a specific command. During resting-state fMRI, patients in MCS or EMCS demonstrate higher levels of connectivity within large-scale networks than those in VS, suggesting greater degrees of integration within corticocortical and corticothalamic systems responsible for maintaining conscious awareness (Rodriguez Moreno et al., 2010; Vanhaudenhuyse et al., 2010; Soddu et al., 2012; Demertzi et al., 2015; Monti et al., 2015; Di Perri et al., 2016). In the subacute to chronic stages of brain injury, fMRI correlates of increasing auditory and language discrimination were predictive of the degree of behavioral recovery (Coleman et al., 2009). In patients with DOC, innovative experimental paradigms can examine the performance of one or more cognitive tasks during the fMRI acquisition. Thus, near-normal fMRI patterns of cortical processing have been demonstrated in behaviorally unresponsive (VS or MCS) patients who were asked to perform motor and spatial mental imagery tasks (Owen et al., 2006; Monti et al., 2010). The utility of resting or task-based fMRI for prognostication in the acute phase of brain injury may be severely confounded by sedation or metabolic derangements seen in this period.

An association has been described between consciousness and both global and regional brain metabolic activity measured using fluorodeoxyglucose (FDG)-positron emission tomography (PET) (Shulman et al., 2009; Hyder et al., 2013; Stender et al., 2015, 2016). This relationship is most conspicuous within frontoparietal structures believed to be the networks responsible for conscious awareness (Stender et al., 2015). In a recent study, FDG-PET was found to be more sensitive for the detection of patients in MCS than mental-imagery fMRI, and also correctly predicted 12-month functional outcome in a higher percentage of patients (Stender et al., 2014).

## Neurophysiologic testing

### ELECTROENCEPHALOGRAPHY

EEG is a versatile point-of-care monitor which may help detect seizures and cerebral ischemia in patients with SBI (Sutter et al., 2013). Seizure activity and status epilepticus are common following SBI and may be difficult to detect clinically, due to the frequent onset of a nonconvulsive phenotype. Moreover, seizure activity may be associated with worse short- and long-term functional outcome in patients with TBI (Vespa et al., 1999, 2007, 2010; Claassen and Vespa, 2014), AIE (Legriel et al., 2009; Rossetti et al., 2010b; Foreman et al., 2012; Mani et al., 2012; Rittenberger et al., 2012; Knight et al., 2013; Crepeau et al., 2014, 2015; Amorim et al., 2015; Youn et al., 2015), SAH (Claassen et al., 2005, 2006; Kondziella et al., 2015; De Marchis et al., 2016), and ICH (Vespa et al., 2003). For these reasons, consideration for serial or continuous EEG monitoring has been recommended in comatose patients following SBI (Claassen et al., 2013; Claassen and Vespa, 2014).

In patients with TBI, seizures are associated with dramatic physiologic disturbances, including increased cerebral metabolic rate, blood flow, and blood volume, resulting in an elevation of intracranial pressure (Vespa et al., 2007). Seizures in severe TBI could be associated with long-term morphologic changes in the brain, as indicated in a report in which brain MRI at 6 months postinjury demonstrated asymmetric hippocampal atrophy that was more prominent ipsilateral to the seizure focus (Vespa et al., 2010). EEG in TBI patients allows the detection of a range of other abnormal patterns, such as periodic epileptiform discharges; however, the relationship between such patterns and TBI outcomes is unclear (Claassen and Vespa, 2014).

A large body of evidence supports EEG in the prognostic evaluation of comatose survivors of cardiac arrest (Sandroni et al., 2013; Claassen and Vespa, 2014; Golan et al., 2014). The presence of "malignant patterns" – burst suppression, low-voltage output pattern, alpha/theta coma, focal or generalized seizures, generalized periodic epileptiform discharges, status epilepticus – are predictive of survival and functional outcome (Young et al., 2005; Fugate et al., 2010b; Amorim et al., 2015; Youn et al., 2015; Lamartine Monteiro

et al., 2016; Westhall et al., 2016). The predictive value of malignant EEG patterns is, however, reduced in patients who have been treated with TTM (Rossetti et al., 2010a; Bouwes et al., 2012). It is unclear if successful treatment of seizures seen on EEG actually improves outcomes following AIE (Rossetti et al., 2010b; Crepeau et al., 2013). Recently, a convergence of results indicates that the presence of background EEG reactivity to stimulation is an independent predictor of favorable outcome that is less susceptible to confounding by hypothermia or timing of EEG (Rossetti et al., 2009, 2010b, 2012; Fugate et al., 2010b; Cloostermans et al., 2012; Noirhomme et al., 2014; Lamartine Monteiro et al., 2016).

### SOMATOSENSORY EVOKED POTENTIALS

The prognostic value of somatosensory evoked potentials (SSEPs) has been most extensively studied in patients with AIE (Young et al., 2005; Rossetti et al., 2010a; Cronberg et al., 2011; Bouwes et al., 2012; Kamps et al., 2013; Sandroni et al., 2013; Golan et al., 2014; Rothstein, 2014a, b; Endisch et al., 2015, 2016). The bilateral absence of cortical (N20) signals is consistently reported to be the most accurate and reliable predictor of poor outcome, with false-positive rates of 0–5% across multiple studies in AIE patients managed with TTM (Rossetti et al., 2010a; Kamps et al., 2013; Sandroni et al., 2013; Rothstein, 2014b; Dragancea et al., 2015). The significance of SSEP in predicting death or disability following severe TBI was recognized in several early studies (Hume and Cant, 1981; Anderson et al., 1984; Judson et al., 1990; Claassen and Hansen, 2001; Robinson et al., 2003). More recently, Houlden et al. (2010) found a relationship between presence and bilaterality of SSEP abnormalities on day 3 after injury and 1-year functional outcome and cognitive performance.

### LONG-LATENCY EVOKED POTENTIALS

Evoked potentials can be elicited by sensory, cognitive, or motor paradigms. EPs that peak early, within 100 ms of stimulus presentation, depend largely on the physical parameters of the stimulus and integrity of primary sensory pathways (e.g., SSEP). Longer-latency event-related potentials (ERPs) (>100 ms latency) are believed to reflect cortical responses to, and processing of, the presented information. Long-latency evoked potentials (EPs) are very-low-voltage EEG signals generated in response to specific mental events or external stimuli (Kane et al., 1996; Bekinschtein et al., 2009). In patients with DOC, a common method of eliciting ERPs relevant to auditory processing is the "oddball" paradigm, in which different stimuli are presented in a series, such that one of them, the "oddball" or "deviant" stimulus, is perceived as unexpected within a sequence of "standard" stimuli. "Mismatch negativity" (MMN) is generated by the brain's response to stimulus deviation from preceding repetitive stimuli. It is expressed numerically by subtracting ERP to a standard stimulus from ERPs to a deviant stimulus detected at 100–300 ms (Naatanen et al., 2007). MMN is believed to represent a form of memory trace and predictive capacity, which develops regardless of whether stimuli are attended to or not (i.e., it is preattentive), and its presence has been associated with improved recovery trajectories in patients with SBI (Fischer et al., 1999, 2004, 2006; Jones et al., 2000; Wijnen et al., 2007; Qin et al., 2008; Vanhaudenhuyse et al., 2008; Tzovara et al., 2013, 2015, 2016; Rossetti et al., 2014).

The P300 wave (P3) is generated when there is higher-order processing of a stimulus, in particular, recruitment of attentional mechanisms (Polich, 2007). This is most commonly elicited using an auditory-oddball paradigm as a positive ERP after 300 ms. Instructing the subject to respond to, or increasing the salience of, the deviant stimulus elicits a higher amplitude of P300 response with shorter latencies, thought to be indicative of greater mental performance relative to longer latencies. Patients in MCS may be differentiated from VS patients using stimulus paradigms that distinguish conscious processing from unconscious responses (Boly et al., 2011). Presence of P300 has been associated with a higher probability, and faster recovery, of consciousness following SBI (Perrin et al., 2006; Schnakers et al., 2008; Vanhaudenhuyse et al., 2008; Faugeras et al., 2011; Steppacher et al., 2013; Li et al., 2015).

## Brain-specific serum markers

The potential value of a serum biomarker in the realm of SBI detection, diagnosis, and neuroprognostication ultimately depends on several key variables, including: organ-specificity (e.g., brain vs. other organs), cell origin (e.g., neurons vs. glia), molecular species (protein, lipid, nucleic acid, or low-molecular-weight organic compound), cellular mechanism leading to release of the marker (e.g., necrosis, apoptosis, inflammation), etiologic process (e.g., ischemia, axonal stretching, or immunologic activation), time elapsed after injury, and integrity of the blood–brain barrier. The discussion here is limited to TBI and AIE, in which the majority of the validation work has been conducted.

### TRAUMATIC BRAIN INJURY

A number of serum-based biomarkers have been evaluated in regard to prognosis after TBI. Serum levels of the protein S100β increase following TBI and have been associated with unfavorable functional outcome in the short, mid, and long term (Mussack et al., 2002; Dimopoulou et al., 2003, 2004; Vos et al., 2004, 2010; Korfias et al., 2007; Bohmer et al., 2011; Czeiter et al., 2012; Metting et al., 2012; Mercier et al., 2013). However, cutoff serum values for optimal discrimination between outcome categories have not been defined (Mercier et al., 2013). The protein neuron-specific enolase (NSE) is increased in serum following TBI and predicts mortality and neurologic outcome following moderate and severe TBI (Vos et al., 2004, 2010; Bohmer et al., 2011). However, uncertainty persists regarding the best postinjury timing for NSE sampling and also the cutoff values to maximize discrimination (Cheng et al., 2014). Glial fibrillary acidic protein (GFAP) is released by astrocytes and oligodendrocytes, and increased levels are detectable in the serum of patients with brain injury (Vos et al., 2004, 2010; Bohmer et al., 2011). Serum GFAP levels correlate with clinical and neuroradiologic TBI severity, and are significantly higher in patients who die or have poor functional outcome (Nylén et al., 2006; Mondello et al., 2011; Raheja et al., 2016). Studies in small populations of severe TBI patients have demonstrated increased serum levels of the axonal tau protein (Rubenstein et al., 2015), and serum tau levels correlate with mortality and functional outcomes (Liliang et al., 2010).

Alpha-II spectrin (280 kDa) is a structural component of the neuronal membrane cytoskeleton and is particularly abundant in axons and presynaptic terminals; it is a substrate for the cell-death enzymes, including calpains and caspases. In a study of 40 patients with severe TBI, alpha-II spectrin breakdown products were significantly higher in patients with severe TBI who died compared to survivors (Mondello et al., 2010).

Ubiquitin C-terminal hydrolase-L1 (UCHL1) is involved in the processing of ubiquitin precursors and ubiquitinated proteins and is abundant in neurons. UCHL1 levels are elevated in serum and CSF of patients with severe TBI, and preliminary studies suggest it may be useful in predicting outcomes (Brophy et al., 2011; Mondello et al., 2012a). Recent work has also suggested the potential predictive value of microtubule-associated protein (MAP-2), considered to be a dendritic marker of both acute damage and neuronal regeneration after injury. Early increased levels in CSF were found to correlate with worse outcomes in severe TBI (Papa et al., 2015). However, persistently high levels chronically tend to correlate with improved outcomes (Mondello et al., 2012b).

### ANOXIC-ISCHEMIC ENCEPHALOPATHY

In patients with AIE, elevated serum levels of NSE and S100β have been shown to robustly correlate with the likelihood of death or poor functional outcome in the short and long term following cardiac arrest (Mussack et al., 2002; Fugate et al., 2010b; Rossetti et al., 2010a; Cronberg et al., 2011; Mörtberg et al., 2011; Kamps et al., 2013; Sandroni et al., 2013). Preliminary studies have also suggested a role for elevated serum GFAP and procalcitonin levels as predictors of poor outcome (Mörtberg et al., 2011; Engel et al., 2013). Recent work indicates that the accuracy of serum NSE elevation in patients who received TTM is significantly reduced (Rossetti et al., 2010a; Bouwes et al., 2012; Kamps et al., 2013; Sandroni et al., 2013; Golan et al., 2014). In one study of patients treated with TTM, S100β performed better than NSE as a predictor of poor outcome, while GFAP and brain-derived neurotrophic factor did not adequately discriminate between outcome categories (Mörtberg et al., 2011). Other candidate biomarkers that have been associated with AIE outcome include interleukin-6, serum tau levels, and brain-enriched microRNAs (Randall et al., 2013; Gilje et al., 2014; Vaahersalo et al., 2014; Devaux et al., 2016).

## MULTIVARIABLE MODELS

While single clinical features or biomarker variables may correlate with outcome probabilities, the accuracy of SBI outcome prediction is increased when classifiers are integrated using multivariable logistic regression modeling techniques, or evidence-based algorithms and decision-tree methods. Here again, the discussion is limited to TBI and AIE.

### Traumatic brain injury

There have been several efforts to build prognostic models of severe TBI by combining clinical features, cranial CT scan imaging, and physiologic or biochemical abnormalities (Perel et al., 2006). The International Mission for Prognosis and Analysis of Clinical Trials in TBI (IMPACT) and Corticosteroid Randomisation After Significant Head Injury (CRASH) models were developed by pooling data from large randomized trials conducted in patients with severe TBI (Murray et al., 2007; Perel et al., 2008; Lingsma et al., 2010). Both of these models have been validated internally and externally (Steyerberg et al., 2008; Gomez et al., 2014; Han et al., 2014; Harrison et al., 2015; Lingsma et al., 2015; Castano-Leon et al., 2016). Variables used in these models include demographic characteristics, neurologic exam findings (GCS, pupil reactivity), neuroanatomic descriptors from cranial CT (midline shift and encroachment of basilar cisterns), physiologic derangements (hypoxia and hypotension), presence or absence of extracranial injuries, and select laboratory values (serum hemoglobin and glucose). Both models discriminate outcomes with areas under the receiver operating characteristic curve (AUC) of 0.6–0.8 (Steyerberg et al., 2008; Roozenbeek et al., 2012; Han et al., 2014; Castano-Leon et al., 2016; Zador et al., 2016). While useful for population-based assessments, these systems do not have the degree of accuracy that would be meaningful for individual patient care. Discrimination might be enhanced by multimodality prediction systems; thus, in one recent report, the AUC of the IMPACT score for 1-year functional outcome prediction was increased significantly using a model which combined IMPACT with a DTI measure of white-matter integrity (Galanaud et al., 2012).

### Anoxic-ischemic encephalopathy

Prognostic scoring systems supported by very large patient datasets such as IMPACT and CRASH have not been established for AIE. The out-of-hospital cardiac arrest (OHCA) score is based on five independent predictors to estimate the likelihood of poor outcome at hospital discharge: initial rhythm, no flow interval, low flow interval, serum creatinine, and serum lactate (Adrie et al., 2006); however, the accuracy of discrimination using this score is moderate, with AUC in the 0.7–0.8 range (Adrie et al., 2006; Sunde et al., 2007; Skrifvars et al., 2012; Bisbal et al., 2014). The Pittsburgh Cardiac Arrest Category illness severity score classifies cardiac arrest patients into four categories based on a combination of features derived from the FOUR score and sequential organ failure assessment (Coppler et al., 2015); internal validation indicates that this score correlates with the likelihood of survival and favorable functional status at hospital discharge (Coppler et al., 2015). The Good Outcome Following Attempted Resuscitation score was developed to predict the likelihood of survival with good neurologic function after in-hospital cardiac arrest (Ebell et al., 2013); it includes 13 variables – age, neurologic deficits on admission, history of trauma, stroke, metastatic cancer, septicemia, any medical noncardiac diagnosis, hepatic insufficiency, renal insufficiency, respiratory insufficiency, hypotension or hypoperfusion, pneumonia, and admission from a skilled nursing facility; model performance was fair, with an AUC of 0.78 in the validation set (Ebell et al., 2013).

A widely used prediction algorithm, based on extensive analysis of available literature, is the American Academy of Neurology practice parameter, published in 2006 (Wijdicks et al., 2006). Variables used in this algorithm to predict poor outcome are absence of brainstem reflexes at any time postinjury, myoclonic status epilepticus on day 1, bilaterally absent N20 response or serum NSE > 33 μg/L on day 1–3, or poor neurologic status (absent pupil/corneal, extensor posturing/absent motor response) on day 3.

In current daily practice prediction is based on likely (meaning more often than not) expectations of permanent disability and how the patient would cope with it physically and mentally. This limitation might be addressed via more precise models that integrate biologic features which are the true drivers of post-SBI recovery trajectories. Such models might require computational approaches to analyze and integrate multilayer datasets, including gene and protein expression, metabolomics, advanced imaging, and detailed trajectory analysis (Topol, 2014).

## REFERENCES

Adrie C, Cariou A, Mourvillier B et al. (2006). Predicting survival with good neurological recovery at hospital admission after successful resuscitation of out-of-hospital cardiac arrest: the OHCA score. Eur Heart J 27 (23): 2840–2845.

Albensi BC, Knoblach SM, Chew BG et al. (2000). Diffusion and high resolution MRI of traumatic brain injury in rats: time course and correlation with histology. Exp Neurol 162 (1): 61–72.

Alsop DC, Murai H, Detre JA et al. (1996). Detection of acute pathologic changes following experimental traumatic brain injury using diffusion-weighted magnetic resonance imaging. J Neurotrauma 13 (9): 515–521.

Amorim E, Rittenberger JC, Baldwin ME et al. (2015). Malignant EEG patterns in cardiac arrest patients treated with targeted temperature management who survive to hospital discharge. Resuscitation 90: 127–132.

Anderson DC, Bundlie S, Rockswold GL (1984). Multimodality evoked potentials in closed head trauma. Arch Neurol 41 (4): 369–374.

Bates D, Caronna JJ, Cartlidge NE et al. (1977). A prospective study of nontraumatic coma: methods and results in 310 patients. Ann Neurol 2 (3): 211–220.

Bekinschtein TA, Dehaene S, Rohaut B et al. (2009). Neural signature of the conscious processing of auditory regularities. Proc Natl Acad Sci U S A 106 (5): 1672–1677.

Bisbal M, Jouve E, Papazian L et al. (2014). Effectiveness of SAPS III to predict hospital mortality for post-cardiac arrest patients. Resuscitation 85 (7): 939–944.

Bohmer AE, Oses JP, Schmidt AP et al. (2011). Neuron-specific enolase, S100B, and glial fibrillary acidic protein levels as outcome predictors in patients with severe traumatic brain injury. Neurosurgery 68 (6): 1624–1630. discussion 30–31.

Boly M, Garrido MI, Gosseries O et al. (2011). Preserved feedforward but impaired top-down processes in the vegetative state. Science (New York, NY) 332 (6031): 858–862.

Bouwes A, Binnekade JM, Kuiper MA et al. (2012). Prognosis of coma after therapeutic hypothermia: a prospective cohort study. Ann Neurol 71 (2): 206–212.

Brain Resuscitation Clinical Trial I Study Group (1986). A randomized clinical study of cardiopulmonary-cerebral resuscitation: design, methods, and patient characteristics. Am J Emerg Med 4 (1): 72–86.

Brophy GM, Mondello S, Papa L et al. (2011). Biokinetic analysis of ubiquitin C-terminal hydrolase-L1 (UCH-L1) in severe traumatic brain injury patient biofluids. J Neurotrauma 28 (6): 861–870.

Brown EN, Lydic R, Schiff ND (2010). General anesthesia, sleep, and coma. N Engl J Med 363 (27): 2638–2650.

Carmichael ST, Saper C, Schlaug G (2016). Emergent properties of neural repair: elemental biology to therapeutic concepts. Ann Neurol. http://dx.doi.org/10.1002/ana. 24653.

Carpentier A, Galanaud D, Puybasset L et al. (2006). Early morphologic and spectroscopic magnetic resonance in severe traumatic brain injuries can detect "invisible brain stem damage" and predict "vegetative states". J Neurotrauma 23 (5): 674–685.

Castano-Leon AM, Lora D, Munarriz PM et al. (2016). Predicting outcomes after severe and moderate traumatic brain injury: an external validation of Impact and crash prognostic models in a large Spanish cohort. J Neurotrauma. http://dx.doi.org/10.1089/neu.2015.4182.

Cheng F, Yuan Q, Yang J et al. (2014). The prognostic value of serum neuron-specific enolase in traumatic brain injury: systematic review and meta-analysis. PLoS One 9 (9): e106680.

Ching S, Cimenser A, Purdon PL et al. (2010). Thalamocortical model for a propofol-induced alpha-rhythm associated with loss of consciousness. Proc Natl Acad Sci U S A 107 (52): 22665–22670.

Choi SP, Park KN, Park HK et al. (2010). Diffusion-weighted magnetic resonance imaging for predicting the clinical outcome of comatose survivors after cardiac arrest: a cohort study. Crit Care 14 (1): R17.

Claassen J, Hansen HC (2001). Early recovery after closed traumatic head injury: somatosensory evoked potentials and clinical findings. Crit Care Med 29 (3): 494–502.

Claassen J, Vespa P (2014). Electrophysiologic monitoring in acute brain injury. Neurocrit Care 21 (Suppl 2): S129–S147.

Claassen J, Mayer SA, Hirsch LJ (2005). Continuous EEG monitoring in patients with subarachnoid hemorrhage. J Clin Neurophysiol 22 (2): 92–98.

Claassen J, Hirsch LJ, Frontera JA et al. (2006). Prognostic significance of continuous EEG monitoring in patients with poor-grade subarachnoid hemorrhage. Neurocrit Care 4 (2): 103–112.

Claassen J, Taccone FS, Horn P et al. (2013). Recommendations on the use of EEG monitoring in critically ill patients: consensus statement from the neurointensive care section of the ESICM. Intensive Care Med 39 (8): 1337–1351.

Cloostermans MC, van Meulen FB, Eertman CJ et al. (2012). Continuous electroencephalography monitoring for early prediction of neurological outcome in postanoxic patients after cardiac arrest: a prospective cohort study. Crit Care Med 40 (10): 2867–2875.

Cocchi MN, Lucas JM, Salciccioli J et al. (2010). The role of cranial computed tomography in the immediate post-cardiac arrest period. Intern Emerg Med 5 (6): 533–538.

Coleman MR, Davis MH, Rodd JM et al. (2009). Towards the routine use of brain imaging to aid the clinical diagnosis of disorders of consciousness. Brain 132 (9): 2541–2552.

Cooray C, Mazya M, Bottai M et al. (2016). External validation of the ASTRAL and DRAGON scores for prediction of functional outcome in stroke. Stroke 47 (6): 1493–1499.

Coppler PJ, Elmer J, Calderon L et al. (2015). Validation of the Pittsburgh Cardiac Arrest Category illness severity score. Resuscitation 89: 86–92.

Cramer SC (2008). Repairing the human brain after stroke: I. Mechanisms of spontaneous recovery. Ann Neurol 63 (3): 272–287.

Crepeau AZ, Rabinstein AA, Fugate JE et al. (2013). Continuous EEG in therapeutic hypothermia after cardiac arrest: prognostic and clinical value. Neurology 80 (4): 339–344.

Crepeau AZ, Fugate JE, Mandrekar J et al. (2014). Value analysis of continuous EEG in patients during therapeutic hypothermia after cardiac arrest. Resuscitation 85 (6): 785–789.

Crepeau AZ, Britton JW, Fugate JE et al. (2015). Electroencephalography in survivors of cardiac arrest: comparing pre- and post-therapeutic hypothermia eras. Neurocrit Care 22 (1): 165–172.

Cristia C, Ho ML, Levy S et al. (2014). The association between a quantitative computed tomography (CT) measurement of cerebral edema and outcomes in post-cardiac arrest – a validation study. Resuscitation 85 (10): 1348–1353.

Cronberg T, Rundgren M, Westhall E et al. (2011). Neuron-specific enolase correlates with other prognostic markers after cardiac arrest. Neurology 77 (7): 623–630.

Cruse D, Chennu S, Chatelle C et al. (2011). Bedside detection of awareness in the vegetative state: a cohort study. Lancet (London, England) 378 (9809): 2088–2094.

Czeiter E, Mondello S, Kovacs N et al. (2012). Brain injury biomarkers may improve the predictive power of the IMPACT outcome calculator. J Neurotrauma 29 (9): 1770–1778.

Degos V, Apfel CC, Sanchez P et al. (2012). An admission bioclinical score to predict 1-year outcomes in patients undergoing aneurysm coiling. Stroke 43 (5): 1253–1259.

Dehaene S, Changeux JP (2011). Experimental and theoretical approaches to conscious processing. Neuron 70 (2): 200–227.

Dehaene S, Naccache L (2001). Towards a cognitive neuroscience of consciousness: basic evidence and a workspace framework. Cognition 79 (1–2): 1–37.

Delcourt C, Huang Y, Arima H et al. (2012). Hematoma growth and outcomes in intracerebral hemorrhage: the INTERACT1 study. Neurology 79 (4): 314–319.

Delgado Almandoz JE, Yoo AJ, Stone MJ et al. (2010). The spot sign score in primary intracerebral hemorrhage identifies patients at highest risk of in-hospital mortality and poor outcome among survivors. Stroke 41 (1): 54–60.

De Marchis GM, Pugin D, Meyers E et al. (2016). Seizure burden in subarachnoid hemorrhage associated with functional and cognitive outcome. Neurology 86 (3): 253–260.

Demchuk AM, Dowlatshahi D, Rodriguez-Luna D et al. (2012). Prediction of haematoma growth and outcome in patients with intracerebral haemorrhage using the CT-angiography spot sign (PREDICT): a prospective observational study. Lancet Neurol 11 (4): 307–314.

Demertzi A, Antonopoulos G, Heine L et al. (2015). Intrinsic functional connectivity differentiates minimally conscious from unresponsive patients. Brain 138 (Pt 9): 2619–2631.

Devaux Y, Dankiewicz J, Salgado-Somoza A et al. (2016). Association of circulating microRNA-124-3p levels with outcomes after out-of-hospital cardiac arrest: a substudy of a randomized clinical trial. JAMA Cardiol 1 (3): 305–313.

Dimopoulou I, Korfias S, Dafni U et al. (2003). Protein S-100b serum levels in trauma-induced brain death. Neurology 60 (6): 947–951.

Dimopoulou I, Tsagarakis S, Korfias S et al. (2004). Relationship of thyroid function to post-traumatic S-100b serum levels in survivors of severe head injury: preliminary results. Intensive Care Med 30 (2): 298–301.

Di Perri C, Bahri MA, Amico E et al. (2016). Neural correlates of consciousness in patients who have emerged from a minimally conscious state: a cross-sectional multimodal imaging study. Lancet Neurol. http://dx.doi.org/10.1016/s1474-4422(16)00111-3.

Dragancea I, Horn J, Kuiper M et al. (2015). Neurological prognostication after cardiac arrest and targeted temperature management 33°C versus 36°C: Results from a randomised controlled clinical trial. Resuscitation 93: 164–170.

Ebell MH, Jang W, Shen Y et al. (2013). Development and validation of the Good Outcome Following Attempted Resuscitation (GO-FAR) score to predict neurologically intact survival after in-hospital cardiopulmonary resuscitation. JAMA Intern Med 173 (20): 1872–1878.

Endisch C, Storm C, Ploner CJ et al. (2015). Amplitudes of SSEP and outcome in cardiac arrest survivors: a prospective cohort study. Neurology 85 (20): 1752–1760.

Endisch C, Waterstraat G, Storm C et al. (2016). Cortical somatosensory evoked high-frequency (600Hz) oscillations predict absence of severe hypoxic encephalopathy after resuscitation. Clin Neurophysiol 127 (7): 2561–2569.

Engel H, Ben Hamouda N, Portmann K et al. (2013). Serum procalcitonin as a marker of post-cardiac arrest syndrome and long-term neurological recovery, but not of early-onset infections, in comatose post-anoxic patients treated with therapeutic hypothermia. Resuscitation 84 (6): 776–781.

Faugeras F, Rohaut B, Weiss N et al. (2011). Probing consciousness with event-related potentials in the vegetative state. Neurology 77 (3): 264–268.

Fields JA, Ferman TJ, Boeve BF et al. (2011). Neuropsychological assessment of patients with dementing illness. Nat Rev Neurol 7 (12): 677–687.

Finlayson O, John V, Yeung R et al. (2013). Interobserver agreement of ASPECT score distribution for noncontrast CT, CT angiography, and CT perfusion in acute stroke. Stroke 44 (1): 234–236.

Fischer C, Morlet D, Bouchet P et al. (1999). Mismatch negativity and late auditory evoked potentials in comatose patients. Clin Neurophysiol 110 (9): 1601–1610.

Fischer C, Luaute J, Adeleine P et al. (2004). Predictive value of sensory and cognitive evoked potentials for awakening from coma. Neurology 63 (4): 669–673.

Fischer C, Luaute J, Nemoz C et al. (2006). Improved prediction of awakening or nonawakening from severe anoxic coma using tree-based classification analysis. Crit Care Med 34 (5): 1520–1524.

Foreman B, Claassen J, Abou Khaled K et al. (2012). Generalized periodic discharges in the critically ill: a case-control study of 200 patients. Neurology 79 (19): 1951–1960.

Forkel SJ (2014). Thiebaut de Schotten M, Dell'Acqua F et al. Anatomical predictors of aphasia recovery: a tractography study of bilateral perisylvian language networks. Brain 137 (Pt 7): 2027–2039.

Fugate JE, Rabinstein AA, Claassen DO et al. (2010a). The FOUR score predicts outcome in patients after cardiac arrest. Neurocrit Care 13 (2): 205–210.

Fugate JE, Wijdicks EF, Mandrekar J et al. (2010b). Predictors of neurologic outcome in hypothermia after cardiac arrest. Ann Neurol 68 (6): 907–914.

Galanaud D, Perlbarg V, Gupta R et al. (2012). Assessment of white matter injury and outcome in severe brain trauma: a prospective multicenter cohort. Anesthesiology 117 (6): 1300–1310.

Galanaud D, Perlbarg V, Gupta R et al. (2013). Assessment of white matter injury and outcome in severe brain trauma. A prospective multicenter cohort. Surv Anesthesiol 57 (4): 171–172.

Garnett MR, Blamire AM, Corkill RG et al. (2000a). Early proton magnetic resonance spectroscopy in normal-appearing brain correlates with outcome in patients following traumatic brain injury. Brain 123 (Pt 10): 2046–2054.

Gebel Jr JM, Jauch EC, Brott TG et al. (2002). Relative edema volume is a predictor of outcome in patients with hyperacute spontaneous intracerebral hemorrhage. Stroke 33 (11): 2636–2641.

Gentsch A, Storm C, Leithner C et al. (2015). Outcome prediction in patients after cardiac arrest: a simplified method for determination of gray-white matter ratio in cranial computed tomography. Clin Neuroradiol 25 (1): 49–54.

Geurts M, Macleod MR, van Thiel GJ et al. (2014). End-of-life decisions in patients with severe acute brain injury. Lancet Neurol 13 (5): 515–524.

Giacino JT, Kezmarsky MA, DeLuca J et al. (1991). Monitoring rate of recovery to predict outcome in minimally responsive patients. Arch Phys Med Rehabil 72 (11): 897–901.

Giacino JT, Ashwal S, Childs N et al. (2002). The minimally conscious state: definition and diagnostic criteria. Neurology 58 (3): 349–353.

Giacino JT, Kalmar K, Whyte J (2004). The JFK Coma Recovery Scale-Revised: measurement characteristics and diagnostic utility. Arch Phys Med Rehabil 85 (12): 2020–2029.

Giacino JT, Fins JJ, Laureys S et al. (2014). Disorders of consciousness after acquired brain injury: the state of the science. Nat Rev Neurol 10 (2): 99–114.

Gilje P, Gidlof O, Rundgren M et al. (2014). The brain-enriched microRNA miR-124 in plasma predicts neurological outcome after cardiac arrest. Crit Care 18 (2): R40.

Godoy DA, Pinero G, Di Napoli M (2006). Predicting mortality in spontaneous intracerebral hemorrhage: can modification to original score improve the prediction? Stroke 37 (4): 1038–1044.

Golan E, Barrett K, Alali AS et al. (2014). Predicting neurologic outcome after targeted temperature management for cardiac arrest: systematic review and meta-analysis. Crit Care Med 42 (8): 1919–1930.

Gomez PA, de-la-Cruz J, Lora D et al. (2014). Validation of a prognostic score for early mortality in severe head injury cases. J Neurosurg 121 (6): 1314–1322.

Gosseries O, Di H, Laureys S et al. (2014). Measuring consciousness in severely damaged brains. Annu Rev Neurosci 37: 457–478.

Granziera C, Daducci A, Meskaldji DE et al. (2012). A new early and automated MRI-based predictor of motor improvement after stroke. Neurology 79 (1): 39–46.

Greer D, Scripko P, Bartscher J et al. (2011). Serial MRI changes in comatose cardiac arrest patients. Neurocrit Care 14 (1): 61–67.

Greer DM, Yang J, Scripko PD et al. (2012). Clinical examination for outcome prediction in nontraumatic coma. Crit Care Med 40 (4): 1150–1156.

Grefkes C, Fink GR (2011). Reorganization of cerebral networks after stroke: new insights from neuroimaging with connectivity approaches. Brain 134 (Pt 5): 1264–1276.

Han J, King NK, Neilson SJ et al. (2014). External validation of the CRASH and IMPACT prognostic models in severe traumatic brain injury. J Neurotrauma 31 (13): 1146–1152.

Hanning U, Bernhard Sporns P, Lebiedz P et al. (2016). Automated assessment of early hypoxic brain edema in non-enhanced CT predicts outcome in patients after cardiac arrest. Resuscitation 104: 91–94.

Haring HP, Dilitz E, Pallua A et al. (1999). Attenuated corticomedullary contrast: an early cerebral computed tomography sign indicating malignant middle cerebral artery infarction. A case-control study. Stroke 30 (5): 1076–1082.

Harrison DA, Griggs KA, Prabhu G et al. (2015). External validation and recalibration of risk prediction models for acute traumatic brain injury among critically ill adult patients in the United Kingdom. J Neurotrauma 32 (19): 1522–1537.

Hemphill 3rd JC, Bonovich DC, Besmertis L et al. (2001). The ICH score: a simple, reliable grading scale for intracerebral hemorrhage. Stroke 32 (4): 891–897.

Hemphill 3rd JC, Farrant M, Neill Jr TA (2009). Prospective validation of the ICH Score for 12-month functional outcome. Neurology 73 (14): 1088–1094.

Hill MD, Demchuk AM, Tomsick TA et al. (2006). Using the baseline CT scan to select acute stroke patients for

IV-IA therapy. AJNR Am J Neuroradiol 27 (8): 1612–1616.

Hill CS, Coleman MP, Menon DK (2016). Traumatic axonal injury: mechanisms and translational opportunities. Trends Neurosci 39 (5): 311–324.

Hirsch KG, Mlynash M, Eyngorn I et al. (2016). Multi-center study of diffusion-weighted imaging in coma after cardiac arrest. Neurocrit Care 24 (1): 82–89.

Hoffmann M, Lefering R, Rueger JM et al. (2012). Pupil evaluation in addition to Glasgow Coma Scale components in prediction of traumatic brain injury and mortality. Br J Surg 99 (Suppl 1): 122–130.

Houlden DA, Taylor AB, Feinstein A et al. (2010). Early somatosensory evoked potential grades in comatose traumatic brain injury patients predict cognitive and functional outcome. Crit Care Med 38 (1): 167–174.

Hume AL, Cant BR (1981). Central somatosensory conduction after head injury. Ann Neurol 10 (5): 411–419.

Huttner HB, Schellinger PD, Hartmann M et al. (2006). Hematoma growth and outcome in treated neurocritical care patients with intracerebral hemorrhage related to oral anticoagulant therapy: comparison of acute treatment strategies using vitamin K, fresh frozen plasma, and prothrombin complex concentrates. Stroke 37 (6): 1465–1470.

Hyder F, Fulbright RK, Shulman RG et al. (2013). Glutamatergic function in the resting awake human brain is supported by uniformly high oxidative energy. J Cereb Blood Flow Metab 33 (3): 339–347.

Immonen RJ, Kharatishvili I, Niskanen JP et al. (2009). Distinct MRI pattern in lesional and perilesional area after traumatic brain injury in rat – 11 months follow-up. Exp Neurol 215 (1): 29–40.

Inamasu J, Miyatake S, Suzuki M et al. (2010). Early CT signs in out-of-hospital cardiac arrest survivors: temporal profile and prognostic significance. Resuscitation 81 (5): 534–538.

Inamasu J, Miyatake S, Nakatsukasa M et al. (2011). Loss of gray–white matter discrimination as an early CT sign of brain ischemia/hypoxia in victims of asphyxial cardiac arrest. Emerg Radiol 18 (4): 295–298.

Jennett B, Bond M (1975). Assessment of outcome after severe brain damage. Lancet (London, England) 1 (7905): 480–484.

Jennett B, Plum F (1972). Persistent vegetative state after brain damage. A syndrome in search of a name. Lancet (London, England) 1 (7753): 734–737.

Jennett B, Snoek J, Bond MR et al. (1981). Disability after severe head injury: observations on the use of the Glasgow Outcome Scale. J Neurol Neurosurg Psychiatry 44 (4): 285–293.

Jones SJ, Vaz Pato M, Sprague L et al. (2000). Auditory evoked potentials to spectro-temporal modulation of complex tones in normal subjects and patients with severe brain injury. Brain 123 (Pt 5): 1007–1016.

Judson JA, Cant BR, Shaw NA (1990). Early prediction of outcome from cerebral trauma by somatosensory evoked potentials. Crit Care Med 18 (4): 363–368.

Kamps MJ, Horn J, Oddo M et al. (2013). Prognostication of neurologic outcome in cardiac arrest patients after mild therapeutic hypothermia: a meta-analysis of the current literature. Intensive Care Med 39 (10): 1671–1682.

Kane NM, Curry SH, Rowlands CA et al. (1996). Event-related potentials – neurophysiological tools for predicting emergence and early outcome from traumatic coma. Intensive Care Med 22 (1): 39–46.

Kasprowicz M, Burzynska M, Melcer T et al. (2016). A comparison of the Full Outline of UnResponsiveness (FOUR) score and Glasgow Coma Score (GCS) in predictive modelling in traumatic brain injury. Br J Neurosurg 30 (2): 211–220.

Katz DI, Polyak M, Coughlan D et al. (2009). Natural history of recovery from brain injury after prolonged disorders of consciousness: outcome of patients admitted to inpatient rehabilitation with 1–4 year follow-up. Prog Brain Res 177: 73–88.

Khong PL, Tse C, Wong IY et al. (2004). Diffusion-weighted imaging and proton magnetic resonance spectroscopy in perinatal hypoxic-ischemic encephalopathy: association with neuromotor outcome at 18 months of age. J Child Neurol 19 (11): 872–881.

Kim C, Becker L, Eisenberg MS (2000). Out-of-hospital cardiac arrest in octogenarians and nonagenarians. Arch Intern Med 160 (22): 3439–3443.

Kim JT, Park MS, Choi KH et al. (2010). The CBV-ASPECT Score as a predictor of fatal stroke in a hyperacute state. Eur Neurol 63 (6): 357–363.

Kim SH, Choi SP, Park KN et al. (2013). Early brain computed tomography findings are associated with outcome in patients treated with therapeutic hypothermia after out-of-hospital cardiac arrest. Scand J Trauma Resusc Emerg Med 21: 57.

Knight WA, Hart KW, Adeoye OM et al. (2013). The incidence of seizures in patients undergoing therapeutic hypothermia after resuscitation from cardiac arrest. Epilepsy Res 106 (3): 396–402.

Kondziella D, Friberg CK, Wellwood I et al. (2015). Continuous EEG monitoring in aneurysmal subarachnoid hemorrhage: a systematic review. Neurocrit Care 22 (3): 450–461.

Korfias S, Stranjalis G, Boviatsis E et al. (2007). Serum S-100B protein monitoring in patients with severe traumatic brain injury. Intensive Care Med 33 (2): 255–260.

Kraus MF, Susmaras T, Caughlin BP et al. (2007). White matter integrity and cognition in chronic traumatic brain injury: a diffusion tensor imaging study. Brain 130 (Pt 10): 2508–2519.

Lamartine Monteiro M, Taccone FS, Depondt C et al. (2016). The prognostic value of 48-h continuous EEG during therapeutic hypothermia after cardiac arrest. Neurocrit Care 24 (2): 153–162.

Langkjaer S, Hassager C, Kjaergaard J et al. (2015). Prognostic value of reduced discrimination and oedema on cerebral computed tomography in a daily clinical cohort of out-of-hospital cardiac arrest patients. Resuscitation 92: 141–147.

Laureys S, Faymonville ME, Luxen A et al. (2000). Restoration of thalamocortical connectivity after recovery from persistent vegetative state. Lancet (London, England) 355 (9217): 1790–1791.

Laureys S, Owen AM, Schiff ND (2004). Brain function in coma, vegetative state, and related disorders. Lancet Neurol 3 (9): 537–546.

Laureys S, Celesia GG, Cohadon F et al. (2010). Unresponsive wakefulness syndrome: a new name for the vegetative state or apallic syndrome. BMC Med 8: 68.

Lee BK, Jeung KW, Song KH et al. (2015). Prognostic values of gray matter to white matter ratios on early brain computed tomography in adult comatose patients after out-of-hospital cardiac arrest of cardiac etiology. Resuscitation 96: 46–52.

Legriel S, Bruneel F, Sediri H et al. (2009). Early EEG monitoring for detecting postanoxic status epilepticus during therapeutic hypothermia: a pilot study. Neurocrit Care 11 (3): 338–344.

Levy DE, Caronna JJ, Singer BH et al. (1985). Predicting outcome from hypoxic-ischemic coma. JAMA 253 (10): 1420–1426.

Li R, Song W-q, Du J-b et al. (2015). Connecting the P300 to the diagnosis and prognosis of unconscious patients. Neural Regen Res 10 (3): 473–480.

Liliang PC, Liang CL, Weng HC et al. (2010). Tau proteins in serum predict outcome after severe traumatic brain injury. J Surg Res 160 (2): 302–307.

Lingsma HF, Roozenbeek B, Steyerberg EW et al. (2010). Early prognosis in traumatic brain injury: from prophecies to predictions. Lancet Neurol 9 (5): 543–554.

Lingsma HF, Yue JK, Maas AI et al. (2015). Outcome prediction after mild and complicated mild traumatic brain injury: external validation of existing models and identification of new predictors using the TRACK-TBI pilot study. J Neurotrauma 32 (2): 83–94.

Llinas RR, Steriade M (2006). Bursting of thalamic neurons and states of vigilance. J Neurophysiol 95 (6): 3297–3308.

Longstreth Jr WT, Cobb LA, Fahrenbruch CE et al. (1990). Does age affect outcomes of out-of-hospital cardiopulmonary resuscitation? JAMA 264 (16): 2109–2110.

Luyt CE, Galanaud D, Perlbarg V et al. (2012). Diffusion tensor imaging to predict long-term outcome after cardiac arrest: a bicentric pilot study. Anesthesiology 117 (6): 1311–1321.

Maas AI, Hukkelhoven CW, Marshall LF et al. (2005). Prediction of outcome in traumatic brain injury with computed tomographic characteristics: a comparison between the computed tomographic classification and combinations of computed tomographic predictors. Neurosurgery 57 (6): 1173–1182. discussion 1182.

Mac Donald CL, Dikranian K, Bayly P et al. (2007). Diffusion tensor imaging reliably detects experimental traumatic axonal injury and indicates approximate time of injury. J Neurosci 27 (44): 11869–11876.

Mahoney FI, Barthel DW (1965). Functional evaluation: the Barthel index. Md State Med J 14: 61–65.

Majdan M, Steyerberg EW, Nieboer D et al. (2015). Glasgow coma scale motor score and pupillary reaction to predict six-month mortality in patients with traumatic brain injury: comparison of field and admission assessment. J Neurotrauma 32 (2): 101–108.

Mani R, Schmitt SE, Mazer M et al. (2012). The frequency and timing of epileptiform activity on continuous electroencephalogram in comatose post-cardiac arrest syndrome patients treated with therapeutic hypothermia. Resuscitation 83 (7): 840–847.

Marmarou A, Lu J, Butcher I et al. (2007). Prognostic value of the Glasgow Coma Scale and pupil reactivity in traumatic brain injury assessed pre-hospital and on enrollment: an IMPACT analysis. J Neurotrauma 24 (2): 270–280.

Marshall LF, Marshall SB, Klauber MR et al. (1992). The diagnosis of head injury requires a classification based on computed axial tomography. J Neurotrauma 9 (Suppl 1): S287–S292.

McNett M, Amato S, Gianakis A et al. (2014). The FOUR score and GCS as predictors of outcome after traumatic brain injury. Neurocrit Care 21 (1): 52–57.

Mercier E, Boutin A, Lauzier F et al. (2013). Predictive value of S-100β protein for prognosis in patients with moderate and severe traumatic brain injury: systematic review and meta-analysis. BMJ (Clinical research ed): 346.

Metting Z, Wilczak N, Rodiger LA et al. (2012). GFAP and S100B in the acute phase of mild traumatic brain injury. Neurology 78 (18): 1428–1433.

Minnerup J, Wersching H, Ringelstein EB et al. (2011). Prediction of malignant middle cerebral artery infarction using computed tomography-based intracranial volume reserve measurements. Stroke 42 (12): 3403–3409.

Mlynash M, Campbell DM, Leproust EM et al. (2010). Temporal and spatial profile of brain diffusion-weighted MRI after cardiac arrest. Stroke 41 (8): 1665–1672.

Mondello S, Robicsek SA, Gabrielli A et al. (2010). αII-Spectrin breakdown products (SBDPs): diagnosis and outcome in severe traumatic brain injury patients. J Neurotrauma 27 (7): 1203–1213.

Mondello S, Papa L, Buki A et al. (2011). Neuronal and glial markers are differently associated with computed tomography findings and outcome in patients with severe traumatic brain injury: a case control study. Crit Care 15 (3): R156.

Mondello S, Linnet A, Buki A et al. (2012a). Clinical utility of serum levels of ubiquitin C-terminal hydrolase as a biomarker for severe traumatic brain injury. Neurosurgery 70 (3): 666–675.

Mondello S, Gabrielli A, Catani S et al. (2012b). Increased levels of serum MAP-2 at 6-months correlate with improved outcome in survivors of severe traumatic brain injury. Brain Inj 26 (13–14): 1629–1635.

Monti MM, Vanhaudenhuyse A, Coleman MR et al. (2010). Willful modulation of brain activity in disorders of consciousness. N Engl J Med 362 (7): 579–589.

Monti MM, Rosenberg M, Finoia P et al. (2015). Thalamo-frontal connectivity mediates top-down cognitive functions in disorders of consciousness. Neurology 84 (2): 167–173.

Mörtberg E, Zetterberg H, Nordmark J et al. (2011). S-100B is superior to NSE, BDNF and GFAP in predicting outcome of resuscitation from cardiac arrest with hypothermia treatment. Resuscitation 82 (1): 26–31.

Multi-Society Task Force on PVS (1994a). Medical aspects of the persistent vegetative state (2). N Engl J Med 330 (22): 1572–1579.

Multi-Society Task Force on PVS (1994b). Medical aspects of the persistent vegetative state (1). N Engl J Med 330 (21): 1499–1508.

Murray GD, Butcher I, McHugh GS et al. (2007). Multivariable prognostic analysis in traumatic brain injury: results from the IMPACT study. J Neurotrauma 24 (2): 329–337.

Murthy SB, Moradiya Y, Dawson J et al. (2015). Perihematomal edema and functional outcomes in intracerebral hemorrhage: influence of hematoma volume and location. Stroke 46 (11): 3088–3092.

Mushkudiani NA, Engel DC, Steyerberg EW et al. (2007). Prognostic value of demographic characteristics in traumatic brain injury: results from the IMPACT study. J Neurotrauma 24 (2): 259–269.

Mussack T, Biberthaler P, Kanz KG et al. (2002). Serum S-100B and interleukin-8 as predictive markers for comparative neurologic outcome analysis of patients after cardiac arrest and severe traumatic brain injury. Crit Care Med 30 (12): 2669–2674.

Naatanen R, Paavilainen P, Rinne T et al. (2007). The mismatch negativity (MMN) in basic research of central auditory processing: a review. Clin Neurophysiol 118 (12): 2544–2590.

Nakase-Richardson R, Whyte J, Giacino JT et al. (2012). Longitudinal outcome of patients with disordered consciousness in the NIDRR TBI model systems programs. J Neurotrauma 29 (1): 59–65.

Noirhomme Q, Lehembre R, Lugo Zdel R et al. (2014). Automated analysis of background EEG and reactivity during therapeutic hypothermia in comatose patients after cardiac arrest. Clin EEG Neurosci 45 (1): 6–13.

Nylén K, Öst M, Csajbok LZ et al. (2006). Increased serum-GFAP in patients with severe traumatic brain injury is related to outcome. J Neurol Sci 240 (1): 85–91.

Ogilvy CS, Carter BS (1998). A proposed comprehensive grading system to predict outcome for surgical management of intracranial aneurysms. Neurosurgery 42 (5): 959–968. discussion 68–70.

Owen AM, Coleman MR, Boly M (2006). Detecting awareness in the vegetative state. Science (New York, NY) 313 (5792): 1402.

Papa L, Robertson C, Wang KW et al. (2015). Biomarkers improve clinical outcome predictors of mortality following non-penetrating severe traumatic brain injury. Neurocrit Care 22 (1): 52–64.

Parvizi J, Damasio AR (2003). Neuroanatomical correlates of brainstem coma. Brain 126 (Pt 7): 1524–1536.

Perel P, Edwards P, Wentz R et al. (2006). Systematic review of prognostic models in traumatic brain injury. BMC Med Inform Decis Mak 6: 38.

Perel P, Arango M, Clayton T et al. (2008). Predicting outcome after traumatic brain injury: practical prognostic models based on large cohort of international patients. BMJ (Clinical research ed) 336 (7641): 425–429.

Perrin F, Schnakers C, Schabus M et al. (2006). Brain response to one's own name in vegetative state, minimally conscious state, and locked-in syndrome. Arch Neurol 63 (4): 562–569.

Polich J (2007). Updating P300: an integrative theory of P3a and P3b. Clin Neurophysiol 118 (10): 2128–2148.

Posner JB, Plum F (2007). Plum and Posner's diagnosis of stupor and coma. 4th edn. Oxford University Press, Oxford, p. xiv. 401 p.

Purrucker JC, Haas K, Rizos T et al. (2016). Early clinical and radiological course, management, and outcome of intracerebral hemorrhage related to new oral anticoagulants. JAMA Neurol 73 (2): 169–177.

Qin P, Di H, Yan X et al. (2008). Mismatch negativity to the patient's own name in chronic disorders of consciousness. Neurosci Lett 448 (1): 24–28.

Raheja A, Sinha S, Samson N et al. (2016). Serum biomarkers as predictors of long-term outcome in severe traumatic brain injury: analysis from a randomized placebo-controlled phase II clinical trial. J Neurosurg 1–11.

Randall J, Mörtberg E, Provuncher GK et al. (2013). Tau proteins in serum predict neurological outcome after hypoxic brain injury from cardiac arrest: results of a pilot study. Resuscitation 84 (3): 351–356.

Rappaport M, Hall KM, Hopkins K et al. (1982). Disability rating scale for severe head trauma: coma to community. Arch Phys Med Rehabil 63 (3): 118–123.

Rea TD, Eisenberg MS, Becker LJ et al. (2003). Temporal trends in sudden cardiac arrest: a 25-year emergency medical services perspective. Circulation 107 (22): 2780–2785.

Rittenberger JC, Popescu A, Brenner RP et al. (2012). Frequency and timing of nonconvulsive status epilepticus in comatose post-cardiac arrest subjects treated with hypothermia. Neurocrit Care 16 (1): 114–122.

Robinson LR, Micklesen PJ, Tirschwell DL et al. (2003). Predictive value of somatosensory evoked potentials for awakening from coma. Crit Care Med 31 (3): 960–967.

Rodriguez Moreno D, Schiff ND, Giacino J et al. (2010). A network approach to assessing cognition in disorders of consciousness. Neurology 75 (21): 1871–1878.

Roozenbeek B, Chiu YL, Lingsma HF et al. (2012). Predicting 14-day mortality after severe traumatic brain injury: application of the IMPACT models in the Brain Trauma Foundation TBI-trac(R) New York state database. J Neurotrauma 29 (7): 1306–1312.

Rordorf G, Koroshetz W, Efird JT et al. (2000). Predictors of mortality in stroke patients admitted to an intensive care unit. Crit Care Med 28 (5): 1301–1305.

Rosanova M, Gosseries O, Casarotto S et al. (2012). Recovery of cortical effective connectivity and recovery of consciousness in vegetative patients. Brain 135 (Pt 4): 1308–1320.

Rosengart AJ, Schultheiss KE, Tolentino J et al. (2007). Prognostic factors for outcome in patients with aneurysmal subarachnoid hemorrhage. Stroke 38 (8): 2315–2321.

Rossetti AO, Oddo M, Liaudet L et al. (2009). Predictors of awakening from postanoxic status epilepticus after therapeutic hypothermia. Neurology 72 (8): 744–749.

Rossetti AO, Oddo M, Logroscino G et al. (2010a). Prognostication after cardiac arrest and hypothermia: a prospective study. Ann Neurol 67 (3): 301–307.

Rossetti AO, Urbano LA, Delodder F et al. (2010b). Prognostic value of continuous EEG monitoring during therapeutic hypothermia after cardiac arrest. Crit Care 14 (5): R173.

Rossetti AO, Carrera E, Oddo M (2012). Early EEG correlates of neuronal injury after brain anoxia. Neurology 78 (11): 796–802.

Rossetti AO, Tzovara A, Murray MM et al. (2014). Automated auditory mismatch negativity paradigm improves coma prognostic accuracy after cardiac arrest and therapeutic hypothermia. J Clin Neurophysiol 31 (4): 356–361.

Rost NS, Smith EE, Chang Y et al. (2008). Prediction of functional outcome in patients with primary intracerebral hemorrhage: the FUNC score. Stroke 39 (8): 2304–2309.

Rothstein TL (2014a). Therapeutic hypothermia does not diminish the vital and necessary role of SSEP in predicting unfavorable outcome in anoxic-ischemic coma. Clin Neurol Neurosurg 126: 205–209.

Rothstein TL (2014b). Therapeutic hypothermia does not diminish the vital and necessary role of SSEP in predicting unfavorable outcome in anoxic-ischemic coma. Clin Neurol Neurosurg 126: 205–209.

Rubenstein R, Chang B, Davies P et al. (2015). A novel, ultrasensitive assay for tau: potential for assessing traumatic brain injury in tissues and biofluids. J Neurotrauma 32 (5): 342–352.

Saika A, Bansal S, Philip M et al. (2015). Prognostic value of FOUR and GCS scores in determining mortality in patients with traumatic brain injury. Acta Neurochir 157 (8): 1323–1328.

Sandroni C, Cavallaro F, Callaway CW et al. (2013). Predictors of poor neurological outcome in adult comatose survivors of cardiac arrest: a systematic review and meta-analysis. Part 2: Patients treated with therapeutic hypothermia. Resuscitation 84 (10): 1324–1338.

Saper CB, Scammell TE, Lu J (2005). Hypothalamic regulation of sleep and circadian rhythms. Nature 437 (7063): 1257–1263.

Sato S, Arima H, Hirakawa Y et al. (2014). The speed of ultra-early hematoma growth in acute intracerebral hemorrhage. Neurology 83 (24): 2232–2238.

Scheel M, Storm C, Gentsch A et al. (2013). The prognostic value of gray–white-matter ratio in cardiac arrest patients treated with hypothermia. Scand J Trauma Resusc Emerg Med 21: 23.

Schefold JC, Storm C, Kruger A et al. (2009). The Glasgow Coma Score is a predictor of good outcome in cardiac arrest patients treated with therapeutic hypothermia. Resuscitation 80 (6): 658–661.

Schnakers C, Perrin F, Schabus M et al. (2008). Voluntary brain processing in disorders of consciousness. Neurology 71 (20): 1614–1620.

Seet RC, Lim EC, Wilder-Smith EP (2005). Spindle coma from acute midbrain infarction. Neurology 64 (12): 2159–2160.

Shulman RG, Hyder F, Rothman DL (2009). Baseline brain energy supports the state of consciousness. Proc Natl Acad Sci U S A 106 (27): 11096–11101.

Sidaros A, Engberg AW, Sidaros K et al. (2008). Diffusion tensor imaging during recovery from severe traumatic brain injury and relation to clinical outcome: a longitudinal study. Brain 131 (Pt 2): 559–572.

Skandsen T, Kvistad KA, Solheim O et al. (2011). Prognostic value of magnetic resonance imaging in moderate and severe head injury: a prospective study of early MRI findings and one-year outcome. J Neurotrauma 28 (5): 691–699.

Skrifvars MB, Varghese B, Parr MJ (2012). Survival and outcome prediction using the Apache III and the out-of-hospital cardiac arrest (OHCA) score in patients treated in the intensive care unit (ICU) following out-of-hospital, in-hospital or ICU cardiac arrest. Resuscitation 83 (6): 728–733.

Soddu A, Vanhaudenhuyse A, Bahri MA et al. (2012). Identifying the default-mode component in spatial IC analyses of patients with disorders of consciousness. Hum Brain Mapp 33 (4): 778–796.

Soize S, Barbe C, Kadziolka K et al. (2013). Predictive factors of outcome and hemorrhage after acute ischemic stroke treated by mechanical thrombectomy with a stent-retriever. Neuroradiology 55 (8): 977–987.

Stender J, Gosseries O, Bruno MA et al. (2014). Diagnostic precision of PET imaging and functional MRI in disorders of consciousness: a clinical validation study. Lancet (London, England) 384 (9942): 514–522.

Stender J, Kupers R, Rodell A et al. (2015). Quantitative rates of brain glucose metabolism distinguish minimally conscious from vegetative state patients. J Cereb Blood Flow Metab 35 (1): 58–65.

Stender J, Mortensen KN, Thibaut A et al. (2016). The minimal energetic requirement of sustained awareness after brain injury. Curr Biol 26 (11): 1494–1499.

Steppacher I, Eickhoff S, Jordanov T et al. (2013). N400 predicts recovery from disorders of consciousness. Ann Neurol 73 (5): 594–602.

Stevens RD, Sutter R (2013). Prognosis in severe brain injury. Crit Care Med 41 (4): 1104–1123.

Steyerberg EW, Mushkudiani N, Perel P et al. (2008). Predicting outcome after traumatic brain injury: development and international validation of prognostic scores based on admission characteristics. PLoS Med 5 (8): e165. discussion e165.

Sunde K, Kramer-Johansen J, Pytte M et al. (2007). Predicting survival with good neurologic recovery at hospital admission after successful resuscitation of out-of-hospital cardiac arrest: the OHCA score. Eur Heart J 28 (6): 773. author reply 774.

Sutter R, Stevens RD, Kaplan PW (2013). Continuous electroencephalographic monitoring in critically ill patients: indications, limitations, and strategies. Crit Care Med 41 (4): 1124–1132.

Teasdale G, Jennett B (1974). Assessment of coma and impaired consciousness. A practical scale. Lancet (London, England) 2 (7872): 81–84.

Timofeev I, Grenier F, Bazhenov M et al. (2000). Origin of slow cortical oscillations in deafferented cortical slabs. Cereb Cortex 10 (12): 1185–1199.

Titulaer MJ, McCracken L, Gabilondo I et al. (2013). Treatment and prognostic factors for long-term outcome in patients with anti-NMDA receptor encephalitis: an observational cohort study. Lancet Neurol 12 (2): 157–165.

Tokutomi T, Miyagi T, Ogawa T et al. (2008). Age-associated increases in poor outcomes after traumatic brain injury: a report from the Japan Neurotrauma Data Bank. J Neurotrauma 25 (12): 1407–1414.

Tollard E, Galanaud D, Perlbarg V et al. (2009). Experience of diffusion tensor imaging and 1H spectroscopy for outcome prediction in severe traumatic brain injury: preliminary results. Crit Care Med 37 (4): 1448–1455.

Topol EJ (2014). Individualized medicine from prewomb to tomb. Cell 157 (1): 241–253.

Torbey MT, Selim M, Knorr J et al. (2000). Quantitative analysis of the loss of distinction between gray and white matter in comatose patients after cardiac arrest. Stroke 31 (9): 2163–2167.

Tu TW, Williams RA, Lescher JD et al. (2016). Radiological-pathological correlation of diffusion tensor and magnetization transfer imaging in a closed head traumatic brain injury model. Ann Neurol 79 (6): 907–920.

Tzovara A, Rossetti AO, Spierer L et al. (2013). Progression of auditory discrimination based on neural decoding predicts awakening from coma. Brain 136 (Pt 1): 81–89.

Tzovara A, Simonin A, Oddo M et al. (2015). Neural detection of complex sound sequences in the absence of consciousness. Brain 138 (Pt 5): 1160–1166.

Tzovara A, Rossetti AO, Juan E et al. (2016). Prediction of awakening from hypothermic post anoxic coma based on auditory discrimination. Ann Neurol. http://dx.doi.org/10.1002/ana.24622.

Vaahersalo J, Skrifvars MB, Pulkki K et al. (2014). Admission interleukin-6 is associated with post resuscitation organ dysfunction and predicts long-term neurological outcome after out-of-hospital ventricular fibrillation. Resuscitation 85 (11): 1573–1579.

Vanhaudenhuyse A, Laureys S, Perrin F (2008). Cognitive event-related potentials in comatose and post-comatose states. Neurocrit Care 8 (2): 262–270.

Vanhaudenhuyse A, Noirhomme Q, Tshibanda LJ et al. (2010). Default network connectivity reflects the level of consciousness in non-communicative brain-damaged patients. Brain 133 (Pt 1): 161–171.

van Heuven AW, Dorhout Mees SM, Algra A et al. (2008). Validation of a prognostic subarachnoid hemorrhage grading scale derived directly from the Glasgow Coma Scale. Stroke 39 (4): 1347–1348.

van Swieten JC, Koudstaal PJ, Visser MC et al. (1988). Interobserver agreement for the assessment of handicap in stroke patients. Stroke 19 (5): 604–607.

Vespa PM, Nuwer MR, Nenov V et al. (1999). Increased incidence and impact of nonconvulsive and convulsive seizures after traumatic brain injury as detected by continuous electroencephalographic monitoring. J Neurosurg 91 (5): 750–760.

Vespa PM, O'Phelan K, Shah M et al. (2003). Acute seizures after intracerebral hemorrhage: a factor in progressive midline shift and outcome. Neurology 60 (9): 1441–1446.

Vespa PM, Miller C, McArthur D et al. (2007). Nonconvulsive electrographic seizures after traumatic brain injury result in a delayed, prolonged increase in intracranial pressure and metabolic crisis. Crit Care Med 35 (12): 2830–2836.

Vespa PM, McArthur DL, Xu Y et al. (2010). Nonconvulsive seizures after traumatic brain injury are associated with hippocampal atrophy. Neurology 75 (9): 792–798.

Vos PE, Jacobs B, Andriessen TM et al. (2010). GFAP and S100B are biomarkers of traumatic brain injury: an observational cohort study. Neurology 75 (20): 1786–1793.

Vos PE, Lamers KJ, Hendriks JC et al. (2004). Glial and neuronal proteins in serum predict outcome after severe traumatic brain injury. Neurology 62 (8): 1303–1310.

Wada R, Aviv RI, Fox AJ et al. (2007). CT angiography "spot sign" predicts hematoma expansion in acute intracerebral hemorrhage. Stroke 38 (4): 1257–1262.

Wahlgren N, Ahmed N, Eriksson N et al. (2008). Multivariable analysis of outcome predictors and adjustment of main outcome results to baseline data profile in randomized controlled trials: Safe Implementation of Thrombolysis in Stroke-MOnitoring STudy (SITS-MOST). Stroke 39 (12): 3316–3322.

Wartenberg KE, Patsalides A, Yepes MS (2004). Is magnetic resonance spectroscopy superior to conventional diagnostic tools in hypoxic-ischemic encephalopathy? J Neuroimaging 14 (2): 180–186.

Weiss N, Galanaud D, Carpentier A et al. (2008). A combined clinical and MRI approach for outcome assessment of traumatic head injured comatose patients. J Neurol 255 (2): 217–223.

Westhall E, Rossetti AO, van Rootselaar AF et al. (2016). Standardized EEG interpretation accurately predicts prognosis after cardiac arrest. Neurology 86 (16): 1482–1490.

Wijdicks EF, Bamlet WR, Maramattom BV et al. (2005). Validation of a new coma scale: the FOUR score. Ann Neurol 58 (4): 585–593.

Wijdicks EFM, Hijdra A, Young GB et al. (2006). Practice parameter: prediction of outcome in comatose survivors after cardiopulmonary resuscitation (an evidence-based review): report of the Quality Standards Subcommittee of the American Academy of Neurology. Neurology 67 (2): 203–210.

Wijman CA, Mlynash M, Caulfield AF et al. (2009). Prognostic value of brain diffusion-weighted imaging after cardiac arrest. Ann Neurol 65 (4): 394–402.

Wijnen VJ, van Boxtel GJ, Eilander HJ et al. (2007). Mismatch negativity predicts recovery from the vegetative state. Clin Neurophysiol 118 (3): 597–605.

Wu O, Sorensen AG, Benner T et al. (2009). Comatose patients with cardiac arrest: predicting clinical outcome with diffusion-weighted MR imaging. Radiology 252 (1): 173–181.

Wuerz RC, Holliman CJ, Meador SA et al. (1995). Effect of age on prehospital cardiac resuscitation outcome. Am J Emerg Med 13 (4): 389–391.

Yaghi S, Bianchi N, Amole A et al. (2014). ASPECTS is a predictor of favorable CT perfusion in acute ischemic stroke. Journal of Neuroradiology/Journal de Neuroradiologie 41 (3): 184–187.

Yanagawa Y, Tsushima Y, Tokumaru A et al. (2000). A quantitative analysis of head injury using T2*-weighted gradient-echo imaging. J Trauma Acute Care Surg 49 (2): 272–277.

Youn CS, Callaway CW, Rittenberger JC (2015). Combination of initial neurologic examination and continuous EEG to predict survival after cardiac arrest. Resuscitation 94: 73–79.

Young GB, Doig G, Ragazzoni A (2005). Anoxic-ischemic encephalopathy: clinical and electrophysiological associations with outcome. Neurocrit Care 2 (2): 159–164.

Zador Z, Sperrin M, King AT (2016). Predictors of outcome in traumatic brain injury: new insight using receiver operating curve indices and Bayesian network analysis. PLoS One 11 (7): e0158762.

*Handbook of Clinical Neurology*, Vol. 140 (3rd series)
*Critical Care Neurology, Part I*
E.F.M. Wijdicks and A.H. Kramer, Editors
http://dx.doi.org/10.1016/B978-0-444-63600-3.00022-2

Chapter 22

# Family discussions on life-sustaining interventions in neurocritical care

M.M. ADIL[1]* AND D. LARRIVIERE[2]

[1]*Ochsner Neuroscience Center, New Orleans, LA, USA*

[2]*Division of Neuromuscular Medicine, Ochsner Neuroscience Center, New Orleans, LA, USA*

## Abstract

Approximately 20% of all deaths in the USA occur in the intensive care unit (ICU) and the majority of ICU deaths involves decision of de-escalation of life-sustaining interventions. Life-sustaining interventions may include intubation and mechanical ventilation, artificial nutrition and hydration, antibiotic treatment, brain surgery, or vasoactive support. Decision making about goals of care can be defined as an end-of-life communication and the decision-making process between a clinician and a patient (or a surrogate decision maker if the patient is incapable) in an institutional setting to establish a plan of care. This process includes deciding whether to use life-sustaining treatments. Therefore, family discussion is a critical element in the decision-making process throughout the patient's stay in the neurocritical care unit. A large part of care in the neurosciences intensive care unit is discussion of proportionality of care. This chapter provides a step-wise approach to hold these conferences and discusses ways to do it effectively.

## INTRODUCTION

Patients admitted to the neurocritical care unit (NCCU) often lack the ability to participate in their own treatment decisions as a result of aphasia, neglect, delirium, physical or cognitive impairments. Approximately 20% of all deaths in the USA occur in the intensive care unit (ICU) (Angus et al., 2004) and the majority of ICU deaths involve decisions of de-escalation of life-sustaining interventions (Curtis et al., 1995; Prendergast and Luce, 1997). Life-sustaining interventions may include intubation and mechanical ventilation (MV), artificial nutrition and hydration, antibiotic treatment, brain surgery, or vasoactive support. Family discussions with the care team are essential to help relieve anxiety and prepare for the withdrawal of care and the dying process (Truog et al., 2008). Families have identified communication with healthcare providers and decision making about goals of care as high priorities for improving end-of-life care in Canada (Heyland et al., 2006a, 2010). Decision making about goals of care can be defined as an end-of-life communication and the decision-making process between a clinician and a patient (or a surrogate decision maker if the patient is incapable) in an institutional setting to establish a plan of care. This process includes deciding whether to use life-sustaining treatments (Sinuff et al., 2015). Therefore family discussion is a critical element in the decision-making process throughout the patient's stay in the NCCU.

## COMMON NEUROLOGIC DISORDERS FREQUENTLY REQUIRING ASSESSMENT OF LIFE-SUSTAINING INTERVENTIONS

The decision of de-escalation of life-sustaining treatments is the most common cause of death in critical care (Diringer et al., 2001; Verkade et al., 2012). The past decade has seen a noteworthy growth in palliative care; the number of palliative care teams within US hospitals with ≥50 beds has nearly tripled to over 60% since 2000 (National Palliative Care Registry, 2014). A recent study

*Correspondence to: Malik M. Adil, MD, Department of Neurology Ochsner Neuroscience Center 1514 Jefferson Hwy, New Orleans LA 70118, USA. E-mail: malikmuhammad.adil@gmail.com

found that 80% of older patients hospitalized with a critical illness desire a less aggressive and more comfort care plan that does not include cardiopulmonary resuscitation (Heyland et al., 2013).

Acute stroke constitutes a major proportion of the NCCU population. Stroke patients seen by palliative care specialists are more functionally impaired, less likely to have decision-making capacity, and more likely to die in hospital (Holloway et al., 2010). Compared with nonstroke patients receiving palliative care consultations, stroke patients are more often referred to palliative care for end-of-life and de-escalation of life-sustaining treatment decisions (Holloway et al., 2010; Eastman et al., 2013). Approximately 1 in 15 stroke patients use MV on admission. Compared to ischemic stroke, a higher percentage of intracerebral hemorrhage (ICH) patients require MV and tracheostomy. (Roch et al., 2003; Huttner et al., 2006).

Our current practices are based on results of clinical trials with restricted use of withdrawal of care among treated patients (NINDS, 1995). Patients with serious or terminal illness were excluded from participating trials (NINDS, 1995; Broderick et al., 2013). Studies from the prethrombolytic era found that do-not-resuscitate (DNR) orders were used in 12–32% of patients with acute stroke and the risk of mortality was substantially higher in patients with DNR orders (Alexandrov et al., 1995; Shepardson et al., 1997, 1999). In acute ischemic stroke patients treated with thrombolytics, withdrawal of care was instituted in 3.3% of patients. The annual rates of withdrawal of care increased from 0.4% in 2002 to 5% in 2010 (Qureshi et al., 2013). In other stroke subtypes, such as ICH, relatively high rates of withdrawal of care are already considered important factors of the observed high mortality (Qureshi, 2011).

Our current understanding of variations in use of DNR and withdrawal of care in stroke patients is based on studies performed in patients with ICH. A review during 1999 and 2000 reported that the proportion of patients with DNR orders within the first 24 hours of hospitalization varied from 0% to 70% across hospitals (Hemphill et al., 2004). However, there are limited data regarding withdrawal of care in patients with subarachnoid hemorrhage (SAH) (Kowalski et al., 2013). Patients with SAH have greater than twofold higher odds of withdrawal of MV compared with other patients admitted in an NCCU (Diringer et al., 2001). Withdrawal of care during hospitalization was instituted in 3.4% of SAH patients and annual rates increased from 1.3% in 2002 to 6.4% in 2010 (Qureshi et al., 2014).

Early deaths are common in stroke, and most occur as a result of brain death or in the setting of de-escalation of life-sustaining interventions when prognosis for recovery is believed to be poor; (Shepardson et al., 1999; Centers for Disease Control and Prevention, 2001; Zurasky et al.,

2005; Jaren and Selwa, 2006; Naidech et al., 2009; Kelly et al., 2012). Traumatic brain injury (TBI) is the leading cause of death and disability in patients less than 45 years of age, with mortality rates of 40% and approximately 30% left with serious neurologic outcome. There is noteworthy inconsistency in reported mortality and decisions to withdraw care which results in variances in early de-escalation of life-sustaining treatment (MacKenzie et al., 2006; Turgeon et al., 2013).

## SURROGATE DECISION MAKERS

Patients often lack the ability to participate in decision making, requiring the involvement of surrogate decision makers. These surrogates, generally family members, may be well informed about the patient's values and preferences or have the assistance of a written living will that summarizes the patient's wishes. However, in practice, the patient's previously expressed views, either oral or written, are frequently inadequate and limited to general statements, such as, "If I have no chance for recovery, I do not want to be kept alive on machines." This can lead to more questions than answers for the family members and the care team. What does "recovery" mean? And what level of disability is acceptable to the patient? Similarly, what does it mean to be "kept alive on machines"?

Although surrogate decision makers are unable to predict perfectly patient treatment choices, they provide insight into the patient's former values (Shalowitz et al., 2006). It is important to keep in mind that surrogate decision makers count on multiple sources of information when estimating their patient's prognosis and seldom rely solely on the physician's prognostic estimate (Boyd et al., 2010). In addition, like patients, surrogates are often overly optimistic in predicting how well their patient will do over time (Zier et al., 2012). Surrogate decision makers consistently overestimated the chances of survival of their patients, even when clinicians offered minimal chance for recovery. In one study, when told, "It is very unlikely that your patient will survive," the median chance of survival reported by 80 surrogates was still above 30%. When the chance of survival was quantified specifically by the provider to be 5%, the chance of survival assigned by surrogates was a significantly higher median value of 15%, with a maximum value of 40% (Zier et al., 2012). It is important for physicians to recognize some of these limitations inherent in the use of surrogate decision makers. Patients should make their wishes known as much as possible, so that designated surrogates can be best prepared should their services be needed.

## GENERAL PRINCIPLES OF EFFECTIVE COMMUNICATION

Fragmented communication between providers (neurointensivists, neurologists, physiatrists, neurosurgeons, and palliative care specialists), across interdisciplinary departments (ICU, emergency department, and acute rehabilitation unit) and family members can compromise overall care. Effective communication is fundamental to a team approach.

Most physicians receive limited training in communication skills. Data suggest that physicians often do not talk to patients and families about their options, risks, and benefits (Levinson et al., 2010). Studies have demonstrated that communication between physicians and surrogate decision makers is often poor (Malacrida et al., 1998; Azoulay et al., 2004). Another study reported that 35% of surrogate decision makers did not understand the physician's description about the diagnosis or choices for further care (Azoulay et al., 2004). Similarly, another study demonstrated that almost half of surrogate decision makers reported that physician–family communication was incomplete in the ICU (Azoulay et al., 2005). Dissatisfaction with decision making among family members may not only affect patients' care in ICU, but also the psychologic health of the surrogate decision makers. One study reported that 73% of surrogate decision makers experienced anxiety and 35% experienced depression during their patient ICU stay (Pochard et al., 2005). Another study suggested that 33% of family members had symptoms of posttraumatic stress disorder and also reported that family members had a higher burden of symptoms if they were involved in making decisions about de-escalation of life-sustaining interventions and end-of-life care (Azoulay et al., 2005). These effects can be lessened by clinician communication and behaviors (Lautrette et al., 2007). Other factors, like chart documentation of physician recommendations to withdraw life support; discussions of families' wishes to withdraw life support; and discussions of families' spiritual needs, are associated with family satisfaction with decision making (Gries et al., 2008). Family or patient demographics such as age; race and ethnicity; education level; gender; and patient comorbidities were not associated with family member satisfaction in end-of-life decision making (Gries et al., 2008).

Members of the care team should approach communication with decision makers thoughtfully. In one study, specific communication strategies were associated with increased satisfaction and included: assurances of comfort, providing written information, support for shared decision making, expressions of empathy, specific patient care measures like extubation before death, and family presence at time of death (Hinkle et al., 2015). Prognostic disclosure during withdrawal-of-care discussions is associated with increased satisfaction with decision making (Heyland et al., 2009). Doubt and uncertainty about the prognosis may result in vague recommendations from the physician about end-of-life

decisions (Christakis and Asch, 1993; Christakis and Iwashyna, 1998) and family members could lose trust in the physician and this could also lead to worse family satisfaction in decision making (Reynolds et al., 2005). In such difficult situations physicians can consider the trail of treatment.

The broad scope of family discussions is complex and the multifaceted needs of patients and their families require an interdisciplinary team of health professionals, including physicians, nurses, therapists, pharmacists, spiritual care providers, social workers, and others. The members of the care team should strive to develop a trusting relationship with the patients and their families. The first meeting should focus on developing a trust and working on a model of care, balancing hope for the best with preparing for the worst (Back et al., 2003). The family and healthcare team must simultaneously prepare for survival or decline to death (Lynn, 1997).

The first meeting can be used to attempt to achieve four essential goals. The first is to collect information from the family. This allows the providers to determine the extent of the family knowledge and their expectations. The second goal is for the providers to provide intelligible information in accordance with the family needs and desires. The third goal is to support the family by helping them cope with the emotional impact of the present circumstances. The final goal is to cultivate a strategy in the form of a treatment plan with the participation of the family.

Proactive and periodic meetings with the family may help increase family satisfaction and decision making (Epstein and Street, 2011). These meetings provide an opportunity to collect evidence about a patient's level of function, critical abilities, and tolerable health states. Family members vary as to how much information they wish to know and how active they wish to be in the decision-making process, with some decision makers preferring physicians to take more responsibility for decisions (Heyland et al., 2006b; Curtis and Vincent, 2010). Members of the healthcare team should be aware of the burden that surrogate decision makers carry, and tailor their communication styles to their needs and frequently reassure the family members that they have the support of the healthcare team (Curtis and White, 2008).

The complexity of the interaction can sometimes create serious miscommunications (Taylor, 1988; Lind et al., 1989; Miyaji, 1993; Ptacek and Eberhardt, 1996), such as patient misunderstanding about the prognosis of the illness or purpose of care (Eidinger and Schapira, 1984; Mackillop et al., 1988; Siminoff et al., 1989; Quirt et al., 1997; Haidet et al., 1998; Weeks et al., 1998). In addition to providing the family with adequate information about the patient's illness and prognosis, physicians and the other members of the healthcare team should assess the family's understanding of the information delivered after each care conference or when there has been an exchange of significant information (e.g., when there has been a change in the patient's clinical status). Time limitations have spurred clinicians' fear of the open-ended question and a tendency to interrupt quickly. But the skill to engage realistically with the family, to listen empathically, and to join with them in their suffering helps construct a respectful and effective partnership between the provider team and the family. Decision makers usually want to know the prognostic information early in the course of critical illness, even if this prognostic information includes a high degree of uncertainty, yet physicians are often hesitant to offer this information (LeClaire et al., 2005; Anderson et al., 2015). Given the fact that many surrogate decision makers count on multiple sources of information to inform their own view of prognosis, not just the physicians' estimates (Boyd et al., 2010), physicians and the members of the care team may wish to outline the diagnostic uncertainty, including the variables that drive the uncertainty, with the family as a part of building the relationship of trust and mutual respect.

## COMMUNICATION STRATEGIES IN THE ICU

The process of family discussions can be improved by understanding the process involved, approaching it as a stepwise procedure, and using well-established principles of communication and counseling. Canadian guidelines recommend that healthcare providers can consider addressing few key elements when discussing goals of care with patients and families (Clayton et al., 2007; Harle et al., 2008).

The five most important elements to discuss were preferences for care in the event of life-threatening illness, values, prognosis, fears or concerns, and additional questions about goals of care. One study found that these elements are infrequently discussed. These findings may perhaps be used to ascertain important opportunities to improve communication and decision making. Use of these elements in family discussions is associated with greater concordance between preferred and prescribed goals of care, and with greater satisfaction. Family members rated prognostic disclosure as highly important (You et al., 2014).

Members of the healthcare team must also be prepared to convey bad news to patients and their families. Bad news can be defined as any information which seriously or adversely affects an individual's view of his or her future. How bad news is discussed and disclosed can affect the patient's and family's comprehension of information, level of satisfaction with care (Butow et al., 1995; Ford et al., 1996), level of hopefulness (Sardell

and Trierweiler, 1993), and consequent psychologic adjustment (Slavin et al., 1982; Roberts et al., 1994; Last and van Veldhuizen, 1996). On the other hand, breaking bad news is also a complex communication task. In addition to the verbal component of disclosing the bad news, it necessitates other skills: responding to family emotional reactions, involving the family in decision making, dealing with the expectation for cure, the involvement of multiple family members, and the dilemma of how to give hope when a poor outcome is likely. Physicians and other members of the healthcare team can minimize the complexity and risks associated with conveying unfavorable information by understanding the process involved and applying standardized principles of communication and counseling. SPIKES, a six-step strategy, was developed as a method for this purpose (Baile et al., 2000).

### Step 1: S – setting up the interview

Arrange for some privacy, involve family members, sit down (sitting down relaxes the patient and is also a sign that you will not rush), make connection with the patient (maintaining eye contact may be uncomfortable but it is an important way of establishing rapport; touching the patient or family members on the arm or holding a hand is another way to accomplish this), manage time constraints and interruptions (set your pager on silent or ask a colleague to respond to your pages).

### Step 2: P – assessing the patient or patient's family perception

What have you been told about your family member medical situation so far?

### Step 3: I – obtaining the patient or family invitations

Most patients and family members express a desire for complete information about their diagnosis, prognosis, and details of their illness; some patients and family members do not. When a clinician perceives a patient and family express clearly a desire for information, it may decrease the anxiety associated with the bad news.

### Step 4: K – giving knowledge and information to the patient and family

Provide medical information using vocabulary that the patient and their family can understand. Try to use non-technical words. Avoid excessive bluntness and give information in small pieces and check intermittently as to the patient's and family's understanding. When the prognosis is poor, avoid using phrases such as "There is nothing more we can do for you."

## Step 5: E – addressing the patient's emotions with empathic responses

Learning to respond to the full spectrum of the patient's and family's emotions is one of the most difficult challenges physicians face when delivering bad news. Emotional reactions may vary from silence to disbelief, crying, denial, or anger. Observe for any emotion on the part of the patient or families. This may be tearfulness, a look of sadness, silence, or shock. Use open questions to query the patient and families as to what they are thinking or feeling.

## Step 6: S – strategy and summary

Before discussing a treatment plan, it is important to ask patients or families if they are ready at that time for such a discussion.

Family physician disagreement is another challenge that physicians encounter and have to deal with effectively in order to maintain their trust with families. In some studies, family–physician disagreement was documented in only 5% of cases. Other studies have reported that, when precisely asked about conflict, family members report family–physician conflict in 40% of cases. Family–physician conflict was most commonly associated with poor communication (33%) or unprofessional behavior of the staff (15%) (Abbott et al., 2001).

## ROLE OF PROGNOSTIC MODELS AND FACTORS ASSOCIATED WITH DE-ESCALATION OF LIFE-SUSTAINING INTERVENTIONS

Physicians must accurately assess and clearly communicate prognosis in order for patients to make fully informed decisions about their care. As a part of this process, physicians must correctly order and interpret ancillary data collected in the course of care. Studies have suggested clinical, radiographic, and laboratory factors associated with outcomes, and various prediction models exist. It is central to recognize the strengths and weaknesses of various methods of formulating prognostic estimates, mainly when they are used to guide decisions about palliative, end-of-life treatments and de-escalation of life-sustaining interventions. No prognostic model has been scientifically assessed in a controlled study to define its efficacy in guiding decisions about end-of-life treatment and de-escalation of life-sustaining interventions (Baird, 2009).

Prognostic models and clinical experience may be biased by the frequent de-escalation of life-sustaining treatments, leading to a self-fulfilling prophecy in which the true prognosis is difficult to ascertain (Becker et al., 2001; Zahuranec et al., 2010; Creutzfeldt et al., 2011). The physician's prognosis of survival and poor outcome is one of the strongest predictors of withdrawal of life-sustaining treatments (Fried et al., 2002; Cook et al., 2003). In addition, "favorable outcomes" differ between patients and the definition varies across models, with several focusing on risk of short-term mortality. However, long-term outcome and quality of life are likely more important to many patients and families. Therefore, it is vital for clinicians to be confident that a selected model has been developed with suitable methodology and validation of accuracy in diverse populations (Counsell and Dennis, 2001; Moons et al., 2009; Teale et al., 2012). Furthermore, there are challenges in applying probability estimates derived from a population-based statistical model to an individual's risk of death or disability, even when each individual model is well calibrated (Lemeshow et al., 1995; Stern, 2012). These difficulties raise some concerns and some studies suggest that model-predicted probabilities should not be used as the primary basis for decisions regarding de-escalation of life-sustaining treatments (Lemeshow et al., 1995; Ariesen et al., 2005; Gabbay et al., 2010).

An alternative to model-based estimate for prognosis is to utilize clinician experience with prior similar cases and predictable neurologic outcome from knowledge of neuroanatomy. However, clinician prognostic estimates are also imperfect and flawed, because they can differ significantly among physicians (Becker et al., 2001; Racine et al., 2009) and are subject to both optimistic and pessimistic outcome predictions (Christakis and Lamont, 2000; Finley Caulfield et al., 2010; Meadow et al., 2011; Navi et al., 2012). Literature from withdrawal of care suggests that obtaining a second opinion from an experienced multidisciplinary team of experts or colleague may benefit and reduce the influence of individual biases on prognostic estimates (Christakis and Lamont, 2000; Glare and Sinclair, 2008), but it is unclear how to handle diversity of opinion.

In spite of the potential limitations of prognostic models, precisely validated models can provide useful information for the healthcare team. For example, studies have suggested various prediction models for each stroke type (Morgenstern et al., 2010; Jauch et al., 2013), although the value of current stroke prognostic models differs widely (Counsell and Dennis, 2001; Ariesen et al., 2005; Rosen and Macdonald, 2005; Teale et al., 2012). Most stroke prognostic models include the patient's age and initial stroke severity, with severity being the main predictor of subsequent disability or death (Duncan et al., 1992; Frankel et al., 2000; Smith et al., 2010; Saposnik et al., 2011; Fonarow et al., 2012). Studies have identified other predictive factors for ischemic stroke, including comorbid illness, laboratory values such as initial glucose, and stroke subtype (Frankel et al., 2000; Johnston et al., 2007; Saposnik et al., 2011). In one study predictors of withdrawal of care among thrombolytic-treated ischemic stroke patients were female gender, presence of atrial fibrillation, aphasia, presence of hemiplegia/hemiparesis, postthrombolytic ICH, All Patient Refined-Diagnosis-Related Group (APR-DRG) severity scale (extreme loss of function), hospital location (west region), and teaching hospitals (Qureshi et al., 2013). In one study, the iScore has been shown to be more accurate than physician estimate alone at predicting short-term outcome (Saposnik et al., 2013). Another study reviewed patients with ischemic stroke who died or were discharged to hospice during their hospitalization over 1 year. All but one of 37 deaths and hospice discharges involved a decision by the patient or surrogate to withdraw or withhold life-sustaining interventions. The authors concluded that these deaths were related to patient and family preferences and occurred in spite of evidence-based care (Xian et al., 2011). Similar findings were reported in a study in patients with early DNR orders compared to patients without DNR orders. The higher mortality in DNR patients was felt to reflect underlying stroke severity as well as patient and family preferences (Reeves et al., 2012).

Because early decisions of de-escalation of life-sustaining interventions in ICH are more common, the potential for withdrawal bias is likely far higher in ICH than in other stroke types (Hemphill et al., 2004; Hemphill, 2007; Zahuranec et al., 2007). ICH score (incorporating age, Glasgow Coma Scale (GCS), hemorrhage volume, presence of intraventricular hemorrhage, and infratentorial origin: Cheung and Zou, 2003; Ruiz-Sandoval et al., 2007) is one of the most frequently reported models that has been associated with both 30-day mortality and 12-month modified Rankin scale (Hemphill et al., 2001, 2009; Clarke et al., 2004).

For aneurysmal SAH, the Hunt–Hess scale and the World Federation of Neurological Surgeons scale are reportedly prognostic models, although several issues with these scales have been identified and additional validation studies are needed (Rosen and Macdonald, 2005). Other clinical factors commonly reported to be associated with poor outcome after SAH include hyperglycemia, aneurysm size and location, amount of blood, and late complications such as rebleeding and delayed cerebral ischemia (Rosen and Macdonald, 2005; Ogilvy et al., 2006; van Norden et al., 2006; Bederson et al., 2009; Kruyt et al., 2009). In one study predictors of withdrawal of care among SAH patients were age >65, female gender, African American race, Hispanic ethnicity, renal failure, ICH, APR-DRG severity score

of extreme loss of function, and southern hospital region (Qureshi et al., 2014).

TBI is the leading cause of death and disability in patients less than 45 years of age, with mortality rates of 40% and approximately 30% of patients left with serious neurologic outcome or vegetative state. There is noteworthy inconsistency in reported mortality and decisions to withdraw care (Turgeon et al., 2013). Inaccurate early assessment of neurologic severity in head injury may misguidedly assign poor prognosis to patients who go on to recover. This risk is particularly prevalent in younger patients (Stocchetti et al., 2004). Well-known poor prognostic factors after TBI include initial motor score on GCS of 1 or 2 (extensor posturing), lack of pupil reactivity, hypoxia and hypotension, and head computed tomography (CT) characteristics fulfilling the Marshall criteria (e.g., mass lesion, SAH, or signs of raised intracranial pressure) (Steyerberg et al., 2008). In addition, the GCS has lost its predictive power for TBI since the late 1990s (Balestreri et al., 2004). Various predictive models and scores have been recommended to help predict the patient's outcome with TBI. These include Acute Physiology and Chronic Health Evaluation (APACHE), Simplified Acute Physiology Score (SAPS), Glasgow Outcome Scale/Extended (GOS, GOSE), and Mortality Prediction Model (MPM). Two prognostic models were developed recently: the International Mission on Prognosis and Analysis of Clinical Trials in Traumatic brain injury (IMPACT) database and the Corticosteroid Randomization After Significant Head injury (CRASH) trials (Turgeon et al., 2013). Surprisingly, despite extensive validation of IMPACT and CRASH scoring systems, there is still lack of accuracy. Serum biomarkers such as S100 protein, neuron-specific enolase, and glial fibrillary acidic protein may be helpful in predicting outcomes after TBI; however, the specificity and sensitivity of these biomarkers are questionable (Stevens and Sutter, 2013). Lack of reliable prognostic models to precisely predict outcomes for TBI patients results in variances in early withdrawal of life-sustaining treatment (MacKenzie et al., 2006). Similar to other examples provided in this chapter, caution should be taken with early withdrawal of life-sustaining treatment after TBI as self-fulfilling prophecy (Turgeon et al., 2013).

The outcome of patients with sudden cardiac arrest (SCA) is generally poor. The cause of mortality after SCA is primarily related to effects of anoxic brain injury and not necessarily from cardiac complications. In 1985, Levy, et al. identified detailed clinical findings that predicted recovery (or death) in patients from hypoxia-ischemia post cardiac arrest. The presence of pupillary light reflexes, motor flexor to noxious stimuli, and spontaneous eye movements from day 1 predicted good outcomes; no patients recovered who had absent pupillary response on day 1 post arrest. In 2006 the American Academy of Neurology published predictors of poor neurologic outcome post cardiac arrest. These predictors were absent papillary or corneal reflexes and motor responses at day 3, absent N20 responses to somatosensory evoked potentials beginning on day 1, serum neuron-specific enolase > 33 ng/mL on days 1–3, and presence of myoclonic status epilepticus within 24 hours of arrest (Wijdicks et al., 2006). Biomarkers that appear to be associated with severe brain injury after SCA are serum S100B and interleukin-8. Increased S100B values measured at 12 hours after insult are associated with unfavorable neurologic outcome at 12 months. Outcome in patients treated with therapeutic hypothermia (targeted temperature management) may be different and recommendations are in flux.

## DISCUSSION ON ILLNESS TRAJECTORIES

Four illness trajectories have been recommended to conceptualize how function declines as diseases advance to death. These illness trajectories allow patients, family members, healthcare providers, and healthcare planners to prepare for next steps and to make more informed and critical decisions about care. Four illness trajectories are: (1) for cancer: a short decline; (2) for heart failure: an episodic decline; (3) for dementia: a prolonged decline; and (4) for acute brain injury: patients who survive the acute stage enter a chronic stage of recovery. In this case, survivors' trajectories are reset and they may survive for long periods. The pattern of their illness may follow any of the other trajectories at another point in time (Lynn and Adamson, 2003; Murray et al., 2005; Creutzfeldt et al., 2015). This distinct pattern of trajectory for patients with brain injury can be used during discussion with family members to make decisions about goals of care, treatment options, and outcomes.

## DISCUSSION OF SIGNIFICANCE OF MECHANICAL VENTILATION

Approximately 1 in 15 stroke patients require MV on admission. Compared to ischemic stroke, a greater percentage of ICH patients require MV and tracheostomy (Roch et al., 2003; Huttner et al., 2006). During a trial of MV, organized communication with surrogate decision makers is important to assist decision making. Overall mortality among mechanically ventilated stroke patients is high, with a 30-day death rate ranging from 46% to 75% (Roch et al., 2003; Rabinstein and Wijdicks, 2004; Holloway et al., 2005). In ischemic stroke, 40–70% of patients who receive prolonged MV have poor functional outcomes (Rabinstein and Wijdicks, 2004) and this association is particularly strong in patients older than 60 years of age, those presenting with a GCS score <10, and patients with preexisting brain injury (Rabinstein and Wijdicks, 2004; Golestanian et al., 2009). There is significant disparity in rates of withdrawal of life-sustaining therapies that is not entirely explained by disease severity and patient preferences (Wunsch et al., 2005; Cooper et al., 2009). Although difficult to estimate precisely, withdrawal of MV occurs in up to 35–60% of all deaths in patients with stroke, which makes it one of the most common modes of death (Mayer and Kossoff, 1999; Diringer et al., 2001; Cooper et al., 2009), although >50–70% patients survive <24 hours after extubation (Mayer and Kossoff, 1999; Prendergast and Puntillo, 2002). Physicians should counsel family members about anticipated signs and symptoms after extubation and prepare family members for the fact that death may not necessarily occur shortly after extubation. Up to 60% of patients may exhibit labored breathing after extubation (Mayer and Kossoff, 1999). General guidelines are available to make this transition as comfortable as possible for the patient and family (Quill et al., 2014). Discussing the goals of care with family members requires the physician to inform the family about the likelihood of the patient surviving and the quality of life with intubation and MV compared with noninvasive treatment approaches. These prognostic estimates need to be tailored to the individual patient based on clinical and other parameters. It is equally important to discuss the benefits and risks of intubation and MV in those patients at risk for respiratory compromise.

## CONFLICT AND CONFLICT RESOLUTION

Conflicts may result from emotions, mistrust, genuine value differences, information breaches, and treatment goal confusion (Back and Arnold, 2005). Conflict can occur within families, between staff and families, and among treatment teams. Most conflict revolves around differences of opinion, an intervention desired by a surrogate, and understanding of the facts. It's important to understand why a family member is asking for something the care team does not believe to be helpful. This understanding can be used as a part of the discussion of why the requested treatment is inconsistent with the overall goals of care or will not provide the patient with the outcome the family is seeking. Time spent by the physician in listening to the family's request and the reasons for it is often more helpful that trying to convince the family of the care team's position (Quill et al., 2009). These discussions can be emotionally charged and may require significant time. However, they should not become confrontational.

## RELIGIOUS AND SPIRITUAL SUPPORT

Although clinicians are not expected to be experts in various cultural or religious practices, it is essential that they are respectful of these preferences and aware of the influence they may have in decision making. Awareness of cultural and religious preferences and practices can facilitate understanding of family choices when discussing options, particularly when families demand or decline evidence-based therapy (Barclay et al., 2007). It is reasonable to consider asking families about their possible spiritual or religious beliefs and to offer referral to a chaplain or spiritual care provider.

## BRAIN DEATH AND ORGAN DONATION

Brain death determination and participation in the process of organ donation are common in the NCCU. Although all US states have similar legal definition of brain death, there are some state- and hospital-based differences in the process for determining brain death. The American Academy of Neurology recently updated the 1995 American Academy of Neurology guideline for the diagnosis of brain death in patients older than 18 years (Wijdicks et al., 2010). Each year, the estimated number of donors after brain death is 10 500–13 800, and stroke accounts for a large percentage of patients declared brain-dead who become potential organ donors (Organ Procurement and Transplantation Network, 2003; Sheehy et al., 2003). In the USA, hospitals are mandated by law to involve organ procurement agencies in the assessment of these cases for possible organ donation and to offer the option to the families of suitable candidates. Available estimates indicate that >50% of families provide consent for organ donation (Sheehy et al., 2003), but donation rates indicate that donation only occurs in one-third of appropriate cases (Gortmaker et al., 1996). This gap can be reduced by separating the communication of brain death from the discussion of organ donation (von Pohle, 1996), improving the identification of potential donors (Cloutier et al., 2006), and ensuring well-timed communication with the organ procurement agency (Brown et al., 2010). Programs that incorporate an in-house presence of the coordinator from the organ procurement agency can be effective in achieving these goals (Salim et al., 2011).

## CONCLUSIONS

The current medical system – geared towards shorter hospital stays and quicker discharges – places a tremendous premium on early decision making. However, physicians require time for a clearer prognosis to emerge and families require time to fully understand the illness and its implications. Hospitals and care teams should be prepared to provide this time to the populations they serve.

Viewed from a contemporary perspective, supporting family members through the decision to de-escalate life-sustaining interventions when survival is unlikely could be an important target for improving satisfaction. We recommend that decisions about de-escalating life-sustaining interventions should not be made until sufficient time has elapsed to allow for better assessment of prognosis and for the patient and family members to fully understand the illness and its implications. It is important to revisit family and medical team discussions frequently during the acute and postacute phases of the illness to endorse or revise goals and treatment preferences.

### REFERENCES

Abbott KH, Sago JG, Breen CM et al. (2001). Families looking back: one year after discussion of withdrawal or withholding of life-sustaining support. Crit Care Med 29: 197–201.

Alexandrov AV, Bladin CF, Meslin EM et al. (1995). Do-not-resuscitate orders in acute stroke. Neurology 45: 634–640.

Anderson WG, Cimino JW, Ernecoff NC et al. (2015). A multicenter study of key stakeholders' perspectives on communicating with surrogates about prognosis in intensive care units. Ann Am Thorac Soc 12: 142–152.

Angus DC, Barnato AE, Linde-Zwirble WT et al. (2004). Use of intensive care at the end of life in the United States: an epidemiologic study. Crit Care Med 32: 638–643.

Ariesen MJ, Algra A, Van Der Worp HB et al. (2005). Applicability and relevance of models that predict short term outcome after intracerebral hemorrhage. J Neurol Neurosurg Psychiatry 76: 839–844.

Azoulay E, Pochard F, Chevret S et al. (2004). Half the family members of intensive care unit patients do not want to share in the decision-making process: a study in 78 French intensive care units. Crit Care Med 32: 1832–1838.

Azoulay E, Pochard F, Kentish-Barnes N et al. (2005). Risk of post-traumatic stress symptoms in family members of intensive care unit patients. Am J Respir Crit Care Med 171: 987–994.

Back AL, Arnold RM (2005). Dealing with conflict in caring for the seriously ill: "it was just out of the question". JAMA 293: 1374–1381.

Back AL, Arnold RM, Quill TE (2003). Hope for the best, and prepare for the worst. Ann Intern Med 138: 439–443.

Baile WF, Buckman R, Lenzi R et al. (2000). SPIKES – a six-step protocol for delivering bad news: application to the patient with cancer. Oncologist 5: 302–311.

Baird AE (2009). Improving stroke prognosis. Neurology 73: 1084–1085.

Balestreri M, Czosnyka M, Chatfield DA et al. (2004). Predictive value of Glasgow Coma Scale after brain trauma: change in trend over the past ten years. J Neurol Neurosurg Psychiatry 75: 161–162.

Barclay JS, Blackhall LJ, Tulsky JA (2007). Communication strategies and cultural issues in the delivery of bad news. J Palliat Med 10: 958–977.

Becker KJ, Baxter AB, Cohen WA et al. (2001). Withdrawal of support in intracerebral hemorrhage may lead to self-fulfilling prophecies. Neurology 56: 766–772.

Bederson JB, Connolly Jr ES, Batjer HH et al. (2009). Guidelines for the management of aneurysmal subarachnoid hemorrhage: a statement for healthcare professionals from a special writing group of the Stroke Council, American Heart Association. Stroke 40: 994–1025.

Boyd EA, Lo B, Evans LR et al. (2010). "It's not just what the doctor tells me:" factors that influence surrogate decision-makers' perceptions of prognosis. Crit Care Med 38: 1270–1275.

Broderick JP, Palesch YY, Demchuk AM et al. (2013). Endovascular therapy after intravenous t-PA versus t-PA alone for stroke. N Engl J Med 368: 893–903.

Brown CV, Foulkrod KH, Dworaczyk S et al. (2010). Barriers to obtaining family consent for potential organ donors. J Trauma 68: 447–451.

Butow PN, Dunn SM, Tattersall MH (1995). Communication with cancer patients: does it matter? J Palliat Care 11: 34–38.

Centers For Disease Control And Prevention (2001). Technical appendix from Vital Statistics of the United States, National Vital Statistics System, mortality, 2001. Work Table 307: deaths from 39 selected causes by place of death, status of decedent when death occurred in hospital or medical center, and age: United States, 2011. Available online at: http://www.cdc.gov/nchs/data/statab/mortfinal2001_work307.pdf. (accessed 15 October 2015).

Cheung RT, Zou LY (2003). Use of the original, modified, or new intracerebral hemorrhage score to predict mortality and morbidity after intracerebral hemorrhage. Stroke 34: 1717–1722.

Christakis NA, Asch DA (1993). Biases in how physicians choose to withdraw life support. Lancet 342: 642–646.

Christakis NA, Iwashyna TJ (1998). Attitude and self-reported practice regarding prognostication in a national sample of internists. Arch Intern Med 158: 2389–2395.

Christakis NA, Lamont EB (2000). Extent and determinants of error in doctors' prognoses in terminally ill patients: prospective cohort study. BMJ 320: 469–472.

Clarke JL, Johnston SC, Farrant M et al. (2004). External validation of the ICH score. Neurocrit Care 1: 53–60.

Clayton JM, Hancock KM, Butow PN et al. (2007). Clinical practice guidelines for communicating prognosis and end-of-life issues with adults in the advanced stages of a life-limiting illness, and their caregivers. Med J Aust 186: S77. S79, S83–108.

Cloutier R, Baran D, Morin JE et al. (2006). Brain death diagnoses and evaluation of the number of potential organ donors in Quebec hospitals. Can J Anaesth 53: 716–721.

Cook D, Rocker G, Marshall J et al. (2003). Withdrawal of mechanical ventilation in anticipation of death in the intensive care unit. N Engl J Med 349: 1123–1132.

Cooper Z, Rivara FP, Wang J et al. (2009). Withdrawal of life-sustaining therapy in injured patients: variations between trauma centers and nontrauma centers. J Trauma 66: 1327–1335.

Counsell C, Dennis M (2001). Systematic review of prognostic models in patients with acute stroke. Cerebrovasc Dis 12: 159–170.

Creutzfeldt CJ, Becker KJ, Weinstein JR et al. (2011). Do-not-attempt-resuscitation orders and prognostic models for intraparenchymal hemorrhage. Crit Care Med 39: 158–162.

Creutzfeldt CJ, Longstreth WT, Holloway RG (2015). Predicting decline and survival in severe acute brain injury: the fourth trajectory. BMJ 351: h3904.

Curtis JR, Vincent JL (2010). Ethics and end-of-life care for adults in the intensive care unit. Lancet 376: 1347–1353.

Curtis JR, White DB (2008). Practical guidance for evidence-based ICU family conferences. Chest 134: 835–843.

Curtis JR, Park DR, Krone MR et al. (1995). Use of the medical futility rationale in do-not-attempt-resuscitation orders. JAMA 273: 124–128.

Diringer MN, Edwards DF, Aiyagari V et al. (2001). Factors associated with withdrawal of mechanical ventilation in a neurology/neurosurgery intensive care unit. Crit Care Med 29: 1792–1797.

Duncan PW, Goldstein LB, Matchar D et al. (1992). Measurement of motor recovery after stroke. Outcome assessment and sample size requirements. Stroke 23: 1084–1089.

Eastman P, McCarthy G, Brand CA et al. (2013). Who, why and when: stroke care unit patients seen by a palliative care service within a large metropolitan teaching hospital. BMJ Support Palliat Care 3: 77–83.

Eidinger RN, Schapira DV (1984). Cancer patients' insight into their treatment, prognosis, and unconventional therapies. Cancer 53: 2736–2740.

Epstein RM, Street Jr RL (2011). Shared mind: communication, decision making, and autonomy in serious illness. Ann Fam Med 9: 454–461.

Finley Caulfield A, Gabler L, Lansberg MG et al. (2010). Outcome prediction in mechanically ventilated neurologic patients by junior neurointensivists. Neurology 74: 1096–1101.

Fonarow GC, Saver JL, Smith EE et al. (2012). Relationship of national institutes of health stroke scale to 30-day mortality in Medicare beneficiaries with acute ischemic stroke. J Am Heart Assoc 1: 42–50.

Ford S, Fallowfield L, Lewis S (1996). Doctor–patient interactions in oncology. Soc Sci Med 42: 1511–1519.

Frankel MR, Morgenstern LB, Kwiatkowski T et al. (2000). Predicting prognosis after stroke: a placebo group analysis from the National Institute of Neurological Disorders and Stroke rt-PA Stroke Trial. Neurology 55: 952–959.

Fried TR, Bradley EH, Towle VR et al. (2002). Understanding the treatment preferences of seriously ill patients. N Engl J Med 346: 1061–1066.

Gabbay E, Calvo-Broce J, Meyer KB et al. (2010). The empirical basis for determinations of medical futility. J Gen Intern Med 25: 1083–1089.

Glare PA, Sinclair CT (2008). Palliative medicine review: prognostication. J Palliat Med 11: 84–103.

Golestanian E, Liou JI, Smith MA (2009). Long-term survival in older critically ill patients with acute ischemic stroke. Crit Care Med 37: 3107–3113.

Gortmaker SL, Beasley CL, Brigham LE et al. (1996). Organ donor potential and performance: size and nature of the organ donor shortfall. Crit Care Med 24: 432–439.

Gries CJ, Curtis JR, Wall RJ et al. (2008). Family member satisfaction with end-of-life decision making in the ICU. Chest 133: 704–712.

Haidet P, Hamel MB, Davis RB et al. (1998). Outcomes, preferences for resuscitation, and physician-patient communication among patients with metastatic colorectal cancer. SUPPORT Investigators. Study to Understand Prognoses and Preferences for Outcomes and Risks of Treatments. Am J Med 105: 222–229.

Harle I, Johnston J, Mackay J et al. (2008). Advance Care Planning with Cancer Patients: Evidentiary Base. Program in Evidence-Based Care; Cancer Care Ontario, Toronto. Available online at: http://WWW.CANCERCARE.ON.CA/COMMON/PAGES/USERFILE.ASPX?FILEID=269020. (accessed 15 October 2015).

Hemphill 3rd JC (2007). Do-not-resuscitate orders, unintended consequences, and the ripple effect. Crit Care 11: 121.

Hemphill 3rd JC, Bonovich DC, Besmertis L et al. (2001). The ICH score: a simple, reliable grading scale for intracerebral hemorrhage. Stroke 32: 891–897.

Hemphill 3rd JC, Newman J, Zhao S et al. (2004). Hospital usage of early do-not-resuscitate orders and outcome after intracerebral hemorrhage. Stroke 35: 1130–1134.

Hemphill 3rd JC, Farrant M, Neill Jr TA (2009). Prospective validation of the ICH Score for 12-month functional outcome. Neurology 73: 1088–1094.

Heyland DK, Dodek P, Rocker G et al. (2006a). What matters most in end-of-life care: perceptions of seriously ill patients and their family members. CMAJ 174: 627–633.

Heyland DK, Frank C, Groll D et al. (2006b). Understanding cardiopulmonary resuscitation decision making: perspectives of seriously ill hospitalized patients and family members. Chest 130: 419–428.

Heyland DK, Allan DE, Rocker G et al. (2009). Discussing prognosis with patients and their families near the end of life: impact on satisfaction with end-of-life care. Open Med 3: e101–e110.

Heyland DK, Cook DJ, Rocker GM et al. (2010). Defining priorities for improving end-of-life care in Canada. CMAJ 182: E747–E752.

Heyland DK, Barwich D, Pichora D et al. (2013). Failure to engage hospitalized elderly patients and their families in advance care planning. JAMA Intern Med 173: 778–787.

Hinkle LJ, Bosslet GT, Torke AM (2015). Factors associated with family satisfaction with end-of-life care in the ICU: a systematic review. Chest 147: 82–93.

Holloway RG, Benesch CG, Burgin WS et al. (2005). Prognosis and decision making in severe stroke. JAMA 294: 725–733.

Holloway RG, Ladwig S, Robb J et al. (2010). Palliative care consultations in hospitalized stroke patients. J Palliat Med 13: 407–412.

Huttner HB, Kohrmann M, Berger C et al. (2006). Predictive factors for tracheostomy in neurocritical care patients with spontaneous supratentorial hemorrhage. Cerebrovasc Dis 21: 159–165.

Jaren O, Selwa L (2006). Causes of mortality on a university hospital neurology service. Neurologist 12: 245–248.

Jauch EC, Saver JL, Adams Jr HP et al. (2013). Guidelines for the early management of patients with acute ischemic stroke: a guideline for healthcare professionals from the American Heart Association/American Stroke Association. Stroke 44: 870–947.

Johnston KC, Wagner DP, Wang XQ et al. (2007). Validation of an acute ischemic stroke model: does diffusion-weighted imaging lesion volume offer a clinically significant improvement in prediction of outcome? Stroke 38: 1820–1825.

Kelly AG, Hoskins KD, Holloway RG (2012). Early stroke mortality, patient preferences, and the withdrawal of care bias. Neurology 79: 941–944.

Kowalski RG, Chang TR, Carhuapoma JR et al. (2013). Withdrawal of technological life support following subarachnoid hemorrhage. Neurocrit Care 19: 269–275.

Kruyt ND, Biessels GJ, De Haan RJ et al. (2009). Hyperglycemia and clinical outcome in aneurysmal subarachnoid hemorrhage: a meta-analysis. Stroke 40: e424–e430.

Last BF, Van Veldhuizen AM (1996). Information about diagnosis and prognosis related to anxiety and depression in children with cancer aged 8–16 years. Eur J Cancer 32A: 290–294.

Lautrette A, Darmon M, Megarbane B et al. (2007). A communication strategy and brochure for relatives of patients dying in the ICU. N Engl J Med 356: 469–478.

Leclaire MM, Oakes JM, Weinert CR (2005). Communication of prognostic information for critically ill patients. Chest 128: 1728–1735.

Lemeshow S, Klar J, Teres D (1995). Outcome prediction for individual intensive care patients: useful, misused, or abused? Intensive Care Med 21: 770–776.

Levinson W, Lesser CS, Epstein RM (2010). Developing physician communication skills for patient-centered care. Health Aff (Millwood) 29: 1310–1318.

Levy DE, Caronna JJ, Singer BH et al. (1985). Predicting outcome from hypoxic-ischemic coma. JAMA 253: 1420–1426.

Lind SE, Delvecchio Good MJ, Seidel S et al. (1989). Telling the diagnosis of cancer. J Clin Oncol 7: 583–589.

Lynn J (1997). An 88-year-old woman facing the end of life. JAMA 277: 1633–1640.

Lynn J, Adamson DM (2003). Living well at the end of life. Adapting health care to serious chronic illness in old age. Available online at http://pacificinstitute.org/pdf/Living_Well_at_the_End_of_Life.pdf. (Accessed 6 November 2016).

Mackenzie EJ, Rivara FP, Jurkovich GJ et al. (2006). A national evaluation of the effect of trauma-center care on mortality. N Engl J Med 354: 366–378.

Mackillop WJ, Stewart WE, Ginsburg AD et al. (1988). Cancer patients' perceptions of their disease and its treatment. Br J Cancer 58: 355–358.

Malacrida R, Bettelini CM, Degrate A et al. (1998). Reasons for dissatisfaction: a survey of relatives of intensive care patients who died. Crit Care Med 26: 1187–1193.

Mayer SA, Kossoff SB (1999). Withdrawal of life support in the neurological intensive care unit. Neurology 52: 1602–1609.

Meadow W, Pohlman A, Frain L et al. (2011). Power and limitations of daily prognostications of death in the medical intensive care unit. Crit Care Med 39: 474–479.

Miyaji NT (1993). The power of compassion: truth-telling among American doctors in the care of dying patients. Soc Sci Med 36: 249–264.

Moons KG, Royston P, Vergouwe Y et al. (2009). Prognosis and prognostic research: what, why, and how? BMJ 338: b375.

Morgenstern LB, Hemphill 3rd JC, Anderson C et al. (2010). Guidelines for the management of spontaneous intracerebral hemorrhage: a guideline for healthcare professionals from the American Heart Association/American Stroke Association. Stroke 41: 2108–2129.

Murray SA, Kendall M, Boyd K et al. (2005). Illness trajectories and palliative care. BMJ 330: 1007–1011.

Naidech AM, Bernstein RA, Bassin SL et al. (2009). How patients die after intracerebral hemorrhage. Neurocrit Care 11: 45–49.

National Palliative Care Registry (2014). Annual Survey Summary. Palliative Care Growth in U.S. Hospitals. https://registry.capc.org/cms/portals/1/Reports/%20Registry_Summary%20Report_2014.pdf. Accessed April 22, 2015.

Navi BB, Kamel H, McCulloch CE et al. (2012). Accuracy of neurovascular fellows' prognostication of outcome after subarachnoid hemorrhage. Stroke 43: 702–707.

NINDS (1995). Tissue plasminogen activator for acute ischemic stroke. The National Institute of Neurological Disorders and Stroke rt-PA Stroke Study Group. N Engl J Med 333: 1581–1587.

Ogilvy CS, Cheung AC, Mitha AP et al. (2006). Outcomes for surgical and endovascular management of intracranial aneurysms using a comprehensive grading system. Neurosurgery 59: 1037–1042. discussion 1043.

Organ Procurement and Transplantation Network (2003). Data reports. Available online at http://optn.transplant.hrsa.gov/latestData/viewDataReports.asp. (accessed 15 October 2015).

Pochard F, Darmon M, Fassier T et al. (2005). Symptoms of anxiety and depression in family members of intensive care unit patients before discharge or death. A prospective multicenter study. J Crit Care 20: 90–96.

Prendergast TJ, Luce JM (1997). Increasing incidence of withholding and withdrawal of life support from the critically ill. Am J Respir Crit Care Med 155: 15–20.

Prendergast TJ, Puntillo KA (2002). Withdrawal of life support: intensive caring at the end of life. JAMA 288: 2732–2740.

Ptacek JT, Eberhardt TL (1996). Breaking bad news. A review of the literature. JAMA 276: 496–502.

Quill TE, Arnold R, Back AL (2009). Discussing treatment preferences with patients who want "everything". Ann Intern Med 151: 345–349.

Quill TEBK, Holloway RG, Shah MS et al. (2014). Goal setting, prognosticating, surrogate decision making: Primer of Palliative Care. 6th edn. American Academy of Hospice and Palliative Medicine, Chicago, IL.

Quirt CF, Mackillop WJ, Ginsburg AD et al. (1997). Do doctors know when their patients don't? A survey of doctor-patient communication in lung cancer. Lung Cancer 18: 1–20.

Qureshi AI (2011). Intracerebral hemorrhage specific intensity of care quality metrics. Neurocrit Care 14: 291–317.

Qureshi AI, Adil MM, Suri MF (2013). Rate of utilization and determinants of withdrawal of care in acute ischemic stroke treated with thrombolytics in USA. Med Care 51: 1094–1100.

Qureshi AI, Adil MM, Suri MF (2014). Rate of use and determinants of withdrawal of care among patients with subarachnoid hemorrhage in the United States. World Neurosurg 82: e579–e584.

Rabinstein AA, Wijdicks EF (2004). Outcome of survivors of acute stroke who require prolonged ventilatory assistance and tracheostomy. Cerebrovasc Dis 18: 325–331.

Racine E, Dion MJ, Wijman CA et al. (2009). Profiles of neurological outcome prediction among intensivists. Neurocrit Care 11: 345–352.

Reeves MJ, Myers LJ, Williams LS et al. (2012). Do-not-resuscitate orders, quality of care, and outcomes in veterans with acute ischemic stroke. Neurology 79: 1990–1996.

Reynolds S, Cooper AB, Mckneally M (2005). Withdrawing life-sustaining treatment: ethical considerations. Thorac Surg Clin 15: 469–480.

Roberts CS, Cox CE, Reintgen DS et al. (1994). Influence of physician communication on newly diagnosed breast patients' psychologic adjustment and decision-making. Cancer 74: 336–341.

Roch A, Michelet P, Jullien AC et al. (2003). Long-term outcome in intensive care unit survivors after mechanical ventilation for intracerebral hemorrhage. Crit Care Med 31: 2651–2656.

Rosen DS, MacDonald RL (2005). Subarachnoid hemorrhage grading scales: a systematic review. Neurocrit Care 2: 110–118.

Ruiz-Sandoval JL, Chiquete E, Romero-Vargas S et al. (2007). Grading scale for prediction of outcome in primary intracerebral hemorrhages. Stroke 38: 1641–1644.

Salim A, Berry C, Ley EJ et al. (2011). In-house coordinator programs improve conversion rates for organ donation. J Trauma 71: 733–736.

Saposnik G, Kapral MK, Liu Y et al. (2011). IScore: a risk score to predict death early after hospitalization for an acute ischemic stroke. Circulation 123: 739–749.

Saposnik G, Cote R, Mamdani M et al. (2013). JURaSSiC: accuracy of clinician vs risk score prediction of ischemic stroke outcomes. Neurology 81: 448–455.

Sardell AN, Trierweiler SJ (1993). Disclosing the cancer diagnosis. Procedures that influence patient hopefulness. Cancer 72: 3355–3365.

Shalowitz DI, Garrett-Mayer E, Wendler D (2006). The accuracy of surrogate decision makers: a systematic review. Arch Intern Med 166: 493–497.

Sheehy E, Conrad SL, Brigham LE et al. (2003). Estimating the number of potential organ donors in the United States. N Engl J Med 349: 667–674.

Shepardson LB, Youngner SJ, Speroff T et al. (1997). Variation in the use of do-not-resuscitate orders in patients with stroke. Arch Intern Med 157: 1841–1847.

Shepardson LB, Youngner SJ, Speroff T et al. (1999). Increased risk of death in patients with do-not-resuscitate orders. Med Care 37: 727–737.

Siminoff LA, Fetting JH, Abeloff MD (1989). Doctor–patient communication about breast cancer adjuvant therapy. J Clin Oncol 7: 1192–1200.

Sinuff T, Dodek P, You JJ et al. (2015). Improving end-of-life communication and decision making: the development of a conceptual framework and quality indicators. J Pain Symptom Manage 49: 1070–1080.

Slavin LA, O'Malley JE, Koocher GP et al. (1982). Communication of the cancer diagnosis to pediatric patients: impact on long-term adjustment. Am J Psychiatry 139: 179–183.

Smith EE, Shobha N, Dai D et al. (2010). Risk score for in-hospital ischemic stroke mortality derived and validated within the Get With the Guidelines-Stroke Program. Circulation 122: 1496–1504.

Stern RH (2012). Individual risk. J Clin Hypertens (Greenwich) 14: 261–264.

Stevens RD, Sutter R (2013). Prognosis in severe brain injury. Crit Care Med 41: 1104–1123.

Steyerberg EW, Mushkudiani N, Perel P et al. (2008). Predicting outcome after traumatic brain injury: development and international validation of prognostic scores based on admission characteristics. PLoS Med 5: e165. discussion e165.

Stocchetti N, Pagan F, Calappi E et al. (2004). Inaccurate early assessment of neurological severity in head injury. J Neurotrauma 21: 1131–1140.

Taylor KM (1988). "Telling bad news": physicians and the disclosure of undesirable information. Sociol Health Illn 10: 109–132.

Teale EA, Forster A, Munyombwe T et al. (2012). A systematic review of case-mix adjustment models for stroke. Clin Rehabil 26: 771–786.

Truog RD, Campbell ML, Curtis JR et al. (2008). Recommendations for end-of-life care in the intensive care unit: a consensus statement by the American College [corrected] of Critical Care Medicine. Crit Care Med 36: 953–963.

Turgeon AF, Lauzier F, Burns KE et al. (2013). Determination of neurologic prognosis and clinical decision making in adult patients with severe traumatic brain injury: a survey of Canadian intensivists, neurosurgeons, and neurologists. Crit Care Med 41: 1086–1093.

Van Norden AG, Van Dijk GW, Van Huizen MD et al. (2006). Interobserver agreement and predictive value for outcome of two rating scales for the amount of extravasated blood after aneurysmal subarachnoid haemorrhage. J Neurol 253: 1217–1220.

Verkade MA, Epker JL, Nieuwenhoff MD et al. (2012). Withdrawal of life-sustaining treatment in a mixed intensive care unit: most common in patients with catastropic brain injury. Neurocrit Care 16: 130–135.

Von Pohle WR (1996). Obtaining organ donation: who should ask? Heart Lung 25: 304–309.

Weeks JC, Cook EF, O'Day SJ et al. (1998). Relationship between cancer patients' predictions of prognosis and their treatment preferences. JAMA 279: 1709–1714.

Wijdicks EF, Hijdra A, Young GB et al. (2006). Practice parameter: prediction of outcome in comatose survivors after cardiopulmonary resuscitation (an evidence-based review): report of the Quality Standards Subcommittee of the American Academy of Neurology. Neurology 67: 203–210.

Wijdicks EF, Varelas PN, Gronseth GS et al. (2010). Evidence-based guideline update: determining brain death in adults: report of the Quality Standards Subcommittee of the American Academy of Neurology. Neurology 74: 1911–1918.

Wunsch H, Harrison DA, Harvey S et al. (2005). End-of-life decisions: a cohort study of the withdrawal of all active treatment in intensive care units in the United Kingdom. Intensive Care Med 31: 823–831.

Xian Y, Holloway RG, Noyes K et al. (2011). Racial differences in mortality among patients with acute ischemic stroke: an observational study. Ann Intern Med 154: 152–159.

You JJ, Dodek P, Lamontagne F et al. (2014). What really matters in end-of-life discussions? Perspectives of patients in hospital with serious illness and their families. CMAJ 186: E679–E687.

Zahuranec DB, Brown DL, Lisabeth LD et al. (2007). Early care limitations independently predict mortality after intracerebral hemorrhage. Neurology 68: 1651–1657.

Zahuranec DB, Morgenstern LB, Sanchez BN et al. (2010). Do-not-resuscitate orders and predictive models after intracerebral hemorrhage. Neurology 75: 626–633.

Zier LS, Sottile PD, Hong SY et al. (2012). Surrogate decision makers' interpretation of prognostic information: a mixed-methods study. Ann Intern Med 156: 360–366.

Zurasky JA, Aiyagari V, Zazulia AR et al. (2005). Early mortality following spontaneous intracerebral hemorrhage. Neurology 64: 725–727.

*Handbook of Clinical Neurology*, Vol. 140 (3rd series)
*Critical Care Neurology, Part I*
E.F.M. Wijdicks and A.H. Kramer, Editors
http://dx.doi.org/10.1016/B978-0-444-63600-3.00023-4

Chapter 23

# Organ donation protocols

C.B. MACIEL[1], D.Y. HWANG[1], AND D.M. GREER[2]*

[1]*Division of Neurocritical Care and Emergency Neurology, Department of Neurology, Yale School of Medicine, New Haven, CT, USA*

[2]*Department of Neurology, Yale School of Medicine, New Haven, CT, USA*

## Abstract

Organ transplantation improves survival and quality of life in patients with end-organ failure. Waiting lists continue to grow across the world despite remarkable advances in the transplantation process, from the creation of public engagement campaigns to the development of critical pathways for the timely identification, referral, approach, and treatment of the potential organ donor. The pathophysiology of dying triggers systemic changes that are intimately related to organ viability. The intensive care management of the potential organ donor optimizes organ function and improves the donation yield, representing a significant step in reducing the mismatch between organ supply and demand. Different beliefs and cultures reflect diverse legislations and donation practices amongst different countries, creating a challenge to standardized practices. Maintaining public trust is necessary for continued progress in organ donation and transplantation, hence the urge for a joint effort in creating uniform protocols that ensure transparent practices within the medical community.

## BACKGROUND

Organ donation (OD) is an altruistic act with a significant impact on society by reducing healthcare costs associated with supporting patients with end-organ failure and by improving the survival and quality of life of recipients (Wolfe et al., 1999; Pinson et al., 2000). Accumulating evidence supports additional benefits of OD to grieving families, such as averting delayed regret for missing the opportunity to donate organs (Oliver et al., 2001) and helping them deal with their grief (Cleiren and Van Zoelen, 2002; Bellali and Papadatou, 2006; Merchant et al., 2008; Tavakoli et al., 2008).

### Defining deceased organ donors

Deceased donors are the main source of solid organs for transplantation (European Directorate for the Quality of Medicines and Healthcare, 2014). At the very beginning of the transplantation era, all organs from deceased donors were retrieved from patients soon after cardiorespiratory arrest; this practice continued until the concept of brain death (BD) was accepted by the medical community (Ethics Committee, 2001). The "dead donor rule" (DDR), established by the Uniform Anatomical Gift Act, mandates that the removal of organs must not lead to the donor's death; therefore, it is imperative that death determination precede organ retrieval (Robertson, 1999). Advances in medicine have allowed for extraordinary organ support measures, making necessary the derivation of a legal standard for the definition of biologic death. In the USA, this was achieved by the Uniform Determination of Death Act (UDDA), which establishes the permanent biologic end of life as either the irreversible cessation of spontaneous respiratory and circulatory functions ("circulatory determination of death") or irreversible cessation of all detectable brain function ("neurologic determination of death"); either one is assessed by utilizing accepted medical standards (Uniform Law Commission, 1980; Medical Consultants, 1981). Despite these definitions, declaring death can be challenging without precise guidelines and

*Correspondence to: David M. Greer, MD, Department of Neurology, Yale School of Medicine, P.O. Box 208018, New Haven CT 06520, USA. Tel: +1-203-785-5947, Fax: +1-203-785-2238, E-mail: david.greer@yale.edu

a stepwise approach, which leaves room for questioning the legitimacy of death determination, especially in the context of donation (Shemie et al., 2014). In fact, despite uniform state laws, the states of New Jersey and New York have exceptions in place to accommodate personal objections to death declaration by neurologic criteria on religious grounds (Iltis and Cherry, 2010). Importantly, although no major organized religion strictly prohibits donation or receipt of organs, it is frequent for families to seek guidance from their community regarding the morality of the donation process according to their own faith (Oliver et al., 2011). The majority of religious arguments against OD are based on fully and accurately ascertaining the death of the donor. A consultation with a respected religious scholar may be advisable when discussing specific conflicting points with families during the processes of death determination and OD.

In order to address concerns regarding the generalizability of death definitions, an invitational forum organized by Canadian Blood Services in conjunction with the World Health Organization has developed an international guideline for the determination of death (Shemie et al., 2014). The following effective definition was agreed upon:

> *Death is the permanent loss of capacity for consciousness and all brainstem functions. This may result from permanent cessation of circulation or catastrophic brain injury.*

This definition implies that the permanence of the circulatory arrest will meet the irreversibility criteria, a requirement by the UDDA, as the reversibility potential is nonexistent once interventions to counteract the loss of circulatory function are purposefully withheld (Bernat et al., 2010).

## Demand and supply mismatch

According to the United Network for Organ Sharing (UNOS), 6 people are added to the waiting list every hour and 22 die every day while waiting for an organ in the USA (OPTN/UNOS, 2015). The mismatch between supply and demand of transplantable solid organs is expected to worsen as the prevalence of chronic diseases with end-stage organ dysfunction continues to increase (Levitt, 2015). There are several barriers to diminishing this mismatch: cultural reservations regarding deceased OD; legal barriers to implementation of policies aimed at expanding the donor pool; lack of efficient protocols for identification, referral, and management of potential donors; suboptimal quality of retrieved organs; and high discard rates.

In the USA, the Department of Health and Human Services partnered with national transplant leaders and practitioners to launch the Organ Donation and Transplantation Breakthrough Collaborative to increase the organ supply and number of transplants. Between 1999 and 2007, there was an increase in number of deceased donors, particularly from 2003 to 2006, reaching a 24% increment in organ availability (Sung et al., 2008). Nevertheless, recent reports show that organ availability has declined since 2008, reflecting an alarming decrease in the total numbers of living and deceased donations (Klein et al., 2010; NHS Blood and Transplant, 2014; Israni et al., 2015). Proposed explanations for this decline include loss of momentum obtained when the Organ Donation and Transplantation Breakthrough Collaborative was launched, concerns regarding economic and practical implications of utilizing high-risk donors, and failure to obtain public engagement in the OD process (Klein et al., 2010). Attempts to solve this worldwide public health challenge have included public education, expanded eligibility criteria for utilization of organs, monetary incentives to living donors to make donation a cost-neutral process, presence of in-house transplant coordinators, changes in donation policies and enrollment methods, as well as development of goal-directed OD protocols.

Some of these measures have raised important ethical issues, inciting avid debates in this field. Scant high-quality data are available assessing the impact of such policies in organ transplantation, probably due to the difficulty in designing such studies. Recently, a study was able to provide a large-scale overview of the effect of the following state policies implemented from 1988 to 2010 in the USA: public education programs and dedicated revenue pools for living and deceased donor recruitment efforts; first-person consent laws and donor registries; and paid leaves of absence and tax benefits for living donors. Surprisingly, among all studied policies, only the establishment of revenue pools had an effect (however modest) on the number of transplants during the analyzed period (Chatterjee et al., 2015). As such measures are quite heterogeneous and could have led to a positive effect in one organ type or in one state versus another, this finding does not imply that all state policies studied were futile (Matas and Hays, 2015).

Importantly, simply increasing the supply of organs might not be the only answer in solving the organ shortage problem; combined approaches also targeting prevention of end-stage organ diseases and reducing, or at least stabilizing, the demand should be also considered (Levitt, 2015). The establishment of local organ donor councils with interdisciplinary collaborative work among clinical, administrative, and community representatives to develop and implement quality improvement and staff education measures is also a promising way to improve donation outcomes (Kong et al., 2010).

# Neurointensive care unit and organ donation

Patients with neurologic catastrophes are commonly admitted to an intensive care unit (ICU); such catastrophes may render relatively young and otherwise healthy individuals dependent on mechanical ventilation and other organ support. Families have the delicate mission of speaking on their loved one's behalf, and may opt for removal of aggressive measures when chances of acceptable functional recovery are dismal. Other neurologic tragedies may progress further, leading to BD. Consequently, the ICU staff is commonly involved in the care of potential organ donors and has a key role in preserving the option of OD. This preservation can be achieved by promptly notifying the organ procurement organization (OPO) following the identification of a potential donor, implementing donor goal-directed therapies, and fostering an environment in which the dignity of the deceased person is maintained, while promoting an atmosphere of peace and tranquility for grieving families. Accumulating evidence suggests that providing intensive care and organ support to the potential organ donor may positively impact the yield of retrieved organs by systematically meeting donor management goals (Angel et al., 2006; Salim, 2006b; Singbartl, 2011; Malinoski et al., 2012; Callahan et al., 2014; Patel et al., 2014; Abuanzeh, 2015). Importantly, families' dissatisfaction with care provided during a hospitalization that involved OD has been associated with further complicated adaptation to the loss of a loved one (Cleiren and Van Zoelen, 2002; Merchant et al., 2008), which may complicate donation efforts.

## DONATION AFTER CIRCULATORY DETERMINATION OF DEATH

Before the concept of death by neurologic criteria was introduced, donation after circulatory death (DCD) was the conventional method used for organ procurement; however, only a few DCD programs existed at that time, and criteria for declaration of death were inconsistent. During subsequent years, this practice declined as donation after brain death (DBD) was prioritized by several programs, mainly due to higher yield rates of organ procurement, and possibly better outcomes when compared with DCD (Foley et al., 2005; Reich et al., 2009). The recent need to expand the donor pool fueled the development of new DCD programs, and the University of Pittsburgh was a pioneer in the USA (DeVita and Snyder, 1993). DCD has become an increasingly important source of solid organs, as the cultural challenges surrounding the acceptance of the BD concept limit the number of DBD donors in some regions (Bendorf et al., 2013).

## Categories of donors

The Maastricht classification separated DCD or "nonheart-beating" organ donors into four different categories, each having its own peculiarities regarding pathophysiology of organ damage after death determination, organ preservation and viability, and ethical aspects (Kootstra, 1995; Ridley, 2005). Further development of DCD programs led to modifications in this classification, which now includes five different types of donors (Table 23.1). Uncontrolled DCD (uDCD) involves patients in whom cardiopulmonary resuscitation (CPR) could not be attempted or was unsuccessful (categories I and II), entails a substantial workload to promote organ preservation (Institute of Medicine, 2000), and is associated with lower yield rates (Fieux et al., 2009; Ortega-Deballon et al., 2015; Wall et al., 2016). There are several barriers limiting OD with category I and II donors: estimating the true ischemic time with available information is challenging, and contacting families in a timely fashion is difficult. uDCD is only performed in a limited number of countries. Category III is traditionally considered "controlled" donation, as it includes patients who are awaiting death by circulatory criteria, and remains the preferred category of DCD donors (cDCD) in most regions. Patients who suffer a cardiac arrest during BD evaluation, or following declaration of BD before organ procurement, represent category IV, which some authors also classify as cDCD (Intensive Care Society, 2004). In order to preserve organ viability in category IV donors, some authors recommend that equipment for initiation of cooling be maintained at the bedside of every potential donor undergoing BD evaluation (Kootstra et al., 2002). The Eurotransplant Organization has now recognized donation after medically assisted circulatory arrest, or euthanasia, in the Netherlands, Belgium, and Luxembourg, representing category V of donors, which is also considered cDCD (Evrard, 2014).

## Death determination

As stated by the UDDA, death by circulatory criteria must be irreversible, and a potential restoration of spontaneous circulation, either spontaneously or as a result of an intervention, precludes death pronouncement. Outside of an ICU or emergency department, clinicians do not have access to a cardiac monitor to assess electric function when pronouncing the death of a patient; the absence of a pulse, a heart beat and respiratory incursions suffices under these circumstances. However, in the DCD context (in which the cardiac rhythm is usually known), some institutions require that the cessation of cardiac contractility and circulation be accompanied by absence of cardiac electric activity during death

*Table 23.1*

**Modified Maastricht classification of nonheart-beating donors**

| Category | Description | Particularities |
|---|---|---|
| I | Dead on arrival at hospital<br>Resuscitation attempts not possible | Not widely used. Organs need to be tested first for viability prior to initiation of preservation methods. Time from circulatory arrest and organ preservation must be <45 minutes |
| II | Unsuccessful resuscitation<br>(a) Out-of-hospital refractory cardiac arrest: CPR initiated by EMS and taken over by hospital staff on arrival<br>(b) In-hospital refractory cardiac arrest: CPR initiated by hospital personnel | Not widely used. Preparatory handlings* may be used as bridge until consent for donation is obtained in some regions, depending on local legislation |
| III | Awaiting death by cardiorespiratory arrest<br>Hospitalized patients with terminal condition or who are critically ill planned for withdrawal of life support | Most commonly used. Cardiac arrest is anticipated while life support measures are withdrawn; most commonly, this occurs in the OR. The time elapsed between removal of support and mechanical asystole is one of the main determinants of organ suitability for retrieval and transplantation |
| IV | Death by cardiorespiratory arrest during or after brain death diagnostic procedure<br>Unexpected cardiac arrest occurring either during the process of brain death evaluation or immediately after its determination but before organ retrieval | Unusual circumstance. Resuscitation efforts may be permitted according to family's wishes. Preparatory handlings may be started during resuscitation attempts until body is moved to OR. If circulatory function is restored and brain death confirmed, donation protocols following DBD are pursued, or the protocol is switched to DCD if resuscitation attempts are unsuccessful |
| V | Medically assisted cardiorespiratory arrest in a terminally ill patient | Not recognized in the majority of countries since it involves euthanasia |

Adapted from Kootstra (1995); Detry et al. (2012); Organización Nacional de Trasplantes (2012); and Evrard (2014).
*Preparatory handlings are interventions aimed at promoting organ preservation and include, but are not limited to, cardiac massage, artificial ventilation, and hypothermia.
CPR, cardiopulmonary resuscitation; EMS, emergency medicine services; OR, operating room; DBD, donation after brain death; DCD, donation after circulatory death.

determination. The invitational forum that is currently attempting to derive international guidelines for death determination agreed on minimal acceptable standards for the cessation of circulation and breathing (pulseless apnea): absent palpable pulse, breath sounds, heart sounds, and respiratory effort, as well as loss of pulsatile arterial blood pressure, together with coma and fixed pupils (Shemie et al., 2014). Electric asystole was not a mandatory requirement, but may be still considered necessary in some institutions (Fugate et al., 2011).

In order to fulfill these requirements during cDCD, pulseless apnea is observed for a few minutes, while resuscitation measures are withheld. An observation period is necessary, as on some occasions forward circulation is reachieved spontaneously, a phenomenon called autoresuscitation. In a recent pilot study, transient restoration of blood pressure was observed in 4 out of 30 patients (Dhanani and Shemie, 2014). Initially, the proposed observation time was as long as 10 minutes (Kootstra et al., 2002). The minimal duration of observation can vary according to local institutional protocols, and is widely accepted to range between 2 and 5 minutes, although there is not universal agreement regarding whether this should refer to lack of blood pressure or electric asystole (Institute of Medicine, 1997).

Autoresuscitation has never been observed beyond 5 minutes without blood pressure in the setting of OD. In fact, autoresuscitation in the absence of preceding unsuccessful CPR has never been reported (Hornby et al., 2010; Sheth et al., 2012). Up to 2008, all 32 reported cases of autoresuscitation following failed CPR reported times ranging from seconds to 33 minutes in cases with inconsistent hemodynamic monitoring, but none beyond 7 minutes with continuous monitoring

(Hornby et al., 2010). The practice variability in pulse-less apneic observation times is a reflection of a lack of high-quality data to steer uniform guidelines. All documented cases of autoresuscitation are from case reports, letter to editors, or small case series, with documentation in varying scenarios with highly inconsistent hemodynamic monitoring methods (Hornby et al., 2010). This phenomenon was not reported in a retrospective study of 73 patients being considered for cDCD while being monitored with continuous arterial catheters (Sheth et al., 2012). However, in a prospective study, restoration of blood pressure after absence for as long as 170 seconds (possibly with one intervening second of blood pressure after 80 seconds) was observed (Dhanani et al., 2014).

Given the increased risk of autoresuscitation in uDCD due to prior CPR, an observational period of at least 10 minutes may be prudent. Usually, an experienced clinician performs the clinical evaluation for cessation of circulatory and respiratory functions, but there is significant practice variation, and in some places, up to three clinicians are required to independently assess the donor's death (Joris, 2011).

## Identification of potential cDCD candidates

The candidacy of potential donors for organ procurement also depends on the total amount of time from withdrawal of life-sustaining therapies (WLST) to death, since a prolonged withdrawal phase may compromise organ function. To allow for a successful DCD, this time should ideally be less than 60 minutes and no more than 120 minutes (Bernat et al., 2006). However, these thresholds are based on little supportive data, and some centers are using longer time intervals. The time from onset of severe hypotension to declaration of death is likely a more important variable. Patients with devastating neurologic injuries whose goals of care are transitioned to comfort measures are often potential cDCD donors; however, many survive the initial hour following WLST (Yee et al., 2010). Reliable prediction of time from WLST to death is a challenging task, but crucial for logistical planning in cDCD. Multiple prediction models have been proposed (Lewis et al., 2003; DeVita et al., 2008; Yee et al., 2010; de Groot et al., 2012; Rabinstein et al., 2012; He et al., 2015b):

- The University of Wisconsin DCD Evaluation Tool is a scoring system that stratifies patients into high-, moderate-, and low-risk groups for maintaining spontaneous breathing once ventilatory support is removed. In its original description, it was able to accurately predict suitability for OD in more than 80% of cases (Lewis et al., 2003). This score includes vasopressor requirements and body mass index, in addition to relying on respiratory performance during a 10-minute interval from the discontinuation of ventilatory support. Some centers do not use this tool because of the need to temporarily discontinue ventilatory support. Furthermore, other OD programs have not found its performance to necessarily be as favorable.

- The UNOS set of criteria includes the requirement of mechanical and hemodynamic support, in addition to respiratory parameters. The cumulative presence of more than one criterion increases the odds ratio of death within 60 minutes of WLST; in one multicenter study, this tool was associated with a positive predictive value of 63% (DeVita et al., 2008).

- The DCD-N score was the first to be validated specifically in neurocritical care patients, who constitute the vast majority of DCD donors, and includes markers of severe neurologic dysfunction. This score has also been independently validated, and performs well in predicting death within 60 minutes (area under receiver operating characteristic curve of 0.81 in one study) (Rabinstein et al., 2012). This score attributes points to elements constituting poor neurologic exams – absence of corneal (1 point) and cough reflexes (2 points), no motor response or presence of extensor posturing (1 point), and a high oxygenation index (1 point if >3). Notably, DCD-N was not able to identify all patients who could be successful DCD donors (who died within 60 minutes).

- A nomogram for time of death prediction following WLST in neurologically devastated patients was recently developed as an alternative tool. It provides in a simple graphic representation the numeric probability of a clinical event based on a statistical predictive model. A comprehensive list of radiologic and clinical neurologic variables, with their respective weighted scores, is used to assign points, and the total sum is plotted in the nomogram, where probabilities for 30-, 60-, 120-, and 240-minute mortalities are given (He et al., 2015b). Further validation of this nomogram in a large, multicenter cohort is under way (He et al., 2015a).

Death determination in refractory out-of-hospital cardiac arrest uDCD may be established in the field, as allowed in New York City protocols (Wall et al., 2016), or upon hospital arrival in countries such as Spain, France, and Scotland (Sanchez-Fructuoso et al., 2006; Fondevila et al., 2007, 2012; Suarez et al., 2008; Fieux et al.,

2009; Mateos-Rodríguez, 2010; Gomez-de-Antonio, 2011; Rodriguez et al., 2011; Hanf et al., 2012). There is significant variation amongst protocols in the clinical findings representative of death (e.g., whether electric asystole or documentation of neurologic examination is required or not), in addition to lack of uniformity regarding the duration of cardiac arrest necessary for being considered refractory (Dhanani et al., 2014; Ortega-Deballon et al., 2015).

## Pathophysiology

Warm ischemia time (WIT) for a particular organ is the interval during which that organ is vulnerable to an ischemic insult; this interval includes the time frame during which there is still circulation, but not enough to adequately deliver oxygen to organs and tissues (Institute of Medicine, 2000). The total WIT is considered the interval from removal of artificial ventilation to initiation of cold organ perfusion (Reich et al., 2009). The true WIT, or functional ischemia time, is the total amount of time from hypotension (with variable thresholds ranging from mean arterial pressure ≤60 mmHg to systolic blood pressure 35–50 mmHg) and/or severe hypoxemia (oxygen saturation thresholds ranging from 25 to 70%) to initiation of organ perfusion (Reich et al., 2009; Detry et al., 2012; NHS Blood and Transplant, 2013). The rates of graft complications are directly proportionate to true WIT, and remain a fundamental problem with DCD; thus, organ protection strategies during WLST and organ retrieval are largely targeted to reduce WIT as much as possible. Tolerance of WIT is organ-specific, and particular attention to the duration of WIT is important when assessing organ suitability for donation (Abt et al., 2003; Foley et al., 2005; Bernat et al., 2006; Lee et al., 2006; Locke et al., 2007). Cold ischemia time (CIT) is the interval from organ perfusion until transplantation with restoration of circulation, regardless of *in situ* preservation (Institute of Medicine, 2000).

Uncontrolled DCD is unique for its variable periods of no flow and low flow, which makes the estimation of WIT difficult. The potential donor starts off with refractory cardiac arrest (no flow); CPR is resumed for organ preservation (low flow); a "no touch" period is observed for death determination (no flow); and finally, cannulation is started with selected perfusion (low flow) (Ortega-Deballon et al., 2015).

The complex mechanisms involved in the pathophysiology of dying play an important role in overall organ status. There are several types of organ-specific dysfunction post transplantation, invariably related to ischemic times and reperfusion injury. Definitions vary across studies, making comparison of incidence rates and risk factors challenging.

### KIDNEYS

Delayed graft function (DGF) is usually defined as need for dialysis during the first week post transplant (Yarlagadda et al., 2008) and may lead to increased allograft immunogenicity and a higher risk of acute rejection episodes, as well as decreased long-term recipient survival (Perico, 2004). DGF results from immunologic and nonimmunologic factors related to ischemia-reperfusion injury, as well as donor and recipient factors (Irish et al., 2003; Ponticelli, 2014). Rates of DGF in recipients of grafts from cDCD donors are consistently higher than with DBD. However, rates of DGF may fall to rates approaching those of DBD donors when CIT is limited to less than 12 hours (Locke et al., 2007).

### HEART

Primary allograft dysfunction in heart recipients is evidenced by hypotension, low cardiac output, and high filling pressures, even in the absence of secondary causes of graft failure (Russo et al., 2010). The circulatory arrest followed by reperfusion in DCD heart donors is associated with a dramatic rise in circulating catecholamines (epinephrine and norepinephrine), which are associated with the inflammatory response potentially implicated in rejection mechanisms (Ali et al., 2009). Additionally, the catecholamine surge has been implicated in the pathophysiology of right ventricular impairment (Ali et al., 2009), in a similar fashion to what is observed in DBD (Stoica et al., 2006). Prolonged ischemia is the major determinant of graft dysfunction and death in heart transplants (Banner et al., 2008; Russo et al., 2010).

### LUNGS

Primary graft dysfunction (PGD) in lung recipients happens in the initial 72 hours post transplant, and is characterized by hypoxia and impaired ventilation, usually due to noncardiogenic pulmonary edema from capillary leak (King et al., 2000; Lee et al., 2010; Munshi et al., 2013). The formation of reactive oxygen species inherent to ischemia-reperfusion injury leads to direct injury to pulmonary endothelium and epithelium, signaling cellular influx and inflammation (Lee et al., 2010; Ferrari and Andrade, 2015; Porteous et al., 2015). The underlying endothelial damage associated with procurement and preservation, as well as recipient factors, is involved in the development of PGD (King et al., 2000; Lee et al., 2010). PGD is the main contributor to early mortality after transplantation, and can be associated with the systemic inflammatory response syndrome and multisystem organ failure (King et al., 2000; Lee et al., 2010).

## LIVER

Cold preservation also leads to impairment in the sinusoidal endothelial cells, with accumulation of leukocytes and platelets in liver grafts (Suarez et al., 2008). The bile duct epithelial cells are exquisitely sensitive to reperfusion injury compared with hepatocytes, and intrahepatic strictures, following prolonged cold ischemia, may significantly affect graft survival (Suarez et al., 2008). The incidence of biliary complications and graft failure is somewhat higher with DCD than DBD.

## PANCREAS

Graft pancreatitis is a major complication arising from ischemia-reperfusion injury, and it is associated with the development of vascular thrombosis, graft failure, and death (Humar et al., 2004; Barlow et al., 2015). The microcirculatory failure from endotheliitis and arteritis associated with the necrotic endothelial cells as a result of ischemic reperfusion injury underpins the lymphocytic infiltration that leads to posttransplant pancreatitis (Nadalin et al., 2013). Donor body mass index, older age, and increased CIT are thought to increase the risk of graft pancreatitis (Benz et al., 2001; Humar et al., 2004; Nadalin et al., 2013).

## Epidemiology

Rates of DCD are increasing over time by an average of 0.3% per year, according to a recent study analyzing data from 82 countries (Bendorf et al., 2013). DCD accounts for more than 20% of all deceased organ donors worldwide (Munshi et al., 2013), and over 60% in Japan (Bendorf et al., 2013). In the USA, approximately 10% of all organ transplantations (living and deceased) are from DCD (Blackstock and Ray, 2014).

The UK witnessed an increase of more than 800% in DCD activity from 2000–2001 to 2009–2010 (NHS Blood and Transplant, 2010); however, for the first time since 2007–2008 there was a decline in the number of DCD donors by 6%, according to the 2014–2015 report (NHS Blood and Transplant, 2014). Despite this overall decrease, there was a slight increase in DCD of double-lung, combined kidney and pancreas, and liver transplants in the UK over the same period (NHS Blood and Transplant, 2014). In fact, use of DCD livers in transplants increased 10-fold in the past decade (Klein et al., 2010). There is reluctance in using DCD donor hearts for transplantation, and reported cases have been mainly in the pediatric population (Morrissey and Monaco, 2014).

## Organ support

The critical care management of the potential DCD organ donor includes several interventions to optimize organ viability that may occur prior to, during, or after death. The administration of specific medications targeting the microcirculatory disturbances associated with ischemic-reperfusion injury to enhance organ perfusion, such as vasodilators (e.g., phentolamine), inotropes, or heparinoids, remains controversial since their purpose is solely to benefit the potential recipient, and they should be given prior to death to maximize their effectiveness (Phua et al., 2007). Further controversies afflict practices of antemortem administration of thrombolytics and femoral cannulation in preparation for cold preservation solution administration.

The use of chest compressions, either mechanical or manual, is not universally recommended despite being used in some centers following cessation of circulation for organ support. This recommendation is due to the increased risk of achieving return of spontaneous circulation (ROSC) in some patients, a concern which raises the question of irreversibility of their circulatory arrest (Mateos-Rodríguez, 2010). Whenever employed as a method of organ preservation, both extracorporeal membrane oxygenation (ECMO) and mechanical chest compressions should be preceded by a careful elucidation to donor families of the possibility of restoration of brain perfusion before irreversible cessation of all functions or return of spontaneous circulation (Bernat et al., 2010; Akoh, 2012).

Upon death determination, the trachea may be reintubated and, after at least 10 minutes of cessation of circulation, the lungs may be re-expanded with continuous positive pressure as a single recruitment maneuver. However, cyclic ventilation must not occur until the cerebral circulation has been isolated to avoid brain oxygenated reperfusion (Manara, 2012). Importantly, after procurement is concluded, several important steps during preservation may impact organ viability. Relevant factors include the method and type of preservation solution, storage temperature, flow perfusion parameters, lung inflation techniques, transportation mode, pharmacologic agents, and overall ischemic times (Ali et al., 2009; Munshi et al., 2013). Several institutional specific protocols are available, but no formal comparisons have been performed.

### COLD STORAGE VERSUS MACHINE PERFUSION

Static cold storage is the most common method of organ preservation following retrieval; however, hypothermic preservation strategies have been associated with necrosis and apoptosis of the cells (Watts et al., 2013). Recent advances in machine perfusion techniques (either normothermic or hypothermic) are promising for their additional benefit of providing a means for the administration of cytopreservatives and energy substrates, as well as removing toxic waste and improving the microcirculation, thus improving organ viability and potentially expanding the donor pool and CIT limits (Ko, 2000; Magliocca et al., 2005; Bumgardner, 2007; Collins et al., 2008; Ali et al., 2009; Munshi et al., 2013; White et al., 2013; Barlow et al., 2015; Bejaoui et al., 2015; Van Raemdonck et al., 2015). Additionally, *ex vivo* machine perfusion allows for organ-specific measurements to assess function prior to transplantation (Bumgardner, 2007; Collins et al., 2008; Bejaoui et al., 2015). Some protocols include abdominal *in situ* thrombolysis through the perfusion circuit in addition to hemodilution and leukofiltration for removal of leukocytes and platelet aggregates in uDCD in order to treat the microcirculatory failure (Reznik et al., 2013).

## Protocols and guidelines

The considerable variation among OPOs and local institutions motivated the Institute of Medicine to release a report in 1997 with recommendations for a national policy for uniformity of deceased OD practices. Subsequently, a committee recruited by the same institute steered an effort to facilitate the adoption of DCD protocols by all OPOs that were consistent with available scientific evidence and ethical guidelines, patient and family options (e.g., right to attend life support withdrawal), and public trust. As a result, in the USA since 2007, all OPOs and transplant healthcare institutions are required to have a protocol in place for DCD. Nevertheless, a national survey demonstrated lack of standardized recommendations within protocols, with a lack of clear specific methodologic approaches and definitions in key aspects of cDCD, including death determination (Fugate et al., 2011). In Europe, ethical and legal restrictions preclude several countries from this type of OD. In addition, there is significant variation in the type of registration system: opt-in systems require active enrollment as registered donors, whereas an opt-out system requires active registration to not be a donor, and is referred to as presumed consent. Such heterogeneity in policies across Europe sets the stage for further variability in DCD practices, including aspects of death determination (Wind et al., 2013).

### CONTROLLED DCD PROTOCOLS AND PRACTICE GUIDELINES

The rising demand for expanding donor pools and the consequent requirement to streamline the process of organ procurement and transplantation in cDCD have steered the American Society of Transplant Surgeons to develop practice guidelines, aligned with the report from the Institute of Medicine, to be adopted by transplant centers and to be individualized to fit local institutional policies (Reich et al., 2009). Similarly, the UK, Canada, and Australia have developed guidelines that share the same key concepts (Institute of Medicine, 2000; Ethics Committee, 2001; Intensive Care Society, 2004; Shemie et al., 2006; Australian Government Organ and Tissue Authority, 2010). These guidelines provide recommendations pertinent to each stage of the process, including the development of local protocols, the approach used with families and surrogates when obtaining informed consent, limitations of specific roles by transplant team personnel, WLST, death determination, maintenance of an adequate grieving environment, organ procurement and *ex vivo* perfusion techniques, and organ-specific particularities (Reich et al., 2009). The most relevant aspects of these recommendations to critical care professionals are summarized here.

It is advisable that local institutional protocols have prior approval of the respective OPO and transplant center, in addition to being well known and easily accessible to members of transplant team, and even open to the public (Institute of Medicine, 1997). Importantly, transplant team members should be well versed on relevant ethical principles related to cDCD and should not be involved in any decision making related to patient prognosis, WLST, or death determination, thus avoiding potential conflicts of interest. In fact, in the UK, it is recommended that two senior clinicians share the decision of WLST, as its implications are similar to that of diagnosing BD in that country (Academy of Medical Royal Colleges, 2011).

A transplant team member who initially provided care for a potential organ donor in a different role (as an intensivist or a trauma specialist), and subsequently transferred the care of the patient to another practitioner to avoid conflicts of interest, may still be part of the team involved in the organ procurement after death determination, as at that point there are no further conflicts of interest (Institute of Medicine, 1997). In addition, whenever obtaining informed consent from families, it is important to inform them, before the process is initiated, about the possibilities that the patient may not die after removal of support, or may not ultimately provide the intended organs (Institute of Medicine, 1997, 2000; Ethics Committee, 2001; Bernat et al., 2006).

In order to minimize WIT and streamline the process of organ procurement, some centers perform WLST in the operating room. Other centers prefer to perform WLST in the ICU, since it is a better-suited environment for the provision of optimal end-of-life care. In this case, the patient is moved to the operating room as rapidly as possible after death is declared. Families should be respected and given the opportunity to spend time with the patient as much as possible, particularly prior to removal of support until pulseless apnea is appreciated (Institute of Medicine, 1997). Heparin and phentolamine mesylate administration should be considered prior to WLST after specific informed consent is obtained, unless the patient has a clinical condition in which these drugs are expected to hasten death or if their administration is prohibited by local protocols (Bernat et al., 2006). However, there is little high-quality evidence to guide the actual need for these drugs, let alone the optimal dose and timing. Premortem anticoagulation is considered illegal in some countries, including some (e.g., U.K.) that have a sizable experience with cDCD.

The use of end-of-life medications aimed to provide comfort is permitted and necessary, even if the unintended consequence is the potential hastening of death (commonly referred to as the rule of double effect); however, the practitioner prescribing such interventions should not be involved in the procurement process (Bernat et al., 2006). Ideally, institutions would have protocols in place to standardize use of end-of-life medications, irrespective of whether the patient is a potential organ donor.

The procurement team members may be present in some institutions prior to WLST to prepare and drape the patient; however, they should not be present at the time of withdrawal of support and not until death has been determined. It is important to note that the death declaration is the responsibility of the treating care team and should be determined using acceptable medical standards and institutional policies. The OPO coordinator should document the hemodynamic measurements on a minute-to-minute basis, as well as times for WLST, pulseless apnea occurrence, waiting period, death declaration, incision and perfusion of each organ. This information is of paramount importance for the assessment of ischemic injury (Bernat et al., 2006). In case the patient survives for longer than the period stipulated by the OPO, the donation process is aborted and the patient is returned to the appropriate clinical setting (ward or ICU) for continuation of end-of-life care (Institute of Medicine, 1997; Intensive Care Society, 2004; Shemie et al., 2006). Figure 23.1 summarizes the key points in the clinical pathway for cDCD.

### UNCONTROLLED DCD PROTOCOLS AND PRACTICE GUIDELINES

Lack of uniformity is also the hallmark of protocols and guidelines for uDCD, according to a recent meta-analysis (Ortega-Deballon et al., 2015). This includes the location of refractory cardiac arrest (out of hospital versus in hospital); age limits for the potential donor; duration of refractory cardiac arrest for death determination (ranging from 5 to 30 minutes); duration of the hands-off interval required

prior to declaration of death (ranging from 5 to 20 minutes); timing of initiation of organ preservation measures (antemortem or not); need for consent for initiation of organ preservation; method of organ preservation; and maximum permissible times for cardiac arrest prior to CPR for organ preservation (ranging from 15 to 30 minutes), CPR to cannulation (ranging from 90 to 120 minutes), and cannulation to organ procurement (ranging from 120 to 360 minutes). Nevertheless, all studied guidelines recommend the use of ECMO for organ preservation, and some centers add *in situ* cooling with the administration of cold preservatives into the abdominal wall. Despite high discard rates for liver, reported positive outcomes for liver, lung, and kidney transplantations demonstrate that uDCD may be a feasible alternative to increase the donor pool (Blackstock and Ray, 2014; Ortega-Deballon et al., 2015). At present, not all active protocols include recommendations for all organs. Available outcome data are from observational studies. Randomized clinical trials comparing different approaches to uDCD protocols would be helpful to guide future practices in jurisdictions that permit uDCD.

Figure 23.2 summarizes the key points in the clinical pathway for uDCD.

## Ethical considerations

OD in DCD programs raises several unique ethical issues related to the determination of death, timing and type of organ support interventions, possible conflicts of interest in selected team members participating in different stages of the donation process, methods of obtaining consent, and adequacy of the environment and atmosphere for grieving families when saying goodbye to their loved one (Ethics Committee, 2001).

### ORGAN RECOVERY PRIOR TO DEATH

Strict observation of the DDR may result in most dying patients missing the opportunity to donate their organs (Cochrane, 2009). Specific directives regarding observation of the DDR in living wills have been proposed, thereby granting permission to procure vital organs before death declaration according to the argument that the DDR hinders the donor's interest by preventing a wish from being fulfilled (Cochrane and Bianchi, 2011). If the decision was made to forgo life-sustaining therapy, then the death of the potential donor is imminent, inevitable, and intentional regardless of the donation, and violation of DDR would not lead to any harm to the dying patient (Cochrane, 2009; Cochrane and Bianchi, 2011; Wilkinson and Savulescu, 2012). In this setting, protocols for antemortem bilateral kidney harvesting in the operating room under general anesthesia followed by WLST in the ICU have been proposed, with the argument that

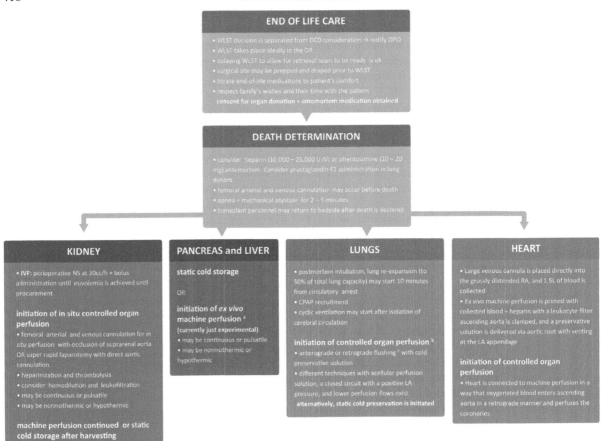

**Fig. 23.1.** Clinical pathway for controlled donation after circulatory death (cDCD). This flowchart was created based on work from Foley et al. (2005); Reich et al. (2009); Wind (2011); Barlow et al. (2013); Reznik et al. (2013); Morrissey and Monaco (2014); Bejaoui et al. (2015); Dhital et al. (2015); Chaumont et al. (2015). The most commonly used cold storage solution for the majority of organs is the University of Wisconsin (UW) solution, which was developed in 1980, and remains the gold standard (Dikdan et al., 2012). Anti-ischemic drugs, hormones, proteasome inhibitors, carbonic anhydrase II, statins, and anti-inflammatory agents are being studied as potential additives to preservative solutions (Bejaoui et al., 2015).

[a]Machine perfusion in pancreas transplantation is currently an investigational procedure. The delicate structure of the pancreas, particularly its endothelium, challenges this technique requiring strict pressure and flow limits. It has been associated with pancreatic graft edema and congestion, raising the risk of early thrombosis and graft failure. Encouraging results are demonstrated with its use for islet isolation and transplantation, but it may also disrupt the whole-organ architecture, being less useful for whole-organ transplantation. Normothermic perfusion allows assessment of exocrine and endocrine responses in pancreas grafts (Barlow et al., 2013), and viability assessment in liver grafts (Bejaoui et al., 2015). In liver transplantation, machine perfusion also assists with decreasing both glutathione depletion and superoxide anion release, thus, reducing ischemic-reperfusion injury. In contrast to kidneys, in which successful machine perfusion is independent of oxygenation, oxygenated perfusion of liver has been beneficial in maintaining the functional integrity of hepatocytes during ischemia (Bejaoui et al., 2015).

[b] Normothermic lung perfusion is preferred. Machine perfusion in lungs has additional organ-specific advantages: it allows for the administration of antimicrobial therapy, thrombolytics, and gene therapies (Munshi et al., 2013). Additionally, it allows for organ function assessment prior to transplantation.

[c]Anterograde flushing is accomplished by infusing the preservative solution through the pulmonary artery and draining through the pulmonary vein (atrial), and is the traditional approach. Retrograde flushing overcomes the difficulty of distributing the solution completely across the vascular bed (limited by hypoxic vasoconstriction). Additionally, it achieves better clearance of clots and other embolic material, and has better ability to reach restricted vascular beds (Munshi et al., 2013).

CPAP, continuous positive airway pressure; DCD, donation after circulatory death; IVF, intravenous fluid; LA, left atrium; NS, normal saline; OPO, organ procurement organization; OR, operating room; RA, right atrium; WLST, withdrawal of life-sustaining therapy.

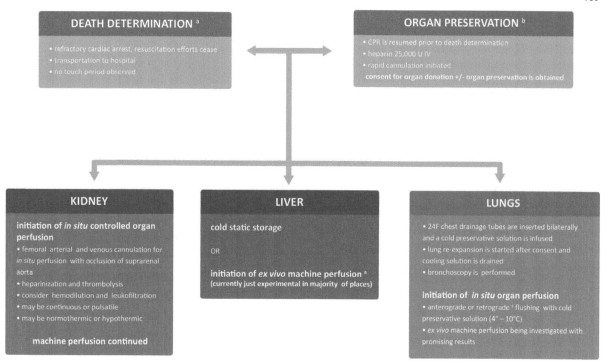

**Fig. 23.2.** Clinical pathway for uncontrolled donation after circulatory death. This flowchart was created based on the work from Fieux et al. (2009); Fondevila et al. (2012); Gomez-de-Antonio et al. (2012); Wall et al. (2016).

[a]In New York City death is declared in the field; in Spain and France it happens in the hospital. The "no touch" period is not clearly defined.

[b]In countries where patients are presumed donors unless they have actively opted out, such as Spain and France, invasive measures for organ preservation may start even before consent for donation and cannulation is obtained. Therefore, organ preservation may be initiated prior to arrival to a hospital and prior to death declaration. However, postmortem *in situ* perfusion may only commence after consent is obtained. Interestingly, in New York City death is pronounced in the field, but such organ preservation measures may only start after full consent is obtained at the hospital. CPR, cardiopulmonary resuscitation; IV, intravenous.

such patients would have their autonomy fulfilled by donating their organs in optimal conditions and their dignity respected with the institution of end-of-life care away from the traditional DCD hassle (Morrissey, 2012). The major argument against such practice is based on the potential catastrophic consequences of an inaccurate neurologic prognosis leading to the decision of WLST, rendering now anephric patients even more vulnerable to a complicated death (Wertin et al., 2012).

There is significant debate on public views facing situations where the cause of death is organ procurement. A recent questionnaire evaluating American public attitudes towards OD showed that almost three-quarters of the respondents agreed that it should be legal for donation to be the cause of death in a potential donor in a hypothetic case of irreversible coma (Nair-Collins et al., 2015). Nevertheless, the compliance of medical professionals with the set of rules that represent the values and interests of each society (in this case, the DDR) is imperative to maintain public trust in OD and other end-of-life practices. Practices allowing for death

by OD or assisted suicide during DCD should not be promoted without accompanying modifications in the set of rules that guide the donation process.

### ORGAN PRESERVATION: ISSUES WITH CONSENT AND TIMING OF INTERVENTIONS

In some European countries, invasive organ preservation interventions, such as femoral cannulation, are sometimes initiated well before donation consent is obtained, in some cases after legal permission is obtained from a judge (Gomez-de-Antonio, 2011; Reznik et al., 2013). However, this approach is not universally accepted and incites two ethical issues: (1) the initiation of measures that have the sole purpose of facilitating donation, without any direct benefit to the potential donor (who has not yet died); and (2) doing so before obtaining the family's consent for such intervention. In the UK, antemortem physical interventions are not permitted, and in the USA, having surrogate decision makers' explicit consent for such interventions is a requirement (Reich et al., 2009; Wall et al.,

2011; Blackstock and Ray, 2014). Additionally, some argue that antemortem organ preservation measures benefit solely the recipient and are thus not ethically appropriate. On the other hand, the practice of OD is crafted on the pillars of altruism, and the benefit to the potential donor is to have his/her autonomy respected, although many individuals who have expressed an intent to donate organs after death may not have considered the possibility of antemortem interventions (Dalal, 2015).

### CONTINUATION OF RESUSCITATION EFFORTS VERSUS DONATION IN uDCD

Another ethical consideration specific to uDCD is the conflict of interest in discontinuation of resuscitation and initiation of organ preservation measures (Mateos-Rodríguez, 2010; Ortega-Deballon et al., 2015). On the one hand, the medical community is challenged with the need to increase the donor pool and consequent development of donation protocols that can increase the yield of organs. However, without resolving the ethical controversies in uDCD, resultant public mistrust may make those efforts counterproductive. Advances in medicine, particularly in the field of resuscitation, blur the fine line between a potential organ donor and a potential survivor, thus challenging the DDR and unveiling a possible conflict of interest in implementing organ-preserving measures instead of continuing life-saving interventions. Centering clinical efforts on the latter until those are exhausted and exploring donation options only afterwards would alleviate this conflict of interest, in addition to earning public confidence (Doig and Zygun, 2008; Manara and Thomas, 2010; Hanto and Veatch, 2011; Rodriguez-Arias and Deballon, 2012; Rodriguez-Arias et al., 2013; Reed and Lua, 2014).

### Future trends

The heterogeneity of views and protocols in cDCD and uDCD is a reflection of the complexity of this process, which involves delicate ethical nuances and controversies. Continuation of the public debate on the acceptable boundaries of DCD while maintaining legal standards for death determination is a necessary step for the creation of social and political consensus and further development of successful DCD programs (Harrington, 2009). Additionally, the derivation of a uniform medical standard for the methodology of death determination, with clearly recommended waiting times to be incorporated in guidelines amongst medical institutions, is an urgent next step to facilitate and improve the transparency of the donation process as DCD programs continue to grow.

There is also a need for further studies to hone predictive models of death, following WLST across different patient populations. While recently proposed nomograms and scores are promising bedside tools, further refinement and validation in the potential donor population are required (He et al., 2015b).

Advances in organ support and preservation techniques are pushing the limits of WIT by improving already available procedures but also developing new therapeutic interventions to improve organ function and methods to assess organ viability and minimize discard rates. Finally, further public and political discussions are needed regarding acceptable strategies to include death by OD as a possible amendment to the DDR, should society agree that this practice is morally acceptable.

# DONATION AFTER BRAIN DETERMINATION OF DEATH

## Evolution of the definition of brain death

The development of advanced resuscitation techniques in the late 1950s, specifically positive-pressure mechanical ventilation and alternating-current cardiac defibrillation, allowed for a new neurologic process to be recognized: *coma dépassé* or irretrievable coma (Mollaret and Goulon, 1959). Patients with no discernible central nervous system (CNS) activity, rendered unresponsive to any stimulation, and susceptible to further systemic complications by the absence of all brainstem functions, were able to have spontaneous circulation of oxygenated blood maintained by mechanical support. The rising need to modify the death definition in order to provide closure to families and prioritize use of scarce medical resources in the setting of cessation of all brain function led researchers and clinicians to characterize the concept of BD (Wertheimer et al., 1959) and unveil its association with electric silence on electroencephalography (EEG) (Jouvet, 1959). Concurrently, advances in organ transplantation techniques resulted in successful outcomes, and the need for a modern definition of death, congruent with the medical developments of that time, became further evident.

In 1968, an Ad Hoc Committee at Harvard Medical School published criteria on the new clinical definition of irreversible coma and consequent death of the brain which, in the absence of hypothermia or sedatives, included a state of complete unawareness and unresponsiveness to any externally applied stimuli, total absence of spontaneous breathing, and no brainstem reflexes; a flat EEG was of confirmatory value. Notably, the Harvard criteria also included the complete absence of spontaneous motor movements and brainstem reflexes. Finally, in 1980, the UDDA incorporated the neurologic concept of death in the USA, but did not delineate minimal standards for its determination nor establish an algorithmic approach (Uniform Law Commission, 1980).

The American Academy of Neurology (AAN) identified the need for guiding physicians in assessing BD and introduced the first practice parameters for its determination in 1995, summarizing available evidence and clarifying the importance of the distinction of BD (including the brainstem) from the complete absence of CNS activity; the occurrence of reflexes and motor responses originating in the spinal cord was made permissible in BD determination (Wijdicks, 1995). Subsequently, in 2010, an updated statement was released by AAN with the intention of standardizing the practice and ensuring that BD determination is accurately performed 100% of the time, summarizing available evidence and providing a stepwise approach to BD determination, including checklists, prerequisites, clinical and ancillary testing, as well as documentation (Wijdicks et al., 2010).

Of note, a patient with a primary brainstem process could fulfill all of the necessary clinical features of BD, including coma, brainstem areflexia, and apnea. Controversy regarding the equivalence of "brainstem" death to "whole-brain" death remains; in the USA, there is not a formal stance as to whether a patient with a primary brainstem process can, or cannot, be declared dead by neurologic criteria. However, the absence of all brainstem functions is a cardinal sign of the cessation of all brain functions (Wijdicks, 2015a). Despite a potential conceptual difference between whole-BD and brainstem death, the practical process of clinical determination of brain(stem) death is the same, and in practice, only the role of ancillary testing is potentially different (Smith, 2015). In other words, a patient with evidence of cortical electric activity or with residual cerebral blood flow may still be considered brain-dead by clinical criteria in countries that endorse the brainstem death concept, such as the UK, Hong Kong, and India, whereas in jurisdictions that utilize the whole-BD approach they would not be considered dead.

## Identification of likely BD candidates

Donation following BD quickly became the preferred method of organ procurement in the countries where BD is culturally and legally accepted (NHS Blood and Transplant, 2014). The American Society of Transplant Surgeons recommends the pursuit of DBD over DCD in situations where the potential organ donor is, or will likely become, brain-dead (Reich et al., 2009). For patients in whom BD is considered "imminent," and if the family is in agreement, some clinicians believe the opportunity to wait for progression of neurologic injury should be considered (Reich et al., 2009). However, the ethics of "elective" or "nontherapeutic ventilation," where a patient with a dismal prognosis continues to receive "life-sustaining" interventions entirely for the possibility of progression to BD and OD, remains controversial (McGee and White, 2013). In these patients, it may be advisable to include the possibility of conversion to DBD from DCD when consenting for OD. The Organ Procurement and Transplantation Network proposed the term "imminent neurologic death" for patients who are ≤70 years old, requiring ventilatory support, and with the absence of ≥3 brainstem reflexes as a result of a severe neurologic injury, but who have not yet progressed to BD (OPTN/UNOS, 2008). Subsequently, in an attempt to reliably identify these patients for a timely referral to OPOs and to provide a reliable estimation of the number of potential donors, a study compared two validated coma scales (the Full Outline of Unresponsiveness (FOUR) score and the Glasgow Coma Scale (GCS)) coupled with the absence of ≥3 brainstem reflexes as a marker of brainstem injury. The accuracy of the lowest possible score using the FOUR score (which includes respiration in its calculation algorithm) for identifying imminently brain-dead patients seemed superior to a combination of the lowest possible GCS with the absence of three brainstem reflexes (de Groot et al., 2010).

## Death determination

Physicians' recognition of patients' potential for progressing to BD may significantly affect OD rates. The diagnosis of BD relies on medical providers having a high index of suspicion; without the prompt recognition of clinical signs suggestive of BD, further evaluation is delayed or may not happen at all, which in turn may preclude an OD opportunity from families (Procaccio et al., 2010; Lustbader et al., 2011). Alarmingly, a study in Poland found that, in areas of low OD rates, physicians were twice as reluctant to initiate diagnostic assessment of BD than in areas with high rates (Kosieradzki et al., 2014). The remaining wide variation in international standards for BD determination calls into question the possibility of a worldwide consensus (Wahlster et al., 2015). In fact, even in the USA, where national standards were set by the AAN practice parameters, there remains a lack of consensus amongst institutions (Greer et al., 2008, 2015; Wijdicks et al., 2010; Da Silva and Frontera, 2015), and even amongst board-certified neurologists (Joffe et al., 2012).

### CLINICAL TESTING

The diagnosis of BD is based on clinical findings, and is supported by ancillary testing in situations where the complete clinical examination is not possible or not entirely reliable. Having a known and irreversible cause for the apneic, unresponsive state and brainstem areflexia is a prerequisite for BD assessment. Exclusion of medication effects and severe metabolic, endocrine, or toxicologic derangements is necessary, although these have been inconsistently defined in guidelines around the world. In fact, having absolute certainty that any possible confounders have no lingering effects clouding the clinical assessment is of utmost importance. Allowing for at least five times the half-life of sedatives and analgesics to pass before BD assessment is recommended, possibly longer if there is abnormal hepatic and renal function. Additionally, normothermia and normotension are necessary for BD assessment. Neuroimaging demonstrating expected structural damage corresponding to etiology of brain injury is recommended. In hypoxic-ischemic patients, the initial imaging may be unrevealing; however, evidence of diffuse cerebral edema should be present in subsequent imaging. Repeatedly normal neuroimaging is a red flag, and further BD determination should not be performed (Wijdicks, 2015b). Table 23.2 provides a checklist for the clinical assessment of BD, including apnea testing.

Several clinical complications have been associated with apnea tests: acidemia and hypoxemia, with resultant hemodynamic instability, barotrauma (pneumothorax or pneumomediastinum), and even cardiac arrest (Saposnik et al., 2004). Placement of pressure tubing with an outside diameter of 3 mm instead of the standard 6-mm $O_2$ tubing has been shown to reduce the potential complications of air trapping (Denny et al., 2015); this approach should be considered, particularly in patients with endotracheal tubes of $\leq 7.0$ mm inner diameter. Apnea testing may also cause atelectasis and worsening oxygenation (Paries et al., 2012). A single recruitment maneuver following apnea test (e.g., sustained positive pressure of 35 cm $H_2O$ for 40 seconds) has been shown to prevent decrements in the $Pao_2/Fio_2$ ratio (Paries et al., 2012). It is important to ensure euvolemia prior to recruitment maneuvers, and for physicians to remain present at the bedside, as the consequent decrease in venous return, albeit transient, may lead to significant hypotension. Continuous positive airway pressure (CPAP) during apnea testing is also helpful in avoiding derecruitment, and can be applied in different ways: directly by the ventilator, by means of a CPAP valve with a reservoir (Ambu), or through a T-piece system (Solek-Pastuszka et al., 2015; Wieczorek and Gaszynski, 2015). The safety and feasibility of using CPAP during apnea testing followed by recruitment maneuvers seem promising even in patients being supported by ECMO (Giani, 2016). Further studies replicating the feasibility and safety of these approaches are required.

## ANCILLARY TESTING

Ancillary testing is pursued when apnea testing is contraindicated or inconclusive, to shorten observation times between exams (Hoffmann and Masuhr, 2015), or when there is a question regarding the reliability of clinical exam findings (Wijdicks et al., 2010). In some countries, however, ancillary testing is mandatory for BD diagnosis in adults and children (Orban et al., 2015). Importantly, these tests should never replace the clinical assessment of BD (Wijdicks, 2010), and the potential pitfalls of false-positive and false-negative results with any of these tests should encourage caution (Busl and Greer, 2009; Wijdicks, 2010; Hwang et al., 2013; Wijdicks, 2015b). Supportive evidence for BD is usually obtained by demonstration of absent brain blood flow or electric silence on EEG. Most experience assessing blood flow comes from use of catheter angiography, transcranial Doppler, or radionuclide imaging. Studies using computed tomography (CT) angiography have applied variable definitions for absence of blood flow, resulting in a wide range of estimates for sensitivity (Kramer and Roberts, 2014; Taylor, 2014). Use of CT angiography is considered acceptable in some countries, with the highest sensitivity occurring when the criteria for BD are absence of opacification of distal vasculature and internal cerebral veins (Kramer and Roberts, 2014). MR angiography has not been well validated. A systematic review of ancillary testing for the neurologic determination of death is under way and should further guide the creation of international guidelines for its use and interpretation (Chasse et al., 2013). Table 23.3 provides an overview of the most commonly used ancillary tests in clinical practice.

## Pathophysiology

Similar to DCD donors, organs procured from DBD donors are susceptible to ischemia-reperfusion injury, inherent in transplantation. This process is intimately related to ischemia times and the generation of reactive oxygen species that drive the inflammatory process, and may culminate with rejection and graft failure. In addition, severe brain injury leads to a systemic proinflammatory response, leading to leukocyte recruitment to major organs, release of inflammatory mediators, generation of reactive oxygen species, leaky capillaries, and ultimately organ dysfunction (Anthony et al., 2012; Watts et al., 2013). Massive autonomic storm and release of cytokines in BD states, coupled with coagulopathy, hemodynamic instability, and endocrine dysfunction, potentiate inflammation and secondary ischemic injury (Watts et al., 2013). Alpha-adrenergic discharge is

*Table 23.2*

**Brain death determination**

**Checklist for the clinical assessment of brain death**

**Step 1: Prerequisites for initiation of clinical assessment (all must be fulfilled)**

Establishment of irreversible and proximal cause of the unresponsive state

Neuroimaging supportive of unresponsive state

Exclude CNS – depressant effect: calculation of drug clearance using five half-lives if normal renal and hepatic functions (longer if preceding therapeutic hypothermia), negative blood and urine toxicology screen, blood alcohol level $\leq 0.08\%$

Exclude residual neuromuscular blockade effect: four twitches on train-of-four testing is required if recent paralytics were administered

Exclude severe metabolic acidosis or laboratory values markedly deviated from the norm

Achieve normal core temperature ($>36°C$) with the use of warming blankets if necessary

Correct hypotension (target systolic blood pressure $\geq 100$ mmHg) with the use of intravenous fluid targeting euvolemia and vasopressors if necessary

Be certain that an adequate amount of time has elapsed since onset of brain injury to exclude the possibility of recovery*

**Step 2: Clinical examination (all must be fulfilled)**

Absence of responsiveness: no eye opening/movement or facial movement to noxious stimulation, no blink to visual threat, no motor response to noxious stimulation other than spinally mediated reflexes[‡]

Absent pupillary light reflex bilaterally. Pupils should be 4–9 mm in diameter; constricted pupils may suggest residual drug effect. When uncertainty exists, the use of magnifying glass or pupilometer may be helpful

Absent ocular movements including absent oculocephalic[§] and oculovestibular[¶¶] reflexes bilaterally

Absent corneal reflex bilaterally[¶]

Absent gag[**] bilaterally and cough[††] reflexes

**Step 3: Prerequisites for initiation of apnea testing (all must be fulfilled)**

Achieve euvolemia and maintain systolic blood pressure target $\geq 100$ mmHg Abort testing if systolic blood pressure is sustained below 90 mmHg

Maintain core temperature $>36°C$

Achieve eucapnia ($Paco_2$ 35–40 mmHg) by reducing ventilation frequency to 10 breaths per minute. No prior $CO_2$ retention is also required

Absence of hypoxemia is required. Preoxygenate for 10 minutes with $Fio_2$ 100% for a target $Pao_2 > 200$ mmHg. Abort testing if oxygen saturation is $<85\%$ for $>30$ seconds[‡‡]

Consider reducing PEEP to 5 cmH$_2$O to assess for desaturation, which may preclude apnea testing

**Step 4: Apnea testing[§§] (all must be fulfilled)**

Obtain a baseline arterial blood gas

Disconnect patient from the ventilator. Preserve oxygenation by inserting an insufflation catheter through the endotracheal tube, advance it to the level of the carina, and deliver O$_2$ at 6 L/min

Observe closely for any respiratory movements (abdominal and chest excursions) during subsequent 8–10 minutes

If no respiratory effort noted, repeat arterial blood gas after approximately 8 minutes. Keep patient disconnected from the ventilator if clinical status permits.

*Continued*

# Table 23.2

## Continued

A positive test includes $Paco_2 \geq 60$ mmHg or 20 mmHg increase in arterial $Pco_2$ from baseline and no respiratory effort was noted

Repeated arterial blood gases may be necessary while maintaining observation for longer periods of time (up to 15 minutes) if the test is inconclusive and clinical status permits.

or

Apnea test is aborted or contraindicated, and patient will require ancillary testing (only one needs to be performed): cerebral angiogram, electroencephalogram, transcranial Doppler, or cerebral scintigraphy

Adapted from Wijdicks et al. (2010). This assessment refers to adults ($\geq$18 years old).

*In the majority of countries, the amount of time necessary to exclude confounding factors is already adequate to be sure of the irreversibility of coma. In Australia, it is recommended to wait at least 4 hours before proceeding with clinical testing. One exception is hypoxic-ischemic encephalopathy following cardiac arrest: the majority of countries recommend waiting at least 24 hours after arrest (Youn and Greer, 2014).

†In the majority of the USA, one examination is required by law (although local institutional practices may require more than one), and a second examination is needed in the following states: California, Connecticut, Florida, Iowa, Kentucky, and Louisiana (Wijdicks, 2015b). In Europe, one examination is required in Belgium, Finland, the Netherlands, Norway, and Switzerland; Hungary and Lithuania require three separate examinations; the remaining countries require two examinations (Citerio and Murphy, 2015). Additionally, in some institutions, certain expertise is required from the examiner (having an active medical license or faculty position, or even a certain specialty).

‡Spinally mediated reflexes other than triple flexion of lower extremities may be complex and require expertise for an accurate differentiation from brainstem-initiated motor reflexes.

§Oculocephalic testing requires the confirmation of cervical spine integrity; therefore, it should not be tested in patients who need a hard cervical collar. The head is briskly rotated horizontally and vertically and the absence of eye movement relative to the head movement is observed.

¶Oculovestibular testing requires the confirmation of the external ear canal patency and the integrity of the tympanic membrane. The head of the bed should be elevated to 30° for maximal stimulation of the horizontal canal. The administration of 40–60 cc of ice water (4°C) over 60 seconds is performed while the eyes are held open and observed for lack of any movement (slow and fast components must be absent) for an additional 60 seconds. It is recommended that a waiting period of 3–5 minutes is observed before testing the other side to allow rewarming of the previously tested ear.

‖Different stimulation methods are suggested to test the corneal reflex. However, the absence of eye blink with saline squirt requires confirmation with maximal stimulation (e.g., gentle pressure with a cotton swab).

**Bilateral stimulation of the pharynx with a tongue blade or suctioning device is performed and absent gag reflex appreciated. The movement of an endotracheal tube is not routinely recommended due to the potential displacement of the device.

††A suctioning device is advanced to the level of the carina (for maximal stimulation) and absent cough reflex is observed after 1–2 passes.

‡‡In case of sustained hypoxemia with oxygen saturations <85%, the procedure is aborted until saturation recovers with further increase in oxygen supply. Another attempt is permitted with a T-piece, continuous positive airway pressure 10 cm $H_2O$, and 12 L/min of oxygen.

§§The following are recommendations for the standard apnea testing. Different methods have been proposed and described in other sections of this chapter.

CNS, central nervous system; PEEP, positive end-expiratory pressure.

*Table 23.3*

**Overview of ancillary testing for brain death determination**

| Test | Key technical aspects | Test performance | Limitations |
|---|---|---|---|
| Conventional cerebral angiogram (Wijdicks, 1995; Wijdicks et al., 2010) Gold standard for the assessment of cerebral circulation arrest | The contrast medium should be injected in the aortic arch under high pressure and reach bilateral anterior and posterior cerebral circulations (four vessels) No intracerebral filling should be detected at the level of entry of the vertebral and carotid arteries to the skull. However, contrast stasis in the intracranial arteries may be seen as an early finding of BD Extracranial vessels should demonstrate flow Possible demonstration of delayed filling of the superior sagittal sinus | Interobserver studies have not been published The procedure has the potential to yield conflicting results, as no guidelines for interpretation have been developed | High cost Limited availability Requires iodinated contrast Requires highly trained staff Requires transportation to the angiography suite |
| Transcranial Doppler (TCD) (Sloan et al., 2004) Flow-related study | There should be bilateral insonation. The probe is placed at the temporal bone above the zygomatic arch or the vertebrobasilar arteries through the suboccipital transcranial window Insonation via orbital window is an acceptable approach The identification of reverberating flow, or small systolic peaks in early systole, in bilateral anterior and posterior circulations, is diagnostic of BD Absent acoustic flow in the major intracranial vessels is not reliable for the diagnosis of BD, as false-positive results may occur in patients with inadequate windows (Youn and Greer, 2014) | Noninvasive, relatively inexpensive, and independent of contrast media Overall TCD specificity of 99% and sensitivity of 89% for BD (Monteiro et al., 2006) False-positive results (when compared with clinical examination) warrants caution when interpreting results in patients with ventriculostomy or skull defects (Thompson et al., 2014) | Heavily dependent on operator skills Approximately 10% of patients lack adequate acoustic windows |
| Computed tomography angiography (CTA) Flow-related study | Involves at least three acquisitions for BD diagnosis (Sawicki et al., 2014):<br>1. a nonenhanced reference scan<br>2. an early postcontrast scan demonstrating no IC but positive EC vessel filling 20 seconds after initiation of contrast bolus | Different CTA evaluation scales have been proposed with varying sensitivities (Sawicki et al., 2014):<br>• 4-point IC vessel nonfilling 86–96%<br>• 7-point IC vessel nonfilling 52–100%<br>• 10-point IC vessel nonfilling and 54–70% | No widely accepted CTA criteria exist (Taylor, 2014) Requires iodinated contrast Requires transportation to the CT scanner Requires validation comparing these findings with nonbrain-dead patients with intracranial hypertension as controls |

*Continued*

*Table 23.3*

Continued

| Test | Key technical aspects | Test performance | Limitations |
|---|---|---|---|
| | 3. a late postcontrast scan assessing IC vessel filling 60 seconds after initiation of contrast bolus confirming absence of flow and ruling out delayed filling due to intracranial hypertension | Agreement between readers (Sahin and Pekcevik, 2015): <br> • 4-point scale 88% <br> • 7-point scale 100% <br> • 10-point scale 100% <br> Potential false negatives in cases of HIE, ventriculostomy, multiple skull fractures, decompressive craniectomy (Escudero 2009) <br> False positives with hypotension (Greer et al., 2009) and delayed contrast bolus (Shankar and Vandolpe, 2013) | Provides only anatomic information The addition of brainstem perfusion techniques may add functional information, but further studies are required to validate findings (Shankar and Vandolpe, 2013; Shankar and Banfield, 2015) <br> Variation in the quantitative perfusion analysis by using different postprocessing software is a possible limitation of CTP techniques |
| Magnetic resonance angiography (MRA) Flow-related study | Absent cerebral blood flow distal to supraclinoid internal carotid arteries on brain gadolinium-enhanced MRA is consistent with BD (Luchtmann et al., 2014) | The procedure has the potential to yield conflicting results, as no guidelines for interpretation have been developed <br> No large studies or meta-analysis are available reporting sensitivity and specificity of this test for BD diagnosis | No widely accepted MRA criteria exist <br> Requires validation comparing these findings with conventional angiography <br> Requires transportation to the MRI scanner <br> Requires administration of gadolinium |
| Radionuclide cerebral perfusion scan Flow-related study | The tracer $^{99m}$Tc-labeled HMPAO is administered and subsequent imaging with SPECT brain scintigraphy is obtained at several time points: immediately, 30–60 minutes following tracer administration, and at 2 hours. The tracer penetrates in the brain proportionally to regional blood flow <br> Hollow skull phenomenon is diagnostic for BD and represents the absence of uptake in the brain (no brain perfusion). <br> Both anterior and lateral views should be obtained to avoid false-positive results | Comparable accuracy to conventional cerebral angiography (Munari et al., 2005) <br> Sensitivity for the diagnosis of BD reported to range from 94.7 to 98.5% (Flowers and Patel, 1997; Venkatram et al., 2015) <br> If performed too soon, residual intracerebral blood flow may be seen given its high sensitivity for blood flow. Repeat testing is recommended in such cases <br> Recent false-positive reports despite anterior and lateral views suggest caution in the interpretation of this test (Venkatram et al., 2015) | Requires transportation to the nuclear scanner <br> Limited availability |
| Electroencephalography (Szurhaj et al., 2015) | Minimum of eight scalp electrodes (standard scalp or needle) with minimum interelectrode distance of 10 cm and | No large studies or meta-analysis are available reporting sensitivity and specificity of this test for BD diagnosis | Affected by temperature, hemodynamic parameters, drug administration, and metabolic disorders; therefore, should not |

| | | | |
|---|---|---|---|
| Gold standard for cerebral isoelectric activity Cerebral electric activity study | impedance between 100 and 10 000 Ohms The integrity of the entire recording system should be confirmed<br><br>Sensitivity should be increased to 2 mV for 30 minutes, with inclusion of appropriate calibrations, and demonstration of cerebral electric silence is required in two different recordings<br><br>Frequency filters should be set to allow 0.53–70 Hz frequencies. Notch filters are allowed<br><br>Standardized activating procedures should be performed to document lack of reactivity | No recent data on the reproducibility of digital EEG in the context of BD | be used as ancillary testing if those confounders cannot be ruled out<br><br>Electric noise common in the ICU setting may produce artifact limiting EEG interpretation.<br><br>A waiting period of 12 hours is recommended prior to performing EEG in patients who suffered a cardiac arrest. |
| Evoked potentials Cerebral electric activity study | SSEP: Median nerve is stimulated bilaterally and evoked potentials recorded by scalp electrodes: bilaterally absent N20–P22 responses are supportive of BD diagnosis<br><br>BAER: Absent waves III–V in the presence of cochlear response (wave I) is required for BD diagnosis<br><br>Evoked potentials evaluate specific pathways and may be negative in conditions with preservation of other brainstem function that were not evaluated by these tests<br><br>Performed at bedside | No large studies or meta-analysis are available reporting sensitivity and specificity of this test for BD diagnosis<br><br>No recent data on the reproducibility of evoked potentials in the context of BD | Requires validation<br>Affected by temperature and drug administration |

This table was created based on the review work from Youn and Greer (2014).

BD, brain death; IC, intracranial; EC, extracranial; HIE, hypoxic-ischemic encephalopathy; CTP, computed tomography perfusion; MRI, magnetic resonance imaging; HMPAO, hexamethylpropylenea-mineoxime; SPECT, single-photon emission computed tomography; EEG, electroencephalogram; ICU, intensive care unit; SSEP, somatosensory evoked potential; BAEP, brainstem auditory evoked potential.

thought to be a major factor triggering neurogenic pulmonary edema by causing pulmonary vasoconstriction and consequent high intravascular pressures, in turn leading to increased capillary permeability (Busl and Bleck, 2015).

Dysautonomia with BD is a result of unopposed sympathetic input due to loss of vagal parasympathetic nucleus function (Schrader et al., 1985; Watts et al., 2013). The catecholamine surge may occur as a compensatory response to overcome markedly increased intracranial pressure and maintain cerebral blood flow, but has serious systemic effects: end-organ vasoconstriction and tissue hypoperfusion; neurogenic stunned myocardium with both systolic and diastolic dysfunction; and neurogenic pulmonary edema (Berman et al., 2010). Eventual loss of sympathetic drive contributes to ensuing hypotension, which also results from the concurrent hormonal failure (e.g., relative hypothyroid state, adrenal insufficiency, and diabetes insipidus) and metabolic acidosis (Salim, 2006a; Munshi et al., 2013; Watts et al., 2013). The addition of microthrombi formation exacerbates the microcirculatory failure, with further ischemic injury (Avlonitis et al., 2005). The release of tissue thromboplastin by the ischemic brain promotes activation of the coagulation cascade which, coupled with endothelial disruption, may lead to disseminated intravascular coagulation (Smith, 2004). Hypothermia from hypothalamic failure contributes to coagulopathy.

As neuronal cell death progresses in a rostrocaudal manner, there is concurrent hypothalamic-hypophyseal failure leading to a severe endocrinopathy that is variable in timing and severity. An early sign of endocrine failure is the depletion of antidiuretic hormone, resulting in massive diuresis, hyperosmolality, hypernatremia, and volume depletion. There is also decreased thyroid-stimulating hormone secretion which, in combination with decreased peripheral conversion of tetraiodothyronine ($T_4$), results in a rapid decline in free triiodothyronine ($T_3$) (Chen et al., 1996). This contributes to decreased cardiac contractility related especially to depletion of high-energy phosphates (Smith, 2004). The accompanying fall in insulin levels and resulting decrease in intracellular glucose contribute to lactic acidosis. Hyperglycemia is further exacerbated by the catecholamine storm and promotes osmotic. Finally, donor stress responses are blunted due to adrenal insufficiency frequently encountered in BD; the decreased levels of cortisol and adrenocorticotropic hormone contribute to the hypotension and cardiovascular instability (Chen et al., 1996). Table 23.4 provides an overview of systemic complications in BD.

*Table 23.4*

**Prevalence of systemic complications in brain-dead donors**

| Complication | Prevalence |
| --- | --- |
| Neurogenic pulmonary edema (Smith, 2004; Salim, 2006a) | 13–18% |
| Thrombocytopenia (Salim, 2006a) | 56% |
| Disseminated intravascular coagulation (Smith, 2004; Salim, 2006a) | 28–55% |
| Hypotension (Smith, 2004) | 80% |
| Cardiac arrhythmias (Dujardin et al., 2001; Smith, 2004) | 25–32% |
| Systolic myocardial dysfunction (Smith, 2004) | 42% |
| Diabetes insipidus (Gramm et al., 1992; Salim, 2006b) | 46–86% |

## Epidemiology

The USA witnessed a slight increase in the total number of deceased organ donors in 2014 compared to 2013, reflecting an increase in the total number of both DCD and DBD (Healthcare EDftQoM, 2013; European Directorate for the Quality of Medicines and Healthcare, 2014). Conversely, the UK experienced a decrease by 1% in the number of DBD donors, in addition to a fall in living and DCD donors in 2015 compared to 2014, resulting in a reduction of 5% in the total number of transplants (NHS Blood and Transplant, 2014). This fall is a reflection of the decrease in all forms of OD; however, there was a small increase in DBD kidneys and pancreas (NHS Blood and Transplant, 2014). Interestingly, a trend towards older and nontraumatic donors was observed, which may reflect efforts in increasing the donor pool by expanding eligibility criteria for donation.

## Organ support

Organ preservation begins with optimal management of the potential organ donor, and continues during procurement and storage, with the goal of increasing the yield of transplantable organs per donor, and improving graft function after transplantation (Klein et al., 2010). The cascade of multisystem changes resulting from BD warrants a systematic approach to the potential DBD donor.

### ENDOCRINE SUPPORT

The collapse of the hypothalamic–pituitary axis leads to significant hormonal derangements, potentially impacting organs at molecular, cellular, and tissue levels. The implementation of protocols for hormonal support seems intuitive, but its efficacy has not been completely elucidated, and practices vary across the USA (Klein et al., 2010). Retrospective studies have demonstrated improvement in hemodynamics, procurement yield, and posttransplant cardiac graft function with use of thyroid hormones, while a meta-analysis of randomized trials failed to support this conclusion (Dikdan et al., 2012; Macdonald et al., 2012). Recently, a large retrospective review of over 60 000 donors showed an increase of approximately 15% in the procurement yield with T3/T4 therapy (Novitzky et al., 2014). Regimens vary widely, with oral and intravenous formulations appearing equivalent (Sharpe et al., 2013). Combining thyroid replacement with vasopressin and corticosteroids is recommended for patients with refractory shock, or in potential heart donors with a left ventricular ejection fraction < 45% (Kotloff et al., 2015). The most commonly used corticosteroid regimen is high-dose methylprednisolone (15 mg/kg), although lower doses may have comparable effects with less hyperglycemia (Dhar, 2013). Use of corticosteroids reduces vasopressor requirements, which may be important in maximizing organ usage (Pinsard et al., 2014). Similarly, vasopressin use has been associated with greater organ procurement and reduces the need for other vasoactive drugs (Dikdan et al., 2012), in addition to its value in the treatment of diabetes insipidus and hypernatremia. A target sodium concentration < 155 mEq/L is recommended, given an association between hypernatremia and worsened liver graft survival (Kotloff et al., 2015; Mi et al., 2015).

### HEMODYNAMIC SUPPORT

Assessing volume status in the potential brain-dead organ donor is challenging. Frequently, coexisting comorbidities such as neurogenic pulmonary edema, diabetes insipidus, distributive shock, hormonal failure, and dysautonomia may cloud the interpretation of hemodynamic parameters and urinary output, which are often used for this assessment. Moreover, patients with severe neurologic injury preceding BD were often given osmotherapy, which may further affect volume status. Minimally invasive methods for the assessment of cardiac output and fluid responsiveness may be helpful (Hadian et al., 2010). However, a large, multicenter, randomized trial failed to show a significant increase in the number of transplanted organs by using a protocol-guided therapy targeting cardiac index, mean arterial pressure, and pulse pressure variation (Al-Khafaji et al., 2015).

Low-dose dopamine infusion (4 µg/kg/min) in brain-dead donors has been shown in one study to reduce the need for dialysis posttransplant (Schnuelle et al., 2009); a possible mechanism of renal protection is the attenuation

of ischemia-reperfusion injury by stimulation of D3 receptors (Wang et al., 2015). However, this study did not demonstrate any improvement in long-term graft survival with dopamine. In another recent randomized trial, targeting mild kidney donor hypothermia to 34–35°C resulted in less DGF among recipients. The results of this study were confounded by longer CITs in the control group and relatively high overall rates of DGF, which may not be broadly generalizable at all centers (Niemann et al., 2015). Further studies assessing the optimum temperature management of potential organ donors are warranted.

## Ventilatory support

The lungs of brain-dead donors can frequently not be transplanted, due to impaired gas exchange from aspiration, neurogenic pulmonary edema, and acute respiratory distress syndrome (Munshi et al., 2013). In a multicenter randomized controlled trial, the implementation of a lung donor management protocol consisting of lung-protective ventilation, apnea testing with CPAP, optimal positioning of the patient, optimization of volume status, and frequent recruitment maneuvers for potential donors who did not meet the required $Pao_2/Fio_2$ threshold doubled the lung donation rate without an increase in PGD (Mascia et al., 2010; Minambres et al., 2015). Some concern has been raised regarding the possible negative effect of a restrictive fluid balance with goal central venous pressures < 8 mmHg on kidney grafts; however, accumulating evidence suggests that this approach is safe (Minambres et al., 2010; Miñambres, 2013; Munshi et al., 2013).

Observational research has reported an association between increased lung recovery and treatment with corticosteroids in donors (Follette et al., 1998; Dhar, 2013). Conversely, β-agonist inhalers were associated with higher rates of tachycardia, without improvement of oxygenation or donation yields, and their routine use is not recommended (Ware et al., 2014).

### ORGAN SUPPORT AFTER PROCUREMENT

Similar to DCD organs, methods of organ preservation following DBD vary. Cold static storage remains the most common approach. Use of *ex vivo* lung perfusion is expanding across institutions. Machine perfusion may be less important in DBD organs, where WIT is less of a concern.

## DBD protocols and practice guidelines

There is significant variation across the world in BD determination. Hospitals in lower-income countries are less likely to have protocols (Wahlster et al., 2015).

Similar variation is seen in protocols for management of organ donors. However, improvement in procurement yields without a negative impact on graft function has been observed with protocols targeting early goal-directed management of potential donors (Rosendale et al., 2002; Angel et al., 2006; Salim, 2006b; DuBose, 2008; Venkateswaran et al., 2008; Singbartl, 2011; Miñambres, 2013; Abuanzeh, 2015). Acknowledging this variability in practice and the importance of intensivists' role in OD, the Society of Critical Care Medicine and American College of Chest Physicians commissioned the creation of a consensus document to guide practices related to OD (Kotloff et al., 2015). The most relevant aspects of these recommendations to the neurointensivist are summarized here.

Hospitals and OPOs are responsible for the development of local protocols for BD determination, which should be in accordance with national practice parameters (Wijdicks et al., 2010). Clinicians and OPO members should be aware that, in some jurisdictions, patients' previous authorization for donation through a registry may be available, and knowing this status can be valuable in conveying their wishes to families. The prompt identification of potential donors and timely notification (within 1 hour) of OPOs is an expectation of clinicians. It is recommended that conversations with surrogate decision makers should generally be carried out by designated requestors with sufficient training and experience, using a collaborative approach with ICU staff.

Hemodynamic goals to be targeted in the management of brain-dead donors include the following: maintenance of euvolemia and adequate perfusion pressures (mean arterial pressure $\geq 60$–$70$ mmHg); urine output $> 1$ mL/kg/h, left ventricular ejection fraction $> 45\%$ (Kotloff et al., 2015). Ideally, these goals would be achieved while utilizing the lowest possible vasopressor support. Hemodynamic monitoring to assist in volume management should be considered. Initial volume resuscitation with either crystalloid or colloids is acceptable, although starch solutions should be avoided (Patel et al., 2015). If vasopressors are needed, consideration of dopamine and vasopressin as first-line agents is recommended, leaving norepinephrine, phenylephrine, dobutamine, and epinephrine for severe shock. Additionally, specific scenarios may require prioritization of one agent versus others: in primary cardiogenic shock, dobutamine, dopamine, and epinephrine are preferred; in distributive shock, norepinephrine and phenylephrine are recommended. Hormonal replacement is indicated when hemodynamic goals are not met with initial fluid resuscitation and inotrope/vasopressor needs escalate above the desired doses (dopamine or dobutamine $> 10$ µg/kg/min; or norepinephrine or epinephrine $> 0.05$ µg/kg/min), or left ventricular ejection fraction remains $< 45\%$.

Of note, functional assessments from early echocardiography in BD donors may not accurately reflect true myocardial function and suitability of the heart for transplantation, and repeat assessments may be necessary following aggressive donor management. Maintenance of enteric nutrition is recommended to increase glycogen stores, with the potential to optimize allograft function. Serial assessment of lactate levels, central venous oxygen saturation, acid–base status, and invasive or noninvasive hemodynamic measurements are recommended to guide further therapy. Coronary arteriography should be recommended for any potential heart donor above 40 years of age. Bronchoscopy should be performed in all potential lung donors.

Figure 23.3 summarizes the key points in the clinical pathway for DBD.

## Ethical considerations

### ACCEPTANCE OF BRAIN DEATH BY FAMILIES

Conflicts between patients' first-person authorization (previously stated decision to donate) and families' perspectives may occur. These conflicts are addressed on a case-by-case basis, and involve substantial collaboration between OPO staff and leadership, healthcare providers, hospital administration, and families (Kotloff et al., 2015). The adoption of personalized OD directives – an audiovisual record of the individual's OD intention – has been suggested as a potential solution (Shaw, 2014).

Family objection to a conclusion of death by neurologic criteria constitutes another potential challenge. Most BD protocols in the USA do not provide guidance on how to navigate such a scenario (Lewis et al., 2016). Some protocols allow for prolongation of organ support after BD declaration based on religious and moral objection grounds, as well as for social reasons, or for awaiting family arrival. Among recommendations in some hospitals, there were maintenance of organ support until cardiac arrest, counseling, offering a second opinion, transferring care to another facility, and even removal of support against family wishes. Regardless of the actions taken, such situations have a high potential for distress among families and hospital staff, and should be handled in a collaborative way to avoid further confrontation.

### BRAIN DEATH CONCEPT AND CONTROVERSIES

One of the barriers holding back the expansion of DBD programs is public acceptance of the concept of BD. Even in the USA (a country where BD is culturally acceptable), one population survey demonstrated more willingness to donate organs in the case of both uDCD and cDCD as opposed to DBD (Volk et al., 2010).

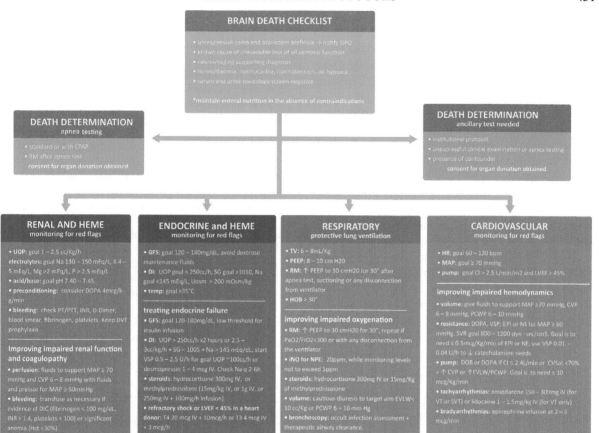

**Fig. 23.3.** Clinical pathway and algorithm for the potential donation after brain death organ donor management. This flowchart was created based on Wood et al. (2004); Schnuelle et al. (2009); Dikdan et al. (2012); Paries et al. (2012); Munshi et al. (2013); Chaumont et al. (2015); Kotloff et al. (2015); Citerio et al. (2016). Organ preservation techniques are similar to the ones demonstrated in the donation after circulatory death flowcharts. CI, cardiac index; CPAP, continuous positive airway pressure; CVP, central venous pressure; DI, diabetes insipidus; DIC, disseminated intravascular coagulation; DOB, dobutamine; DOPA, dopamine; DVT, deep venous thrombosis; EPI, epinephrine; EVLW, extravascular lung water; GFS, glucose fingerstick; Hct, hematocrit; HOB, head of bed; HR, heart rate; iNO, inhaled nitric oxide; INR, international normalized ratio; IV, intravenous; LVEF, left ventricular ejection fraction; MAP, mean arterial pressure; NE, norepinephrine; NPE, neurogenic pulmonary edema; OPO, organ procurement organization; PCWP, pulmonary capillary wedge pressure; PEEP, positive end-expiratory pressure; PT, prothrombin time; PTT, partial thromboplastin time; RM, recruitment maneuver; SG, specific gravity; SVR, systemic vascular resistance; SVT, supraventricular tachycardia; T3, triiodothyronine; T4, thyroxine; TV, tidal volume; UOP, urinary output; VSP, vasopressin; VT, ventricular tachycardia.

A similar finding was reported in a survey of a Spanish population (Andres et al., 2009). Possible explanations include familiarity of families' conception of death with cardiac criteria and the "certainty" of outcomes in cases where the heart is no longer beating. A careful explanation of the irreversibility of BD along with an explanation regarding the patient's beating heart may help address families' concerns (Andres et al., 2009; Volk et al., 2010). One randomized study suggested that families were more accepting of the concept of BD when it was explained in terms of cerebral circulatory arrest (Soldatos et al., 2010). Unfortunately, donor families may be afflicted by the emotional distress surrounding

the concept of BD (Merchant et al., 2008; Tavakoli et al., 2008), and provision of clear and comprehensive education may alleviate such distress (Cleiren and Van Zoelen, 2002). Moreover, it is important to clarify to families that death is declared regardless of willingness to donate organs when an individual is determined dead by neurologic criteria (Barron, 2015).

## Future trends

The creation of international standards for the details of clinical assessment and ancillary testing regarding BD determination would facilitate uniform practice and further development of DBD programs worldwide. Specifically, the standardization of BD criteria for the use of new imaging modalities, once validated, and the establishment of clear clinical settings in which ancillary testing is mandatory would represent progress. Exploring new methods of apnea testing could improve the safety of this test and expand its use, thus avoiding further ancillary testing and delays in BD diagnosis. As endocrine support is widely used despite conflicting data (particularly in the case of thyroxine), further large studies comparing different dosing and combinations of endocrine supplementation are needed. The effects of mild hypothermia in transplantation outcomes should be further investigated, particularly in the light of the recent data supporting its use in renal donors (Niemann et al., 2015). Studies targeting inhibition of the inflammatory response induced by BD may be promising in improving transplant outcomes (Westendorp et al., 2011; Carlessi, 2015). Finally, the discovery of serum biomarkers for prediction of graft failure may optimize the use of resources in DBD, improving the yield of procurement.

## CONCLUSION

Significant variability in all steps of management of the potential organ donor exists across the world; hence, there is a need for global standards. Since complicated grief may affect up to 50% of donor families, pursuing professional bereavement support may have a significantly positive impact in the donation experience (Soriano-Pacheco et al., 1999; Merchant et al., 2008). The implementation of specific psychologic support services for families of brain-dead patients may assist in dealing with the impact of unexpected and devastating news, thus helping to focus on the next step in decision making (Adanir et al., 2014). Progress in the management of potential organ donors is a result of efforts that focus also on outcomes in potential recipients (Dhanani and Shemie, 2014).

Efforts to mitigate the mismatch between organ supply and demand include improving individual healthcare providers' familiarity with the donation process; optimizing management of the potential organ donor; developing strategies to rehabilitate marginal organs and improve procurement yields; instituting clear protocols guiding OD processes; implementing strategies to improve organ allocation; increasing authorization rates; and improving policies to facilitate donation with the assistance of societal engagement.

### REFERENCES

Abt P, Crawford M, Desai N et al. (2003). Liver transplantation from controlled non-heart-beating donors: an increased incidence of biliary complications. Transplantation 75: 1659–1663.

Abuanzeh RR (2015). Early donor management increases the retrieval rate of hearts for transplantation in marginal donors. Eur J Cardio-Thorac Surg 47: 72–77.

Academy of Medical Royal Colleges (2011). An ethical framework for controlled donation after circulatory death, accessed. Available: http://www.aomrc.org.uk/index.php/publications/reports-a-guidance.

Ad Hoc Committee (1968). A definition of irreversible coma. Report of the Ad Hoc Committee of the Harvard Medical School to examine the definition of brain death. JAMA 205: 337–340.

Adanir T, Erdogan I, Hunerli G et al. (2014). The effect of psychological support for the relatives of intensive care unit patients on cadaveric organ donation rate. Transplant Proc 46: 3249–3252.

Akoh JA (2012). Kidney donation after cardiac death. World J Nephrol 1: 79–91.

Ali A, White P, Dhital K et al. (2009). Cardiac recovery in a human non-heart-beating donor after extracorporeal perfusion: source for human heart donation? J Heart Lung Transplant 28: 290–293.

Al-Khafaji A, Elder M, Lebovitz DJ et al. (2015). Protocolized fluid therapy in brain-dead donors: the multicenter randomized MOnIToR trial. Intensive Care Med 41: 418–426.

Andres A, Morales E, Vazquez S et al. (2009). Lower rate of family refusal for organ donation in non-heart-beating versus brain-dead donors. Transplant Proc 41: 2304–2305.

Angel LF, Levine DJ, Restrepo MI et al. (2006). Impact of a lung transplantation donor-management protocol on lung donation and recipient outcomes. Am J Respir Crit Care Med 174: 710–716.

Anthony DC, Couch Y, Losey P et al. (2012). The systemic response to brain injury and disease. Brain Behav Immun 26: 534–540.

Australian Government Organ and Tissue Authority (2010). National protocol for donation after cardiac death, accessed. Available: http://www.donatelife.gov.au/national-protocol-donation-and-cardiac-death.

Avlonitis VS, Wigfield CH, Kirby JA et al. (2005). The hemodynamic mechanisms of lung injury and systemic inflammatory response following brain death in the transplant donor. Am J Transplant 5: 684–693.

Banner NR, Thomas HL, Curnow E et al. (2008). The importance of cold and warm cardiac ischemia for survival after heart transplantation. Transplantation 86: 542–547.

Barlow AD, Hosgood SA, Nicholson ML (2013). Current state of pancreas preservation and implications for DCD pancreas transplantation. Transplantation 95: 1419–1424.

Barlow AD, Hamed MO, Mallon DH et al. (2015). Use of ex vivo normothermic perfusion for quality assessment of discarded human donor pancreases. Am J Transplant 15: 2475–2482.

Barron RS (2015). Death: past, present, and future. J Crit Care 30: 214–215.

Bejaoui M, Pantazi E, Folch-Puy E et al. (2015). Emerging concepts in liver graft preservation. World J Gastroenterol 21: 396–407.

Bellali T, Papadatou D (2006). Parental grief following the brain death of a child: does consent or refusal to organ donation affect their grief? Death Stud 30: 883–917.

Bendorf A, Kelly PJ, Kerridge IH et al. (2013). An international comparison of the effect of policy shifts to organ donation following cardiocirculatory death (DCD) on donation rates after brain death (DBD) and transplantation rates. PLoS One 8: e62010.

Benz S, Bergt S, Obermaier R et al. (2001). Impairment of microcirculation in the early reperfusion period predicts the degree of graft pancreatitis in clinical pancreas transplantation. Transplantation 71: 759–763.

Berman M, Ali A, Ashley E et al. (2010). Is stress cardiomyopathy the underlying cause of ventricular dysfunction associated with brain death? J Heart Lung Transplant 29: 957–965.

Bernat JL, D'Alessandro AM, Port FK et al. (2006). Report of a National Conference on Donation after cardiac death. Am J Transplant 6: 281–291.

Bernat JL, Capron AM, Bieck TP et al. (2010). The circulatory-respiratory determination of death in organ donation. Critical Care Medicine 38: 963–970.

Blackstock MJ, Ray DC (2014). Organ donation after circulatory death: an update. Eur J Emerg Med 21: 324–329.

Bumgardner GL (2007). Pulsatile perfusion: a preservation strategy to optimize the use and function of transplanted kidneys. Curr Opin Organ Transplant 12: 345–350.

Busl KM, Bleck TP (2015). Neurogenic pulmonary edema. Crit Care Med 43: 1710–1715.

Busl KM, Greer DM (2009). Pitfalls in the diagnosis of brain death. Neurocrit Care 11: 276–287.

Callahan DS, Kim D, Bricker S et al. (2014). Trends in organ donor management: 2002 to 2012. J Am Coll Surg 219: 752–756.

Carlessi RR (2015). Exendin-4 attenuates brain death-induced liver damage in the rat. Liver Transplantation 21: 1410–1418.

Chasse M, Glen P, Doyle MA et al. (2013). Ancillary testing for diagnosis of brain death: a protocol for a systematic review and meta-analysis. Syst Rev 2: 100.

Chatterjee P, Venkataramani AS, Vijayan A et al. (2015). The effect of state policies on organ donation and transplantation in the United States. JAMA Intern Med 175: 1323–1329.

Chaumont M, Racape J, Broeders N et al. (2015). Delayed graft function in kidney transplants: time evolution, role of acute rejection, risk factors, and impact on patient and graft outcome. J Transplant 2015: 163757.

Chen EP, Bittner HB, Kendall SW et al. (1996). Hormonal and hemodynamic changes in a validated animal model of brain death. Crit Care Med 24: 1352–1359.

Citerio G, Murphy PG (2015). Brain death: the European perspective. Semin Neurol 35: 139–144.

Citerio G, Cypel M, Dobb GJ et al. (2016). Organ donation in adults: a critical care perspective. Intensive Care Med 42: 305–315.

Cleiren MP, Van Zoelen AA (2002). Post-mortem organ donation and grief: a study of consent, refusal and well-being in bereavement. Death Stud 26: 837–849.

Cochrane TI (2009). Wanted, dead or alive. Hastings Cent Rep 39: 5. author reply 6.

Cochrane T, Bianchi MT (2011). "Take my organs, please": a section of my living will. Am J Bioeth 11: 56–58.

Collins MJ, Moainie SL, Griffith BP et al. (2008). Preserving and evaluating hearts with ex vivo machine perfusion: an avenue to improve early graft performance and expand the donor pool. Eur J Cardiothorac Surg 34: 318–325.

Da Silva IR, Frontera JA (2015). Worldwide barriers to organ donation. JAMA Neurol 72: 112–118.

Dalal AR (2015). Philosophy of organ donation: review of ethical facets. World J Transplant 5: 44–51.

de Groot YJ, Jansen NE, Bakker J et al. (2010). Imminent brain death: point of departure for potential heart-beating organ donor recognition. Intensive Care Med 36: 1488–1494.

de Groot YJ, Lingsma HF, Bakker J et al. (2012). External validation of a prognostic model predicting time of death after withdrawal of life support in neurocritical patients. Crit Care Med 40: 233–238.

Denny JT, Burr A, Tse J et al. (2015). A new technique for avoiding barotrauma-induced complications in apnea testing for brain death. J Clin Neurosci 22: 1021–1024.

Detry O, Le Dinh H, Noterdaeme T et al. (2012). Categories of donation after cardiocirculatory death. Transplant Proc 44: 1189–1195.

DeVita MA, Snyder JV (1993). Development of the University of Pittsburgh Medical Center policy for the care of terminally ill patients who may become organ donors after death following the removal of life support. Kennedy Inst Ethics J 3: 131–143.

DeVita MA, Brooks MM, Zawistowski C et al. (2008). Donors after cardiac death: validation of identification criteria (DVIC) study for predictors of rapid death. Am J Transplant 8: 432–441.

Dhanani S, Shemie SD (2014). Advancing the science of organ donor management. Crit Care 18: 612.

Dhanani S, Hornby L, Ward R et al. (2014). Vital signs after cardiac arrest following withdrawal of life-sustaining therapy: a multicenter prospective observational study. Crit Care Med 42: 2358–2369.

Dhar RR (2013). Comparison of high- and low-dose corticosteroid regimens for organ donor management. J Crit Care 28: 111.e111–111.e117.

Dhital KK, Iyer A, Connellan M et al. (2015). Adult heart transplantation with distant procurement and ex-vivo preservation of donor hearts after circulatory death: a case series. Lancet 385: 2585–2591.

Dikdan GS, Mora-Esteves C, Koneru B (2012). Review of randomized clinical trials of donor management and organ preservation in deceased donors: opportunities and issues. Transplantation 94: 425–441.

Doig CJ, Zygun DA (2008). (Uncontrolled) donation after cardiac determination of death: a note of caution. J Law Med Ethics 36: 760–765. 610.

DuBose JJ (2008). Aggressive organ donor management protocol. J Intensive Care Med 23: 367–375.

Dujardin KS, McCully RB, Wijdicks EF et al. (2001). Myocardial dysfunction associated with brain death:

clinical, echocardiographic, and pathologic features. J Heart Lung Transplant 20: 350–357.

Escudero DD (2009). Diagnosing brain death by CT perfusion and multislice CT angiography. Neurocritical Care 11: 261–271.

Ethics Committee (2001). Recommendations for nonheart-beating organ donation. A position paper by the Ethics Committee, American College of Critical Care Medicine, Society of Critical Care Medicine. Crit Care Med 29: 1826–1831.

European Directorate for the Quality of Medicines and Healthcare (2014). International Figures on Donation and Transplantation 2014, accessed. Available: https://www.edqm.eu/sites/default/files/newsletter_transplant_2015.pdf.

Evrard P (2014). Belgian modified classification of Maastricht for donors after circulatory death, Transplant Proc 46: 3138–3142.

Ferrari RS, Andrade CF (2015). Oxidative stress and lung ischemia-reperfusion injury. Oxidative Medicine and Cellular Longevity 2015: 1–14.

Fieux F, Losser MR, Bourgeois E et al. (2009). Kidney retrieval after sudden out of hospital refractory cardiac arrest: a cohort of uncontrolled non heart beating donors. Crit Care 13: R141.

Flowers Jr WM, Patel BR (1997). Radionuclide angiography as a confirmatory test for brain death: a review of 229 studies in 219 patients. South Med J 90: 1091–1096.

Foley DP, Fernandez LA, Leverson G et al. (2005). Donation after cardiac death: the University of Wisconsin experience with liver transplantation. Ann Surg 242: 724–731.

Follette DM, Rudich SM, Babcock WD (1998). Improved oxygenation and increased lung donor recovery with high-dose steroid administration after brain death. J Heart Lung Transplant 17: 423–429.

Fondevila C, Hessheimer AJ, Ruiz A et al. (2007). Liver transplant using donors after unexpected cardiac death: novel preservation protocol and acceptance criteria. Am J Transplant 7: 1849–1855.

Fondevila C, Hessheimer AJ, Flores E et al. (2012). Applicability and results of Maastricht type 2 donation after cardiac death liver transplantation. Am J Transplant 12: 162–170.

Fugate JE, Stadtler M, Rabinstein AA et al. (2011). Variability in donation after cardiac death protocols: a national survey. Transplantation 91: 386–389.

Giani MM (2016). Apnea test during brain death assessment in mechanically ventilated and ECMO patients. Intensive care med 42: 72–81.

Gomez-de-Antonio DD (2011). Non-heart-beating donation in Spain. General Thoracic and Cardiovascular Surgery 59: 1–5.

Gomez-de-Antonio D, Campo-Canaveral JL, Crowley S et al. (2012). Clinical lung transplantation from uncontrolled non-heart-beating donors revisited. J Heart Lung Transplant 31: 349–353.

Gramm HJ, Meinhold H, Bickel U et al. (1992). Acute endocrine failure after brain death? Transplantation 54: 851–857.

Greer DM, Varelas PN, Haque S et al. (2008). Variability of brain death determination guidelines in leading US neurologic institutions. Neurology 70: 284–289.

Greer DM, Strozyk D, Schwamm LH (2009). False positive CT angiography in brain death. Neurocritical Care 11: 272–275.

Greer DM, Wang HH, Robinson JD et al. (2015). Variability of brain death policies in the United States. JAMA Neurol 1–6.

Hadian M, Kim HK, Severyn DA et al. (2010). Cross-comparison of cardiac output trending accuracy of LiDCO, PiCCO, FloTrac and pulmonary artery catheters. Crit Care 14: R212.

Hanf W, Codas R, Meas-Yedid V et al. (2012). Kidney graft outcome and quality (after transplantation) from uncontrolled deceased donors after cardiac arrest. Am J Transplant 12: 1541–1550.

Hanto DW, Veatch RM (2011). Uncontrolled donation after circulatory determination of death (UDCDD) and the definition of death. Am J Transplant 11: 1351–1352.

Harrington MM (2009). The thin flat line: redefining who is legally dead in organ donation after cardiac death. Issues Law Med 25: 95–143.

He X, Liang W, Xu G et al. (2015a). The development and validation of a nomogram for identification of potential donation after cardiac death donors. Am J Transplant 15: 2531–2532.

He X, Xu G, Liang W et al. (2015b). Nomogram for predicting time to death after withdrawal of life-sustaining treatment in patients with devastating neurological injury. Am J Transplant 15: 2136–2142.

Healthcare EDftQoM (2013). International figures on donation and transplantation 2013. Available: (accessed 1/8/2016), https://www.edqm.eu/sites/default/files/newsletter_transplant_2015.pdf.

Hoffmann O, Masuhr F (2015). Use of observational periods or ancillary tests in the determination of brain death in Germany. Eur Neurol 74: 11–17.

Hornby K, Hornby L, Shemie SD (2010). A systematic review of autoresuscitation after cardiac arrest. Crit Care Med 38: 1246–1253.

Humar A, Ramcharan T, Kandaswamy R et al. (2004). Technical failures after pancreas transplants: why grafts fail and the risk factors – a multivariate analysis. Transplantation 78: 1188–1192.

Hwang DY, Gilmore EJ, Greer DM (2013). Assessment of brain death in the neurocritical care unit. Neurosurg Clin N Am 24: 469–482.

Iltis AS, Cherry MJ (2010). Death revisited: rethinking death and the dead donor rule. J Med Philos 35: 223–241.

Institute of Medicine (1997). Non-heart-beating organ transplantation: medical and ethical issues in procurement, National Academy of Sciences, Washington, DC.

Institute of Medicine (2000). Non-heart-beating organ transplantation: practice and protocols, National Academy of Sciences, Washington, DC.

Intensive Care Society (2004). Guidelines for the adult organ and tissue donation, accessed. Available: http://www.ics.ac.uk/ics-homepage/guidelines-and-standards/.

Irish WD, McCollum DA, Tesi RJ et al. (2003). Nomogram for predicting the likelihood of delayed graft function in adult cadaveric renal transplant recipients. J Am Soc Nephrol 14: 2967–2974.

Israni AK, Zaun DA, Rosendale JD et al. (2015). OPTN/SRTR 2013 Annual data report: deceased organ donation. Am J Transplant 15 (Suppl 2): 1–13.

Joffe AR, Anton NR, Duff JP et al. (2012). A survey of American neurologists about brain death: understanding the conceptual basis and diagnostic tests for brain death. Ann Intensive Care 2: 4.

Joris JJ (2011). End of life care in the operating room for non-heart-beating donors: organization at the University Hospital of Liège. Transplantation Proceedings 43: 3441–3444.

Jouvet M (1959). Electro-subcorticographic diagnosis of death of the central nervous system during various types of coma. Electroencephalogr Clin Neurophysiol 11: 805–808.

King RC, Binns OA, Rodriguez F et al. (2000). Reperfusion injury significantly impacts clinical outcome after pulmonary transplantation. Ann Thorac Surg 69: 1681–1685.

Klein AS, Messersmith EE, Ratner LE et al. (2010). Organ donation and utilization in the United States, 1999–2008. Am J Transplant 10: 973–986.

Ko WJW (2000). Extracorporeal membrane oxygenation support of donor abdominal organs in non-heart-beating donors. Clinical Transplantation 14: 152.

Kong AP, Barriso C, Salim A et al. (2010). A multidisciplinary organ donor council and performance improvement initiative can improve donation outcomes. Am Surg 76: 1059.

Kootstra GG (1995). Categories of non-heart-beating donors. Transplantation Proceedings 27: 2893.

Kootstra G, Kievit J, Nederstigt A (2002). Organ donors: heartbeating and non-heartbeating. World J Surg 26: 181–184.

Kosieradzki M, Jakubowska-Winecka A, Feliksiak M et al. (2014). Attitude of healthcare professionals: a major limiting factor in organ donation from brain-dead donors. J Transplant 2014: 296912.

Kotloff RM, Blosser S, Fulda GJ et al. (2015). Management of the potential organ donor in the ICU: Society of Critical Care Medicine/American College of Chest Physicians/Association of Organ Procurement Organizations consensus statement. Crit Care Med 43: 1291–1325.

Kramer AH, Roberts DJ (2014). Computed tomography angiography in the diagnosis of brain death: a systematic review and meta-analysis. Neurocrit Care 21: 539–550. http://dx.doi.org/10.1007/s12028-014-9997-4.

Lee KW, Simpkins CE, Montgomery RA et al. (2006). Factors affecting graft survival after liver transplantation from donation after cardiac death donors. Transplantation 82: 1683–1688.

Lee JC, Christie JD, Keshavjee S (2010). Primary graft dysfunction: definition, risk factors, short- and long-term outcomes. Semin Respir Crit Care Med 31: 161–171.

Levitt M (2015). Could the organ shortage ever be met? Life Sci Soc Policy 11: 23.

Lewis J, Peltier J, Nelson H et al. (2003). Development of the University of Wisconsin donation after cardiac death evaluation tool. Prog Transplant 13: 265–273.

Lewis A, Varelas P, Greer D (2016). Prolonging support after brain death: when families ask for more. Neurocritical Care 24: 481–487.

Locke JE, Segev DL, Warren DS et al. (2007). Outcomes of kidneys from donors after cardiac death: implications for allocation and preservation. Am J Transplant 7: 1797–1807.

Luchtmann M, Beuing O, Skalej M et al. (2014). Gadolinium-enhanced magnetic resonance angiography in brain death. Sci Rep 4: 3659.

Lustbader D, O'Hara D, Wijdicks EF et al. (2011). Second brain death examination may negatively affect organ donation. Neurology 76: 119–124.

Macdonald PS, Aneman A, Bhonagiri D et al. (2012). A systematic review and meta-analysis of clinical trials of thyroid hormone administration to brain dead potential organ donors. Crit Care Med 40: 1635–1644.

Magliocca JF, Magee JC, Rowe SA et al. (2005). Extracorporeal support for organ donation after cardiac death effectively expands the donor pool. Journal of Trauma: Injury, Infection, and Critical Care 58: 1095.

Malinoski DJ, Patel MS, Daly MC et al. (2012). The impact of meeting donor management goals on the number of organs transplanted per donor: results from the United Network for Organ Sharing Region 5 prospective donor management goals study. Crit Care Med 40: 2773–2780.

Manara ARA (2012). Donation after circulatory death. Br J Anaesth 108 (Suppl 1): i108–i121.

Manara AR, Thomas I (2010). The use of circulatory criteria to diagnose death after unsuccessful cardiopulmonary resuscitation. Resuscitation 81: 781–783.

Mascia L, Pasero D, Slutsky AS et al. (2010). Effect of a lung protective strategy for organ donors on eligibility and availability of lungs for transplantation: a randomized controlled trial. JAMA 304: 2620–2627.

Matas AJ, Hays RE (2015). Transplantation: little effect of state policies on organ donation in the USA. Nat Rev Nephrol 11: 570–572.

Mateos-Rodríguez AA (2010). Kidney transplant function using organs from non-heart-beating donors maintained by mechanical chest compressions. Resuscitation 81: 904–907.

Medical Consultants (1981). Guidelines for the determination of death. Report of the medical consultants on the diagnosis of death to the President's Commission for the Study of Ethical Problems in Medicine and Biomedical and Behavioral Research. JAMA 246: 2184–2186.

Merchant SJ, Yoshida EM, Lee TK et al. (2008). Exploring the psychological effects of deceased organ donation on the families of the organ donors. Clin Transplant 22: 341–347.

McGee AJ, White BP (2013). Is providing elective ventilation in the best interests of potential donors? J Med Ethics 39: 135–138. http://dx.doi.org/10.1136/medethics-2012-100991. Epub 2013 Jan 15.

Mi Z, Novitzky D, Collins JF et al. (2015). The optimal hormonal replacement modality selection for multiple organ procurement from brain-dead organ donors. Clin Epidemiol 7: 17–27.

Miñambres EE (2013). Aggressive lung donor management increases graft procurement without increasing renal graft loss after transplantation. Clinical Transplantation 27: 52–59.

Minambres E, Rodrigo E, Ballesteros MA et al. (2010). Impact of restrictive fluid balance focused to increase lung procurement on renal function after kidney transplantation. Nephrol Dial Transplant 25: 2352–2356.

Minambres E, Perez-Villares JM, Chico-Fernandez M et al. (2015). Lung donor treatment protocol in brain dead-donors: a multicenter study. J Heart Lung Transplant 34: 773–780.

Mollaret P, Goulon M (1959). The depassed coma (preliminary memoir). Rev Neurol (Paris) 101: 3–15.

Monteiro LM, Bollen CW, van Huffelen AC et al. (2006). Transcranial Doppler ultrasonography to confirm brain death: a meta-analysis. Intensive Care Med 32: 1937–1944.

Morrissey PE (2012). The case for kidney donation before end-of-life care. Am J Bioeth 12: 1–8.

Morrissey PE, Monaco AP (2014). Donation after circulatory death: current practices, ongoing challenges, and potential improvements. Transplantation 97: 258–264.

Munari M, Zucchetta P, Carollo C et al. (2005). Confirmatory tests in the diagnosis of brain death: comparison between SPECT and contrast angiography. Crit Care Med 33: 2068–2073.

Munshi L, Keshavjee S, Cypel M (2013). Donor management and lung preservation for lung transplantation. Lancet Respir Med 1: 318–328.

Nadalin S, Girotti P, Konigsrainer A (2013). Risk factors for and management of graft pancreatitis. Curr Opin Organ Transplant 18: 89–96.

Nair-Collins M, Green SR, Sutin AR (2015). Abandoning the dead donor rule? A national survey of public views on death and organ donation. J Med Ethics 41: 297–302.

NHS Blood and Transplant (2010). Transplant activity in the UK. Activity report 2009/10. Available: https://nhsbtmediaservices.blob.core.windows.net/organ-donation-assets/pdfs/activity_report_2009_10.pdf (accessed 12/20/2015).

NHS Blood and Transplant (2013). National standards for organ retrieval from deceased donors. Available: http://www.bts.org.uk/Documents/9.1.13%20Retrieval%20Standards%20Document%20v2%206%20effective%20010113.pdf (accessed 8/22/2016).

NHS Blood and Transplant (2014). Transplant activity in the UK. Activity report 2014/15. Available http://nhsbtmediaservices.blob.core.windows.net/organ-donation-assets/pdfs/activity_report_2014_15.pdf (accessed 12/17/2015).

Niemann CU, Feiner J, Swain S et al. (2015). Therapeutic hypothermia in deceased organ donors and kidney-graft function. N Engl J Med 373: 405–414.

Novitzky D, Mi Z, Sun Q et al. (2014). Thyroid hormone therapy in the management of 63,593 brain-dead organ donors: a retrospective analysis. Transplantation 98: 1119–1127.

Oliver RC, Sturtevant JP, Scheetz JP et al. (2001). Beneficial effects of a hospital bereavement intervention program after traumatic childhood death. J Trauma 50: 440–446. discussion 447–448.

Oliver M, Woywodt A, Ahmed A et al. (2011). Organ donation, transplantation and religion. Nephrol Dial Transplant 26: 437–444.

OPTN/UNOS (2008). OPTN/UNOS OPO Committee Report. accessed. Available: http://optn.transplant.hrsa.gov/converge/committeereports/board_main_opocommittee_2_26_2008_12_20.pdf.

OPTN/UNOS (2015). The Organ Procurement and Transplantation Network data. [Online]. Available: http://optn.transplant.hrsa.gov (accessed November 10, 2015).

Orban J-C, Ferret E, Jambou P et al. (2015). Confirmation of brain death diagnosis: a study on French practice. Anaesthesia Critical Care & Pain Medicine 34: 145–150.

Organización Nacional de Trasplantes (2012). Donation after circulatory death in Spain: current situation and recommendations. National Consensus document. Available: http://www.ont.es/infesp/Paginas/DocumentosdeConsenso.aspx (accessed 12/21/2015).

Ortega-Deballon I, Hornby L, Shemie SD (2015). Protocols for uncontrolled donation after circulatory death: a systematic review of international guidelines, practices and transplant outcomes. Crit Care 19: 268.

Paries M, Boccheciampe N, Raux M et al. (2012). Benefit of a single recruitment maneuver after an apnea test for the diagnosis of brain death. Crit Care 16: R116.

Patel MS, Zatarain J, De La Cruz S et al. (2014). The impact of meeting donor management goals on the number of organs transplanted per expanded criteria donor: a prospective study from the UNOS Region 5 Donor Management Goals Workgroup. JAMA Surg 149: 969–975.

Patel MS, Niemann CU, Sally MB et al. (2015). The impact of hydroxyethyl starch use in deceased organ donors on the development of delayed graft function in kidney transplant recipients: a propensity-adjusted analysis. Am J Transplant 15: 2152–2158.

Perico NN (2004). Delayed graft function in kidney transplantation. The Lancet (British edition) 364: 1814–1827.

Phua J, Lim TK, Zygun DA et al. (2007). Pro/con debate: in patients who are potential candidates for organ donation after cardiac death, starting medications and/or interventions for the sole purpose of making the organs more viable is an acceptable practice. Crit Care 11: 211.

Pinsard M, Ragot S, Mertes PM et al. (2014). Interest of low-dose hydrocortisone therapy during brain-dead organ donor resuscitation: the CORTICOME study. Crit Care 18: R158.

Pinson CW, Feurer ID, Payne JL et al. (2000). Health-related quality of life after different types of solid organ transplantation. Ann Surg 232: 597–607.

Ponticelli C (2014). Ischaemia-reperfusion injury: a major protagonist in kidney transplantation. Nephrol Dial Transplant 29: 1134–1140.

Porteous MK, Diamond JM, Christie JD (2015). Primary graft dysfunction: lessons learned about the first 72 h after lung transplantation. Curr Opin Organ Transplant 20: 506–514.

Procaccio F, Rizzato L, Ricci A et al. (2010). Do "silent" brain deaths affect potential organ donation? Transplant Proc 42: 2190–2191.

Rabinstein AA, Yee AH, Mandrekar J et al. (2012). Prediction of potential for organ donation after cardiac death in patients in neurocritical state: a prospective observational study. Lancet Neurol 11: 414–419.

Reed MJ, Lua SB (2014). Uncontrolled organ donation after circulatory death: potential donors in the emergency department. Emerg Med J 31: 741–744.

Reich DJ, Mulligan DC, Abt PL et al. (2009). ASTS recommended practice guidelines for controlled donation after cardiac death organ procurement and transplantation. Am J Transplant 9: 2004–2011.

Reznik ON, Skvortsov AE, Reznik AO et al. (2013). Uncontrolled donors with controlled reperfusion after sixty minutes of asystole: a novel reliable resource for kidney transplantation. PLoS One 8e64209.

Ridley SS (2005). UK guidance for non-heart-beating donation. Br J Anaesth : BJA 95: 592.

Robertson JAJ (1999). The dead donor rule. The Hastings Center Report 29: 6.

Rodriguez DA, Del Rio F, Fuentes ME et al. (2011). Lung transplantation with uncontrolled non-heart-beating donors. Transplantation. Donor prognostic factor and immediate evolution post transplant. Arch Bronconeumol 47: 403–409.

Rodriguez-Arias D, Deballon IO (2012). Protocols for uncontrolled donation after circulatory death. Lancet 379: 1275–1276.

Rodriguez-Arias D, Ortega-Deballon I, Smith MJ et al. (2013). Casting light and doubt on uncontrolled DCDD protocols. Hastings Cent Rep 43: 27–30.

Rosendale JD, Chabelewski FL, McBride MA et al. (2002). Increased transplanted organs from the use of a standardized donor management protocol. Am J Transplant 2: 761.

Russo MJ, Iribarne A, Hong KN et al. (2010). Factors associated with primary graft failure after heart transplantation. Transplantation 90: 444–450.

Sahin H, Pekcevik Y (2015). CT angiography as a confirmatory test in diagnosis of brain death: comparison between three scoring systems. Diagn Interv Radiol 21: 177–183.

Salim AA (2006a). Complications of brain death: frequency and impact on organ retrieval. The American Surgeon 72: 377.

Salim AA (2006b). The effect of a protocol of aggressive donor management: implications for the national organ donor shortage. Journal of Trauma: Injury, Infection, and Critical Care 61: 429–435.

Sanchez-Fructuoso AI, Marques M, Prats D et al. (2006). Victims of cardiac arrest occurring outside the hospital: a source of transplantable kidneys. Ann Intern Med 145: 157–164.

Saposnik G, Rizzo G, Vega A et al. (2004). Problems associated with the apnea test in the diagnosis of brain death. Neurol India 52: 342–345.

Sawicki M, Bohatyrewicz R, Walecka A et al. (2014). CT angiography in the diagnosis of brain death. Pol J Radiol 79: 417–421.

Schnuelle P, Gottmann U, Hoeger S et al. (2009). Effects of donor pretreatment with dopamine on graft function after kidney transplantation: a randomized controlled trial. JAMA 302: 1067–1075.

Schrader H, Hall C, Zwetnow NN (1985). Effects of prolonged supratentorial mass expansion on regional blood flow and cardiovascular parameters during the Cushing response. Acta Neurol Scand 72: 283–294.

Shankar JJ, Banfield JC (2015). Comments on Shemie et al.: international guideline development for the determination of death. Intensive Care Med 41: 571.

Shankar JJ, Vandolpe R (2013). CT perfusion for confirmation of brain death. Am J Neuroradiol : AJNR 34: 1175–1179.

Sharpe MD, van Rassel B, Haddara W (2013). Oral and intravenous thyroxine (T4) achieve comparable serum levels for hormonal resuscitation protocol in organ donors: a randomized double-blinded study. Canadian Journal of Anesthesia 60: 998–1002.

Shaw D (2014). Personalized organ donation directives: saving lives with PODDs. Crit Care 18: 141.

Shemie SD, Baker AJ, Knoll G et al. (2006). National recommendations for donation after cardiocirculatory death in Canada: donation after cardiocirculatory death in Canada. CMAJ 175: S1.

Shemie SD, Hornby L, Baker A et al. (2014). International guideline development for the determination of death. Intensive Care Med 40: 788–797.

Sheth KN, Nutter T, Stein DM et al. (2012). Autoresuscitation after asystole in patients being considered for organ donation. Crit Care Med 40: 158–161.

Singbartl KK (2011). Intensivist-led management of brain-dead donors is associated with an increase in organ recovery for transplantation. Am J Transplant 11: 1517–1521.

Sloan MA, Alexandrov AV, Tegeler CH et al. (2004). Assessment: transcranial Doppler ultrasonography: report of the Therapeutics and Technology Assessment Subcommittee of the American Academy of Neurology. Neurology 62: 1468–1481.

Smith M (2004). Physiologic changes during brain stem death – lessons for management of the organ donor. J Heart Lung Transplant 23: S217–S222.

Smith M (2015). Brain death: the United Kingdom perspective. Semin Neurol 35: 145–151.

Soldatos T, Karakitsos D, Wachtel M et al. (2010). The value of transcranial Doppler sonography with a transorbital approach in the confirmation of cerebral circulatory arrest. Transplant Proc 42: 1502–1506. http://dx.doi.org/10.1016/j.transproceed.2010.01.074.

Solek-Pastuszka J, Saucha W, Iwanczuk W et al. (2015). Evolution of apnoea test in brain death diagnostics. Anaesthesiol Intensive Ther 47: 363–367.

Soriano-Pacheco JA, Lopez-Navidad A, Caballero F et al. (1999). Psychopathology of bereavement in the families of cadaveric organ donors. Transplant Proc 31: 2604–2605.

Stoica SC, Satchithananda DK, White PA et al. (2006). Brain death leads to abnormal contractile properties of the human donor right ventricle. J Thorac Cardiovasc Surg 132: 116–123.

Suarez F, Otero A, Solla M et al. (2008). Biliary complications after liver transplantation from maastricht category-2 non-heart-beating donors. Transplantation 85: 9–14.

Sung RS, Galloway J, Tuttle-Newhall JE et al. (2008). Organ donation and utilization in the United States, 1997–2006. Am J Transplant 8: 922–934.

Szurhaj W, Lamblin MD, Kaminska A et al. (2015). EEG guidelines in the diagnosis of brain death. Neurophysiol Clin 45: 97–104.

Tavakoli SA, Shabanzadeh AP, Arjmand B et al. (2008). Comparative study of depression and consent among brain death families in donor and nondonor groups from March 2001 to December 2002 in Tehran. Transplant Proc 40: 3299–3302.

Taylor TT (2014). Computed tomography (CT) angiography for confirmation of the clinical diagnosis of brain death. Cochrane Database of Systematic Reviews 3. CD009694.

Thompson BB, Wendell LC, Potter NS et al. (2014). The use of transcranial Doppler ultrasound in confirming brain death in the setting of skull defects and extraventricular drains. Neurocritical Care 21: 534–538.

Uniform Law Commission (1980). Determination of death act summary. [Online]. Available: http://www.uniformlaws.org/ActSummary.aspx?title=Determination%20of%20Death%20Act (accessed November 10, 2015).

Van Raemdonck D, Neyrinck A, Cypel M et al. (2015). Ex-vivo lung perfusion. Transpl Int 28: 643–656.

Venkateswaran RV, Patchell VB, Wilson IC et al. (2008). Early donor management increases the retrieval rate of lungs for transplantation. The Annals of Thoracic Surgery 85: 278–286.

Venkatram S, Bughio S, Diaz-Fuentes G (2015). Clinical brain death with false positive radionuclide cerebral perfusion scans. Case Rep Crit Care 2015: 630430.

Volk ML, Warren GJ, Anspach RR et al. (2010). Attitudes of the American public toward organ donation after uncontrolled (sudden) cardiac death. Am J Transplant 10: 675–680.

Wahlster S, Wijdicks EF, Patel PV et al. (2015). Brain death declaration: practices and perceptions worldwide. Neurology 84: 1870–1879.

Wall SP, Kaufman BJ, Gilbert AJ et al. (2011). Derivation of the uncontrolled donation after circulatory determination of death protocol for New York city. Am J Transplant 11: 1417–1426.

Wall SP, Kaufman BJ, Williams N et al. (2016). Lesson from the New York City out-of-hospital uncontrolled donation

after circulatory determination of death program. Ann Emerg Med 67: 531–537.

Wang Z, Guan W, Han Y et al. (2015). Stimulation of dopamine d3 receptor attenuates renal ischemia-reperfusion injury via increased linkage with Galpha12. Transplantation 99: 2274–2284.

Ware LB, Landeck M, Koyama T et al. (2014). A randomized trial of the effects of nebulized albuterol on pulmonary edema in brain-dead organ donors. Am J Transplant 14: 621.

Watts RP, Thom O, Fraser JF (2013). Inflammatory signalling associated with brain dead organ donation: from brain injury to brain stem death and posttransplant ischaemia reperfusion injury. J Transplant 2013: 1–19.

Wertheimer P, Jouvet M, Descotes J (1959). Diagnosis of death of the nervous system in comas with respiratory arrest treated by artificial respiration. Presse Med 67: 87–88.

Wertin TM, Rady MY, Verjeijde JL (2012). Antemortem donor bilateral nephrectomy: a violation of the patient's best interests standard. Am J Bioeth 12: 17–20.

Westendorp WH, Leuvenink HG, Ploeg RJ (2011). Brain death induced renal injury. Curr Opin Organ Transplant 16: 151–156.

White CW, Ali A, Hasanally D et al. (2013). A cardioprotective preservation strategy employing ex vivo heart perfusion facilitates successful transplant of donor hearts after cardiocirculatory death. J Heart Lung Transplant 32: 734–743.

Wieczorek A, Gaszynski T (2015). Boussignac CPAP system for brain death confirmation with apneic test in case of acute lung injury/adult respiratory distress syndrome – series of cases. Ther Clin Risk Manag 11: 961–965.

Wijdicks EF (1995). Determining brain death in adults. Neurology 45: 1003–1011.

Wijdicks EF (2010). The case against confirmatory tests for determining brain death in adults. Neurology 75: 77–83.

Wijdicks EF (2015). The clinical determination of brain death: rational and reliable. Semin Neurol 35: 103–104.

Wijdicks EF (2015). Determining brain death. Continuum (Minneapolis, Minn.) 21: 1411–1424.

Wijdicks EF, Varelas PN, Gronseth GS et al. (2010). Evidence-based guideline update: determining brain death in adults: report of the Quality Standards Subcommittee of the American Academy of Neurology. Neurology 74: 1911–1918.

Wilkinson D, Savulescu J (2012). Should we allow organ donation euthanasia? Alternatives for maximizing the number and quality of organs for transplantation. Bioethics 26: 32–48.

Wind JJ (2011). Preservation of kidneys from controlled donors after cardiac death. British Journal of Surgery 98: 1260–1266.

Wind J, Faut M, van Smaalen TC et al. (2013). Variability in protocols on donation after circulatory death in Europe. Crit Care 17: R217.

Wolfe RA, Ashby VB, Milford EL et al. (1999). Comparison of mortality in all patients on dialysis, patients on dialysis awaiting transplantation, and recipients of a first cadaveric transplant. N Engl J Med 341: 1725–1730.

Wood KE, Becker BN, McCartney JG et al. (2004). Care of the potential organ donor. N Engl J Med 351: 2730–2739.

Yarlagadda SG, Coca SG, Garg AX et al. (2008). Marked variation in the definition and diagnosis of delayed graft function: a systematic review. Nephrol Dial Transplant 23: 2995–3003.

Yee AH, Rabinstein AA, Thapa P et al. (2010). Factors influencing time to death after withdrawal of life support in neurocritical patients. Neurology 74: 1380–1385.

Youn TS, Greer DM (2014). Brain death and management of a potential organ donor in the intensive care unit. Crit Care Clin 30: 813–831.

# Index

NB: Page numbers in *italics* refer to figures, tables and boxes.